D0093984

MARION MORRA, ScD, is an international expert in health communications. Former associate director of the Yale Cancer Center, she is an associate clinical professor at the Yale School of Nursing in New Haven, CT. Widely published, she is a member of the Board of Directors of the American Cancer Society and of the Board of Directors of the International Cancer Information Services Group. She is a consultant to the National Cancer Institute and many major cancer centers across the country.

EVE POTTS has been writing about medical subjects for more than 30 years. She has served as a medical writer and consultant to the Department of Health and Human Services and to many medically oriented companies and institutions. Her particular area of expertise is in making difficult medical information easily understood. Her interest in historic preservation is represented by authorship of the book, *Westport: A Special Place*.

The two authors, who are sisters, have collaborated on seven books especially written for cancer patients, their friends and families: the first three editions of *Choices* (1980, 1987, and 1994); the *Prostate Cancer Answer Book* (1997), *Triumph: Getting Back to Normal When You Have Cancer* (1990), and *Understanding Your Immune System* (1986).

lulu,
To all our Continued
adventures, hurdles and
wonderful days b
friendship

Marylen &
July 25 2010

CHOICES

Fourth Edition

Marion Morra and Eve Potts

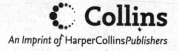

An Imprint of HarperCollins*Publishers*

CHOICES, FOURTH EDITION. Copyright © 1980, 1987, 1994, 2003 by Marion Morra and Eve Potts. All rights reserved. Printed in the United States of America. No part of this book may be used or reproduced in any manner whatsoever without written permission except in the case of brief quotations embodied in critical articles and review. For information, address HarperCollins Publishers Inc., 10 East 53rd Street, New York, NY 10022.

HarperCollins books may be purchased for educational, business, or sales promotional use. For information please write: Special Markets Department, HarperCollins Publishers Inc., 10 East 53rd Street, New York, NY 10022.

Fourth Edition: October 2003
Third Edition: October 1994
Second Edition: March 1987
First Edition published by Avon Books, April 1980

Interior illustrations by Dick Oden, unless otherwise noted.
Map by James Sinclair
Designed by Richard Oriolo

LIBRARY OF CONGRESS CATALOGING-IN-PUBLICATION DATA

Morra, Marion E.
    Choices / Marion Morra and Eve Potts.—4th ed.
       p. cm.—(A HarperResource book)
    "First edition"—T.p. verso.
    Includes bibliographical references and index.
      1. Cancer—Miscellanea.   2. Cancer—Hospitals—United States—Directories.
    I. Potts, Eve.   II. Title.   III. Series.

RC270.8.M67 2003
616.99'4—dc21   2003050947

ISBN   0-06-052124-4

08 09 WBC/RRD 10 9 8 7

This fourth edition of Choices *is dedicated to*
Robert A. Potts,
whose positive attitude inspires us.
First diagnosed with prostate cancer in 1980,
his determination to understand all his choices,
his decision to go through implant seeding
and get on with his life has been a revelation.
He is a good example of the chronic nature of
this disease. Even last year, when a new cancer,
this time a lymphoma, appeared,
he went through the necessary chemo treatments,
got a crew cut and continues to thrive.

Contents

1   FACING THE DIAGNOSIS   1

Survival Statistics ▪ Ten things you need to do before deciding on treatment ▪ How to proceed ▪ Judging your attitude ▪ Thoughts for your mental computer

2   SEARCHING FOR ANSWERS ON THE WEB   11

Finding the right site ▪ Selected cancer information Web sites ▪ Choosing a search engine ▪ Choosing a reliable site ▪ Listservs, newsgroups, and chatrooms ▪ Forums ▪ Latest cancer news ▪ Searching medical journals on the Web ▪ Searching libraries on-line ▪ Checking doctor, hospital, and nursing home credentials ▪ Genetic information ▪ Environment ▪ Insurance and Medicare ▪ Selected Web sites for specific cancers

3   CHOOSING YOUR DOCTOR AND HOSPITAL   33

Basic facts to help in choosing doctor and hospital ▪ Board certification ▪ Major specialties ▪ Judging your doctor ▪ Choosing a surgeon ▪ Getting a second opinion ▪ Role of nurses ▪ Health plans ▪ Judging your hospital ▪ Locations of Comprehensive Cancer Centers ▪ Difference between Comprehensive Cancer Centers and other hospitals ▪ Understanding research and teaching hospitals ▪ Hospital records ▪ Web pages to check out

Preface

THIS IS THE fourth edition of *Choices*. We wrote the first edition 23 years ago because we were struck by the need to answer questions about cancer for the people who needed it most—cancer patients and their families. In 1980, tremendous advances were being made to fight cancer, but useful information about the disease, new technologies, and treatment options were available almost solely to members of the medical community. Most patients then still believed cancer was a death sentence and didn't know how or what to ask about their survival chances and healthcare choices. We decided to write a book that gave people the answers they needed in lay terms so that they could take up the battle "armed" with the right information.

Along the way a great thing happened. We met more and more people who were beating cancer. We saw similarities in survivors' attitudes and the approaches they took to living with and overcoming the disease. In 1990, we wrote *Triumph*, which was dedicated to helping people resume normal lives after cancer, an idea that had barely existed only a few years before.

Now, in 2003, the whole picture has again made a dramatic shift. Most cancer patients today *expect* to survive. The stories of Lance Armstrong, Peggy Fleming, Rudolph Giuliani, and others are well known. More importantly, there are 9 million people in the U.S. who have triumphed over cancer and are going about their lives all around us—in our neighborhoods, at work, and at school.

The lack of information about cancer that spurred us to action almost 25 years ago has now turned to information overload. Type "cancer" into an Internet search engine and you'll literally find millions of Web pages to choose from. The challenge now is to sort through the mountains of information to find out what is real, accurate, timely, and applicable. So, in addition to a chapter on researching on the Internet, each chapter of this book includes a list of selected Web pages—the ones we think are most informative for the specific topics discussed in that chapter.

Choices, Fourth Edition, sticks to the question-and-answer format that we have found helps readers get direct information quickly and allows them to dig as deeply as they want into specific topics. With each edition, the vocabulary has become more sophisticated to keep pace with the public's growing knowledge and awareness of cancer. What struck us particularly in looking back over the past two decades is how much more quickly people who have cancer pick up the nomenclature of their disease and treatment. Because the terminology is what is used in hospitals and doctors' offices, we have tried to clarify language throughout the book so that when you encounter it during treatment, you will understand what the doctor is saying. We have attempted to define the terms, so that in discussions with the medical profession, who use these terms in their daily language, you will be on familiar territory.

We reexamined every piece of information contained in our previous editions, researching, rewriting, reconfirming, and amplifying facts, conferring with patients, nurses, and doctors for their views, and honing the material to include every kernel that we felt would be helpful. As before, much of the information contained in the pages of this book is drawn from the experiences of hundreds of people who have endured treatments and shared with us what they would have liked to have known before starting out on the cancer journey.

If you are reading this, chances are that you, or someone you care about, has been diagnosed with cancer. We also know from our discussions with many of you that you appreciate getting the information that your doctor would never think to tell you, as well as the information that you are told but that you might not understand. While every cancer case is different, every type of cancer is different, and the course of every cancer illness is different from every other, basic information and the questions that need to be explored remain the same.

We hope this book will help you make sense of your situation as you navigate the way back to good health. We have attempted to provide a discussion of a wide range of topics—from the homey to the high-tech—that are the most common and important to the thousands of you whom we have met. We hope this book will make it possible for you to ask more detailed questions and therefore enter into more meaningful discussions, helping you to become a partner with your doctor in dealing with your cancer problem.

Acknowledgments

THIS IS A BOOK that speaks from the souls of the hundreds of people who are involved in dealing with cancer and the women, men, and children and, yes, their families who are living with cancer. It also echoes the experiences of the many caregivers—the doctors, nurses, and researchers who labor day after day trying to understand how better to help others.

This book owes its existence to many who have had cancer and the thousands involved in cancer care who have shaped the medical advances of the last decades. It is impossible to acknowledge all of them or all the books and other sources, such as articles, original scientific writings, pamphlets, oncology seminars, and medical textbooks, that made it possible for us to write this latest edition of *Choices*. The materials from the National Cancer Institute, especially the state-of-the-art statements, articles, and materials from the National Library of Medicine, and the American Cancer Society's textbooks and research reports have been of inestimable value.

Most important to the tone and content of the book have been the insights of the many patients and families who continue to share with us their experiences and the real-life, everyday problems they encounter. From the very start, it has been the amazing people living with cancer on a day-to-day basis who have inspired us. We have been enriched by each encounter, and thanks to their sharing, we have added to our knowledge. We have a special place in our hearts for friends who were especially dear and who lost the good fight, like Ann Marie Howell, Peter DiLeo, Pat Hanley, Trish Greene, and Joan Dickinson, who are always in our thoughts as we write and try to understand. Others like Audrey Hanley, Joanie Willis, and Lisa A. S. Pierot, who continue on their own private journeys, have given us inspiration as has Diane Erdos with her insights on survivorship. From all the many people we have talked with and from their questions, we have gleaned invaluable material that is the heart of this book.

Countless physicians and other health-care professionals in a variety of specialties at major cancer centers, most specifically Yale Medical Center, Memorial Sloane Kettering, M. D. Anderson, Fred Hutchinson, and Mayo Clinic, were invaluable in supplying information. Personal experiences with friends in the profession—Peter Dixon, MD, hematology/oncology, Middlesex Hospital; Bernard Lytton, MD, professor of surgery (Urology), Yale University Medical School; Dr. George P. Pillari, diagnostic radiologist, New Hyde Park, NY; and Karen Andrews and Kathy Giusti of the Multiple Myeloma Foundation—offered special insights. Dr. Tish Knobf, associate professor at the Yale School of Nursing; Chris Thomsen, director, Office of Communications, National Center for Complementary and Alternative Medicine, National Institutes of Health; and Linda Mowad, RN, director, Cancer Information Service of New England were among those who guided us to a better understanding of patients' concerns. We thank Amy Potts for her continuing help with our Web site and David and Dan Donovan for their keen insights. We are grateful to the members of our families—especially Mark, Jane, and Matt Potts, and Abby and Michael Pillari—for their encouragement from beginning to end. To Bob Potts, Eve's husband, who has been down the cancer path himself numerous times with both prostate cancer and lymphoma, and Mollie Donovan, our other sister, we express gratitude for their ongoing assistance and infinite patience.

Last, but not least, we thank Gilbert Maurer of Hearst Publications for his original and continued guidance and the group at HarperCollins, especially Megan Newman and Kathryn Huck, who believed in the value of this book and encouraged us with their faith, trust, and enthusiasm.

Though it is through the help of many, many people that this book came to life, we alone take responsibility for any errors or misinterpretations.

List of Illustrations

One

FACING THE DIAGNOSIS

A CANCER DIAGNOSIS—no matter what kind of cancer it is—makes you feel like you've been left dangling off the cliff of life. Days of testing, bone scans, CT scans, MRIs, x-rays, and blood tests are followed by days of growing fear while you wait for the final answer. Then, the solemn pronouncement that you have cancer and with it the feeling that life will never be the same again. And not only your life—but also the lives of everyone around you.

No one disputes the fact that your life will be changed by your diagnosis. But try not to panic. This is NOT the end of the world. This is not the end of your life. This is the moment when you need to take control and call up your inner will to live and your determination to learn all you can about what is happening to you.

There is so much going on in every kind of cancer treatment that you have every reason to feel positive about the possibility of being cured. We have seen dozens of patients who made dramatic recoveries, when ten years ago they would have had no hope for living another year. We know people who just one year ago would have died were it not for the fact that they received the very newest treatments. We know many who have had chronic cases of cancer, who have been treated, lived a few disease-free years, and then discovered that the cancer returned. They have been treated again. They've gone back into patient mode, gone through another round of treatments, and recovered again. Each time they've survived, they've gained a bit more time to test out newer treatments with fewer side effects and better effectiveness. The bottom line is: **cancer isn't what it used to be.**

We are extremely optimistic about the treatments that continue to come to the marketplace or are on the near horizon. We have researched every resource to give you as much information as possible on the many different kinds of treatments available as well as the very newest thinking and experiments that are presently being tested.

Cancer is a chronic disease with many possibilities for cure. Position yourself to take advantage of every possibility for being one of those who is cured. And always remember, people have survived every type of cancer, at every stage.

What happens now?
This is the moment when you have the **greatest number of choices** concerning the kind of treatment best for you and you are faced with making decisions about how you will proceed. Each decision may make a critical difference in the outcome. The wrong choices close the doors to other options. In order to make informed decisions, you need information, the kind of information that makes it possible for you to seek out the right doctor and hospital as well as sufficient information to make it possible for you to ask the right questions.

You need to put the whole emotional background of having cancer into perspective before you can deal intelligently with the diagnosis of cancer. For many people, the cancer word—the big C—still carries with it the old fears and myths, left over from the days when cancer was incurable. Today, with nearly nine million people alive with a history of cancer, you need to be aware that in the vast majority of cases, cancer is considered and treated as a "chronic" illness that can be managed for many years with proper treatment.

- **Cancer is a major illness but it is not necessarily fatal, contrary to what many people still believe.**
- **You can have cancer and continue to enjoy life.**

There's no question that the diagnosis of cancer is one of the low points in life. The real news is that many people are being cured. For some types of cancer, nine out of ten people diagnosed can be considered cured. Many others will live a very long time before dying of cancer. There is hope for every patient. Some are cured at once, by surgery, chemotherapy, and radiation. Some are never cured, but their disease is controlled so they can expect to live for many, many years. Admittedly, there are some types of cancer where treatments are only able to prolong life for a few months, but those cases are in the minority.

It is important for you to know at the outset what category your type of cancer is so that you will not be worrying unnecessarily and so that you will be dealing with reality when you make decisions about your treatments and how you will be living your life. Specifically, you need to know the type of cancer, the stage of the cancer, whether it has spread to any other site, and if there are tumor markers that are used to track your cancer. You need full information to make certain that you will be getting the very best possible treatment for your cancer as well as for your coping style, personality, and living style.

The best place to begin in collecting information, of course, is with your doctor. But, you need to search out further information on your own if you plan to be an involved consumer. Our favorite first information stop is the National Cancer Institute (NCI), where ongoing research puts cutting-edge information at your fingertips through its Cancer Information Service telephone line, 1-800-4-CANCER, and Web site (www.cancer.gov). Our favorite search engine is Google, where you can put in a few words and get access to a wealth of information. If you are looking for community-oriented information, try the American Cancer Society, 1-800-ACS-2345, and its Web site (www.cancer.org). See Chapter 2, Searching for Answers on the Web, as well as information at the end of each chapter on specific cancers for additional Internet sources.

If you are confused by the stream of statistics that continues to make the front pages you are not alone. We have been involved with a close study of cancer for more than 25 years. First of all, the statistics are not meant to predict what will happen to an individual patient. They are designed to be used as a gauge for the scientific community to help monitor progress in the detection and treatment of cancer and to guide in making decisions about how funds can best be spent—which is a very different perspective. Also, they don't reflect the latest in treatment because they are based on people who were diagnosed and treated at least eight years ago. Additionally, the newest statistics are based on new age adjustments having to do with the 2000 census rather than on the 1970 census as they were before (in the past, some also were based on the 1980 or 1940 census). Be leery of being caught up in the latest statistics game **because it has little to do with you as an individual patient.**

MORE ABOUT SURVIVAL STATISTICS

In discussing your case, your doctor may talk about "five-year survival" rates. Many people misinterpret this to mean that you are expected to live only five years after treatment or that you aren't considered cured even after five years without cancer. Five-year survival is used as a measure by scientists to compare the value of one treatment against another from statistics gathered by state tumor registries. In many forms of cancer, five years without symptoms following treatment is the accepted time to consider a patient cured. Actually, depending on the type of cancer, some patients are considered cured after one or two years, others after three years, while for some it may be longer than five years. One more thing—the statistics are based on treatments that were done eight years or more ago. With the fast pace of change in cancer treatment and with increasing successes, those statistics become outdated quickly.

Facts You Should Know About Cancer

- Over nine million Americans alive today have a history of cancer.
- Over 1.3 million new cases of cancer will be diagnosed this year. This figure excludes those who have basal cell and squamous cell skin cancers, an additional one million cases per year.
- Things have changed. In the early 1900s, most cancer patients had no hope of long-term survival. In the 1930s, less than one in five was alive five years after treatment. In the 1940s, it was one in four and in the 1960s, one in three. Today, statistics show survival rates of over 60 percent.

Once you know you have cancer, you can live in fear, or you can learn to live with the facts and begin to do positive things to help yourself. Knowing the facts and facing them takes a lot of the scare away.

Here are some basics for starters. Check them and see how many coincide with your own thinking.

- The fact that you have cancer cannot be changed. The time that is most important in decision making is right now, at the very start, when numerous choices are open to you.
- You must look at all possible choices and alternatives. If you make a decision to go ahead with surgery without sufficient testing or a second opinion, you limit the possibility for other choices.
- Stay calm and in control. Don't be afraid to say: "I'm going to take the time to learn all I can about this cancer and the options I have available to me before I do anything."

- **CAUTION:** This does not mean postponing taking action. It means postponing starting treatment so you are personally assured that you're taking the right steps.

- You must be an activist. You must become a partner with your doctors in the fight so you can live your life in the way that is best for you.

- You have a right to ask questions just as you would as a consumer of any product or service. However, you need to learn what questions to ask, what the terminology means, and what the realistic possibilities are.

- Hope is not the same as denial. Denying you have cancer closes your mind and your resources to all the possibilities that exist for you. You shut off your inner abilities to deal with reality. Denial closes doors. Hope opens the channels for action.

- Without question, the most difficult time you will experience is at the beginning, when the diagnosis is first presented to you. At that moment, cancer becomes an inescapable fact for you. That is the time when you must mobilize yourself and your resources to plan your future intelligently.

HOW TO PROCEED

- Get a loose-leaf notebook for keeping records. You can divide it into sections in a way that makes sense for you. You may want to have a section for all the information you will gather about your kind of cancer, names and phone, fax and e-mail addresses of doctors, nurses, office personnel, hospitals, Internet addresses, etc.

- Another section may be reserved for all questions that occur to you and notes on what you are told.

- You probably will want additional sections to include information on medications, doctor appointments, travel expenses, insurance, prescription charges, medical deductions, payments made, etc.

- A tape recorder can be handy for reference purposes. With the approval of the person being recorded, you can keep a record of discussions you have with the various medical professionals you will be seeing.

- Many people find it helpful to have a running narrative or personal account of what is happening to them throughout the treatment. Try to enter something at least once a week. Do it when you're waiting in the doctor's office or for your treatments. Try to focus on your feelings and write about them rather than just recording events.

TEN THINGS YOU NEED TO DO BEFORE DECIDING ON TREATMENT

1. Ask the doctor to discuss all the possible alternatives with you. There is more than one treatment choice for almost every single case of cancer.

2. Learn all you can about the kind of cancer you have. Ask your doctor for specific information about the type of cancer and the stage it is in so that when you are researching you are doing so with valid information in hand.

3. Call the Cancer Information Service, toll-free, at 1-800-4-CANCER for the latest up-to-date information and facts on your type of cancer. Making this call is one of the most important things you can do for yourself. Trained information specialists can talk to you about your kind of cancer and help you decide what steps to take, what questions to ask your doctor, and what treatments are available for your kind of cancer. They also will be happy to supply you with detailed information, send printed material, find clinical trials that are being done on your type of cancer, and provide PDQ statements from the National Cancer Institute that give you the latest information on treatments. If you have further questions at a later date, don't hesitate to call again.

4. Go on the Web for information. Do it yourself or get a computer literate friend to help. See Chapter 2, Searching for Answers on the Web. Start with the main Web pages we have discussed in that chapter. Since all information on the Web is not necessarily accurate information, we suggest that you start your search with the Web pages we have discussed and be choosy about where you visit.

5. If a medical library is available to you, look there for information (or get to one via the Web). The Cancer Information Service is a good starting point for information, but you and your friends and family may want to do other research as well. So much new research is being done in so many places that you may find an important clue to a treatment that may be helpful to you.

About your feelings

- Expect to feel depressed at times.
- Expect to find that many of your emotions will be on the surface.
- Try to deal with your feelings honestly.
- Don't try to hide your illness and prognosis from your family and friends.
- Accept and welcome the help and concern of others.

6. Meanwhile, make sure you have the right doctor. The kind of treatment you get depends on how much your doctor knows about your particular kind of cancer. Ask about clinical trials and the latest PDQ statement from the National Cancer Institute on your kind of cancer. There are doctors (called oncologists) who specialize in treating cancer. Beyond that there are specialists in every kind of cancer, down to specialists who deal exclusively with one cell type of cancer (1-866-ASK-ABMS will get you information on certification of doctors). Get an opinion on treatment from someone who is treating your type of disease on a daily basis.

7. If during your research you find a doctor who has written a paper on your type of cancer, don't hesitate to call to discuss your case.

8. If at all possible, seek a second opinion before submitting to cancer treatment of any kind. The original diagnosis and treatment plan you were given will probably be confirmed but you deserve the right to have your doctor's diagnosis reconfirmed and any other possible treatments explored and explained to you. Take the time to do your homework. Most treatments are long and difficult. A few extra weeks usually will not make any difference as far as the progress of the cancer is concerned but can make all the difference in your future.

9. In many cases, a second pathological opinion is a good idea. The pathology report is the basis on which all future decisions will be made, and although some cancers are pathologically diagnosed without any question, you need to check to make certain this is true in your case.

10. Check to see if there is a Comprehensive Cancer Center designated by the National Cancer Institute in your area. See Chapters 3 and 28. (You can also ask the Cancer Information Service or check the NCI Web site). These centers attract some of the best doctors, meet high standards set by the NCI, and offer you the chance for promising new treatment. But be an informed consumer: not all hospitals that call themselves "cancer centers" or even "comprehensive cancer centers" have necessarily passed the rigorous standards set by the National Cancer Institute.

■   Think about whether quality or quantity of life—how good and how long— is most important for you. You may be faced with some decisions where the answer to this question will determine what choices you will make.

■   Once you've done all the background work and embarked on a course of treatment, your own ways of coping will help you feel in control. You will be able to face your problems if you know what is being done to you, why it is being done, how it will be done, and what the prognosis is.

- You will undoubtedly be anxious, may not sleep well, and may lose your appetite. This is normal.
- You may be surprised to find that once you have made your decisions, you will experience a sense of relief and a feeling of calmness.

Dealing with doctors

- Keep a list of questions you want answered and bring them with you when you keep appointments with doctors.
- Take notes whenever talking with the doctor, radiologist, physical therapist, or nurse. (Or you may want to ask if it is OK for you to tape record conversations; then you can play them back for yourself or your family at your leisure.)
- Review your notes and save them for future reference.
- Ask the doctor to explain any medical terms you do not understand.
- Try always to have a family member or good friend with you when you visit your doctor. It's helpful to have another person with you who can help you remember and interpret what is being told to you. You may wish to ask that person to take notes for you.
- Don't hesitate to ask for information about tests and other procedures and why they are being done. You are entitled to all information that the doctor has about your case.
- Ask when the test results are going to be ready and how you will get the results. If you do not hear, call to get them.
- Let the doctor know that you are planning on getting other opinions before going any further. This is **not** an **unreasonable or unusual** request. Do not be pressured into proceeding before you are confident about what is being recommended.

Put These Thoughts Into Your Mental Computer

- People have recovered from every type of cancer.
- Cancer is the most curable of all chronic diseases. Cured means that you have the same life expectancy as someone your age who never had cancer.
- It helps to learn about every detail of your kind of cancer.
- A fighting spirit is healthier than stoic acceptance. It also may strengthen your immune response.
- It's better to express your feelings than to bottle them up. Keeping a journal of your feelings is a good way to express them.

JUDGING YOUR OWN ATTITUDE TOWARD CANCER

TRUE OR FALSE	THE REAL ANSWER
____You will die if you have cancer.	**FALSE.** Cancer, especially if discovered at an early stage, is curable in many instances, or chronic in most cases.
____Cancer is contagious.	**FALSE.**
____Cancer can develop in any part of the body.	**TRUE.** All parts of the body are susceptible— bone, lymph, skin, nervous system, etc.
____ Most cancer is inherited.	**FALSE.** Only about 5 or 10 percent of cancers are hereditary, caused by a damaged gene that has been inherited.
____ The outlook for cancer treatment is hopeful.	**TRUE.** Cancer is a different disease than it was just a few years go. Some people are cured. Others are living with a chronic disease. Even with advanced cancer that cannot be cured, there are treatments that you can have. The outlook is very hopeful.
____ The doctor can tell how long you have to live.	**FALSE.** Every case is different and doctors' estimates on how long a patient will live are often guesswork and can do a real disservice to you if you take them as gospel.
____ There are no untreatable cancers.	**TRUE.** There are always treatments that can be prescribed to make a patient more comfortable, although treatments are not always available to effect a cure.
____ Putting off seeing a doctor can forfeit the possibility of a cure.	**TRUE.** The earlier cancer is found, the more curable it may be. Of those who die of cancer each year, a large percentage die needlessly because of late diagnosis and inadequate treatment.

(continued)

- Consider yourself an equal partner with your doctor in achieving recovery.
- Listen to your body.
- Don't make a career of having cancer.
- Don't save up real living for tomorrow. Live your best today.

JUDGING YOUR OWN ATTITUDE TOWARD CANCER (continued)

_____ More people are being diagnosed with cancer than ever before.	**TRUE.** This is mainly because more people are living to an age when cancer occurs more frequently. Also, because diagnostic techniques are better, more cases are being found.
_____ Cancer is more frequent in men and women over 40.	**TRUE.** Cancer is primarily a disease of middle and old age. Less than one percent of all cancers are found in children.
TRUE OR FALSE	**THE REAL ANSWER**
_____ A lump in the breast means you have cancer.	**FALSE.** Eighty percent of all breast lumps are not cancer.
_____ Smoking can cause lung cancer.	**TRUE.** Eighty-seven percent of lung cancers are caused by smoking. Two-pack-a-day smokers die of lung cancer at rates 15 to 25 times greater than nonsmokers.
_____ The sun is good for you.	**FALSE.** Almost all of the one million cases of basal and squamous cell skin cancer each year are sun-related. Sun exposure is also a major factor in melanoma, a cancer that is increasing especially in fair-skinned persons.
_____ Grains, breads, vegetables, and fruits reduce risk of colon cancer.	**TRUE.** High-fiber diets may help reduce risk of colon cancer.

Have you made your call to the
Cancer Information Service?
1-800-4-CANCER
PLEASE DO IT NOW!

Two

SEARCHING FOR ANSWERS ON THE WEB

The World Wide Web offers an incredible amount of information about cancer. It is a seemingly infinite source of materials that were found previously only in books, medical journals, and brochures. But this wealth of materials can make searching on the Web frustrating and overwhelming. Our recent search using the word "cancer" on the Google search engine turned up over 16 million entries. Since anybody can publish on the Internet, some information is naturally biased or inaccurate. So, you need to be aware that you must separate valuable information from the mediocre or the untrue.

THERE ARE SEVERAL different kinds of sites related to cancer—some give basic cancer and treatment information; others concentrate on a specific kind of cancer. There are also on-line discussion groups and support groups. Many hospitals, cancer centers, organizations, and agencies have their own sites that can provide you with referral information.

This chapter has some basic Web information and some selected Web pages that will get you started in each of the categories. The Web pages listed are those that we ourselves have found useful. We also have added some selected Web pages at the end of each chapter in the book that are more specific to the chapter topic. There will be many others that we have not listed, but make sure you understand who is sponsoring the site before you assume that the information on it is accurate and up-to-date.

FINDING THE RIGHT SITE

Help! How can I start getting information from the Internet?
We assume that you already know how to get onto the Web (or have a family member or friend who can get you started) and have a sense of what information you need. Our best advice for finding reliable information is to begin with trusted organizations and cancer centers with national reputations. First try these two Internet sites, both of which offer credible, accurate, and up-to-the minute cancer information. They differ both in character and the kind of information that they have on them, but, in our experience, these are the two most valuable sources for you to start with and to check back on as you find other sites and other information:

- **www.cancer.gov**—this will bring you to the home page for the National Cancer Institute (NCI), where you can find all kinds of cancer information from prevention and screening to diagnosis and supportive care. It will tell you the treatment options for your particular kind of cancer. If you are interested in looking for clinical trials, you can do that here via its PDQ link. Click on its dictionary to find definitions of medical terms. Booklets that are published by the National Cancer Institute can be searched, downloaded, and viewed or ordered on the site (put the words "Publication Locator" into the search window on the site). It has a news center logo on the home page that will give you the latest cancer news. This site gives you access to medical articles, with its links to Medline, to the National Library of Medicine, and to the Web sites of other governmental and nongovernmental organizations. It also has a link to the NCI LiveHelp Service, which provides Internet users with the ability to chat online with an Information Specialist. Information Specialists can help Internet users find information on NCI Web sites and answer questions about cancer.

- **www.cancer.org**—this is the site of the American Cancer Society (ACS). Again, it is filled with a wealth of information that also is from a most credible source. Here you can get treatment guidelines for the major cancers and information about support services that are available in your own area, with a zip search feature. You can look in the cancer drug guide and find the actions and side effects of your drug treatment. The site also houses the Cancer Survivors Network, where you can listen to, read, or download pre-recorded personal stories and discussions among survivors and caregivers, participate in chats and discussions groups, or communicate with other survivors and caregivers via e-mail. Cancer statistics and risk and prevention information are also available on this site, along with addresses of the American Cancer Society local offices and local activities and events. You also can order books it publishes from its Web bookstore. Its "search" feature allows you to look up specific topics. Again, this is a valuable source of credible information.

How can I find out what information is included on individual Web sites?

On most sites, look for the words "site map," "table of contents" or "site index" to get this information. You may need to go to the bottom of the page to find it (or you can put the words in its search box). Click on it and you will get the outline of the site, what it contains, and where.

Are there any other reliable Web sites that feature cancer information?

There are many others. We have listed a selected group of them on the table labeled "Selected Cancer Information Web sites."

SELECTED CANCER INFORMATION WEB SITES

www.cancer.gov	National Cancer Institute Web site. See text for features.
www.cancer.org	American Cancer Society Web site. See text for features.
www.oncolink.com	One of the oldest cancer Web sites with information by cancer site or type, treatment information, book reviews, and news. Site of the University of Pennsylvania Cancer Center.
www.cancercare.org	Cancer Care, Inc. Web site. Special features include audio files from organization's popular teleconferences and searchable site for support services.
www.canceradvocacy.org	National Coalition of Cancer Survivorship. Raises awareness of cancer survivors and advocates for insurance, employment, and legal rights.

(continued)

SELECTED CANCER INFORMATION WEB SITES *(continued)*

www.medicare.gov	Government's Medicare site. You can search it by city and state for doctors, suppliers, drug assistance programs, or nursing homes that participate in the Medicare program. Publications can be ordered.
www.mskcc.org www.mdanderson.org	Web sites of Memorial Sloan-Kettering and of the M. D. Anderson Comprehensive Cancer Centers, two of the oldest NCI-designated centers in the country, who serve only cancer patients. Good information, especially herb, botanical, and other therapies on the first and pain control on the second.
www.cancersource.com	Site for both patients and health professionals with up-to-date information. Sponsored by Jones and Bartlett, publishers of health professional cancer texts.
www.rarediseases.org	National Organization for Rare Disorders. Maintains databases of rare diseases and of orphan drugs.
www.rarediseases.info.gov	Index of rare diseases and orphan drugs.
www.asco.org	Site of the American Society of Clinical Oncologists. Look at its Patients Living With Cancer for information, chat rooms, etc.
www.fda.gov/orphan	Information about drugs used for diseases affecting fewer than 200,000 Americans.

What is a "link"?

A link takes you from one Web site to another. When you get on a Web site you will usually see words such as "links to other sites" or "resources." If you click your mouse onto the title of the other Web pages, you will automatically be brought to those pages. Understand that when you do this, you will leave the original site.

What Web sites are there for specific kinds of cancer?

There are an increasing number of Web sites that are aimed at specific cancer sites. For instance, the National Alliance of Breast Cancer Organizations, the Prostate Cancer Infolink, the Leukemia and Lymphoma Society, and the National Brain Tumor Foundation are all examples of Web sites that discuss only one kind of cancer. These sites not only give you valuable information about the specific type of cancer but many also offer information about supportive services, chat rooms, or discussion areas. See information for each type of cancer in this chapter and listings at the end of the individual chapters.

What if I have a rare cancer?

There are several sites for rare diseases that have good searchable databases. The National Institutes of Health has an Office of Rare Diseases that lists rare (or orphan) diseases that affect fewer than 200,000 people in the United States. Its Web site (www.rarediseases.info.nih.gov) gives you information on rare diseases, information on research studies and how to become a part of them, progress on research, links to support groups and transportation to treatment sites, and information on genetics and genetic testing. The National Organization of Rare Disorders, Inc (www.rarediseases.org) has a site with an index of rare diseases, a database of orphan drugs, and information on medical assistance programs.

Can I get material on cancer on health sites that are not specifically for cancer?

Yes, there are health sites that cover many illnesses, including cancer, that give good cancer information. Here are a few you might wish to look at:

- Family doctor: www.familydoctor.org
- Harvard Center for Cancer Prevention: www.yourcancerrisk.harvard.edu
- HealthFinder: www.healthfinder.gov
- Dr. Koop: www.drkoop.com
- Mayo Clinic: www.mayoclinic.com
- Medscape Health: www.health.medscape.com
- National Women's Health Information Center: www.healthywomen.org
- New York Online Access to Health (NOAH): www.noah-health.org
- WebMD: www.webmd.com

How can I decide on good Web sites to go to?

You need to make sure that the Web site you are on is more than just good graphics and easy to use. And you need to be careful when you are looking for the Web site of a major organization because Web addresses can be similar. Finding the right one can take time. You can use the links that are part of the Web sites belonging to the National Cancer Institute and the American Cancer Society. But you need to know that clicking on the links will take you away from your original site and bring you to a new one. Or you can use search engines—they are similar to the old card catalog in the library, but much faster. A search engine will scan hundreds of sites looking for whatever topic you wish. In seconds, you will get, on your screen, a listing of sites that you can then click on to look at.

How can I be sure that the site is a reliable one and that the information I am getting is accurate and up to date?

There are several clues that will help you determine what kind of site you are on and what kind of information you are getting:

- The most reliable type of a site is one that is run by a government agency (such as the National Cancer Institute) or a well-known health agency (such as the American Cancer Society).

- If the site is not an organization you are familiar with, look on the site itself to see who is sponsoring it and the credentials of those creating the information.

- Always look for dates when the site was created and when it was last updated. A site with a "What's New" button usually has updates created within the last month.

- Be alert to Web addresses that are similar to those of major national organizations or sites that masquerade as national organizations.

- If the site asks you for personal information, be sure you understand what will be done with it. Look at their "privacy policy" to see whether or not your e-mail address will be shared, sold, or used to solicit you for money.

- Look for the words "HONcode" or "we subscribe to the Honor Code principles." This means that the site adheres to the eight principles of the Honor Code, sponsored by Health On Net (www.hon.ch), an organization whose mission is to help people find useful and reliable online medical and health information. Sites that follow these principles carry its symbol on their Web site.

Is there more than one search engine?

There are many search engines to choose from. Search engines have distinct personalities, are compiled in different ways, and look for information differently. Some search the entire Web and give you a listing of all the topics that have the "search word" in them. Others provide categories from which you can choose. Still others will answer a question you ask.

What are some of the search engines I can use for finding cancer information?

There are many. Our all-out favorite is Google (www.google.com), where you can enter a single word or a string of words and will be rewarded with a wealth of sites to browse. Here is a list of a few of the more popular search engines:

Alta Vista	www.altavista.com
Ask Jeeves	www.askjeeves.com
Dog Pile	www.dogpile.com
Excite	www.excite.com
Google	www.google.com
Lycos	www.lycos.com
MSN	www.msn.com
Wisenut	www.wisenut.com
Yahoo	www.yahoo.com

What can I get out of a search?

In order to get the most out of your search, you need to think about what you want before you start. The broader the topic, the more entries you will get. For instance, our search on Google with the word "cancer" found 16,800,000 entries and did it in .07 seconds. When the word "prostate" was entered, 564,000 entries were found. Using a term such as "PSA" will narrow the search even further and combining terms, such as entering "prostate PSA," will bring you even more specific entries.

Should I look at the first entry on the list?

It depends on the search engine. Usually the first few entries on each page are the most desired spots. Be careful if you see terms such as "products" or "services" on the page in a box on top or side of the list or even above the first couple of entries on the list. These terms mean that these spots on the list are being paid for and may not be the most unbiased information. Usually the entries that most closely match your search words are higher up on the page.

How can I find out who is sponsoring the site?

The address itself can tell you. Those ending in .com are paid for by commercial organizations; .gov means they are government sponsored; .org is often a nonprofit agency; and .edu are educational institutions. You should also check sections on the site such as "About Our Company," "Editorial Board," "About Us," "Investors," and "Mission." If you read this material, you will be able to find out who the sponsors are. Read it to see whether or not you are comfortable with it. For example, will it make a difference to you if a company is getting money from drug companies to enroll persons in clinical trials?

QUESTIONS TO ASK YOURSELF ABOUT INTERNET SITES

Whose site is it and what is its purpose?	You need to be sure that the sponsor of the site is credible. The site should make it easy to find out whose site it is. The purpose should be stated. Look for a link to "About Us" or "About this Site."
Where is the information coming from?	What are the credentials of the writers of the material? Has it been reviewed by medical experts? If the information is coming from other Web sites, that should be clear and the original source should be clearly stated, and its policy on getting frequent updates should be included.
Is the information scientifically based?	The site should note where it got its facts. Are they from articles in medical journals? Does an editorial board choose what goes on the site?
Who pays for the site?	You should know how the site is financed. Is it advertising? An agency or a donor? Sometimes sponsors will slant the information in order to sell you something. What and how the content is presented can be affected by who pays the bills.
How often is the material updated?	You need to be sure that the material is reviewed and updated frequently and that the date is posted on the site. If information on when the site has been updated or the site's policy on updating is not on the site, be leery.
Does the site ask for personal information?	If so, check to see what will happen to that information. Look for the privacy policy of the site. You need to know exactly what will be done with the information that is being collected about you.
Is advice or an opinion given on the site?	Opinions should be set apart from scientific material. The qualifications of those offering the advice or opinion should be stated.
Is the Honor Code symbol on the site?	This signifies that the site adheres to the principles of Health on Net.

LISTSERVS, NEWS GROUPS, AND CHATROOMS

Many people use on-line discussion groups for support during their cancer diagnosis and treatment. You can discuss your feelings with people who are facing the same thing and without anybody knowing who you are. If you have a rare cancer, you can probably find someone else who has been treated for it who can give you some information about it. On the other hand, you need to be aware of the disadvantages of Internet support groups. You are getting information based on one person's experience, not on science. There can be a mix of patients, who have had a variety of treatments, whose cancers are different types and at different stages. That means that some of the subjects may not be of interest to you or may even be topics you do not want to discuss, such as recurrence of cancer. Or the information may be misleading, depending on who is involved in presenting it, such as someone promoting an alternative treatment. Unlike a usual face-to-face support group, there is probably no professional leader, although sometimes there are health professionals monitoring the group.

How can I distinguish between the different on-line discussion groups?

It can be very confusing. Among the common terms used for such groups are listserv, mailing list, Web forum, and chat room.

What is a listserv?

A listserv, also called a mailing list, is a database of users who sign up to be included on mass discussion of a topic. In cancer, the discussion would be about a kind of cancer or a treatment. You subscribe by sending an e-mail or filling out a form for the listserv you wish to join. The listserv gives you an e-mail address that you then use to send messages to everybody else on the listserv, and in addition you will receive messages from any other person who wishes to send one to you.

How can I join one?

The simplest way to join is to go to www.acor.com, the home page for the Association for Cancer Online Resources, a nonprofit group that sponsors listservs. This should bring you to a page that lists different mailing lists, as well as frequently asked questions about lists. When you click on the list you are interested in, you will find a description of it along with instructions on how to subscribe. It is worth looking at more than one list, since mailing lists can vary in their content.

What will it cost me to join?
Most groups do not charge you either for joining or for being a member.

What is the difference between a listserv and a Web forum?
They are similar in that they share information from individual users; however, a Web forum is like a giant bulletin board where you send and receive messages. You will not get individual e-mail messages. Your message is posted through a Web site and then immediately appears. It will probably be put in a topic category (thread). Responses to your question or additional questions on the topic are considered part of the same thread. Whatever you post is there for everybody else to read, and it is kept in an archive file so that anyone can refer back to it.

How can I find a Web forum on the subject I'm interested in?
The easiest way is to go to a search engine, such as Google.com, search for Web forums or news groups, and then type in the subject that you are looking for.

How can I join a chat room?
The best way to join a chat room is to go to a heath site that you usually visit and click onto its link for a chat room. They are called by different names on different sites. Try "Cancer Survivor's Network" on the American Cancer Society site (www.cancer.org). On WebMD, look for "Member Communities." On Dr. Koop's site, it's labeled "Community." Some of the sites have open forums. Others use moderators.

Are there Web sites where patients can communicate with other patients with similar problems?
Sometimes good support and advice can come from other patients who have had to face similar problems. Some of the Web sites and groups that might be helpful include:

- Anderson Network: www.manderson.org/andersonnetwork
- Cancer Hope Network: www.cancerhopenetwork.org
- Friends/Health Connection: www.friendshealthconnection.org
- Med Help International Patient Network: www.medhelp.org.network.htm

What about virtual groups?
New types of Internet support groups are being added daily. Cancer Care, for instance, offers not only the regular face-to-face and telephone support groups, but also on-line support groups (www.cancercare.org) and one-hour

teleconferences. Technology already allows you to add a photo or video/audio file, making virtual relationships in cyberspace possible. Many patients have faster modems and cable connections for teleconferencing, allowing support groups to have live video and audio with people from around the world. This means that groups for specific kinds of cancer, for different age groups, and for family members or caregivers are forming.

Are there sites for family members and friends who are caring for cancer patients?
The National Family Caregivers Association (www.nfcacares.org) provides education, support, respite care, and advocacy for caregivers. Several of the sites discussed above also have specific areas for caregivers.

GETTING THE LATEST CANCER NEWS ON THE NET

Are there sites that give the latest news on cancer?
There are several sites that will give you this information. They vary from Cancer News on the Net (www.cancernews.com), which posts the most current articles, books, and research findings, to HemeOncLinx (www.mdlink. hemeonclinx.com), which surveys articles appearing in medical journals. Most of the cancer sites carry some kind of news features. The National Cancer Institute site, for instance, carries the latest cancer research and clinical trials news from the National Cancer Institute as well as other fast-breaking stories in the cancer field.

BOOKS AND JOURNALS YOUR DOCTOR READS

Where can I find the kind of technical medical information available to the health professionals?
A good place to start is PUBMED at the National Institutes of Health (NIH) Web site (www.cancer.gov/search/pubmed). Its "Cancer Literature" page allows searches on more than 100 cancer topics. Another source is the Electronic Journal of Oncology (www.elecjoncol.org), an international, non-profit, university-based e-journal. It contains peer-reviewed original publications in the field of oncology, including "Oncolynx" to help access useful oncology sites on the Internet. This link section includes drugs, organizations, journals, and databases.

Does the government have Internet sites about cancer other than www.cancer.gov?
Although the cancer.gov site is a major way to access current cancer information, there are other sites that could be useful to you, such as the Federal

SELECTED SITES FOR CHECKING THE LATEST NEWS ABOUT CANCER

Cancer News on the Net	www.cancernews.com	Gets cancer news from various resources, with links available.
Medscape	www.medscape.com	Web site for patients and doctors. General medical stories on research, drugs including cancer.
HemeOncLinx	www.mdlink.hemeonclinx. com	Surveys medical journal articles.
National Cancer Institute	www.cancer.gov	Click onto news center icon. Searchable site. Can access NCI site that gives news on cancer trials.

Drug Administration, which regulates drugs and medical devices. Its site (www.fda.gov) gives information about approved oncology drugs, and information about developing drugs and rights of patients. The National Center for Complementary and Alternative Medicine site (www.nccam.nih.gov) has a searchable database for scientific literature on alternative medicine topics.

SEARCHING A LIBRARY ON-LINE

Can I search a library on-line?
There are many libraries that have on-line capabilities, including your own public library. The best health library on the Internet is run by the federal government—the National Library of Medicine (www.medlineplus.gov). Its site is very easy to use and contains helpful information with links to many other sources for you to check. You can look for clinical trials for your type of cancer as well as for research articles in medical journals. This site also will link you to one of the most useful health encyclopedias (www.medlineplus. adam.com), where you can find information on tests and diagnostic procedures, medicines, treatments, side effects, and many other subjects.

CREDENTIALS

Are there any sites that will check credentials or offer comparisons in the healthcare field?

Using the Internet to find comparisons on a range of topics is a growing area. For instance, the Medicare site (www.medicare.gov) will let you compare heath plans, nursing homes, and supplemental insurance plans, and also gives information about doctors who participate in Medicare and about assistance with prescription drugs. HealthGrades (www.healthgrades.com) and the Health Pages (www.thehealthpages.com) are two other sites that offer comparisons of hospitals, mammography centers, nursing homes, doctors, and assisted living facilities. Other sites discussed offer information or comparisons on one or more of the issues. In any of the commercial sites, be aware that you might see a "pop-up" page boasting about a particular hospital or agency—understand that these are ads that are paid for by the hospital or the agency.

SELECTED HEALTH LIBRARIES AND DICTIONARIES ON THE INTERNET

National Library of Medicine www.medlineplus.gov	Most complete, with easy to find materials, links to other related sites, research studies, and research articles.
ADAM Medical Encyclopedia www.nlm.nih.gov/medlineplus.encyclopedia.html	Health encyclopedia. You can search by category or alphabetically.
MedicineNet www.medterms.com	Dictionary of medical terms.
Gray's Anatomy of the Human Body www.bartleby.com/107	More than 1,200 illustrations and 13,000 entries. You can search the site by word or through the table of contents.
Association of Cancer Online Resources www.acor.org	Glossary of more than 1,000 terms; can be searched alphabetically. Definition finder link for immediate answers.
National Cancer Institute www.cancer.gov	Comprehensive dictionary of cancer terms, non-technical and technical. Alphabetical and word searchable.

(continued)

American Cancer Society www.cancer.org	Comprehensive glossary of cancer terms. Alphabetical and word searchable.
PUBMED www.cancer.gov/search/pubmed	From this page, more than 100 cancer topics are searchable.

Checking Your Doctors' Credentials

**Is there any way I can check a doctor's
credentials on the Internet?**

The American Board of Medical Specialists, the national organization that credentials specialty doctors (see Chapter 3, Choosing Your Doctor and Hospital), has a Web site (www.abms.org) but you need medical identification to use it. (You can call 1-866-ASK-ABMS to see if your doctor is board certified or to get names of doctors who are.) The Physician Select Service on the American Medical Association's site (www.ama-assn.org) offers professional information about almost every licensed doctor in the country. Many of the specialty groups have their own sites that give you information about doctors practicing in individual fields. Surgeons who are fellows of the American College of Surgeons (ACOS), their accrediting organization, are listed on the ACOS site (www.web.facs.org). The American Society of Clinical Oncology (www.asco.org) has a listing of doctors who belong to its organization worldwide. You can search by name, institutions, location, or type of specialty. HealthGrades and the Health Pages also give physician information.

**How can I determine whether or not the doctor I
choose accepts Medicare assignment?**

The Medicare site (www.medicare.gov) has a listing of doctors that accept assignment. That means that they will not charge patients more than Medicare will pay for a specific test or treatment.

**Is there a site that discusses doctors who have had
problems with malpractice?**

The Public Citizen Research Group's site (www.questionabledoctors.org) tells you how to get information on doctors who have been disciplined in your state.

How can I check the doctors that are on my HMO list?

First check your insurance company's Web site. Many times it will have information on the doctors who are in your plan. You also can use the information discussed above to see if the doctor is board-certified and to verify medical and educational information. Finally, *U.S. News and World Report* has a listing of best HMOs on its site (www.usnews.com).

CHOOSING A HOSPITAL

How can I find a major cancer center for treatment on the Internet?

If you don't know the name of a major center, you can find the comprehensive cancer centers that have been approved by the National Cancer Institute by going to its site at www.cancer.gov. Many cancer centers have their own Web pages where you can find information about the kind of cancer they treat, the qualifications of their medical personnel, and how to make appointments, along with what clinical trials they are running. The American College of Surgeons (ACOS) accredits cancer programs at hospitals and other treatment facilities. At its searchable Web site (www.facs.org) you can access the names of the 1400 institutions in the United States whose programs have been designated as "Approved Cancer Programs" by the ACOS. Health Web will link you to hospital sites around the country (www.lmgh.harvard. edu/hospitalweb.html). See Chapter 3, Choosing your Doctor and Hospital, and Chapter 28, Where to Get Help, for the listing of the cancer centers designated by the National Cancer Institute, along with their addresses and phone numbers.

Is it possible to find out how one hospital compares to others?

There are several sites on the Web that can help. You may need to dig a little, but you should be able to come up with that information. The Joint Commission on Accreditation of Healthcare Organizations is a major player in this area because it officially evaluates hospitals. The results of its hospital surveys are on line (www.jcaho.org). The American Hospital Association can tell you what the average length of stay and costs are for a variety of services (www.ahd.com). HealthGrades offers a report card that rates hospitals (www.healthgrades.com). Each year, *U.S. News and World Report* rates the top hospitals (www.usnews.com) and its site lists them.

SELECTED SITES FOR FINDING DOCTORS AND THEIR CREDENTIALS ON THE WEB

American Medical Association's Physician Select	www.ama-assn.org	Allows you to select a doctor by location, name, specialty, age, educational institution, and other credentials.
American Society of Clinical Oncology	www.asco.org Go to "People Living With Cancer/Community Center/ASCO Physician" database.	Searchable site of ASCO members.
Medicare	www.medicare.gov Look under search tools for "participating physician directory."	Lists physicians who participate in the Medicare program and who accept assignment. Site also lets you compare health plans, nursing homes, and supplemental insurance plans.
Public Citizen Research Group	www. questionabledoctors.org	Describes how to reach your state's medical board for information on disciplined doctors.
HealthGrades	www.healthgrades.com	Searchable database of over 650,000 physicians for credentials. Tells if doctor has been sanctioned; charge for report on details of sanctioning.
U.S. News and World Report	www.usnews.com	Yearly listing of best HMOs in the U.S.

If I am going to have treatment far away from home are there any special services to help me with my travel expenses?

There are several:

- Air Care Alliance, a national organization of volunteer pilots who arrange patient transport. Their Web site (www.aircarecall.org) offers a central searchable source for all free air transportation services provided by volunteer pilots and charitable aviation groups.

- Corporate Angel Network (www.corpangelnet.org) matches available space on corporate airlines with patients who need transportation to recognized treatment centers.

- National Patient Travel Helpline (www.patienttravel.org) provides information about long-distance medical air transportation and referrals to all programs in the national charitable medical air transportation network.

If I need a nursing home, is there a Web site that compares them?

The Medicare site (www.medicare.gov) has an interactive tool that allows you to get comparison information on every Medicare-and Medicaid-certified nursing home in the country, more than 1,700 nationwide, to use in evaluating nursing homes. Medicare has set up ten qualitative measures (percentage of patients with pressure sores, urinary incontinence, pain, lack of ability to do basic daily tasks, etc.) and compares each individual nursing home on these measures with state and with national averages. It also provides summary information about the nursing home's last state inspection and tells you what deficiencies were found and if they have been corrected. It will tell you the number of beds, types of ownership, how to reach the long-term care ombudsman, and whether or not it participates in Medicare, Medicaid, or both. You can search by county, city, or name of nursing home. You can also call the Medicare toll-free number (1-800-633-4227) to find out more about nursing homes in your area. HealthGrades also has information on nursing homes.

GENETICS

Where can I find basic information about cancer genetics for patients and their families?

A good place to start is at the NCI site (www.cancer.gov, search for "cancer genetics"), where you will find general information including an overview of cancer genetics and a glossary of genetic terms. There also is material to help you understand gene testing; information on specific cancers, such as colon, breast, ovary, and thyroid; risk assessment tools; and the Cancer Genetics Network. You also can access a Cancer Genetics Services directory at this site. Another NCI

FINDING INFORMATION ABOUT MAJOR MEDICAL CENTERS ON THE WEB

National Cancer Institute	www.cancer.gov	Lists cancer centers that have been designated by the NCI as approved "comprehensive" or "clinical" centers.
American College of Surgeons	www.web.facs.org Go to cancer programs then to database of approved programs.	Lists 1,400 institutions in U.S. that have ACOS "approved cancer programs."
American Hospital Directory	www.ahd.com	Lists how much it costs for specific operations and hospital stays.
American Hospital Direct	www.ahd.com	Gives financial and utilization data on over 6,000 hospitals. Search by location.
Joint Commission on Accreditation of Healthcare Organizations	www.jcaho.org	Judges how well hospitals (and other healthcare facilities) meet standards.
U.S. News Best Hospitals	www.usnews.com	Lists best hospitals as determined by their editors.

site with cancer genetics information is www.cancer.gov/cancerinformation/prevention, where there is more information on genetics and specific cancer types. Also see Chapter 11, New Advances and Investigational Treatments.

What is included in the Cancer Genetics Services Directory?
It includes over 300 professionals who provide services related to cancer genetics in cancer risk assessment, genetic counseling, genetic susceptibility testing, and others. You'll find professionals of various disciplines, such as genetic counseling, oncology, nursing, psychology, social work, and clinical genetics. In order to be listed in the directory, each person must be licensed, certified, or eligible for board certification in the profession, have specific training in cancer genetics, and be affiliated with an interdisciplinary team with substantial expertise in cancer genetics. Each person listed must also be a member of one of the professional organizations and be willing to accept referrals. You can

search the directory by cancer type, specialty, and/or name of professional person and get information about the person's background, training, certification, and affiliations.

Are there any sites for genetics that are not sponsored by the government?

There are several. Among them:

- National Alliance of Breast Cancer Organizations (www.nabco.org) publishes ongoing updates on genetics and breast cancer.

- Genetic Alliance (www.geneticalliance.org) educates the public and supports individuals with genetic conditions and their families.

- Facing Our Risk of Cancer Empowered (www.facingourrisk.org), a Web-based, nonprofit organization that offers information, resources, support groups, and on-line chat rooms for women at high risk of developing breast and ovarian cancer.

- Oncolink's (www.oncolink.com) "Ask An Expert" section helps those with questions about inherited cancer and genetic testing. This site is sponsored by the University of Pennsylvania.

ENVIRONMENT

What are the major Web sites for information about environmental causes of cancer?

Many governmental sites are focused on environmental information. Among them:

- National Cancer Institute's site (www.cancer.gov), where you can check the various fact sheets available on cancer causes.

- Atlas of Cancer Mortality in United States: 1950–1994 (www3.cancer.gov/atlasplus/), with color-coded maps for over 3,000 U.S. counties including descriptions of geographical differences in death rates in 40 cancers.

- Long Island Breast Cancer Study Project (www.epi.grants.cancer.gov/LIBCSP) gives details of several studies of possible causes of breast cancer on Long Island.

- NCI's Surveillance, Epidemiology and Ends Result Program (www.seer.cancer.gov), an authoritative source of information on cancer incidence and survival in the U.S.

- National Toxicology Program (www.ehp.niehs.nih.gov/roc/) lists substances that may pose a potential hazard to human health.

- National Institute of Environmental Health Sciences (www.nieh.nih.gov), chief federal agency responsible for research on environment and health.

- Environmental Protection Agency (EPA), responsible for protecting human health and safeguarding the natural environment, offers Envirofacts Warehouse (www.epa.gov/enviro), Enviromapper (www.epa.gov/epahome/comm. htm), and Environmental Atlas (www.epa.gov/ceisweb1/ceishome/atlas).

- Centers for Disease Control and Prevention's National Center for Environmental Health (www.cdc.gov/nceh/) and its National Institute for Occupational Health and Safety (www.cdc.gov/niosh).

INSURANCE AND MEDICARE

What sites can I access to learn more about my health insurance?

Today, there are more choices than ever in health insurance. There are several places to go on the Web to get information that both compares differences among the types and finds insurance plans that will suit your needs. The Agency for Healthcare Research and Quality (AHRQ), a federal agency, offers information on its site (www.ahcpr.gov), along with checklists that will help you. If you need information about Medicare and Medicaid, go to www.medicare.gov. Not only will you get authentic information about benefits on this user-friendly site, but there also is a Personal Plan Finder that shows you the plan choices you have with Medicare. This allows you to compare the different Medicare health plans to determine what is the best plan for you. If you are just looking for information on a particular health insurance company or plan, the Health Insurance Association of America site may be useful for you (www.hiaa.org). In its consumer education area, it gives links to the companies that belong to the association.

Where can I find information that will help me compare my health plan with others?

The independent nonprofit group the National Committee for Quality Assurance (NCQA) sets standards for the quality of care and service that health plans provide to their members and issues report cards on them. Its Web site (www.hprc.ncqa.org) includes an interactive tool designed to help you find the health plan that's right for you. You can get answers to questions such as: Does the health plan provide good customer service? Will you have access to the care you need? Does the plan check doctors' qualifications? If you get sick, which plan will take better care of you? Enter information about your plan on the computer and it will provide a chart showing how your plan rates.

How can I reach the insurance commissioner in my state?

Go to the Web site of the National Association of Insurance Commissioners (www.naic.org). This association is the organization of insurance regulators from the 50 states, the District of Columbia, and the four U.S. territories. Under "Services" you will find a map and state-by-state links to the insurance commissioners. This site also gives information about insurance companies. Also see Chapter 28, Where to Get Help, for information.

SELECTED WEB SITES FOR SPECIFIC CANCERS

(Also see general cancer information Web pages on p. 13–14 and listings at end of individual chapters.)

Breast

- www.bcdg.org: Department of Defense—Breast Cancer Decision Guide.
- www.nabco.org: National Alliance of Breast Cancer Organizations.
- www.susanlovemd.com: Susan Love, MD
- www.nccn.org: National Comprehensive Cancer Network Breast Treatment Guidelines for Patients.
- www.lymphnet.org: National Lymphedema Network.
- www.komen.org: Susan G. Komen Breast Cancer Foundation.
- www.y-me.org: Y-Me National Breast Cancer Organization.
- www.youngsurvival.org: Young Survival Coalition.

Prostate, Testicular, Penis

- www.capcure.org: CaP Cure.
- www.4npacc.org: National Prostate Cancer Coalition.
- www.prostate-cancer.org: Prostate Cancer Research Institute.
- www.ustoo.com: Us Too! International.

Colon and Rectum

- www.ccalliance.org: Colon Cancer Alliance, Inc.
- www.hopkins-coloncancer.org: Johns Hopkins Hereditary Colorectal Cancer Resources.
- www.yourcancerrisk.harvard.edu: Harvard Center for Cancer Prevention.
- www.uoa.org: United Ostomy Association.

Lung

- www.alcase.org: Alliance for Lung Cancer Advocacy, Support and Education.
- www.lungusa.org: American Lung Association.
- www.lungcanceronline.org: Resource compiled by cancer survivor Karen Parles.

Cervix, Uterus, Fallopian Tubes, Ovary

- www.nccc-online.org: National Cervical Cancer Coalition.
- www.ovariancancer.org: Ovarian Cancer National Alliance.

Melanoma and Other Skin Cancers

- www.skincancer.org: Skin Cancer Foundation.

Leukemia, Lymphoma, Multiple Myeloma, Sarcomas

- www.leukemia-lymphoma.org: The Leukemia Society of America & Lymphoma Society.

Bladder, Stomach, Kidney, Liver, Pancreas

- www.afnd.org: American Foundation for Urologic Disease.
- www.pancan.org: Pancreatic Cancer Action Network.

Brain and Spinal Cord

- www.abts.org: American Brain Tumor Association.
- www.tbts.org: Brain Tumor Society.
- www.braintumor.org: National Brain Tumor Foundation.

Head and Neck

- www.spohnc.org: Support for Head and Neck Cancer.

Childhood Cancer

- www.candlelighters.org: Candlelighters Childhood Cancer Foundation.
- www.rmhc.com: Ronald McDonald House Charities (housing).

Cancer Screening Guidelines

- www.guideline.gov: National Guideline Clearinghouse.

Note: Web sites were checked at publication date and were accurate at that time.

Three

CHOOSING YOUR
DOCTOR AND HOSPITAL

Doctors vary depending on their training, experience, and the services they perform. They *differ* in the way they deal with patients. So finding the doctor who is the right one for you *and* your case isn't simple. Most of us do more research in buying a car than we do in choosing our doctor or the hospital where we will be treated. Often this is true because we don't really know exactly what to look for.

WHEN YOU ARE dealing with cancer treatment, it is especially important that you give careful thought to the doctor and the hospital you will be using. With the many changes in health care delivery and with more and more doctors involved in health care organizations, the problem of making decisions about doctors and hospitals has become more important and even more complicated than ever before. However, the facts surrounding your decisions about which doctor and which hospital to choose for your medical care have not changed—even though it might be more difficult to achieve your goal.

A doctor who deals with a specific kind of cancer on a daily basis usually has broader knowledge of the treatment options available than a doctor who sees such a cancer only occasionally. A hospital that specializes in cancer

SOME BASIC FACTS THAT WILL HELP YOU IN
CHOOSING A DOCTOR AND HOSPITAL

- When you have cancer, you need to be under the care of someone who specializes in cancer care. Such doctors are known as **oncologists. There are many different specialists in oncology, such as surgical oncologists, medical oncologists, and radiation oncologists.** The major point to remember right now is that *you should not feel that you are limited to dealing exclusively with your present doctor.*

- Your doctor should be board-certified in the practice specialty.

- It is important to check out your doctor's credentials. A doctor doesn't have to be certified in a field to be listed as a specialist in it. Make sure that if your doctor is listed as an internist or a cancer specialist, the doctor has been certified in that field. Be aware. Don't take the listing in the phone book for granted.

- We recommend that you consider getting a second opinion before making any final decisions on treatment. This is perfectly standard practice and should not offend your doctor.

- If you live near a Comprehensive or Clinical Cancer Center that has been so designated by the National Cancer Institute, you should definitely consider getting treatment, or at least a second opinion, there. These centers attract the best doctors, meeting high standards set by the National Cancer Institute, and offering strong laboratory and clinical research, the ability to put the research into practice, and the chance to be first in line for offering promising treatments. Again, you need to be an informed consumer. Not all hospitals that call themselves "cancer centers" or even "comprehensive cancer centers" have necessarily passed the rigorous standards designated by the National Cancer Institute.

- A referral and a consultation are two different things. A referral means that once you see the specialist, you become a patient of that doctor. A consultation is designed to get another opinion from another doctor. The consulting doctor will not be taking over the responsibility for your care but simply will report the findings to your doctor.

- If your managed care plan and your primary physician seem to be blocking your ability to see a specific specialist, explain that you have a medical necessity. Your health plan has a contractual obligation to pay for "a medical necessity." If it is an emergency, ask for priority scheduling.

treatment has more services for the cancer patient than a small local hospital that is designed to serve broader community needs. In a cancer center with many specialists working under one roof, patients benefit from the combined expertise.

What does board certification mean?

The specialty boards are private, voluntary, nonprofit, autonomous organizations founded to conduct examinations, issue certificates of qualifications, and improve and broaden opportunities for graduate education and training. Once doctors finish their required residency in a particular specialty, they become eligible to be certified by the board. This requires taking a rigorous written and oral examination given by other doctors who practice in this specialty. Many doctors do not become certified after their first examinations by the board. Some boards require recertification after a specified number of years. A fellowship in the "college" of the specialty means that the doctor is qualified to teach others. It is another step up the ladder and earns a more esteemed place among the doctor's colleagues. While board-certification is no assurance of the quality of care you'll receive, it indicates that a doctor has met standards that are higher than those required to obtain a medical license in any state.

Are there good doctors who are not board-certified?

Lack of board-certification may reflect a serious problem with a doctor's training, competence, or character. Board-certification and fellowships are designed to indicate a high level of competence, but there are reasons why competent doctors may not be board-certified. In the field of cancer, especially, there are many good doctors who treat only cancer patients but are not board-certified in oncology. This is because the boards in oncology are relatively new and were not available to older doctors when they started in practice. Some practicing doctors in the large cancer centers who combine research with patient care are not board-certified but are extremely well qualified to treat cancer patients. What's important is to understand the reason behind why a doctor may not be board-certified.

What is the difference between a board-certified and a board-eligible doctor?

A doctor who passes the examination for a given specialty is known as a diplomate of the board and is said to be board-certified. A physician who has completed a formal training program in the specialty but has either chosen not to take the exams or has not completed the exams is called board-eligible (newly trained doctors are board-eligible between the time they finish their residency or fellowship and the time they take their boards and get the results). The American Board of Medical Specialties has a policy that they no longer use the "board-eligible" terminology because some candidates have used the term year after year without making progress toward certification. Instead, their Member Boards respond to specific inquiries about board-certification by stating the doctor's precise position in the certifying process. Of course, there are well-trained specialists who for good, legitimate reasons continue to be board-eligible. These are exceptions. There's no question that it's better to have passed the exams than not to have passed them.

> CALL THIS NUMBER TO SEE
> IF YOUR DOCTOR IS BOARD-CERTIFIED
> OR TO GET NAMES OF DOCTORS
> WHO ARE BOARD-CERTIFIED
> 866-ASK-ABMS
> (866-275-2267)
> or 847-491-9091
> fax: 847-328-3596
>
> (American Board of Medical Specialists)
> NOTE: Phoning is the easiest way to check about board-certification. Going on the Web requires that you log in with a medical identification.

Are there other ways to check out my doctor's credentials?

There are several directories that list doctor credentials. The *Directory of Medical Specialists* and the *American Medical Directory* are two of the most readily available. Our favorite is the *Directory of Medical Specialists* because it lists only those doctors who are board-certified. The listing of doctors in the *American Medical Directory* is a listing of all doctors who belong to the American Medical Association, whether or not they have board-certification. If your library does not have either of these books, you can call 866-ASK-ABMS to check on whether or not the doctor is certified. You could also search doctor's name and location online using a search engine, but the easiest way of checking is to make the call to the ASK-ABMS number. In addition, your state or local department of health or medical society can give you information.

What are the major specialties?

- **Allergy and immunology:** Treatment of primary and secondary immunodeficiency diseases, autoimmune diseases, immunologic aspects of bone marrow and organ transplantation, immune aspects of gene replacement, immune aspects of organ specific inflammatory diseases, and immune aspects of cancer and malignancy.

- **Anesthesiology:** Administration of drugs for relief of pain during surgery or childbirth. During an operation in which general anesthetic is used, the anesthesiologist is responsible for monitoring and maintaining safe levels of the patient's bodily functions. Some anesthesiologists are also certified in pain management.

- **Colon and Rectal Surgery:** Diagnosis and treatment of diseases of the intestinal tract, rectum, and anus.

- **Dermatology:** Treatment of skin diseases and conditions, including skin cancer.

- **Emergency medicine:** All aspects of emergency treatment.

- **Family practice:** Continuing and total care of the family.

- **Internal Medicine:** Covers a wide range of medical problems. Internists who take an additional one or more years of "fellowship" are certified for subspecialties such as:

  Cardiovascular Disease: Diseases of heart, lungs, and blood vessels.

  Endocrinology: Diseases of organs that secrete hormones into the blood stream—such as the thyroid, adrenal glands, and ovaries.

  Diabetes and Metabolism: Diseases of endocrinology.

  Gastroenterology (GI): Diseases of the digestive tract (mouth to anus, including stomach, bowels, liver, gallbladder).

  Hematology: Diseases of the blood and blood-making tissues (bone marrow, spleen, lymph glands).

  Infectious Diseases: Difficult cases of infection.

  Medical Oncology: All types of benign and malignant cancers in any organ of the body, prescribe chemotherapy or may refer patient to radiation oncologists or surgeons.

  Nephrology: Disease of the kidneys, urinary system, and related disorders of metabolism.

Pulmonary: Diseases of the lung.

Rheumatology: Diseases of joints, ligaments, muscles, bones, and tendons.

- **Medical Genetics:** Diseases that are linked with hereditary disorders.

- **Neurological Surgery:** Surgery in the nervous system, including brain, spinal cord, and nerves.

- **Nuclear Medicine:** evaluate functions of all organs in body, treat benign and malignant tumors and radiation exposure.

- **Obstetrics and Gynecology:** Treatment of the female reproductive system; there is a specialty in gynecological oncology.

- **Ophthalmology:** Comprehensive medical and surgical care of eyes and vision.

- **Orthopaedic surgery:** Adult reconstructive surgery, sports medicine, surgery of the spine.

- **Otolaryngology:** Medical and surgical treatment of head and neck; called otolaryngologists, head and neck surgeons, or ear, nose, and throat doctors.

- **Pathology:** Study of body tissues, secretions, and fluids to diagnose disease and gauge how far it has spread. There are subspecialties in this discipline including: dermatopathology (skin), hematology (blood), cytopathology (cancer cells).

- **Pediatrics:** Care for children up to age 16. Subspecialties are similar to internal medicine and include: pediatric hematology-oncology, pediatric endocrinology, pediatric nephrology, etc.

- **Physical Medicine and Rehabilitation:** Evaluation and treatment of patients with impairments and restoring maximal function. Called physiatrists.

- **Plastic Surgery:** Correct functional and cosmetic deformities of face, head, body, and extremities.

- **Preventive Medicine:** Promote, protect, and maintain health and well-being and prevent disease, disability, and premature death. Includes aerospace and undersea medicine, occupational medicine, public health, and general preventive medicine.

- **Psychiatry and Neurology:** Treatment of mental, addictive, and emotional disorders as well as treatment of disorders of nervous system (brain, spinal cord, nerves) and muscles, including tumors.

- **Radiology:** Divided into three categories—radiation oncology (use of radiation in treatment of cancer), diagnostic radiology (use of Xrays, CAT scans and MRI for diagnosis of cancer), and diagnostic radiology with special competence in nuclear radiology (use of radioactive substances in diagnosis of disease).

■ **Surgery:** Manage a broad spectrum of surgical conditions affecting almost any area of the body; specialty in thoracic surgery, including cancers of the lung and esophagus.

■ **Thoracic Surgery:** Surgery on organs within the chest cavity including heart, lung major blood vessels and esophagus.

■ **Urology:** Treatment of urinary system including kidneys, bladder, prostate adrenal gland, and testes.

What other information can I determine from the listings in the medical directories?

You will want to scan the information in the front of the directory, so you will be able to decipher all the information given in each biographical listing. The listings are geographical by specialty, so this is a good time to find out and jot down the names and credentials of other specialists in your area— such as surgeons, anesthesiologists, gynecologists, urologists, etc. If no one in your town is listed, look for names of doctors in nearby towns. (Just a tip: it's easier to check the alphabetical listing in the index of the last volume of the book if you have the name of a specific doctor you want to check. It will give you the page number for the listing.)

What should I look for in analyzing the listings?

■ Does the doctor have a teaching appointment at a medical-school affiliated hospital? This indicates the doctor is up to date and respected by peers.

■ What kind of hospital is the doctor affiliated with? Is it a medical-school-affiliated hospital? Requirements for this sort of hospital are rigid and must be earned through teaching appointments.

■ If the doctor is a surgeon, does he have privileges at three or more hospitals? This sounds impressive but it takes so much of the doctor's time that you might be better served by someone who concentrates on one or two hospitals. The quality of the association with the hospital is more important than the number.

■ How large is the hospital? If you don't live in an area with a university hospital center, the larger the hospital (200 beds or more) the more equipment and facilities it will have.

■ What societies does the doctor belong to? One or more is preferable, for these help keep doctors up to date on the latest information being developed by others in the specialty.

Can doctors list themselves as specialists?

Yes. Doctors, once licensed, can list themselves as they wish. Even physicians with no specialized training beyond medical school and internship can call themselves gynecologists or internists or dermatologists, etc. They can legally perform operations. That is why it is important to determine whether or not your physician has had additional training, is board certified, and is practicing in a legitimate hospital. Four years of medical school after college plus one year of internship allows doctors to be licensed to practice under any title they choose to assume. So be sure to check credentials so that you know for certain that your doctor is qualified to be treating you.

What is a medical oncologist?

A medical oncologist is a doctor who specializes in treating cancer with drugs. In the past, this training was often in the treatment of blood diseases (hematology), particularly leukemia and lymphoma, since these were the first tumors to be treated with drugs. More recently, the medical specialty called medical oncology trains doctors exclusively in the treatment of cancer patients. These specialists are certified by the American Board of Internal Medicine, the

JUDGING YOUR DOCTOR

ASSESSMENT SCORE		SCORE YOUR DOCTOR
	KIND OF PRACTICE	
+5	Hospital-based office	
+5	One-specialty group	
+5	Multi-specialty group	
+2	Loose association with other doctors	
+1	Partner	
− 5	Practices alone	

Generally, a doctor who practices with a group that specializes in a variety of disciplines is better as a family doctor. Specialists who practice in a group or in a hospital are subject to constant review by peers.

	HOSPITAL AFFILIATION	
+10	Practices at an NCI-designated Comprehensive or Clinical Cancer Center	

JUDGING YOUR DOCTOR *(continued)*

ASSESSMENT SCORE		SCORE YOUR DOCTOR
	HOSPITAL AFFILIATION	
+5	Practices at hospital which you prefer	
+5	University or medical school hospital (part or full-time staff member)	
+5	On teaching staff of medical school	
+4	Staff, community hospital with 200 beds or more	
+3	Staff, community hospital with fewer than 200 beds	
+1	Part owner, staff of small private hospital (proprietary)	
−1 or −5	No hospital affiliation (ask why, score depends on answer)	

A doctor who is a part- or full-time staff member at a university or medical school hospital or a larger community hospital has shown his merit.
The doctor who practices in a small for-profit hospital, may be just as qualified, but should be checked more closely for other credentials.

	BOARDS	
+10	Board-certified in his specialty, specialist in oncology	
+5	Board-certified and/or fellow of the board	
+4	Board-certified	
−5	No longer eligible or not listed	

Board-certification is a big plus. It means that beyond training in the specialty field, the doctor has been subjected to the scrutiny of peers in written and oral examinations. A fellowship is an extra flag of distinction. Oncology specialty means that the doctor is skilled in cancer treatment.

	MANNER, PERSONALITY, OFFICE EFFICIENCY	
+5	Warm, concerned, explains procedures and listens well	
+2	Difficulty communicating, impersonal, but efficient	
+5	Efficient, well-run office, pleasant personnel	
+5	Willing to discuss fees and insurance	

(continued)

JUDGING YOUR DOCTOR (continued)

ASSESSMENT SCORE		SCORE YOUR DOCTOR
MANNER, PERSONALITY, OFFICE EFFICIENCY		
+5	Files insurance claims	
+3	On-site lab and x-ray facility	
−10	Poor office practices, inefficient appointment schedules	
NURSING STAFF		
+10	Communicative, willing to discuss problems, gives helpful solutions, supportive, professional, skilled	
−10	Office assistants but no nurses	

Your own observations about your doctor's manner, skills, and office personnel are an important part of your evaluation. The manner in which the physician's office is run tells you a great deal about the doctor's standards and probably also reflects on the doctor's professionalism. While not as vital as professional credentials, when taken in context with other observations, this serves as another guideline for judgment.

American Board of Medical Oncology, and, in the case of doctors who treat children, by the American Board of Pediatrics.

What is a radiation oncologist?
The radiation oncologist treats cancer with radiation. This doctor also may be called a therapeutic radiologist. Qualified radiation oncologists are certified by the American Board of Therapeutic Radiology. There is a difference between a radiation oncologist and a diagnostic radiologist. A diagnostic radiologist is a doctor whose specialty is in performing and interpreting x-rays used in diagnosing illness.

What is an interventional radiologist?
This is a relatively new specialty that was recognized by the American Medical Association and the U.S. Department of Health and Human Services in 1992. Interventional radiologists use x-rays and other imaging techniques that "see" inside the body without surgery. They make tiny incisions (about the size of the tip of a pencil) and insert thin tubes (catheters) and other tiny instruments through blood vessels and other pathways of the body to diag-

nose and treat a wide variety of conditions that once required surgery. They are highly trained doctors who have completed medical school, internship, and four years of post-graduate training in radiology and passed special exams to become board-certified radiologists; and then spent an extra year in an interventional radiology fellowship program. These doctors are certified by the American Board of Radiology in both diagnostic radiology and cardiovascular and interventional radiology.

What is the difference between a medical oncologist and a hematologist?

A medical oncologist is a doctor of internal medicine who specializes in the administration of a variety of drugs needed to treat specific cancers. This doctor may also be referred to as a hematologist (one who specializes in blood diseases). The administration of most chemotherapy drugs is very complex. These drugs need to be given under the supervision of a doctor who specializes in this field.

Can any doctor prescribe chemotherapy for me?

Yes, any doctor can—but some are more skilled than others. Giving chemotherapy is a science and you need to be sure that the doctors and nurses who are giving it to you are well trained and up to date on the latest drugs and techniques. If you are having chemotherapy treatment and are not being treated by a medical oncologist, it is important to make sure that your doctor has consulted with a major cancer center, a medical school, or an oncologist to determine which drugs are best for your case, the dose of drug to be given, and the side effects to be expected. In most areas, doctors, nurses, and pharmacists work as a team in the administration of chemotherapy.

How do I find a surgeon who specializes in cancer?

Some surgeons have special training and limit their practices to cancer surgery. Although there is no certification that denotes this kind of training, it is important to find out what a surgeon's interest and experience are. While medical oncologists and radiation oncologists deal exclusively with cancer patients, many surgeons have practices where they deal with a variety of diseases. Look for a cancer surgeon certified by the American Board of Surgeons or by one of its subspecialty boards such as Neurosurgery, Obstetrics and Gynecology, Orthopedic Surgery, or Urologic Surgery. There are surgical specialists who treat specific parts of the body. You will want to discuss the choice of a surgeon with your primary care physician. You also can get referrals from your local hospital, a major medical center, a medical oncologist, or a radiation oncologist. People with very rare or difficult kinds of cancer—such as in the head and neck area—should realize that the best treatment may be available in only a few major cancer centers where significant numbers of people with similar tumors are treated.

CHECKLIST FOR CHOOSING A SURGEON FOR A CANCER PROBLEM

Ask these questions:

- How many of these procedures have you done?
- How often do you do this procedure? (At least two or three times a week, for major surgery, is a minimum. Studies show that mortality rates are lower at hospitals where surgeons do a procedure frequently.)
- How often is this procedure done in your hospital? (The more often, the more likely it is that other staff members who are assisting and caring for you, will be well trained.)
- What is your success rate with this operation?
- What are the complications and aftereffects?
- What happens if I do nothing?
- If it is a new procedure or method, ask: What are the advantages of this procedure over the old-fashioned way?
- How long have you used this procedure?
- Is it more costly?
- How do you handle emergencies if I should need to reach you after office hours?
- Who covers for you on nights and weekends? Will that person have access to my records?
- What hospital are you affiliated with?
- Are you affiliated with my health plan? If not, what extra costs will I have to pay if you do the procedure?

If my doctor has no hospital affiliation what does that mean?
If your doctor has no hospital affiliation you owe it to yourself to ask for the reason. Some perfectly good family doctors confine themselves to office practices. When their patients need hospitalization, they recommend the specialist they feel has the proper skills. If, however, the doctor was once affiliated with a hospital and no longer has that affiliation, make sure you ask for reasons why. You might check the record with your state medical society.

If a doctor is in practice alone, is that a good sign?
Many doctors practice in rural areas and may have no choice but to work alone. However, in general, the doctor who works with other doctors is

usually a better bet than one who has a solo practice. If you have such a doctor, you should know what arrangements have been made for coverage when the doctor is away or unavailable. If the covering doctor does not have access to your medical records, there is a great limitation on how the covering doctor can treat you in your own doctor's absence or during a medical emergency.

Is it a good idea for a group of one kind of doctor to practice together?

If your doctor is part of a group that consists of several other doctors who practice the same specialty, such as a group of internists, this is a real plus. Usually each has a different area of expertise. This gives them, and you, the advantage of other opinions on a specific case.

How can I find out which doctors practice at which hospitals?

The easiest way is to call the hospital's staff office or patient-referral service and ask if the doctor practices there or for the names of doctors in particular specialties who do practice there.

If I have a choice between an equally qualified young doctor and older doctor, which should I choose?

When choosing a doctor in private practice, many people reason that a younger doctor may be more inclined to keep up on the latest technology but an older doctor will be more experienced. In the academic world an older doctor is probably both more up to date and more experienced, since a teaching physician must be ready to explain to students the wisdom of using a particular procedure or treatment.

Why should I consider getting a second opinion?

There are several reasons for getting a second opinion from another qualified physician. Foremost is reassurance that the first opinion is correct and that you have explored all your choices. A second opinion may also be wanted when surgery has been recommended, when you question the evaluation made by your first doctor, when you think the doctor is underestimating the seriousness of your illness, when the doctor seems unable to find out what is wrong with you, or when you think there may be another form of treatment. Getting a second opinion is common practice.

Won't my doctor be offended if I ask for another opinion?

If your doctor is offended, then you have a good reason for finding another doctor. Most doctors *welcome* a second opinion, and many health plans require a second opinion. A second opinion does not mean you are questioning your

WAYS OF GETTING A SECOND OPINION

- Ask your own doctor to suggest the name of someone to see for a second opinion.

- Make the appointment yourself or ask the doctor to make the appointment for you.

- Always discuss your plans for consultation with your doctor. You will need to bring your original x-rays and tests for the other doctor to use during your consultation. If your doctor is uncooperative, then you have other decisions to make about continuing that relationship.

- Call the toll-free 1-800-4-CANCER number and ask for information about getting an appointment with a specialist in your kind of cancer at an NCI-designated comprehensive or clinical cancer center near you.

- Call your nearest medical school and ask for suggestions. A medical school's outpatient clinic, where some of the country's top specialists practice, is also a good place to check.

- Some hospitals have a special telephone line for physician referral—although many simply give names of all the doctors who have privileges to admit patients to their facilities. You can write the director of the hospital of your choice and ask for suggestions.

- Call the American Board of Medical Specialties at 1-866-ASK-ABMS for names of specialists in your area.

- Check the Directory of Medical Specialists at your library and call the specialist directly.

- Check the Directory of Medical Specialists, get the names of two or three doctors in the area, and ask your doctor to suggest which one you should see.

doctor's competence. If you have cancer, a decision about how you proceed with treatment is probably the most important decision you will make in your life. You need the best advice you can get before proceeding with a course of treatment. Just as you don't hesitate to check out various makes and models of cars when you are buying, you should not hesitate to check out all the possible angles before making a decision about your health and your future. Remember, the choices you make at the very beginning are the most important ones.

How can I tell my doctor I want a second opinion?

If you feel uncomfortable, it may be easier for you if you ask a family member to help you do this. He or she can simply explain to your doctor that before going any further you would like to have a confirming opinion. This is not an unusual or unreasonable request. It is a very necessary step for you to take. When you ask, the doctor may tell you that the x-rays and tests are conclusive as far as he is concerned. Do not let that put you off or pressure you into backing down. Explain again that you want a second opinion, that it will strengthen the conclusions already reached and set your mind at ease. In fact, many insurance companies require a second opinion, and even a third opinion, if the second opinion contradicts the first.

What if I don't feel my physician has given me enough information to select a treatment?

Your doctor must tell you the nature of any recommended treatment, its success rate, and its risks and benefits. The doctor must also tell you about other options as well as any risks if you choose not to be treated. Always be sure to ask the question, "What are my other alternatives?"

What if I decide I want to change doctors?

This is more difficult than asking for a second opinion. If you are not satisfied with your relationship with your doctor, you have every right to choose another doctor. Whatever your reason for wanting to change—whether it is because you want someone with more experience or whether you have lost confidence in the ability of your present doctor, if you wish to make the change for personality reasons, or if you are feeling negative about your doctor—it is in your best interest to make the change. You should not be afraid to be honest with your doctor about wanting to end the relationship. No doctor likes to lose a patient, but every doctor has had that experience. You might handle the discussion diplomatically by thanking the doctor for what has been done and assure the doctor that you appreciate all the help that has been given to you, but that you would prefer to try to find someone else who is more suitable for your particular needs at this time. Your doctor is legally obligated to provide your new doctor with any existing records, x-rays, and test results.

Who will recommend a specialist to me?

This can work in a number of ways. You might want to discuss the results of your own research for a specialist with your primary doctor, who will usually want to make a recommendation. Sometimes your primary doctor will give you more than one name. You should be sure to determine the specialist's credentials and be sure you have the answers to these questions:

- Why are you referring me to this particular doctor?
- Is this doctor a specialist in this operation (or field)?
- How often does this specialist perform the particular operation (or service)?
- Is the doctor board-certified? On the staff of an accredited hospital?

How do I get an appointment for a consultation?

Sometimes the doctor who refers you will make the appointment for you. If you are calling yourself, explain that you have already had a diagnosis and wish to make an appointment for a consultation. Don't make the mistake of trying to let the doctor think you haven't been to another doctor. Using a specialist on a consulting basis means that you will get a straight answer, since that doctor has nothing to gain from recommending one treatment over another.

What is the difference between a referral and a consultation?

If your doctor decides that your illness requires the attention of a specialist, you will be given the names of one or several specialists for you to see. This is called a referral and differs from a consultation. A referral means that once you see the specialist (and agree to be treated by that doctor) you become that doctor's patient. In a consultation, the consulting doctor advises you but does not take over responsibility for treating you.

Can I get copies of my test results if I change doctors?

You have a right to copies of your medical records. The information in these records is yours, and many states have laws guaranteeing patient access to this information within a certain number of days of your request. Previous x-rays and test results are important for comparison and can help prevent unnecessary repeat tests when a diagnosis is being made. In some practices, the records will only be sent directly to another doctor.

Is a medical school's outpatient clinic a good place to go for a second opinion?

This is an excellent place to turn for a second opinion. Physicians who practice there are on the faculty of the medical school and are usually using the latest methods of treatment. Because most outpatient departments are divided into specialties, this is where some of the top specialists in the country practice. You can contact the clinic by calling the medical school and explaining that you are interested in contacting a doctor who specializes in the area of your specific problem. Don't be afraid to explain that you want to get a second opinion and to describe your experience to date. Each clinic, of course, has its own setup— but most have appointment secretaries who are very knowledgeable about the clinic and the doctors in their service and will be most helpful in making arrangements for a consultation.

Does having a consultation at a medical school mean I have to go there for treatment?

You have a free choice in the matter. The decision is yours. Sometimes people shy away from getting expert advice from doctors at a large medical center because they think they have to return there for treatments. Many medical and cancer centers diagnose and recommend treatment for patients to be followed by doctors in local communities. If the medical center is far from your home and you do not want the expense and inconvenience of returning there each time you need treatment, you can take advantage of a consultation yet continue to be treated by your own doctor and at your local hospital.

What will a consultation cost?

You will be amazed to find that some of the finest physicians in the country charge no more—and sometimes considerably less—than doctors with far less experience and expertise. Most of the time, health insurance plans pay for second opinions. However, it is always useful to ask what the consultation will cost before you decide you will go ahead with it. And whether or not your particular insurance will cover it. Especially if you are in a managed care plan, you will need to know whether or not the consultation will be covered, in whole or in part, or whether you will be paying for it yourself.

What if the second opinion differs from the first?

Second opinions can be confusing. If the first doctor recommends a course of treatment different from the second, you may be more puzzled than when you started. You have several alternatives: You can ask the two specialists to discuss the case to see if they can resolve the conflict, you can go back to your family doctor and ask for help in making the judgment, you can seek a third opinion and accept the majority decision, or you can follow your own instincts about what doctor and treatment is best for you.

What if I want a second opinion and I am already hospitalized?

Getting a second opinion when you are already hospitalized is more difficult to arrange, unless your doctor is agreeable to the need for another opinion. Explain to your doctor that before you go ahead with any further treatment you would like to have another consultation. Arranging a consultation will be easier if there is a specialist on the hospital staff who is qualified, rather than if the specialist is located at another hospital. However, don't allow difficulties to deter you from seeking a consultation that will give you further insight into what possibilities are open to you. Even when you are hospitalized, it is still your right to demand that your doctor find another physician—even one from another hospital—to give you an independent opinion. Check to see if the hospital has a patient advocate service or ombudsman to help with this kind of situation.

Do I have a right to see my hospital records?
Though many nurses and doctors are extremely secretive about hospital records, you have a right to see them. You may not be able to understand much of what is in the record, because it is written in medical shorthand. Usually, it's helpful to have the nurse or doctor explain so that you will not misunderstand or misread the information.

Is it appropriate for me to take notes or tape record my conversation with the doctor?
It is perfectly acceptable for patients to take notes or even ask to record discussions with physicians. However, it is best to mention to your doctor that you plan to tape the information. Explain that you want to use it as a refresher when you get home, rather than having to call back to ask the doctor to repeat the information for you or your family members. Some doctors, concerned about malpractice suits, may not be entirely comfortable with this, but a taped record can be very helpful to you in reviewing a consultation or can be used to get feedback from someone who is not present during the appointment.

What is the role of the oncology nurse in cancer care?
The nurse is a very important part of the health team in cancer care. Some nurses work in medical centers with the physicians who are doing investigational work in chemotherapy and radiation therapy. Some work in the offices of oncologists. Others are wound ostomy continence nurses who take care of the needs of patients who have had operations in the gastrointestinal areas. Some nurses give chemotherapy drugs under the doctors' supervision. Others are involved with teaching patients how to take care of themselves after leaving the hospital. Many will evaluate how the patient and the family are coping with the illness and managing symptoms such as pain, nausea, vomiting, fatigue, and loss of appetite.

What kinds of nurses are involved with caring for me in the hospital?
It is useful to understand the functions of the various nurses. In most hospitals, particularly in larger ones, you will find, in order of authority:

- Director of nursing (responsible for entire nursing staff)
- Clinical director (in charge of major nursing areas)
- Nurse manager (responsible for a particular unit or units)
- Clinical nurse specialists (advanced clinical skills for management of patients and families)
- Staff nurses (registered nurse who gives direct nursing care)
- Licensed practical nurses (generalized patient care)
- Aides (assist nurses)

What do staff nurses do?

Staff nurses are registered nurses who have completed a nurses' training program, possess a nursing school diploma or an associate's or bachelor's degree, and are licensed by the state to practice nursing. These nurses have fundamental knowledge of most diseases and know how to observe and manage patients. They handle patient care that requires special knowledge such as giving out medication, adjusting medical devices (such as tubes, drains, respirators, etc.), changing intravenous bottles, giving injections, and recognizing problems that need a doctor's care.

What do the initials OCN mean?

When you see the initials OCN after the nurses' names, you know that these nurses have been certified by the Oncology Nursing Society. This designation is similar to board-certification for physicians and is awarded for special expertise and competence in cancer nursing. Advanced practice nurses, with a master's degree, may have additional certification as certified nurse practitioners. Nurses who are fellows of the American Academy of Nursing have earned this special status for scholarly contributions, practice, and research. Get to know the nurses who are involved with your care. They can be your best allies.

What are the duties of the licensed practical nurse?

The licensed practical nurse (LPN) is usually a graduate of a one-year course. She must pass a state examination to practice, but because her formal training is limited, she cannot take the place of the RN. Her tasks include feeding patients who need help, helping patients get out of bed to go to the bathroom, helping patients move on and off bedpans, and generally assisting patients to feel more comfortable. Today many of the nurses who are working in patient care in hospitals are licensed practical nurses who are taking over many of the former duties of staff nurses.

What are the duties of nursing aides and nursing assistants?

Originally these unlicensed nurses' aides were given tasks that required little training, such as taking temperatures, bathing patients, or helping them move from bed to chair. Some hospitals today, because of shortage of help, take workers from departments such as housekeeping and train them to provide direct patient care, such as removing IVs and taking blood pressure readings. It's important that you be aware of the difference in the training of the various members of hospital personnel. The nametag that says, "patient care associate" or "nursing assistant" probably means that you are not being cared for by a nurse. Be sure to ask for an RN (registered nurse) to:

- insert IVs, catheters, or gastric tubes
- change sterile dressings or treat damaged skin
- give shots
- care for a tracheotomy
- give tube feedings

How do I choose a health plan?

Usually you do not have a choice of health plans—most employers offer one specific health plan with defined benefits. If you have a choice, call your physicians or specialists and speak to the billing manager to see which plans they accept and what arrangement they have with the doctor. If you work independently or are not covered at work, look into associations, alumni organizations, churches, and professional groups. Many offer a health plan at a more reasonable rate than if you were buying an individual plan.

Are most doctors now involved in managed care plans?

Most doctors (more than 80 percent of primary care physicians) are involved in managed care plans. Some doctors are very specific about not accepting any HMO or PPO patients. However, most of the country's best doctors are willing to work with the patient within their managed care plans.

How does an HMO operate?

An HMO is a business arrangement using a network of doctors and hospitals grouped together to deliver comprehensive medical care to its members. (HMO stands for Health Maintenance Organization.) The HMOs often pay a large portion of the fee, often requiring only a small copayment. In most cases, the paperwork is taken care of by the doctor's office. Some use doctors who are employed by the HMO; others contract with doctors for a set monthly fee per patient. The larger HMOs have a large panel of doctors. Many require you to pick a primary-care doctor from the HMO directory.

This doctor is then responsible for your health care and decides what health care you will receive and what specialists you will go to. If you need hospital care, you'll have to use one of the hospitals in the HMO's network. In many cases, if you go outside the HMO network, you will have to pay the bills yourself. Some plans have an opt-out or point of service feature where the employer pays some of the cost, if you obtain care outside the HMO. There are positives and negatives to HMO plans. On the one hand, they can be convenient and cost-effective. On the other hand, they have been faulted for giving less comprehensive care, limiting access to specialists, and making it difficult for people to receive emergency room care. It's a good idea, if possible, to check with others who use the same plan with a condition similar to yours to see how things have worked out.

What is a POS?

POS stands for Point of Service and refers to an option sometimes offered by managed care companies. If you stay within your network, charges paid are the same as in the HMO. But if you choose to go out of the network (that is, to doctors and hospitals not on the approved list) you will be charged more. Your plan will only reimburse providers according to its usual, customary, and reasonable rate (referred to as UCR). The monthly premium for a point of service option is usually higher.

What is a PPO?

A PPO is a network of doctors and hospitals that have agreed to give the sponsoring organization discounts from their usual charges. (PPO stands for Preferred Provider Organization.) The doctors and hospitals may be the same ones used in an HMO or they may be different. In a PPO, you can go to any doctor in the network whenever you want (although in some areas you need a referral from your primary physician to see a specialist). As long as you use the network doctors, your coverage will pay the stated proportion of the bill. If you go outside, the plan will pay a smaller percentage. There are also so-called Gatekeeper PPOs, where the medical services are more tightly controlled. In some of these plans, no benefits are paid if members go outside the network. These are known as exclusive provider organizations.

What is an EPO?

An EPO, which stands for Exclusive Provider Organization, resembles an HMO but is usually not regulated under state insurance laws. As a result, this type of plan may lack some consumer safeguards, such as quality assurance programs and the formal grievance procedures found in the usual HMOs.

What is a PHO?

A Physician Hospital Organization, or PHO, is a partnership between a hospital and its physicians. It allows both to share the risks and incentives of managed care. This allows physicians to work closely with the hospital in negotiating managed care contracts, thus making it possible for them to deliver high-quality care in the most cost-effective manner.

How does a fee for service plan work?

Before managed care became popular, most health insurance programs allowed you to go to any doctor, specialist, or hospital. After you had reached your deductible limit, the insurance company would pay a stated percentage of the bill and you would be responsible for the remainder. These plans are still available, but are hard to find and are more expensive than HMOs or the other health plans.

What about company-funded health insurance plans?

Many large companies fund their own health insurance plans. These plans are regulated by federal laws known as ERISA (Employee Retirement Income Security Act).

What are defined care options?

Defined care options are the latest wrinkle in health care plans. They are being offered within existing HMOs. These plans cover health, dental, vision, and related benefits and allow participants to purchase and select their benefit options. The employer allows a specified amount (say $5000) per year on the employee's medical, dental, and vision benefit package and the employees choose which benefits they will take.

What questions should I ask before signing up for a health plan?

IMPORTANT: Before joining a new plan, find out as much as you can about its benefits and be sure to ask if your favorite doctor participates and, if not, what it will cost if you continue seeing that doctor.

- When must I notify the plan before going to the hospital and how do I do it?

- Will I be penalized for going to a doctor outside the network?

- Is there is a percentage paid for services outside the network? What is the percentage paid and what does it apply to?

- Will the plan pay for a second opinion outside of the network?

- What happens if I see a specialist on my own who is not in the plan?

- Which doctors provide primary care? (Sometimes a highly regarded specialist will join the plan as a consultant in a subspecialty but will not be available to provide primary care.)

- Are all services offered by a doctor in a network covered?

- How is payment made to an outside doctor—am I billed? And who pays if my regular doctor is unavailable and another doctor is covering the service?

- Are doctors in the plan taking any new patients?

- Are the doctors in the plan board-certified? Have you checked their credentials? How long have they been involved in the plan?

- Are the doctors satisfied with their involvement in the plan?

- Are the doctors obligated to continue my treatment in the hospital even if they decide to leave the plan?

- Do I need to get a referral from my assigned doctor to go to a specialist?

- Does my doctor have to get approval before sending me to the hospital or to specialists?

- What hospitals are approved?

- Is there a limit to the number of visits I can have with the specialist once I am referred?

- How long does it take to get an appointment for nonemergency care?

- Are prescription drugs, dental treatment, annual physicals, and eye care covered? (Prescription drug coverage is especially important in cancer care.)

- Is it possible to see nonplan doctors if I am willing to pay some of the out-of-pocket medical costs? What percentage will I be required to pay?

- How are emergencies handled?

- Is there a ceiling on my benefits?

- If you are on Medicare, be sure to ask: Will I still get Medicare benefits if I go outside the plan to a specialist?

What if I am unhappy with the medical care I have received from a doctor or a hospital?

You have a right to complain directly to the hospital where you received treatment or to the local medical society. Usually hospitals have ombudsmen that deal with patient complaints. If you are not happy with the results, you can call your state licensing board. For a free information packet on how to file a complaint, write to the People's Medical Society, 462 Walnut Street, Allentown, PA 18102.

CHOOSING YOUR HOSPITAL

It's not always easy to tell a good hospital from a bad one—and deciding which hospital to use may not be simple for you. Sometimes it isn't even a decision you realize you have a right to make, since so much depends upon where a doctor practices. Many people feel most comfortable going to a hospital that is closest to home. Some people feel that a hospital with a religious affiliation of their choosing is important. Others judge a hospital by its atmosphere and the food it serves.

When you need specialized cancer care, it is essential that you evaluate your hospital's credentials in medical terms to be certain that the hospital delivers the very best and the very latest treatment available. Accomplishing this may take a bit of time and effort—but it is worth thinking about.

It is helpful to know the criteria that distinguish a good hospital from a bad one so that you can evaluate your options in determining where you want to be treated. The hospital's track record in dealing with cancer cases, the range of services offered, the hospital's credentials, its participation in research and education, and overall experience are all important to the kind of care and treatment you will receive.

Measuring quality care is much harder than measuring the merits of the new car you are going to buy. Though it may be difficult, it's worth the effort to investigate the credentials of the organization that will have a direct impact on the outcome of your treatment.

How can I tell a good hospital from a bad one?

There are many ways of judging a hospital. Some hospitals that give loving care but do not offer expanded facilities may be fine for some types of hospital stays. However, when you are choosing a hospital for specialized cancer treatments, there are other considerations. There are over 6,000 hospitals in the United States. Of these, about 500 are medical-school affiliated and another 1,500 have intern/residency teaching programs. On the other end of the spectrum, there are approximately 1,600 hospitals that continue to lack minimum accreditation. Somewhere in the middle is a group of average hospitals that offer care ranging from superior to substandard. Surveys done among hospital professionals usually list 25 to 50 hospitals in the country that are categorized as superior. (Be sure to check out the Web sites listed at the end of this chapter that tell you where you can compare hospitals in your area and find out ratings of hospitals.) In addition, there are 39 comprehensive cancer centers, designated by the National Cancer Institute and reaccredited every five years, where the highest level of expertise is to be found. If there is such a hospital within your reach, you may want to consider taking advantage of it.

What kind of accreditation is required of hospitals?

Hospitals voluntarily submit to being judged by a number of organizations that rate them on a variety of criteria. The American College of Surgeons has set up a multidisciplinary cancer committee that surveys hospitals and approves hospital cancer programs along with other requirements. This credential is an important one for anyone planning to have cancer surgery. Most hospitals are surveyed by the Joint Commission on Accreditation of Healthcare Organizations, a nationwide authority that surveys hospitals. The JCAHO decides whether a hospital gets, keeps, or loses accreditation based on its meeting certain criteria for staffing, equipment, and facility safety. If the hospital that you are considering is not accredited, it is important to know why.

Where can I check to see if a hospital is accredited?

You can call the hospital and ask for this information or you can check with the Joint Commission on Accreditation of Healthcare Organizations on the Web or by phone. Their phone number is 1-630-792-3007.

Do I have a choice of hospitals when I'm in a healthcare plan?

When you choose a health plan or select a doctor, often you're choosing a hospital as well—the hospital that the health plan, doctor, or medical group uses.

How do health plans limit hospital choices?

Health plans often have a network of hospitals from which you and your doctor can choose. Health plans may negotiate contracts with certain hospitals that specify reduced rates for the health plan's members.

Do medical groups limit hospital choice?

Most medical groups not only share office space, but also collaborate in other ways with referrals to hospitals and specialists. So, you should be aware that when you choose a doctor, you also are making a decision about which hospital you will be using.

What can I do if I prefer to use a specific hospital?

If going to a specific hospital is important, it is prudent to choose a health plan and medical group that will allow you to use that hospital. Sometimes, even if the hospital is in your health plan's network, your medical group may not have privileges at the hospital. If your hospital choice suits your needs better, it may be necessary to switch to someone affiliated with your chosen hospital. Last but not least, if you have information that shows a certain hospital has better outcomes for the procedure you need, present that information to your health plan and medical group and ask them to approve the change.

**What is the difference between a Comprehensive
Cancer Center and other hospitals?**

There are 39 Comprehensive Cancer Centers, designated by the National
Cancer Institute (NCI), across the country. Each of the Comprehensive Cancer Centers is devoted to the diagnosis and multidisciplinary treatment of
cancer patients, laboratory research in several scientific fields, a strong program of clinical research, and an ability to transfer research findings into
everyday practice. They are specifically geared to treating cancer with the

JUDGING YOUR HOSPITAL

ASSESSMENT SCORE	TYPE OF HOSPITAL	SCORE YOUR HOSPITAL
+50	Comprehensive Cancer Center designated by National Cancer Institute	
+40	Clinical Cancer Center designated by National Cancer Institute	
+40	Community hospital with a community clinical oncology program grant	
++40	Approved hospital cancer center program sponsored by American College of Surgeons	
+20	Directly affiliated with medical school that uses hospital for internship and residency programs	
+15	Teaching hospital, residency and internship training, medical-school affiliation, but medical school not located in hospital	
+10	Residency and/or internship program, without medical school affiliation	
+10	Accredited by Joint Commission on Accreditation for Healthcare Organizations, but without approved internship and/or residency programs	
0	Not accredited	
0	Government supported (so-called public) hospital (VA, Public Health Service, county, city, or state)	
0 or −10	Proprietary or for-profit hospital, owned by individuals or stockholders, including doctors who practice there.	

JUDGING YOUR HOSPITAL *(continued)*

ASSESSMENT SCORE		SCORE YOUR HOSPITAL
	TYPE OF HOSPITAL	

If at all possible, take advantage of the finest facility within your reach. Use of a Comprehensive Cancer Center, if it is accessible, is a wise choice since that is where the experts are. Hospitals with medical schools generally provide excellent care since they attract top doctors and their range of services is extremely broad. If not directly connected to a medical school, facilities are probably good, but not as wide-ranging. Accreditation is a minimum standard ensuring adequate care. About 25 percent of U.S. hospitals are not accredited, and therefore are not eligible for Medicaid payments. Government-sponsored and proprietary hospitals vary from excellent to substandard. Proprietary hospitals sometimes are not as well equipped because of efforts to keep costs low and profits high. Local reputation is the key to your score on this.

	NUMBER OF BEDS	
+20	Over 500 beds	
+15	100 to 500 beds	
+5	Under 100 beds	

This is a good gauge. Of the more than 3000 hospitals with fewer than 100 beds, only a handful are medical-school affiliated, and less than one percent offer residency programs. Check yours out. There are a few outstanding exceptions in this category.

	LOCATION OF HOSPITAL	
+25	Within 30 miles	
+15	Within 100 miles	
+5	Within 200 miles	

If your local hospital does not seem adequate to provide you with the services you will need, you should ask your doctor to refer you to a specialist who is affiliated with a hospital that is better suited to your needs. You must weigh emotional support and the burden of traveling to your calculation. Remember that you can arrange to be evaluated by one of the specialists, who can then advise your doctor on treatment.

(continued)

JUDGING YOUR HOSPITAL *(continued)*

ASSESSMENT SCORE		SCORE YOUR HOSPITAL
	GENERAL HOSPITAL SERVICES	
+5	Postoperative recovery room	
+5	Intensive care unit	
+10	Pathology lab	
+10	Diagnostic laboratories	
+5	Pharmacy	
+5	Blood bank	
+5	Sophisticated x-ray equipment, CT scanner, MRI	
+5	Radioactive Scanning Equipment	
+5	Brain wave equipment (EEG)	
+10	Tumor committee, tumor registry	
+5	24-hour respiratory therapy	
+5	Physical therapy	
+5	Patient advocate services	
+5	Social services, ethics consultant, follow-up services	
+10	Anesthesiologists (rather than anesthetists) in operating room	
+10	Adequate nursing staff	
+10	Advanced practice nurses as part of staff	
+10	24-hour-a-day physician staffing	

All of these facilities are part of an up-to-date hospital facility. Depending upon your needs and condition, these are all items that make up a well-run and well-equipped hospital that can serve every need. This chart is designed to allow you to check your hospital on its ability to deliver cancer care. It is not meant to be used to judge your hospital on its adequacy for emergency care, general surgery, etc.

Over 250—Excellent

Over 180—Very good

Over 130—Good

Over 100—Adequate

Under 100—Poor

most up-to-date methods. Their credentials and programs have been rigorously peer-reviewed and designated by the National Cancer Institute as "centers of excellence." If you live near a Comprehensive Cancer Center, you should definitely consider going there for your diagnosis and treatment.

WARNING: Many hospitals and cancer centers use the word "Comprehensive" in their titles. However, few of these hospitals have been rigorously reviewed by the National Cancer Institute. In addition, there are for-profit groups in various parts of the country that have added the words "comprehensive cancer center" to their titles. These are *not* the same as the NCI-designated Comprehensive Cancer Centers. Many of these for-profit centers are freestanding, not affiliated with medical schools, and do not participate in research. They do, however, make available standard care, including chemotherapy and radiation therapy, and have oncologists on their staffs. If the hospital you use is not listed below or cited as an approved clinical and laboratory center (see Chapter 28, Where to Get Help), then it is **not** an authentically designated **NCI Comprehensive Cancer Center.**

What is the difference between a hospital designated by the NCI as a Comprehensive Cancer Center and one designated by the NCI as a Clinical Cancer Center or one with the simple designation of Cancer Center?
The **Comprehensive Cancer Center designated by the NCI,** as described above, has the most depth and breadth of research activities in each of the three major areas—basic, clinical, and prevention—and exhibits a strong body of interactive research that bridges these scientific areas. **A Clinical Cancer Center designated by the NCI** has reasonable research activities in clinical oncology, with or without research encompassing the basic or prevention sciences. The unmodified term **Cancer Center designated by the NCI** refers to centers that have a focus on basic research or cancer control research, but do not have clinical oncology programs; therefore they do not see patients. However, all three categories of cancer centers, whatever their designations, have been rigorously reviewed and are in the top tier of hospitals for cancer care in the country.

Where are the NCI-designated Comprehensive Cancer Centers located?
The following hospitals are designated as Comprehensive Cancer Centers by the National Cancer Institute:

Alabama: UAB Comprehensive Cancer Center, University of Alabama at Birmingham
Arizona: Arizona Cancer Center, University of Arizona, Tucson

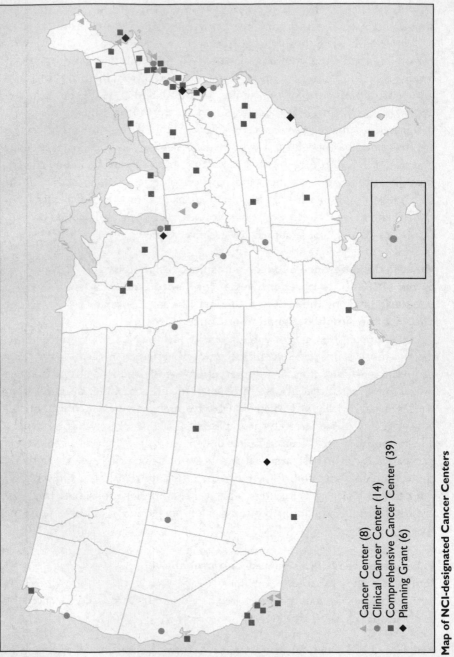

Map of NCI-designated Cancer Centers

△ Cancer Center (8)
● Clinical Cancer Center (14)
■ Comprehensive Cancer Center (39)
◆ Planning Grant (6)

California: City of Hope National Medical Center & Beckman Research Institute, Duarte; Jonnson Comprehensive Cancer Center, University of California, Los Angeles; USC/Norris Comprehensive Cancer Center, University of Southern California, Los Angeles; Chao Family Comprehensive Cancer Center, University of California at Irvine; UCSF Cancer Center & Cancer Research Institute, University of California, San Francisco

Colorado: University of Colorado Cancer Center, University of Colorado Health Science Center, Denver

Connecticut: Yale Comprehensive Cancer Center, Yale University School of Medicine, New Haven

District of Columbia: Lombardi Cancer Research Center, Georgetown University Medical Center, Washington, D.C.

Florida: H. Lee Moffitt Cancer Center & Research Institute at the University of South Florida, Tampa

Illinois: Robert H. Lurie Cancer Comprehensive Center of Northwestern University, Chicago

Iowa: Holden Comprehensive Cancer Center at the University of Iowa, Iowa City

Maryland: The Sidney Kimmel Comprehensive Cancer Center at Johns Hopkins, Baltimore

Massachusetts: Dana-Farber/Harvard Cancer Center, Dana-Farber Cancer Institute, Boston

Michigan: Comprehensive Cancer Center, University of Michigan, Ann Arbor; Barbara Ann Karmanos Cancer Institute, Wayne State University, operating the Meyer L. Prentis Comprehensive Cancer Center of Metropolitan Detroit, Detroit

Minnesota: University of Minnesota Cancer Center, Minneapolis; Mayo Clinic Cancer Center, Mayo Foundation, Rochester

New Hampshire: Norris Cotton Cancer Center, Dartmouth-Hitchcock Medical Center, Hanover.

New Jersey: The Cancer Institute of New Jersey, Robert Wood Johnson University Hospital and Medical School, New Brunswick

New York: Herbert Irving Comprehensive Cancer Center, College of Physicians & Surgeons, Columbia University, New York City; Memorial Sloan-Kettering Cancer Center, New York City; Kaplan Cancer Center, New York University Medical Center, New York City; Roswell Park Cancer Institute, Buffalo

North Carolina: Duke Comprehensive Cancer Center, Duke University Medical Center, Durham; UNC Lineberger Comprehensive Cancer Center, University of North Carolina, Chapel Hill; Comprehensive Cancer Center, Wake Forest University, Winston-Salem

Ohio: Ireland Cancer Center, Case Western Reserve University and University Hospitals of Cleveland; Arthur G. James Cancer Hospital & Richard J. Solve Research Institute, Ohio State University, Columbus

Pennsylvania: Fox Chase Cancer Center, Philadelphia; University of Pennsylvania Cancer Center, Philadelphia; University of Pittsburgh Cancer Institute, Pittsburgh

Tennessee: Vanderbilt-Ingram Cancer Center, Vanderbilt University, Nashville

Texas: M.D. Anderson Cancer Center, Houston

Vermont: Vermont Cancer Center, University of Vermont, Burlington

Washington: Fred Hutchinson Cancer Research Center, Seattle

Wisconsin: Comprehensive Cancer Center, University of Wisconsin, Madison

More information about Comprehensive Cancer Centers, including addresses and telephone numbers, can be found in Chapter 28, Where to Get Help.

Where are National Cancer Institute Clinical Centers located?

California: UC Davis Cancer Center, University of California, Davis

Hawaii: Cancer Research Center of Hawaii, University of Hawaii at Manoa, Honolulu

Illinois: University of Chicago Cancer Research Center, Chicago

Indiana: Indiana University Cancer Center, Indianapolis

Missouri: Siteman Cancer Center, Washington University School of Medicine, St. Louis

Nebraska: University of Nebraska Medical Center/Eppley Cancer Center, Omaha

New York: Cancer Research Center, Albert Einstein College of Medicine, Bronx

Oregon: Oregon Cancer Institute, Oregon Health & Science University, Portland

Pennsylvania: Kimmel Cancer Center, Thomas Jefferson University, Philadelphia

Tennessee: St. Jude Children's Research Hospital, Memphis

Texas: San Antonio Cancer Institute, San Antonio

Utah: Huntsman Cancer Institute, University of Utah, Salt Lake City

Virginia: Massey Cancer Center, Virginia Commonwealth University, Richmond; Cancer Center, University of Virginia, Health Sciences Center, Charlottesville

Where are research facilities designated by the NCI as Cancer Centers located?

There are eight centers or laboratories that have the designation of Cancer Center. They focus on basic research or cancer control research, but do not have clinical oncology programs; therefore they do not see patients.

California: Salk Institute, LaJolla; Burnham Institute, LaJolla
Indiana: Purdue University Cancer Center, West Lafayette
Maine: The Jackson Laboratory, Bar Harbor
Massachusetts: Center for Cancer Research, Massachusetts Institute of Technology, Cambridge
New York: Cold Spring Harbor Laboratory, Cold Spring Harbor; American Health Foundation, New York City
Pennsylvania: The Wistar Institute, Philadelphia

Is it a good idea to go to a Comprehensive Cancer Center for diagnosis and treatment of cancer?

If one of the NCI-designated Cancer Centers is nearby, by all means take advantage of it. You can use its expertise for your care, or you may wish to have your case reviewed by the experts on its staff. If you need help in getting a referral to a comprehensive cancer center, call the Cancer Information Service (1-800-4-CANCER). The information specialist can give you information on how to make an appointment at the centers nearest you.

Is there any way I can benefit from the expertise of a Comprehensive Cancer Center even if I live far away?

You can ask your doctor to refer you for evaluation by one of the center's specialists, who can then confer with your doctor on your treatment. Or, you can ask your doctor to contact one of the doctors who specializes in your type of cancer to discuss your case. This is especially important if you have a rare type of cancer that your doctor does not see very often.

Can I be treated at the Clinical Center at the National Institutes of Health?

The National Institutes of Health, the Federal Government's agency for medical research, has a medical research center and hospital—the Warren Grant Magnuson Clinical Center. You can be treated at the Clinical Center only if your case fits into a research project. The Clinical Center provides nursing and medical care without charge for patients who are being studied in its clinical research program. There is more information on how to get treatment at the clinical center and on clinical trials in Chapter 11, New and Investigational Treatments.

What is a clinical trials cooperative group?

A clinical trials cooperative group, sponsored by the National Cancer Institute, is composed of academic institutions and cancer treatment centers throughout the United States, Canada, and Europe. These groups work with the National Cancer Institute to identify important questions in cancer research and to design carefully controlled clinical trials to answer these questions.

Should I participate in a clinical trial?

Clinical trials are being conducted in most major medical centers as well as through clinical trials cooperative groups. Trials, available for most types of cancer, allow scientists to test new treatment methods and drugs, combinations of drugs, and treatments, as well as different treatment dosages. Although there are advantages and disadvantages to joining a clinical trial, for many people and for many cancers, clinical trials offer one of the best choices for treatment. There is more information about clinical trials in Chapter 11, New Advances and Investigational Treatments.

Is it a good idea to go to a research or teaching hospital?

Naturally, this is a personal decision, based on many factors. Certain demands are made on patients in these hospitals that may be disturbing for some and comforting to others. Physicians, nurses, psychologists, and social workers often interview patients. Members of the medical staff other than the patient's physician may drop by to examine the patient's condition. Of course, patients always have the option of refusing to be examined by or treated by anyone other than their own doctors (except in emergencies where quick decisions are essential). Some people object to being treated by anyone except their own personal physician. If you feel this way, it is important for you to understand how these hospitals operate. The care in research and teaching hospitals can be very attentive, the staff is very competent, and the patient can be assured that the latest and most up-to-date treatment is available.

If I go to a research or teaching hospital will I become a guinea pig for a cancer-research project?

Many people are frightened at the thought of being used in a research project without their consent. Each patient participating in a research project must sign a consent form that explains both the potential value and the possible risks. All research projects must first be approved by the hospital's research committee (sometimes called the human investigations committee), which has strict guidelines it follows in evaluating whether or not the project can be carried out at that hospital. Before consenting to becoming part of a research project, you should consider asking the following questions:

- What is the purpose of the study?

- What kinds of tests and treatments, what will be done to me, and how will it be done?

- What is likely to happen to my cancer with, or without, the new research treatment?

- What are my other possible choices and what are their advantages and disadvantages?

- Are there standard treatments you might recommend for my case and how does the study compare with these standard treatments?

- What side effects might I expect from these research treatments that differ from what I would expect from standard treatments or from the natural course of the disease?

- How long will the study last? Is this longer than standard treatments?

- Will I have to be hospitalized? If so, how often and for how long?

- What will be the cost on my part? Is any of the treatment given free?

- If I should not respond to the new treatment, what further treatment would be possible?

- What type of long-term follow-up care is part of the study?

There is more detailed information on clinical trials in Chapter 11, New Advances and Investigational Treatments.

Why is a teaching hospital considered to be superior to a hospital that does not have an intern/residency program?
In a teaching hospital, there are more professionals on the job—more doctors on site checking up on the competence of other doctors. In a teaching hospital you are seen on regular daily "rounds" by your doctor and other interns and residents. Doctors who receive appointments to these hospitals are usually tops in their fields. Teaching hospitals attract some of the finest medical minds in the country.

If you're in a teaching hospital and feel you're being badgered by too many interns and residents, what can you do?
Some patients find it annoying to be "poked at" by countless interns and residents. If you find this to be a problem, you have a perfect right to discuss this with your doctor, and ask how this practice can be limited. You have the right to know the identity and professional status of anyone who treats you and the purpose of any test or examination.

Can I refuse to be examined by a medical student?

You are within your rights to refuse to be examined. However, many a help-ful diagnosis or insight has been made by a medical student who was doing the job as painstakingly as only a novice will. It may be to your advantage to allow the services of a soon-to-be doctor. Of course, if you are feeling very ill and find the whole process troublesome, you can request that you not be questioned or examined.

Is size an important factor in considering a hospital?

In the checklist, you'll notice we have given greater weight to a hospital with 500 or more beds than we have to one with between 100 and 500 beds or one with fewer than 100 beds. This is a general rule of thumb. We do know of some excellent small hospitals. There are some poor large hos-pitals. Size is not all—but the number of patients with serious illnesses seen by the staff is an important factor. In a larger hospital, in the course of a week, a doctor will probably treat as many patients with a specific ill-ness as the small-hospital doctor will see in a year. **Hospital death rates have been estimated to be 40 percent higher in fewer-than-100-bed hospitals than in larger hospitals.** Although people may complain that large hospitals are impersonal, the overall capabilities of a large hospital are greater than those of a small one.

What if the doctor sends me to a hospital where I do not wish to go for treatment?

You have a right to go to the hospital of your choice. However, if your doc-tor does not have privileges at that hospital, you cannot be treated by that doctor in that hospital. That is why, in choosing a doctor, an important con-sideration is his hospital affiliation. Some doctors have admitting privileges at more than one hospital. Therefore, if you have a specific preference for a hospital, be sure to discuss this with your doctor at the outset.

What is the difference between an anesthesiologist and an anesthetist?

An anesthetist is a person who administers anesthetics. An anesthesiologist is an M.D. whose specialty is the administration of anesthesia. For any operation requiring the use of anesthesia, you should make certain that your anesthesia is administered under the supervision of a board-certified anesthesiologist.

Am I obligated to sign consent forms?

Consent forms are necessary before the doctor can go ahead with any proce-dure that entails any element of risk—surgery, anesthesia, spinal taps, etc. However, do not sign a blank consent form. Do not accept an explanation that there is some uncertainty as to what the surgical procedure will entail and that the consent form will be filled in later. Your doctor has an obligation to inform you of the risks and consequences of any procedure and to state the specific procedure for which you are being asked to give your consent. (Specifications for surgery should include the specific area to be operated on and the specific procedure the surgeon expects to perform.) Do not sign any form unless all your questions have been addressed.

How can I guard against medication errors in the hospital?
You should ask and know what medications your doctor has prescribed for you, what they are designed to do, and what they look like. If you have any question at all about a medication do not take it. Ask the nurse to show you the container from which the pills were taken, to check the order book to make certain the doctor's orders have been followed, or to check back with the doctor in case an error has been made. Many a medical disaster has been averted by a patient who asks, "Is this a new pill?" Be alert to what medications you are taking and why they are being given.

Should I discuss finances with my doctor?
Cancer is a very expensive illness, and you should know what kinds of costs will be involved. You should never be afraid to ask the doctor about office and personal fees, what the laboratory tests will cost, how much the hospital bill will be, and what x-rays and drugs cost. The earlier you have this kind of discussion, the better off you will be. The doctor may not be able to detail all of the costs since office staff usually does the actual billing and accounting. Ask to speak with the person who does the billing, if this is the case. Nurses and social workers can be helpful in some instances since they are knowledgeable about coverage, eligibility, services, programs, and insurance issues.

Web Pages to Check Out

www.cancer.gov: For general up-to-date information, and for clinical trials.
www.cancer.org: For general up-to-date information and community resources.
www.medicalconsumers.org: This site lists the number of times a doctor has performed a particular procedure.
www.ama-assn.org: The American Medical Association's Physician Select Doctor Finder.
www.cancerdirect.com: This is a patient consultation service, which charges a $3,600-a-year fee for coordinating treatment information for specific cancer cases.

www.bestdoctors.com: This is a consultation service with fees ranging from $50 to $500, which helps find the best doctor for a specific condition.

www.healthgrades.com: Database of 650,000 physician credentials.

www.thehealthpages.com: Comprehensive information about more than 500,000 doctors, managed care plans, and other health care providers. You can search for details about a particular provider, compare details about multiple providers in your area, and compare specialists on key criteria such as years of practice, training, plan affiliation, etc. Also allows you to see what others have said about particular health care providers and how they have rated them.

www.jcaho.org: (Joint Commission on Accreditation of Healthcare Organizations.) Click on "general public," where you can insert the name of hospitals and be given their accreditation status and performance reports as well as register any complaints about healthcare organizations.

www.modernmaturity.org: Information on the entire subject of doctors and hospitals.

www.usnews.com: National listing of best hospitals.

Also see Chapter 2, Searching for Answers on the Web, for more information.

Books, Articles, and Other Resources You May Want to Read

- Many of the large city- or state-oriented magazines around the country devote an issue each year to ratings of the top doctors and hospitals in the area. Watch out for these and save them or check your library for a copy.

- *Consumers' Checkbook*, 733 15th Street, NW, Washington, DC, has two books—one on hospitals and one on doctors. They rate 4,500 hospitals nationwide and list 15,000 specialists in major metropolitan areas rated highest by their peers. May also be found on the Web at www.checkbook.org.

Four

WHAT IS CANCER?

Today, we are closer than ever to unraveling the mysteries of cancer that have puzzled scientists for more than 2,000 years. In learning how genes work, the answer to the whys and wherefores of cancer are becoming much clearer. Something in the cell's DNA prevents it from doing its normal job, and instead it starts dividing and forming more cells without control or order. As the cells continue to double themselves, a tumor is formed. All cancers, therefore, are genetic malfunctions of cells that cannot function normally, and are unable to die.

THE HUMAN BODY is made up of some 10 trillion cells. Each cell carries out specialized functions. Most cells have the capacity for infinite multiplication—in a very carefully controlled manner. Cells are constantly dying off and being replaced with new cells. When cancer occurs, the cells escape from the normal mechanism and begin to behave in an uncontrolled fashion. They never stop reproducing themselves and soon there are many more of them than of the healthy cells in the tissue surrounding them. When cells escape from regulatory control, they hand down their independence to their descendants and each continues to reproduce at will, cloning an independent colony in a rebel fashion.

What you need to know about cancer

- Precancerous changes in cells can be detected under the microscope. In healthy tissue, each cell is identically shaped, each with its own sharply defined nucleus.

- In precancerous change, the cells lose their uniformity. Cells of different sizes are interspersed with cells of normal size. In many, the nuclei are irregular. At this point, these irregular cells are no more than that. They show no signs of invasion of other tissue or of movement to other parts of the body.

- When any part of the body needs repair, all cells in the immediate vicinity leap into action, dividing rapidly to repair the defect. If a pathologist looks at tissue from a healing wound, the rapidly dividing, immature cells resemble those from a malignant tumor. However, in the case of ordinary wound healing, the well-controlled cells that are involved revert to their normal pattern when the healing is complete, whereas cancer cells continue their rapid division.

- When cancerous cells begin to reproduce, the distortion of individual cell structure is more pronounced, with a tendency for the cells to appear to be more primitive and with the abnormal cells moving from their normal locations to surrounding tissues. This unconrolled growth of cells is what brings about symptoms—a mass or a lump or bleeding.

- Cancer may behave differently in different people. Learning the basics about cancer will help the person without a medical background to better understand what the doctor is talking about when discussing the diagnosis, treatment, and outcome.

- There are many things you can do to prevent cancer, such as stopping smoking, changing your diet, using sunscreen, or staying out of the sun.

- There are many studies being made to determine the association of environmental issues and cancer, such as DDT, nuclear power plants, and electric power lines.

What new research is being done to learn more about how cancer starts and behaves?

This is an exciting time for scientists who are using the tools of molecular and cellular biology to follow up clues as to why one person gets cancer and another one does not. The current understanding of how various parts of the cellular system develop is almost completely at odds with beliefs that researchers held only a few years ago. Every day, new information is being discovered about how a cell grows and what signals make it divide, as well as how the body rids itself of cancer-causing agents. Words like *cyclins* (proteins that can turn on enzymes stimulating inappropriate cell division) and *adducts* (formed when chemicals stick to DNA; if the damage is not repaired before the cell divides, mutations occur that can cause cancer) are being added to the cancer vocabulary.

What are genes and how are they related to cells?

Genes are the biological units of heredity. It is estimated that humans have anywhere from 30,000 to 100,000 genes. Each gene acts as a blueprint for making a specific enzyme or other protein. A flaw in a gene can result in diseases, including cancer. The genes are arranged on chromosomes—rod-like structures composed of DNA and protein. Each cell, in humans, contains 46 chromosomes (23 pairs) located within a central structure known as the nucleus. Genes that normally direct how often a cell divides are called proto-oncogenes.

What is an oncogene?

An oncogene is a proto-oncogene that has developed a defect. The defect is transmitted on the chromosome. Researchers believe that every person carries oncogenes in each body cell and that the oncogenes remain harmless until triggered by something. Scientists are studying ways to turn off these oncogenes and stop the oncogene from transforming normal cells into malignant ones.

What is a tumor suppressor gene?

This is a gene that protects and slows the division of cells. When this gene is damaged, it stops doing its job and the cancer is allowed to grow. BRCA1, BRCA 2, APC, RB, and p53 are tumor suppressor genes. Mutations in the p53 gene have been linked to over half of the cancers that occur in humans. Although scientists are still not able to correct mutations in tumor suppressor genes, laboratory experiments and some clinical trials are underway using gene therapy to replace defective tumor suppressor genes or to destroy cancer cells that have p53 mutations.

What are tumor growth factors?

Growth factors are the chemical messengers that control cell growth. When they attach to receptors on the cell's surface, vital signals are sent to the vital machinery inside the cell. Some cancer cells produce an unusually high amount of growth factors. Some have too many factor receptors. Others receive more signals to grow and divide by producing too many receptors and excessive levels of growth factors. A great deal of experimental work is being done to determine the best way to prevent growth factors from promoting cancer cell growth.

Does each person's body treat cancer-causing substances in the same manner?

No. New molecular research indicates that people are born with various weak spots in their genetic makeup. Some people, for instance, have genes that allow their bodies to get rid of carcinogens easily, while others, born with genes that are slower-acting, allow the chemicals to bind up with their DNA. Other people have defects on important genes, like the tumor-suppressor p53 gene, that cause them to be more vulnerable to cancer. There are two copies of every gene in most cells. One normal copy of a gene is sufficient to prevent the development of cancer. If both copies are damaged or mutated, however, cancer may develop.

Is cancer inherited?

For many years doctors puzzled over why some families seem to have more cancer than would occur by chance alone. Today scientists are discovering genetic flaws that put some people at higher risk. About five or ten percent of cancers are hereditary, caused by a damaged gene that has been inherited. A gene, called p53, is responsible for an inherited cancer syndrome, known as the Li-Fraumeni syndrome. People with this inherited disorder are at higher risk for breast cancer, colon cancer, soft-tissue sarcomas, bone cancer (osteosarcoma), brain tumors, leukemia, and adrenocortical cancer, all occurring at unusually early ages. The risk of certain other cancers, including melanoma, ovarian, testicular, lung, pancreatic, and prostate, may also be greater, though to a lesser degree. Genes that account for many other illnesses, even those that have complicated genetic patterns, are being discovered at a dizzying rate. This field of research, known as molecular biology, is transforming the way that cancer is detected and diagnosed and also predicting who will get cancer in the first place. (For additional information, see Chapter 11, New Advances and Investigational Treatments.)

Do we know how cancer starts?

Most scientists believe that many cancers come about through a multistep process, called carcinogenisis, in which several events are required to produce cancer. Research in the area of molecular and cellular biology has identified three steps: initiation, promotion, and progression. Cancer-causing agents, known as carcinogens, can contribute to the first two stages.

How does this multistep process work?

It is believed that *initiators* start the damage to the cell, and cause changes that can lead to cancer. The initial damage may be inherited or it may be caused by other factors—tobacco smoke, x-rays, ultraviolet rays, radon gas, and certain chemicals are considered initiators. *Promoters* change the cells already damaged by the initiator from normal cells to cancer cells but usually do not cause cancer. Some substances occurring naturally in the body, such as bile acids, estrogens, and androgens, for instance, are considered promoters. Some substances, such as many found in tobacco, are both initiators and promoters. When cancers first form, cells may not be able to spread to other tissues or organs. But as they continue to grow and mutate, they can become more malignant. This is called *progression*, as tumors spread and metastasize from the initial tumor to other parts of the body.

Do all normal cells look alike?
No, each normal cell has a specialized structure designed to do a particular job in a particular organ. For example, those cells that form the skin tend to be flat. The class of cells that makes up the nerves is long and slender. Within each class, all normal cells are quite uniform in size and almost identical in shape. Each class of cells presents different arrangements when they join each other. Glandular cells, for example, form circles that build upon each other like stones lining a well. Skin cells stretch out in sheetlike layers, row on row, like a brick wall. Each type of cell joins together with other similar cells to form tissues that arrange themselves in orderly patterns to form the various parts of our complex bodies.

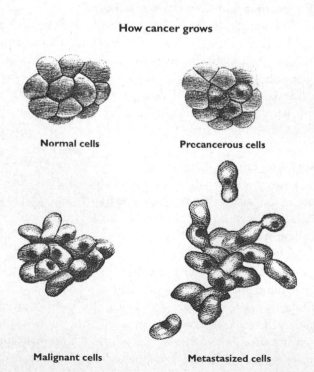

How cancer grows

Normal cells   Precancerous cells

Malignant cells   Metastasized cells

**What's the difference between a benign and a
malignant (cancerous) tumor?**

A benign tumor is a growth that is not cancerous. It can usually be removed
and in most cases does not come back. It does not spread to other parts of
the body. Most benign tumors do not endanger life, unless they are growing
in a confined area such as the brain. Malignant tumors, on the other hand, do
not organize themselves into normal patterns, and even though the tissue
resembles the tissue of the normal cell, the arrangement is imperfect. Sometimes the cancer cells are so dissimilar from the normal structure that it may
be difficult to identify the tissue from which the cancer started. The imper-
fection of the abnormal cells is the failure of the cancer cells to mature (or
differentiate, as the physicians would say). Cancer cells can damage nearby tissues and organs. They also can break away from the malignant tumor and
spread to form new tumors in other parts of the body.

Can benign tumors become cancerous?

In most cases they do not. The tumor that begins as a benign tumor usually
remains a benign tumor. However, there are lesions that are considered precancerous, such as a thickening of the lining of the mouth or cervix. These
should be taken care of before cancer occurs.

Are there fast-growing and slow-growing cancers?

Some cells in the body are normally slow growing; others reproduce and are
shed more rapidly. If a healthy normal cell is one that is slow growing, such
as in the liver, then the cancerous liver cells are also slow growing. There are
also fast-growing and slow-growing types of cancers, which is why different
cancers respond to different kinds of drugs. The important difference is that
cancerous cells never stop reproducing. Cancer cells do die, but their death
rate is lower than their birth rate.

Why are cancerous cells so dangerous?

Cancerous cells deprive normal cells of nourishment and space. In most
types of cancer, the cells build up into a mass of cells that compresses,
invades, and destroys surrounding tissues. This mass is often called a growth,
a tumor, or a neoplasm (new growth).

**Is it true that the more irregular the cells,
the more malignant the cancer?**

As a general rule, the more irregular or abnormal (the doctors call this undifferentiated) the cells look under the microscope, the more malignant the
cancer. The greater the difference in appearance from a normal cell, the more
active the cancer is likely to be and the more uncontrollable its course.

**What does it mean when the doctor refers to
differentiated and undifferentiated cells?**

A differentiated cell is a cancerous cell that resembles a normal cell. An undifferentiated call, as you might expect, is more abnormal. Many types of cancer are graded by how differentiated the cells are, and this factor is considered when treatment is planned.

How many cells are in a cancerous tumor?

The number varies by the size of the tumor and the type of cell. First of all, you should understand that there is considerable variation in the size of cells making up different parts of the human body. The most numerous of the body cells are so small that it would take between 700 and 800 cells to cover the head of a pin. A one-centimeter lump in the breast, a little larger than the size of a pea, is about the smallest lump that you can feel with your fingers. Such a lump contains over a billion cells. This size tumor has undergone about thirty doublings since it first became an abnormal cell.

What does the doctor mean when he says I have a solid tumor?

A solid tumor is a tumor such as carcinoma or sarcoma that forms a mass of growth. Other types (see chart) originate in other types of cells.

DIFFERENT TYPES OF CANCERS

Carcinoma	Originates from tissues that cover a surface or line a cavity of the body. This is the most common type of cancer, accounting for 80–90 percent of all cancers. (Carcinomas are divided into two main subtypes—adenocarcinoma and squamous cell carcinoma.)
Sarcoma	Originates from tissues that connect, support, or surround other tissues and organs. Can be either soft tissue or bone sarcomas. (Includes osteosarcoma, fibrosarcoma, rhabdomyosarcoma, leiomyosarcoma and liposarcoma.)
Myeloma	Originates in the bone marrow in the blood cells that manufacture antibodies.
Lymphoma	Originates in lymph system—the circulatory network of vessels, spaces, and nodes carrying lymph, the almost colorless fluid that bathes the body's cells.
Leukemia	Involves the blood-forming tissues and blood cells.

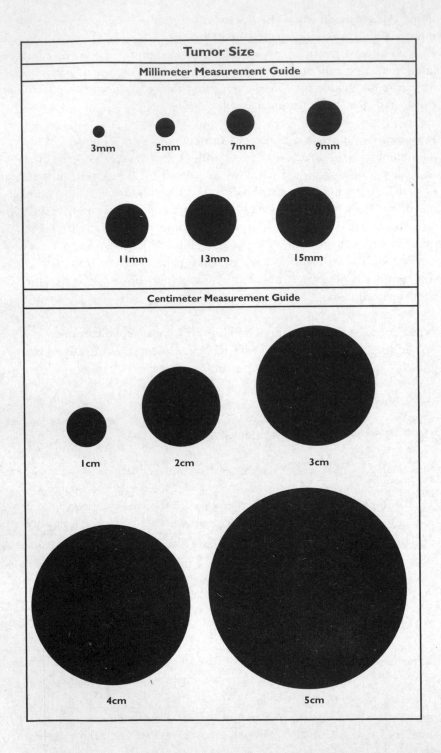

Tumor Size

Millimeter Measurement Guide

3mm 5mm 7mm 9mm

11mm 13mm 15mm

Centimeter Measurement Guide

1cm 2cm 3cm

4cm 5cm

What does the term *in situ* mean?

This term is used to describe an early, noninvasive cancer. One of the most constant characteristics of cancer is the invasion of healthy tissues bordering the tumor. However, there appears to be a period before invasion begins. Such growths are called *in situ*, and the results of removal are more positive than for those cancers that have already begun to spread into neighboring tissues. The term also applies to another group of tumors—usually found on surfaces—which have other characteristics of malignancy but in which normal cells may be completely replaced by tumor cells before there is evidence of cancer in surrounding tissues. In most instances, removal of the *in situ* cancer is considered a cure.

**What does it mean when the
doctor says my cancer has metastasized?**

This means that the cancer is not confined to one area of the body but has spread or has started to spread. (Sometimes the doctor will say that the tumor is disseminated, which means the same as metastasized.) The process by which cancer spreads from where it began (that is, from the primary tumor) to distant parts of the body is called *metastasis*. Tiny clumps of cells break off from the tumor and are carried in the lymphatic vessels or the bloodstream to a distant part of the body. These "seeds" from the original cancer start growing in the new location. The new tumor is said to have metastasized to the new site, and such a tumor is often referred to as a metastatic tumor. The plural of metastasis is metastases. Sometimes you will hear the word *mets* used as a shorthand term for metastases.

Where does cancer usually spread?

Different types of cancer have different spreading patterns. Breast cancer, for instance, generally spreads, or metastasizes, from the breast (primary site) to one or more of four places in the body: liver, bone, lung, and brain. More rarely, it can spread to the spinal cord, to distant lymph nodes, and to other parts of the body. Identifying whether or not a cancer has metastasized is the most decisive factor in the choice of treatment and the success of treatment.

**When a tumor metastasizes or spreads,
is it called by the name of the organ to which it has spread?**

No. This can be quite confusing to most people, but when you understand the way the body works, it makes sense. If the original tumor is in the prostate, for example, and it spreads to the bone, it is not considered or treated like bone cancer. It is prostate cancer that has spread to the bones. The type of cancer cells found in the bones will be the same type as the cancer cells found in the prostate. These cells will grow, reproduce, and behave according to the pattern of metastatic prostate cancer (prostate cancer that has spread to other areas) and not like bone cancer. Because of this fact, metastatic cancer of any kind is generally treated in the way the original cancer responds to best. Cancer that starts in the prostate and spreads to the bones is not treated in the same way as cancer that starts in the bones would be treated. It is still treated as a form of prostate cancer, because that is what it is.

At what age do persons usually get cancer?

Cancer is predominant a disease of middle and old age. In the United States, 77 percent of cancer is diagnosed at age 55 and over. Overall, men and women account for about the same number of new cases of cancer.

Is cancer common in children?

Cancer is quite rare in children and in young adults. However, for children under 15, cancer is the second leading cause of death. Leukemia is the most common form of childhood cancer, followed by tumors of the central nervous system.

Can a person catch cancer?

There is no indication that cancer can be considered contagious in the popular sense of the word. You should not be afraid that you will "catch" cancer from another person. People who care for cancer patients on a daily basis do not have a higher incidence of cancer than the general population. There is no evidence to suggest that living in the same household with a cancer patient over a long period of time, sharing his or her possessions, kissing, or having intercourse with a cancer patient increases the chances of being diagnosed with cancer.

What are the most common warning signs of cancer?

There are seven basic symptoms:

- **Unusual bleeding or discharge.**
- **A lump that does not go away.**
- **A sore that does not heal within two weeks.**
- **Change in bowel or bladder habits.**
- **Persistent hoarseness or cough.**
- **Indigestion or difficulty in swallowing.**
- **Change in a wart or mole.**

Is it possible to have cancer without any warning symptoms?

It is possible. Often symptoms seem so trivial to most people that they may be ignored. For example, coughs are so common that we do not get alarmed when we have one. Usually you can tell yourself that you have been smoking too much, or blame your sinuses, or rationalize that everyone you know has a cough. However, coughing can also be the first visible sign of lung cancer. Irregular vaginal bleeding can be due to a whole list of causes, too, which can lull you into not bothering to see a doctor. But irregular vaginal bleeding can also be the first sign of cancer of the uterus. What is important to remember is that you must learn to pay attention to your body's signals. Any suspicious symptom that persists for longer than two weeks should be investigated by a qualified physician.

Does tobacco play a large role in causing cancer?

Smoking tobacco, chewing tobacco and snuff, and being exposed to tobacco smoke without actually smoking account for about a third of all cancer deaths in the United States each year. Tobacco is the most preventable cause of death in this country. Smoking accounts for more than 85 percent of all lung cancer deaths. Smokers are also more likely than nonsmokers to develop several other types of cancer, such as cancers of the mouth, tongue, lip, larynx, esophagus, pancreas, bladder, kidney, and cervix.

How is alcohol linked to cancer?

Drinking large amounts of alcohol increases the risk of cancer of the mouth, throat, esophagus, and larynx. People who smoke cigarettes or chew tobacco and drink alcohol have an especially high risk of getting those cancers. Alcohol can damage the liver and increase the risk of liver cancer. Alcohol is an example of a classic promoter. It alone does not cause cancer, but it is clearly associated with the development of certain kinds of cancer.

Does diet cause cancer?

Your choice of foods may affect your chance of developing cancer. About a third of cancer deaths each year in the United States are due to poor nutrition and lack of physical activity. Evidence points to a link between a high-fat, low-fiber diet and certain cancers. Physical activity may reduce the risk of some cancers, such as colon, breast, pancreas, and other sites. Being seriously overweight appears to be linked to increased rates of cancer of the endometrium, esophagus, colon, and kidney and to breast cancer in older women. Salt-cured, smoked, and nitrite-cured foods have been linked to cancers of the esophagus and stomach. On the other hand, studies suggest that foods containing fiber and certain nutrients help protect you against some types of cancer.

Is sunlight a cause of cancer?

Ultraviolet radiation from the sun and from sources such as sunlamps and tanning booths damages the skin. Scientists estimate that sunlight is responsible for almost all of the more than 700,000 cases of basal and squamous cell skin cancer every year and is a major factor in the development of melanoma. Repeated exposure to ultraviolet radiation increases the risk of skin cancer, especially if you have fair skin or freckle easily.

Should I be concerned if I am taking hormone replacement drugs?

Many women use estrogen treatment to control the hot flashes, vaginal dryness, and thinning of the bones (osteoporosis) that might occur during menopause. This is a subject of continued debate in the medical community, with conflicting data coming from different studies. Yet recent results from the Women's Health, Trial, a large randomized trial sponsored by the National Institutes of Health, give concern that use of postmenopausal hormones may promote tumor growth. This trial has shown that postmenopausal women who had not had cancer and who had taken estrogen and progestin for five years had an increased risk of breast cancer and cardiovascular disease. The results for use of estrogen alone in this study are not yet known. You need to talk with your doctor about the benefits and risks in this complex issue.

Is a vasectomy linked to the risk for prostate and testicular cancers?

Scientists are continuing to study this issue. A consensus conference that looked at all the data from published and unpublished studies concluded that the research results on the association between vasectomy and prostate cancer are inconsistent. It concluded that since there is no convincing biological explanation for how a vasectomy might cause prostate cancer, additional research is needed. The NCI PLCO Cancer Screening trial and additional research will help clarify the issue. As for testicular cancer, at this time it is believed that there is either no association or a weak association between vasectomy and testicular cancer. Again more research is needed to make a definitive conclusion.

Has exposure to DES during pregnancy proven to be a cancer risk for daughters and sons?

DES is a form of estrogen that doctors prescribed from the early 1940s until 1971 to try to prevent miscarriages. It has been found that when given during the first five months of pregnancy, DES interfered with the development of the reproductive system in a fetus. A link has been found between DES exposure before birth and an increased risk of developing abnormal cells in the tissue of the cervix and vagina. These abnormal cells, sometimes called dysplasia, cervical intraepithelial neoplasia (CIN), and squamous intraepithelial lesions (SIL), resemble cancer cells in appearance. However, they do not invade nearby healthy tissue the way cancer cells do. They usually occur between the ages of 25 and 35 in women whose mothers took DES. Although they are not cancer, they might develop into cancer if not treated.

DES-exposed daughters may also have structural changes in the vagina, uterus, or cervix. Most of these changes do not cause medical problems but some women may have irregular menstruation and an increased risk of miscarriage, premature delivery, and infertility. There is some evidence that DES-exposed sons may have testicular abnormalities, such as undescended testicles or abnormally small testicles, although the risk of testicular or prostate cancer or infertility has not shown an increase. New research looking at grandchildren of the DES-exposed women does not show any evidence that the grandchildren have been affected. They are not developing cancer, although they may have reproductive and urinary system problems.

Are the women who took the DES at higher risk for cancer?

Women who used DES may have a slightly increased risk for breast cancer. If you used DES, it would be useful to know when you started taking it, what amount you were taking, and how you were taking it. You need to make sure your doctor knows this and that you have yearly medical checkups with breast and pelvic exams and a Pap test. You also need to talk with your children so that information about their exposure to DES can be listed on their records.

Has exposure to pesticides been studied as a cause of cancer?

Farmers or workers in industries that are exposed to high doses of pesticides may be at higher risks for some kinds of cancer. DDT, which has now been banned, had been used in farming in the past and has been shown to accumulate in body fat.

What are the findings from the Long Island Breast Cancer Study Project?

The Long Island Breast Cancer Study Project, looking at possible environmental causes of breast cancer, consists of more than 10 studies that include human population studies, a family breast and ovarian cancer registry, and laboratory research designed to explain the development of breast cancer. The main research is a large, population-based study to determine whether polycyclic aromatic hydrocarbons (PAH) and organochloride compounds (such as DDP, DDE, chlordane, dieldrin, and polycholorinated biphendyls [PCB]) are associated with an increased risk for breast cancer. The study's main findings are that organochloride compounds are not associated with the elevated rates of breast cancer on Long Island, and that exposure to PAHs was associated with a modest increased risk for breast cancer. The study did not identify specific environmental factors as a cause for the elevated breast cancer rates in this area. Further studies of the role of the environment in breast cancer are continuing.

Has Agent Orange been tested?
Agent Orange, a mixture of herbicides used during the Vietnam War mainly to defoliate forest trees and destroy crops, continues to be studied. The studies are being conducted by the National Academy of Sciences' Institute of Medicine, a highly respected, independent, non-governmental scientific review organization working on behalf of the Department of Veterans Affairs. A comprehensive search of relevant databases, including public and commercial databases covering biologic, medical, toxicologic, chemical, historical, and regulatory information, are identified and reviewed. Input from veterans and other interested persons at public hearings and in written submissions serves as a valuable source of additional information to the scientific committee studying the data. Four categories, based on the amount and quality of scientific evidence of an association with Agent Orange or other herbicides used in Vietnam, are used to determine whether an association exists: 1) sufficient evidence of an association, 2) limited or suggestive evidence of an association, 3) inadequate or insufficient evidence to determine whether an association exists, and 4) limited/suggestive evidence of *no* association. The first report was issued in 1993, with updates and additional reports issued as new data are received.

Has Agent Orange been associated with any cancers?
Several cancers have been put in the first category where a positive association has been observed between herbicides and the outcomes in studies in which chance, bias, and confounding could be ruled out with reasonable confidence. They are: soft-tissue sarcoma, non-Hodgkin's lymphoma, Hodgkin's disease, and chronic lymphocytic leukemia (CLL). The first three were put into this category in the first report. Chronic lymphocytic leukemia was added in 2002. Prostate cancer, respiratory cancer, and multiple myeloma are in the second category—limited/suggestive evidence of an association. Many cancers were listed in the third category—inadequate or insufficient evidence to determine whether such an association exists: hepatobiliary, nasal or nasopharyngeal, bone, breast, cervical, uterine, ovarian, urinary bladder, renal, testicular, leukemia (other than CLL), skin, childhood cancers in offspring, including acute meylogenous leukemia, and endometriosis. In the fourth category, limited or suggestive evidence of *no* association, are the following cancers: stomach, pancreatic, colon, rectal, and brain tumors. The association between other forms of leukemia and Vietnam herbicide exposure is now being studied.

What do these categories mean to Vietnam veterans?
First of all, the Veterans Administration presumes that all Vietnam veterans were exposed to Agent Orange or other herbicides. If the cancer is listed in category 1, it means that veterans who served in Vietnam don't have to prove

that their illness is related to their military service to qualify for VA disability compensation and the special access to medical care that the VA has offered to Vietnam veterans for health problems from Agent Orange exposure. The conditions are presumed to be service-connected. The cancers in category 2 also have ultimately been recognized as service-connected.

Where can I get additional information?

For complete information on this topic: www.va.gov/agentorange. Copies of reports from the Institute of Medicine are available from the National Academies Press, 500 Fifth Street NW, Lockbox 285, Washington, DC 20055. The telephone numbers are (toll-free) 1-800-624-6242 and (in the Washington, DC, metropolitan area) 202-334-3313. The Web address is www.nap.edu.

Can asbestos and other substances used in the workplace increase cancer risk?

Being exposed to substances such as metals, dust, chemicals, or pesticides at work can increase the risk of cancer. Asbestos, nickel, cadmium, uranium, radon, vinyl chloride, benzidene, and benzene are well-known examples of carcinogens in the workplace. They may act alone or along with another carcinogen, such as cigarette smoke. For example, inhaling asbestos fibers increases the risk of lung diseases, including cancer, and the cancer risk is especially high for asbestos workers who smoke. It is important to follow work and safety rules to avoid contact with dangerous materials.

Is there a danger living near electric power lines?

Electromagnetic fields are routinely produced when electrical current passes through a wire or common household appliance. A large study of residential magnetic field exposures and childhood acute lymphocyte leukemia (ALL) was conducted by the NCI and the Children's Cancer Group. There was little evidence of a relationship between the risk for ALL in children and exposure to magnetic fields. The scientists also concluded that magnetic fields from electrical appliances were unlikely to increase the risk of childhood ALL. The present evidence is not clear.

Do computer screens cause cancer?

Computer screens give off several kinds of radiation, but most of it is of extremely low frequency, far below the standards set by the government. However, research is being done in this area.

Is there any evidence that microwave ovens cause cancer?

There is no evidence of this, if the microwave oven is being used according to directions. There is evidence that sperm can be altered or killed when exposed to high levels of microwave. However, the small amount that can leak from a microwave oven would not cause this problem

Can cell phones cause brain cancer?

Four large studies have been completed that have looked at this question— one each in Sweden and Denmark and two in the United States—comparing the cell phone use of people with brain cancer and people who do not have it. All studies have shown the same results. Cell phone use was not associated with the increased risk of developing brain tumors. This was true whether all brain cancers were considered as a group or different types of brain cancers were looked at individually. Since cell phones are a relatively new technology, longer-term follow-up will need to be done. The phones in question are handheld cellular phones, the kind that have a built-in antenna that is positioned close to the user's head during normal telephone conversations. The safety of so-called "cordless phones," which have a base unit connected to the telephone wiring in a house and which operate at far lower power levels and frequencies, has not been questioned.

Are nuclear facilities responsible for cancer deaths?

There is continuing research underway on this subject by the National Cancer Institute, the Centers for Disease Control and Prevention, various state health departments, and other groups. One major study done by the National Cancer Institute surveyed 62 nuclear facilities, all of which had begun operation before 1982. It examined more than 900,000 deaths, using county mortality records collected from 1950 to 1984. Sixteen types of cancer, with a special focus on childhood leukemia, were studied. The researchers evaluated changes in mortality rates and compared them to counties within the same geographic region that had similar populations but did not have or were not near nuclear facilities. This study showed no general increased risk of death from cancer for the people living in the 107 U.S. counties containing, or closely adjacent to, the nuclear facilities.

Can exposure to radiation from medical x-rays cause cancer?

Your risk of cancer can be increased by exposure to large doses of radiation. X-rays used for diagnosis expose you to very little radiation and the benefits nearly always outweigh the risks. However, repeated exposure can be harmful, so it is a good idea to talk with your doctor and dentist whenever x-rays are suggested about the need for each x-ray. You also should ask about the use of shields to protect other parts of your body.

Does fluoride in the water present cancer risks?

Virtually all water contains fluoride. Currently more than half of all Americans live in areas where fluoride is added to the water supply. The possible relationship between fluoridated water and cancer has been debated at length. The latest survey by the Public Health Service, which reviewed more than 50 human epidemiology studies produced over the past 40 years, led the investigators to conclude that optimal fluoridation of drinking water "does not pose a detectable risk of cancer to humans." In addition, the National Cancer Institute scientists examined more than 2.2 million cancer death records and 125,000 cancer case records in counties using fluoridated water. They found no indication of a cancer risk associated with fluoridated drinking water.

Do viruses cause cancer?

Several viruses of different types can cause cancer or at least play some role in its development. In some cases, viruses may cause the cell to lose its ability to control growth so that it continues to reproduce itself, forming tumors. Other viruses may damage the cells of the immune system itself. In some cases, both processes may be at work.

What viruses are involved with the development of cancer?

There are several viruses that appear to be involved in the development of human cancers. They include: human papillomaviruses (a leading factor in some cervical cancers); hepatitis B and hepatitis C; (which greatly increase the likelihood of developing liver cancers); herpes viruses, such as Epstein-Barr (linked to Burkitt's and other lymphomas and to nasopharyngeal cancer); human T-cell leukemia virus type 1 (HTLV-1—associated with the development of adult T-cell leukemia); and HIV (which can lead to Kaposi's sarcoma, non-Hodgkin's lymphoma, and cancer of the cervix).

Does the cat tumor virus cause cancer in people?

Viruses carried by cats, such as feline leukemia and sarcoma viruses, can cause cancer in other cats. However, there is no evidence that these viruses cause cancer in humans. Research carried out by the National Cancer Institute, using laboratory tests of blood samples of pet owners, veterinarians, research workers who handle these viruses, cancer patients with and without pet cats, and people from the general population, found that none of these groups showed evidence of infection. Therefore, it has been concluded that these viruses are not considered to cause cancer in human beings.

Web Pages to Check Out

www.cancer.gov: For general up-to-date information, and for clinical trials.

www.cancer.org: For general up-to-date information and community resources.

www.genone.gov: Information on genone project.

www.science.gov: Information on new research.

www.va.gov / agentorange: Information on coverage for veterans who have been exposed to Agent Orange.

Also see Chapter 2, Searching for Answers on the Web, for more information.

CANCER CONTROVERSIES: WHAT YOU NEED TO KNOW AND DO

There are many controversies in the cancer field. Some are the result of ongoing research, for new information can challenge what has been an established practice. Others are due to the *lack* of information—decisions need to be made that cannot wait for research that has yet to be completed. Still others have to do with the medical system and how it operates. It is important for you to understand these issues so you and your family can make the right decisions about your diagnosis and treatment. Be aware of the controversies and ask appropriate questions if they apply.

CONTROVERSY #1: WHAT IS THE STORY ON HORMONE REPLACEMENT THERAPY? DOES IT PROTECT AGAINST HEART DISEASE? AGAINST OSTEOPOROSIS? OR IS IT HARMFUL? SHOULD I STOP TAKING IT?

The Issue

There is a great deal of discussion both in the medical profession and in the news about the benefits of hormone replacement therapy, which has been used for decades. It has been widely believed that hormone therapy could prevent heart disease and osteoporosis and prolong youth, sexual vigor, and health.

The latest research totally contradicts that thinking.

Some Facts Around the Controversy

Two relatively new studies have looked at the benefits of using hormone replacement therapy over the long term.

- The findings of the Heart and Estrogen Progestin Replacement Study were first. This study found that not only did hormone combination therapy (estrogen and progestin) not prevent heart attacks and death from heart disease in women who already had a heart problem, but it also created further heart problems for them.

- The Women's Health Initiative, in a large and rigorously conducted clinical trial of 16,000 women, tested estrogen and progestin and abruptly halted the study because the hormones, after five years, caused a small but significant increase in the risk of invasive breast cancer and larger, more advanced cancers. This study also found increases in heart attacks, strokes, and blood clots, but decreases in broken hips and colorectal cancer.

- The part of the Women's Health Initiative that is studying the effects of the use of estrogen alone on heart disease and osteoporosis is still ongoing, with results expected in 2005.

What the latest panel of the United States Preventive Services Task Force concluded was that even though hormones can prevent osteoporosis, broken bones, and colorectal cancer, it is not recommended for those purposes because the hormones can also increase the risk of breast cancer, heart attacks, strokes, gallbladder disease, and blood clots. This task force is an independent panel of experts in primary care and prevention that systematically reviews evidence and develops recommendations. Most organizations with guidelines for the use of postmenopausal hormone replacement therapy are revising them in light of the new findings.

- Both the American College of Obstetricians and Gynecologists and the North American Menopause Society recommend against the use of replacement therapy to prevent heart disease in healthy women or to protect women with pre-existing heart disease.

- Both organizations also recommend caution in the use of hormone therapy solely to prevent osteoporosis. Both organizations consider hormone replacement therapy acceptable treatment for menopausal symptoms but advise caution about the prolonged use for relief of symptoms.

- The American Heart Association recommends against the use of hormones for primary or secondary prevention of cardiovascular disease.

What You Should Do About Taking Hormone Replacement Therapy

- The findings have left many women up in the air about what to do. There is no question that hormone therapy is highly effective in treating certain menopausal symptoms and may still be appropriate for you, depending on your circumstances. However, the results of the latest studies make it a more complicated decision. You will have to evaluate, with your physician, the benefits and risks in your own case. This includes weighing the benefits of using hormone therapy against your own risks for breast cancer and other conditions. Some women choose to manage their symptoms without the use of hormones, either through lifestyle changes alone or with other therapies. Other women, especially those who have severe menopausal symptoms, may conclude that the benefits of using hormones for a short period of time at a low dose is worth the risks to them.

- The task force did not make any recommendations about the use of estrogen alone, without progestin, which is a treatment prescribed for women who have had hysterectomies. There is research, however, that shows that women with a uterus who take only estrogen are at greater risk for endometrial cancer. The results from the Women's Health Initiative on a large group of healthy women using estrogen alone are expected in 2005.

- Future studies on lower hormone doses or different combinations may tell us more, but for now, **all** women taking **all** forms of hormone therapy should be aware of the increased risks found in the latest studies. Research on hormonal therapy and on other therapies continues. Web sites you can check include: www.acog.org and www.ahcpr.gov/clinic.

If you decide to continue to use hormone replacement therapy, you should:

- Take it for the shortest possible time that works for you, in the smallest effective dose. If you have been on hormone therapy for more than five years, you should try to discontinue use. You should understand that there are no data at the present time that establish what is safe for short-term use.

- See your doctor, at least once a year, to review your reasons for taking hormones and to see if you are ready to successfully discontinue use.

- Be sure to have regular breast cancer screenings, physician breast exams, and mammograms.

CONTROVERSY #2: WHY CAN'T DOCTORS AGREE ON WHO SHOULD HAVE A PSA TEST? WHY CAN'T DOCTORS AGREE ON WHICH TREATMENT IS BEST FOR PROSTATE CANCER?

The Issue

Major organizations and doctors disagree widely on who should get a PSA test (blood test used for prostate cancer screening) and when. The American Cancer Society, the American Urological Association, the United States Preventive Services Task Force, and the National Cancer Institute have differing opinions on the value of the test. Some doctors automatically order the blood test as part of a routine physical for any man over 50 or age 45 for African American men, who are at higher risk. Others talk to men about risks and benefits of PSA testing before ordering it, letting men make their own decisions about screening. Furthermore, it is no secret that top experts still cannot agree on what is the best and most effective treatment for prostate cancer.

Some Facts Around the Controversy

- The test is controversial because it is not yet clear whether the benefits of PSA screening outweigh the risks of the follow-up diagnostic tests and cancer treatments. The benefits are still being studied to determine whether this screening test reduces the number of deaths from prostate cancer. Two large clinical trials are expected to report results in the next couple of years.

- Today the PSA test is almost always ordered by the doctor as part of the regular blood test series, and routinely paid for by insurance companies. Most men don't even know they are having the test, usually finding out only when the doctor's office calls a few days after the physical, to say, "Your PSA level is high."

- Even with sophisticated techniques, in many cases doctors are still unable to distinguish patients whose cancers will not progress from those whose cancers will eventually grow and spread. In addition, the diagnostic tests that follow a finding of a high PSA level can be invasive and may cause side effects.

- Compared with most cancers, cancer of the prostate tends to grow very slowly. Many men with prostate cancer die of other causes in the next 10 to 15 years. Since the median age at diagnosis is 72, the question is whether or not men should be put through all the rigors of testing and treatment, with the side effects of potential impotence and incontinence, if they are going to die of something else.

- There is controversy about what treatment should be used if prostate cancer is found as a result of the PSA test. For most men with prostate cancer, there are three long-used methods for treatment: removing the prostate with surgery, external radiation therapy, and watchful waiting (also known as observation). Internal radiation seeding and cryosurgery are other possible treatments that are now available. No clinical trial has compared these treatments with each other.

Work is under way to improve PSA screening or to find new tests, including new biological markers. Several treatment clinical studies are also in progress.

What You Can Do If You Have a High PSA

- If you have a high PSA, be sure you read Chapter 14, Prostate Cancer, before you take any further steps. Some of the early decisions you make will be irreversible. All treatments for prostate cancers often cause incontinence and impotence. Therefore it is important to take this into account. Discuss the pros and cons with your doctor. Be an educated medical patient.

- There are pros and cons for each of the treatments. Your age and the aggressiveness of your tumor should play a part in your decision. Be aware that some treatments will result in more side effects than others.

- At the present time, for men with Stage I and Stage II prostate cancers, five-year data are showing that the results are the same for watchful waiting, surgery, or radiation therapy. Even at the end of ten years, few men will have died from the disease. Ask questions. Be an informed consumer. This is an area where opinions will change as results of new studies come in.

- However, it is important to know that after surgery, pathologists have found that some of the cancers that originally were thought to be Stage I and Stage II have broken through the prostate "capsule," putting them into the Stage III category.

- Don't be in a hurry to make a decision. There is time to explore your choices. Look into the issues and weigh them carefully before you decide on what is right for you. Do your own research. Listen to all sides—

opinions differ among urologists, other surgeons, and radiation oncologists. Since this is usually a very slow-growing cancer you can take the time to make the decision that is best for you.

- Make sure you go to a doctor who has had extensive experience in the newest treatment techniques. Get a second and a third opinion if you need to before you make any decisions.

CONTROVERSY #3: ARE SOME BREAST CANCER PATIENTS GETTING TREATMENT THEY DON'T NEED?

The Issue

Some 50,000 women will be told this year that their mammograms have shown that they have a special type of early breast cancer—ductal carcinoma *in situ* (DCIS), also known as Stage 0, localized, or preinvasive breast cancer. In cancer language "*in situ*" means that it is the earliest stage of cancer, essentially, a 'pre-cancer' that is curable. One would think that this would mean that a lesser treatment would be needed. But that is not what is happening. Because the experts cannot agree on what is the right treatment for DCIS, most women are likely to have a lumpectomy or mastectomy, followed by radiation or hormone therapy—treatment not too different from women treated for invasive, early-stage breast cancer.

Some Facts Around the Controversy

- DCIS, found mainly through mammography, shows up as a pattern of white dots known as microcalcifications. It is an unusual cancer in the milk ducts and cannot spread outside the breast like other cancers.

- Only about 30 percent of DCIS will turn into invasive cancer. The problem is that doctors cannot predict accurately which DCIS will become invasive cancer and which will not. There has been considerable work done to identify cellular patterns, but a staging system has yet to be agreed upon. Researchers are looking for a marker for which of these pre-cancers will become invasive cancer. What is known now is that DCIS can turn into invasive breast cancer but that in the majority of women it does not. As evidence of this, autopsies of women who have died of other causes found 6 to 19 percent had DCIS that had never been diagnosed or treated.

- There have been no large-scale clinical trials that compare all the various treatments for DCIS (several studies are underway comparing parts of different treatments). At present, thousands of women may be having treatment—mastectomies, lumpectomies, and radiation therapy, even having both breasts removed—that may not be needed.

What You Need to Know and Do If You Have Microcalcifications or Are Diagnosed with DCIS

- If you have microcalcifications, ask for a stereotactic core needle biopsy, since 80 percent of the calcifications are benign. This can save you from an unnecessary operation.

- If you have DCIS, these are the treatment options:

  - you can have the breast removed; this may be followed by tamoxifen; or

  - you can have the area of the microcalcification and a wide margin around it removed (called a lumpectomy even though there isn't any lump); this may be followed by radiation and /or tamoxifen.

  Talk with your doctor about the pros and cons of each of the treatments. Get more than one opinion.

- Ask about clinical trials. Unless you have a real preference for one of the treatments, think of participating in a study. There are many under way that will help make the answers to this puzzling disease clearer.

- You don't have to rush into any one treatment because a doctor or someone else wants you to. Take time to make your choice. The decision has to be something that you are comfortable with.

CONTROVERSY #4: DO OLDER PATIENTS GET DIFFERENT TREATMENTS THAN YOUNGER PATIENTS?

The Issue

This is a very interesting question and one that will become thornier as the population continues to age. Although cancer is a disease of older people, studies clearly show that many older patients are getting less effective treatments, such as lower doses of chemotherapy, than younger patients. Compared to younger people, they also have fewer screening tests and less thorough diagnostic testing once cancer is detected.

Some Facts Around the Controversy

- For many years, treatment in clinical trials excluded older people, even though nearly 65 percent of all cancer patients are over 65. It is a relatively recent occurrence that patients 65 and over have been allowed into clinical trials. And it has been only a couple of years since clinical trials have been specially designed for patients over 65, over 75, or over 80 years of age.

- Doctors also have *not* encouraged patients 65 or older to join clinical trials, assuming that the elderly are not interested in treatment clinical trials, that they are unable to tolerate the treatment, or that they have other medical problems that would make them ineligible. One study showed that doctors asked half of their patients who were under 65 to join a clinical study, but only asked a third of those over 65. However, this study also noted that older patients were willing to join clinical trials. Once they were asked, equal percentages of younger and older patients agreed to participate.

- Medicare has also been a roadblock—its regulations have only recently been changed to allow payment for clinical trial treatment.

The Result

Very few older patients have joined treatment clinical trials—although nearly 65 percent of all cancer patients are aged 65 and over, only 25 percent of that age group are patients enrolled in clinical trials. If you look at the number of patients 70 and older, it's even more dramatic—47 percent of all cancer patients are 70 and over, but only 13 percent of that age group are represented in clinical trials. So scientific studies—the gold standard doctors use for making treatment decisions—do not include the people who are most likely to have cancer.

The few studies that have been done on the issue of treatment show that older patients who are in general good health do almost as well on chemotherapy as do younger patients. As a matter of fact, in some areas, older people seem to do better—they have less nausea and vomiting and better quality of life than do younger patients. They are better able to tolerate treatments.

When you look at screening and diagnosis, there also are issues. Compared with younger women, fewer older women have screening tests. And once the cancer is detected, fewer have thorough diagnostic testing.

What You Need to Do If You Are 65 and Over and Are Having Cancer Treatment

- Talk to the doctor about treatment choices. Ask about what the doctor's policy is in giving treatment to your age group.

- Don't let the doctor alone make the decision as to whether or not you should have aggressive treatment. Be a partner with the doctor in making that decision.

- Tell the doctor that you want to be a part of the decision if any changes in doses are made. Ask questions about what will happen if the dosages are lowered. Will the treatment still be effective? Decide for yourself whether or not you are willing to take the full treatment.

CONTROVERSY #5: HOW DO I ASSURE THAT THE DIAGNOSIS IS CORRECT— THAT I REALLY HAVE CANCER?

The Issue

You have been diagnosed with cancer. But then you find out that you really don't have it. Sometimes you find out by asking probing questions. Other times, you find out through a second opinion. But there are some people who are not so lucky and go through treatment that they really did not need to have.

Some Facts Around the Controversy

Here are four of the many true accounts that abound in the cancer field:

- A man in Florida diagnosed with cancer had a lung operation. Half of a lung was taken out and tissue sent to the pathology lab for analysis. It wasn't until a year later that he found out that he had been misdiagnosed. Not only did the post-surgery analysis show that he did not have cancer, but the doctor who operated on him never told him that a mistake had been made. The gentleman was left without one lung through an unnecessary operation.

- A woman in New Jersey, who was a smoker, went to a physician with bronchial symptoms. She had an x-ray. When she returned to the doctor's office, the doctor told her that she had small-cell lung cancer and scheduled her for surgery. When her daughter called the doctor to ask how he could tell the cell type of lung cancer without a biopsy, the doctor told the daughter that he had good news: "Your mother doesn't have cancer." When questioned, the doctor admitted that he had decided, from the pathologist's written description and the woman's symptoms, that small cell lung cancer was a good probability—he had not even looked at the x-ray himself. As it turned out, it was another person's x-ray.

- A breast cancer patient in Connecticut was told that her CT scan showed a recurrence of cancer in her lung and was scheduled to have surgery.

She decided to seek a second opinion at a major medical center. A second CT scan of better quality showed that the so-called "recurrence" was scar tissue.

■ A woman in New York, who had been treated for lung cancer 14 years earlier, was coughing and had pains in her back. X-rays, CT scans, and MRIs were taken, and several specialists at major centers came up with differing opinions of what the "shadows" and "hot spots" were. All tried to hurry her into having surgery on her spine so that a definitive diagnosis could be made. Still not satisfied, she made an appointment with another specialist who decided to start from the beginning and look at the whole picture. He took a medical history, discussed how she was feeling, did a physical exam—something nobody else had done—and studied all the tests, scans, MRIs, and x-ray results. His verdict was that what everybody was seeing was radiation necrosis—scarring from previous radiation treatment. This diagnosis was confirmed by a second specialist, who checked her back and chest for radiation damage and prescribed calcitonin injections to strengthen the bones. That was ten years ago and she is still alive and well with no problems.

The Result

In many cases, cancer is difficult to diagnose. Before you have any treatment, make sure that the diagnosis has been fully explored.

What You Need to Know and Do When You Are Told You Have Cancer

■ Always get a second opinion—and then a third if the first two don't agree.

■ Make sure that your pathology slides have been read by more than one pathologist.

■ Choose your doctors and your medical center carefully (read Chapter 3, Choosing Your Doctor and Hospital).

■ Review the doctors' records as listed in your state's Board of Medical Examiners (see Chapter 28, Where to Get Help). Doctors who have had disciplinary problems are listed with your state board.

■ The first cancer treatment you have is the most important one, so it is essential that you take the time to make sure it is the right one.

■ **Don't be afraid to ask questions. As we have said continuously since we published our first edition of Choices, "If we can leave you with just one piece of good advice, it would be "ask, ask, ask, and ask again.""**

CONTROVERSY #6: WHY DOES INFORMATION ABOUT SCREENING TESTS AND CAUSES OF CANCER CHANGE SO OFTEN? IS MY DOCTOR KEEPING UP TO DATE ON ALL THESE CHANGES?

The Issue

Yesterday the news questioned the value of mammography and of estrogen replacement therapy. Today it is the changing guidelines for detecting cervical cancer. Tomorrow it will be yet another study that shows diet is or is not related to some kind of cancer. The medical community doesn't seem to be able to make up its mind. What's a person to do?

Some Facts Around the Controversy

- Difficulty in obtaining consistent information usually stems from the shortcomings of observational public health studies, where large groups of people and their habits are tracked over a period of time. These studies are very important research tools, for good information can be gleaned from them, but they also can be problematic, since the individuals being tracked may not represent a wide range of behaviors. Is the person who eats five fruits and vegetables a day also more apt to exercise? If so, if you find a lower cancer rate is it due to eating fruits and vegetables or is it due to the exercise? Or maybe both? Or something else you haven't measured?

- Randomized studies, which are more expensive, and usually take a longer time, randomly assign people to a group and then compare the groups against each other. People don't get to choose what group they are going to be in. It's whichever group happens to come up next on the list. Sometimes, as happened with the estrogen studies, the results from the randomized study can be quite different from the observational studies.

- Yet another reason for the controversies is that scientists are taking several older studies and reanalyzing them as a group to make conclusions. Depending on which studies you include to reanalyze, the end results differ. That's what's been happening with mammography studies. The data being reanalyzed are many years old and the procedures for giving mammograms when the studies were done are now outdated.

- And lastly, what you ultimately read or hear on the news is a science writer's interpretation of the data. On the mammography issue, the conclusions differed from one paper to another and from one television network to another.

What You Need to Know and Do When You Are Told You Have Cancer

- Be aware that science is an evolving process. What is true today might not be true tomorrow when new information is discovered.

- Rely on trusted sources when you have questions about the information. Call the NCI Cancer Information Service or the American Cancer Society or go onto their Web sites and see what each organization has to say about the issues.

- Read the original study yourself and make your own decision about the conclusions (see Chapter 2, Searching for Answers on the Web, to find out how to access the medical journals and reliable news sources).

- Check with your heath insurance provider to see whether or not there have been changes as a result of the new data. In the area of Pap tests, for instance, the change in guidelines may mean that you are covered only for one test every three years, rather than yearly tests. If you have the test more often, you may be paying for it yourself.

- Before you change your health practices, stop taking medicine, or have different screening tests, talk with your own doctor. Use the data you have gathered to discuss the pros and cons. Do not make rash changes based on what you are hearing in the media. Be an informed consumer.

CONTROVERSY #7: ARE DOCTORS FOLLOWING THE GUIDELINES FOR TREATING CANCER? WHY ARE THERE DIFFERENCES FROM ONE AREA OF THE COUNTRY TO ANOTHER?

The Issue

Cancer treatment generally has certain guidelines determined by research and reviewed by experts in the field. However, many of these guidelines are not being followed by doctors. Moreover, there seem to be distinct differences and variations in treatment in different parts of the country as well as in major medical and cancer centers vs. community hospitals.

Some Facts Around the Controversy

- The guidelines are established based on clinical trials, on expertise in cancer treatment, and on consensus as to the best treatment.

- Much of the experimental work is done or led by scientists at major medical centers. These medical centers are not evenly distributed across the country.

- The world of cancer treatment is a fast-paced one. New information becomes available every day. However, disseminating the information and changing the habits of medical practice in local communities is a slow process.

- Most cancer patients today are being treated in the community, by community doctors and at community hospitals, where it often takes time before new information is put into practice.

Here are the results of two studies designed to test how patients' treatments differ:

- A study of prostate cancer diagnosis and treatment conducted in Florida found that radiation oncologists and urologists there were more likely to do routine PSA testing in men 75 years and older than were doctors in other parts of the United States. These doctors were more likely to report treating at least 20 percent of their patients with radiation implants. They reported the belief that implants for men with a less than ten-year life expectancy lived longer than those with other treatments. In addition, when surveyed on the subject of external radiation, the Florida urologists had more confidence in the survival benefit of this treatment than urologists in other regions. Radiation oncologists in Florida more often recommended early hormone treatment for men whose PSAs rose after both radiotherapy and surgery than did similar doctors in other regions. The question remains as to why Florida radiation oncologists' and urologists' beliefs and practices differed from their colleagues in other parts of the United States. It seems clear that studies are needed to judge whether the diagnosis and treatment of prostate cancer in Florida results in longer lives or better quality of life than in other parts of the country.

- A study carried out in New Mexico found that recommendations made by the National Institutes of Health Consensus Conferences in 1985, 1990, and 2000 for giving chemotherapy to women with breast cancer were not being carried out by community doctors. The recommended treatment is chemotherapy for premenopausal and postmenopausal women with node-positive tumors or with node-negative tumors greater than one centimeter in size. In this study, only 29 percent of women received chemotherapy. In addition, the use of chemotherapy de-creased substantially as the age of the patients increased. Studies need to be done to determine why treatment guidelines are not being followed and whether the recommendations are overly aggressive or whether practicing oncologists are too conservative in their chemotherapy use.

What You Need to Know and Do When You Are Told You Have Cancer

- Do your own investigation on the recommended treatments. Check sources, such as the NCI and ACS sites, both of which offer information about specific treatment for individual types and stages of cancer.

- Call the Cancer Information Service to verify your understanding of the treatment being recommended.

- If you find that the information differs from what your doctor is recommending, discuss it with your doctor to find out why a different treatment or treatment schedule is being recommended for you.

- Get another opinion on treatment from a physician at a comprehensive cancer center or a major medical center.

Web Pages to Check Out

- Hormone replacement therapy

    www.nlm.nih.gov/medlineplus/hormonereplacementtherapy.html: National Library of Medicine. Latest news, research, links to other sites.

    www.ahcpr.gov/clinic/uspstf/uspspmho.htm: Summary of recommendations including evidence, links to other sites.

    www.acog.org/from_home/publications/press_releases/nr08-30-02.cfm: American College of Obstetricians and Gynecologists. Questions and answers on hormone replacement therapy.

    www.nhlbi.nih.gov/health/women/pht_facts.htm: National Heart, Blood and Lung Institute. Facts about post-menopausal hormone use. Listing of products, schedules, and alternatives.

- Prostate cancer

    www.ahrq.gov/clinic/3rduspstf/prostatescr/prostaterr.htm: U.S. Preventative Services Task Force Screening Guidelines. Includes recommendations and rationale, summary of evidence for PSA screening for prostate cancer.

    www.cancer.org: American Cancer Society's guidelines for PSA screening.

www.cancer.gov/cancerinfo/pdq/screening/prostate/Health-Professional: National Cancer Institute's information and position on PSA screening.

www.urologyhealth.org: American Urological Association patient information on PSA screening.

- Ductal Carcinoma *in situ*

    www.imaginis.com/breasthealth/dcis.asp: General information on ductal carcinoma *in situ*.

    www.minervation.com/cancer/breast/professional/treatment/dcis/index. html: National Electronic Library for Health. Evidence-based treatment summary: ductal carcinoma *in situ*.

    www.cancer.gov/cancerinfo/pdq/screening/breast/: HealthProfessional: National Cancer Institute information on screening for breast cancer, including ductal carcinoma *in situ*.

- Older patients and cancer treatment

    www.new.commentwire.com/commwire_story.asp?commentwire_ID=3558: Older patients and breast cancer treatment.

    www.nci.nih.gov/clinicaltrials/developments/health-exclusions-a-barrier0403: Clinical trials and older patients.

- Diagnosis of cancer

    www.FindCancerExperts.com: Discussion of medical errors and high-risk situations for pathology errors.

    www.upmccancercenters.com/news/reuters/reuters.cfm?article=671: Report on article on breast cancer misdiagnoses published in *Archives of Internal Medicine,* June 24, 2002.

- Screening tests

    www.cancer.gov/cancerinfo/pdq/screening/overview: Information on the science of screening populations, levels of evidence, risks, endpoints.

- Differences in treatment

    www.ncbi.nlm.nih.gov/pubmed: National Library of Medicine to review articles: "United States Radiation Oncologists' and Urologists' Opinions About Screening and Treatment of Prostate Cancer Vary by Region." McNaughton, Collins M. et al. *Urology* 2002, October; 60(4) 628–33; and "Discrepancy Between Consensus Recommendations and Actual Community Use of Adjuvant Chemotherapy in Women with Breast Cancer." Du X.L. et al. in *Annals of Internal Medicine* 2003 January 21; 138(2): 90–7.

www.nccn.org: National Comprehensive Cancer Network, an alliance of major cancer centers. Patient guidelines for treating major cancers and their side effects. Also available on www.cancer.org.

Also see Chapter 2, Searching for Answers on the Web, for more information.

Six

HOW CANCERS ARE DIAGNOSED

In order for your doctor to confirm or establish the diagnosis it is necessary for you to go through a series of tests. The results of laboratory tests are needed to make proper medical decisions. After all the tests are in and a preliminary diagnosis has been made, it's a good idea to seek a multidisciplinary opinion on your case, especially if you are dealing with a less common type of cancer. This allows your doctors to discuss among themselves the best treatment for you, and gives you their combined opinion. If that is not possible, ask your primary doctor to help you sort out the various opinions you have received before making your decisions.

THE ART OF diagnosis has undergone many changes in the past ten years. We are beginning to see 3-D imaging which allows viewing of the organ from every angle, giving a 3-D mockup of the disease process. Many other new techniques that make diagnosis easier and less stressful are in everyday use. With the help of sophisticated computerized equipment, diagnosis has become more accurate. However, it is still important that you understand what tests are being done and what the results mean. Be certain you know who is performing the test, what it will entail and when you will get the results. All necessary tests must be done before treatment starts. The findings from these tests will be the basis for your future treatment. Getting the correct diagnosis is the first step in making certain that your treatment will be as successful as possible. So, don't try to shortcut the process. Take enough time to get all necessary testing done before you start treatment. If the diagnosis is not complete or is uncertain, your treatment may not be appropriate or may be less than satisfactory. Remember, once treatment starts, you shut down many possibilities.

What You Need to Know About Diagnosis

- Many tests for cancer need interpretation by the doctor and are thus subject to different conclusions. Medicine is not an exact science. It is useful to ask for an experienced second opinion on the results of the major diagnostic tests before you begin long-term or difficult treatment.

- Don't be surprised if you get varying opinions from different types of doctors. Doctors who work in specific areas, such as surgeons, medical oncologists, and radiation oncologists, look at cancer and its treatment from different viewpoints and thus may give you a different opinion on what they feel would be best for you.

- Make sure your diagnostic tests are done by competent, qualified physicians and technicians, using up-to-date machines and procedures. This is a sophisticated area that is continually changing.

- It will usually take a few days before the doctor gets the results of your tests. Make sure you have confirmed with the doctor how long it will take to get results of all the tests, and when and how you will be given these results.

- The words *positive* and *negative* are often used in describing test results. *Positive* usually means that something has been found. In most cases, it is something that is not normally supposed to be there. *Negative* means that nothing was found as a result of the test.

- Tumor markers—measurements of substances in the blood, other body fluids or tissues—are playing a larger role in diagnosing cancer. However, at present, they still must be used with other tests since people who do not have cancer also may exhibit the presence of the markers.

- Endoscopy—using a lighted instrument to look into the inside of the body—allows the doctor to diagnose several kinds of cancer without an operation. It is important to have skilled doctors performing these tests, since complications can occur.

- Ultrasound, magnetic resonance imaging, computerized tomography (CT) and nuclear scans, x-rays, PET scans, and cytology also may be used as part of the diagnostic process.

- The biopsy—getting a sample of the tumor—is the only definitive test for cancer. The actual cells must be looked at under the microscope in order for the doctor to make a definite diagnosis.

- Doctors go through a process known as staging in order to plan your treatment. Staging determines how much cancer there is in the body and where it is located. It is vital that tumors are staged to the fullest extent possible during diagnosis in order for you to have the most effective treatment.

Questions You Should Ask Your Doctor When Tests Are Being Ordered

- **What is the test for?**

- **Why do I need this test?**

- **If I have already had this test done can you use the results?**

- **What will be learned from this test?**

- **Is this test necessary to make a treatment decision? How will the results affect my treatment?**

- **What will the test be like? How long will it take? Who will be doing it?**

- **How should I prepare for the test? Will I have to stop taking any of my medicine before I can have this test?**

- **What will the test feel like? Will I be uncomfortable during the test? After the test?**

- **Will I have to be in the hospital for this test? For how long? Can it be done on an outpatient basis instead? Will I need someone to drive me home after it?**

- **How much will the test cost?**

- **What are the risks in doing the test? Is there another test that is less risky?**

- **When will you know the results of the test? When will you tell me?**

- **May I have a copy of the results and diagnosis for my files?**

What are the kinds of tests used to help detect cancer?

This will depend upon what problems you have, what kind of cancer is suspected and the degree to which it might have spread. The tests fall into the following categories:

- A physical examination, including taking a full medical history.

- Laboratory tests, such as blood analyses, including tumor markers, and urine analyses.

- Endoscopy, inserting a lighted instrument into the body.

- Cytology, the examination of sloughed-off cells.

- Imaging techniques, such as ultrasound, magnetic resonance imagine (MRI), nuclear scans, computerized tomography (CT), positron emission tomography (PET), and x-rays.

- Biopsy, taking a piece of tissue to examine under the microscope.

Do doctors do too many diagnostic tests?

Diagnostic tests are a vital part of the workup for any disease, but especially so in the treatment of cancer. Before any treatment is started, it is of major importance for the doctor to determine what kind of cancer you have, the cell type, and where it has spread. Treatment for different kinds of cancer, or different stages of the same type of cancer, vary. If the cancer has spread, surgery may not be the right choice. A good, thorough workup is vital before treatment of any kind is done for cancer.

Is there a risk in waiting to do the surgery until all the diagnostic tests are completed?

There is very little conclusive evidence to show that there is harm in delaying a short time (such as two to three weeks) while you are having the diagnostic tests. Occasionally, of course, it may be necessary to have rapid treatment for some specific type of cancer or specific problems caused by the cancer.

What are some of the things I need to be sure I know about the tests before I have them done?

You need to know what the test is for, what the procedure will be like, what preparations you need to make to take the test, why it is important in light of your symptoms, and how the test will affect the decision your doctor will make about your treatment. You also need to know where you will have the test done, what the test will feel like, what side effects you might have from it, how much the test will cost, and when you will be able to learn the results.

What kinds of risks are there in the tests done for cancer?

The risks depend on the test and the condition of the person on whom the test is being done. Certainly the more simple tests, such as blood counts, involve little or no risk. X-rays, which involve small amounts of radiation, are low-risk tests. However, in some types of x-rays, as well as some of the other procedures, there is risk involved. You need to ask the doctor to discuss the risk versus the benefit of the tests he recommends. Generally, in the area of cancer, the benefits of the tests are worth the risk.

What is an interventional radiologist?
This is a relatively new specialty that was recognized by the American Medical Association and the U.S. Department of Health and Human Services in 1992. Interventional radiologists use x-rays and other imaging techniques to "see" inside the body without surgery. They make tiny incisions (about the size of the tip of a pencil) and insert thin tubes (catheters) and other tiny instruments through blood vessels and other pathways of the body to diagnose and treat a wide variety of conditions that once required surgery. An interventional radiologist is a highly trained doctor who has completed medical school, an internship, four years of post-graduate training in radiology, passed the special exam to become a board-certified radiologist, and then spent an extra year in an interventional radiology fellowship program. These doctors are certified by the American Board of Radiology in both diagostic radiology and cardiovascular and interventional radiology.

Will my doctor be offended if I ask for another opinion?
Most doctors welcome a second opinion. A second opinion does not mean you are questioning your doctor's competence. If you have cancer, a decision about how you proceed with treatment is probably the most important decision you will make in your life. You need the best advice you can get before proceeding with a course of treatment. If your doctor does not want you to get another opinion, you need to think about whether or not you want to change doctors. There is more information on this subject in Chapter 3, Choosing Your Doctor and Hospital.

Will these tests be painful?
Most of these tests are not painful. You may be given a sedative before some of the tests. An area of your body may be numbed, or you may be given local or general anesthesia. In some of the tests, you may have to be in an uncomfortable position for a period of time. You may want to learn a few simple relaxation techniques to help get you through these periods. If you are relaxed, it will be easier for both you and the doctor.

What are some simple relaxation techniques I can use?
Here are three that might be useful. Try practicing them at home before you go for your tests:

■ Slow rhythmic breathing. Stare at an object or close your eyes and concentrate on your breathing. Take a slow, deep breath in, and let it out slowly. Now begin breathing slowly and comfortably, concentrating on your breathing, taking about six to nine breaths a minute. To maintain a slow, even rhythm as you breathe, you can say silently to yourself, In, one, two, Out, one, two.

- Inhale/tense, exhale/relax. Breathe in deeply. At the same time, tense all your muscles or a group of muscles of your choice. For example, you can squeeze your eyes shut, frown, or clench your teeth. Hold your breath and keep your muscles tense for a second or two. Let go. Breathe out and let your body go limp. Relax.

- Think of a favorite scene, such as the beach. Recall the pleasant warmth of the sun and the tranquilizing sound of the waves. Imagine yourself basking in the warmth and let the sound of the waves lull you into relaxation. Try to put yourself into the scene, instead of being on the outside looking in.

Laboratory Tests

What is a complete blood count?

A complete blood count, known as a CBC, is a test to check the number of red cells, white cells, and platelets in a sample of your blood. The CBC also checks your hematocrit (portion of blood value made up of red blood cells), and your hemoglobin (blood's oxygen-carrying capacity), along with the red blood cell indices (size and hemoglobin concentration of red blood cells), and white blood differential (percentage of each type of white blood cells). The CBC, most often used as a screening test for infections and anemia, is also used in the diagnosis and treatment of cancer.

How is a complete blood count done?

Usually blood is taken from a vein in the back of your hand or from your arm. When taking the blood from the vein, the technician will wrap an elastic band around your upper arm, tightly enough to stop the flow of blood through the veins. You will usually be asked to make a fist, to make the veins stand out so the needle can be inserted more easily. Several small vials of blood may be taken at the same time for the different tests that will be performed. A blood smear, which involves spreading blood on a slide which is then stained with a special dye, may be done to identify changes in cell color, size, shape, and type of cells. You will usually feel a small pinch as the needle goes through the skin, but no pain as the blood is drawn. You may have a little bruising (hematoma) at the spot where the needle was placed. If you have bleeding or clotting problems, let the technician know before the test is begun. If there is bruising, apply ice. After 24 hours, use warm, moist compresses. Certain medications may alter CBC test values so be sure to inform your doctor of any medications you take regularly.

QUESTIONS TO THINK ABOUT DURING YOUR DIAGNOSIS

QUESTION	REMARKS
Do I want to know exactly what plans the doctor has for my treatment and what alternative there might be for my type of cancer?	Many people want to participate in the decisions about the treatment of their illness. Knowledge about the treatment plan is important to you if you want to be a part of the decision and how and where you will receive treatment.
Do I want to ask for an independent report from another pathologist?	The pathology report of the biopsy is the basis on which all future decisions will be made. You should think about talking with your doctor about how the pathologist report was done, whether it was reviewed by more than one pathologist, whether the doctor talked with the pathologist, whether or not there is any question or doubt about the diagnosis. You may want to request that the pathology be checked at a large medical center.
Do I want to know specifically what kind of cancer I have and the stage it is in?	These days, most people want to know exactly what they are facing. They like to have all the facts so they can do research on the Web and at the medical library to find out what treatments are being offered. Some want to call the Cancer Information Service and have a search of clinical trials being done on their particular stage of disease. Others may feel they prefer to leave decisions to the doctor. However, if you have a rare type of cancer, you should be informed, because you need to decide whether you want to go to one of the cancer centers or to a medical center specializing in your type of cancer for consultation or treatment. You should at least ask your doctor to have a phone consultation with a doctor doing research in that type of cancer.

(continued)

QUESTIONS TO THINK ABOUT DURING
YOUR DIAGNOSIS (continued)

QUESTION	REMARKS
Do I want my doctor to consult with the nearest NCI-designated cancer center or cooperative group about my case?	There are cancer centers and clinical cooperative groups, designated by the National Cancer Institute, conducting controlled studies to determine the best possible treatments. Your doctor needs the latest information to give you the best possible treatment.
Do I want to go to an NCI-designated cancer center or to a medical school for my treatment?	You need to weigh this decision most carefully. The cancer centers designated by the National Cancer Institute and leading medical schools have doctors on their staffs who are especially trained in the various cancer disciplines. In the course of a week, they will probably be treating more people with your illness than many local doctors see in a year. On the other hand, the practical question of geography and your emotional energy will have to be considered. There are additional details on these issues in Chapter 3, Choosing Your Doctor and Hospital.

What is the cost of a CBC?
The cost varies but should be well under $100.

What does the urinalysis tell the doctor?
The analysis of the urine tells the doctor many things. The degree of concentration of the urine (weight of urine relative to plain water) called specific gravity (SG) indicates urinary obstruction with kidney damage if the count is low, or dehydration if the count is high. Using a simple plastic strip with a series of chemically sensitive patches, the doctor, nurse, or technician can also check the amount of acidity, protein, sugar, and ketones in the urine, to diagnose acidosis or alkalosis, kidney damage, diabetes, and other diseases. The urine sediment exam checks for red cells, white cells, kidney cells, crystals, and microorganisms in the urine that might indicate kidney damage, urinary-tract infection, or gout. The urine sample is frequently analyzed in your doctor's office with special chemical strips that react with substances in the urine and change color. A more detailed analysis, including microscopic examination, may be done in the office or at a pathology laboratory.

Is there a blood or urine test that can detect cancer?

Progress has been made in identifying substances—called tumor markers—that are found in higher amounts than normal in the blood, other body fluids or tissues of people who have cancer. Tumor markers alone are not sufficient to diagnose cancer because levels of these substances can be raised in benign conditions and often are not elevated in persons with cancer. Tumor markers, however, can be used as one of a series of diagnostic tests. For instance, when adults have a higher than normal amount of carcinoembryonic antigen (CEA), in their blood, it may indicate that cancer of the colon or rectum may be present. However, since this protein is also found in the blood of people who do not have cancer, such as smokers and persons with ulcerative colitis, liver disease, and lung infection, it cannot be used alone as a definitive diagnostic tool, but needs to be used along with other tests. There are a few markers that are presently used in cancer diagnosis, including CA–125 in ovarian cancer, calcitonin in thyroid cancer, Philadelphia chromosome in leukemia and PSA in prostate cancer. Many more are being used in clinical trials in an investigational manner. At the present moment, however, there is not one blood or urine test that would tell whether or not you have any kind of cancer in your body. For more information on tumor markers, see Chapter 4, What Is Cancer?

How is the digital rectal examination done?

The doctor, wearing thin gloves, puts a greased finger into the rectum and gently feels for lumps. This examination will detect the presence of any abnormalities in the lowest four inches of the rectum. Any stool on the gloved finger will also be checked for blood.

What is a fecal occult stool test?

The fecal occult stool test (also called the *guaiac test*, pronounced gwī-ak) is a simple, inexpensive method of testing stools for traces of blood. Usually stool samples are taken of three consecutive bowel movements so that if there is intermittent bleeding, this can be discovered. To increase the accuracy of the stool analysis, the doctor may ask you to start a meat-free, high-fiber diet (avoiding such vegetables as radishes and red peppers) 48 hours before the collection of the first stool specimen and continuing through the next three days. Vitamin C, antacids, iron, and aspirin also should be avoided during this time to ensure that the test is accurate. Inaccurate results may also be caused by bleeding gums, hemorrhoids, menstrual blood, or watery stools.

Endoscopies

What is meant by the term *endoscopy*?

This is the medical term for examination of the inside of the body using optical instruments. There are many kinds of instruments used to do these examinations in different parts of the body. Constant improvements are being made on fiber-optic instruments—tiny flexible fibers that carry a powerful light and a telescope that allows the doctor to peer inside the body. In addition, surgical instruments may be inserted, either through the scope or through other small incisions in the area, in order to obtain tissue or fluid samples or to perform therapeutic procedures. Endoscopy allows the diagnosis of various kinds of cancer without doing a major operation. Sometimes endoscopies are used in combination with other tests, such as x-rays to confirm the diagnosis. You can identify these instruments because they end in the term *scope*.

What kind of doctor will perform endoscopies?
Be sure you are in the hands of a specially trained doctor or technician who specializes in this field. Check the credentials of your doctor before submitting to an endoscopy as these tests are delicate, can be difficult to perform, and can lead to complications.

How are the endoscopies done?
Endoscopies are individualized procedures and different institutions have different ways of performing the tests. Today they are most often performed in an outpatient setting. You may start by having blood tests done. Before the endoscopy, you usually are given an injection to relax you. Most of these procedures can usually be done under local anesthesia but some may require spinal or general anesthesia. A large machine may be positioned near you to transmit pictures to a TV monitor. Sometimes, you will be able to see what is on the screen. Many times, lights in the room are dimmed to allow the doctor to see the lighted area more clearly. The TV monitor is used to help your doctor move the scope to different sections of the organ being looked at. A tiny brush or instrument may be inserted through the scope to collect small bits of tissue for analysis under the microscope.

Is there anything I should tell the doctor before having an endoscopy?
There are several things you need to be sure the doctor knows. Your doctor will usually ask if you are allergic to any medicine or anesthetics, if you are taking any medicine, if you have had any kind of bleeding problems, what other kinds of tests you have had recently, and if you might be pregnant.

What should I do to prepare for my endoscopy examination?
It depends on what part of the body is being examined. You may have to fast for eight to 12 hours, stop smoking for 24 hours, and have several blood tests. The day of the examination, you may be given a mild drug to relax you, have an IV line put in your vein and have local or general anesthesia. For

some endoscopic examinations, the preparations are more complex than for others.

What is a bronchoscopy?

A bronchoscopy is used to diagnose tumors in the lung or other lung diseases. The doctor inserts a lighted instrument through your mouth or nose, after giving you local anesthesia so you will be comfortable as the doctor inserts the scope. Be sure to tell the doctor if you have allergies to any medicine or anesthetics, if you are taking any medicine, if you have had bleeding problems, if you have any loose teeth or if you might be pregnant. You will be asked to remove your dentures, glasses, and all your jewelry.

Isn't a bronchoscopy uncomfortable?

The doctor will do everything that can be done to make you comfortable. If the scope is to be put into your throat, the back of your throat probably will be sprayed with anesthetic solution to numb it and to stop you from having a feeling of gagging. Or the anesthesia might be injected into your windpipe. If the scope is going to be put into your nose, the anesthetic is usually swabbed onto your nasal passage. Some people say that their tongues and throats feel swollen and they get the feeling they cannot breathe. Using relaxation techniques from the start, such as taking slow breaths through your nose with your mouth open, can help. The test usually takes 30 to 60 minutes. You will not be able to talk during the test. It might be helpful to discuss with the doctors some hand signals to use should the procedure become uncomfortable. Or you may wish to bring along a pad and pencil to write messages.

Will I have any side effects from my bronchoscopy?

You may have a few. You will need to stay in the hospital or outpatient area for several hours after the test so you can be monitored. Do not eat or drink anything until the numbness in your throat wears off, which will take two hours or more. You may have hoarseness, voice loss, or a sore throat for several days. You may need to gargle a saltwater solution or suck throat lozenges. If a biopsy has been done, you may also spit up some matter with blood in it but signs of bleeding should disappear within 24 hours. If you have heavy bleeding, cannot breathe normally, have chest pain or a fever, you should call your doctor immediately.

What happens if the doctor cannot get an adequate biopsy with the bronchoscopy?

If this happens, the surgeon will use another procedure, making a small incision (about two inches long) to look inside the chest, or lung to determine what treatment should be followed. (See laparoscopy in this chapter.)

COMMON TYPES OF ENDOSCOPIES

PREPARATION FOR TEST	PROCEDURE TYPE
Bronchoscopy Lighted viewing instrument inserted through mouth or nose. No eating or drinking for four to six hours before test. No smoking for prior 24 hours. Several blood tests ordered before procedure is done.	To minimize discomfort topical anesthesia (lidocane) is applied to inside of nostril. May be given medicine to relax and to dry mouth secretions. IV may be placed in vein. Procedure may be done in sitting or lying position. Test usually takes 30 to 60 minutes.
Colonoscopy Lighted instrument inserted in anus and goes through colon. Need to empty colon prior to procedure by one or more of several methods such as liquid diet, laxative, enema, etc.	IV line may be placed in vein, used for sedative and pain reliever. Test takes 30 minutes to two hours depending on whether polyps are removed or a biopsy is done.
Cystoscopy Lighted instrument inserted into ureter and goes into bladder. If being done under local anesthetic, drink plenty of fluids; otherwise no food or drink for four to eight hours before test.	May be given relaxant before test. May have local, spinal, or general anesthetic. IV may be placed in vein for medicines and fluids. Test takes 15 to 45 minutes.
Laparoscopy Lighted instrument inserted through small cut in abdomen to look at organs in the stomach and pelvic area. Sometimes known as "band-aid" surgery because of small incision. Do not eat or drink for four to eight hours before test.	May be given relaxant before test. Catheter may be inserted to empty bladder. Usually done with general anesthesia but local or spinal may be used. Test itself takes 30 to 45 minutes.
Laryngoscopy Flexible instrument inserted in mouth to check base of tongue, epiglottis, larynx, and vocal cords. You will need to take out your dentures. You may need to fast for four to eight hours.	Two types used; one is done in office procedure, other requires operating room facilities. Test takes from ten to 30 minutes.

COMMON TYPES OF ENDOSCOPIES *(continued)*

PREPARATION FOR TEST	PROCEDURE TYPE
Mediastinoscopy Instrument inserted into mediastinum through an incision made in the front of your neck. You will need to fast before the exam.	Done under general anesthesia in an operating room. Tube placed in throat. Procedure takes about an hour.
Sigmoidoscopy Instrument inserted into anus to view lower intestinal tract. Will need enemas, special diet, or a combination of both before the test is done.	Office procedure. Exam takes about ten to 30 minutes depending on whether polyps are removed or biopsy done.
Thoracoscopy Instrument inserted through small incisions made in chest wall. Will have tests to see if lungs function well. You will need to fast before the test.	Usually done under general anesthesia. One lung partially deflated during test so need to be able to breathe with only one lung. Test takes two to four hours. Will need to stay in hospital for two to five days.
Upper GI Endoscopy: Esophagoscopy, Gastroscopy, Dueodenoscopy Lighted instrument inserted into the mouth and threaded into the area to be examined. Must fast for eight hours before test. Iodine contrast dye injected through endoscope. Tell doctor if you are allergic to shellfish or iodine.	Done in special procedure room. IV line put into vein for relaxant and sedative. Test takes 15 to 30 minutes. You will need someone to drive you home.

What is autoflourescence bronchoscopy?

This test allows the doctor to see whether the cells reflect light (flouresce). A dye is injected and is taken up by the tumor cells. If cells do not reflect light, a sample is taken to see whether or not they are cancerous.

What is a colonoscopy?

A colonoscopy is an examination of the colon by means of a flexible, lighted tube, slightly larger in diameter than an enema tube. It lets the doctor view the entire colon as well as the rectum. The doctor uses a colonoscopy to evaluate symptoms in the bowel, to detect cancer, and to check for its recurrence.

It may be used on a routine basis, every ten years, to screen for colon cancer. The instrument allows the doctor to take tissue biopsies or stool samples from any part of the colon. You need to tell your doctor if you are allergic to any medicines, are taking medicine, have had bleeding problems or a history of heart problems, had recent barium x-ray, or might be pregnant. **It is important that the doctor, preferably a gastroenterologist, who does your colonoscopy is skilled in this procedure. Perforation, which requires surgery to repair a hole in the colon, and other complications can occur.**

Do I need to do anything before I have a colonoscopy?

Your colon needs to be cleared before you can undergo a colonoscopy. Several methods are used alone or in combination—being on a liquid diet, taking a laxative, and having enemas to clean the bowel. Your doctor will give you specific instructions on how to do this. Cleansing your colon is an uncomfortable process but is an essential part of this test.

How is the test done?

The colonoscopy is done under local anesthesia or general anesthesia. You will lie on your side, with your knees drawn up. The doctor begins by inserting a gloved, lubricated finger into your rectum. Then, a thin, lubricated tube is inserted into your colon. If you are under local anesthesia, you may be asked to change your position to help the scope go through the twists and turns of your colon. Your doctor looks at the lining of your colon through the scope and on the monitor. During the procedure, the doctor will insert air into your colon to dilate the passage for better viewing. You may get cramping, a feeling of pressure, or the urge to move your bowels. Do not be embarrassed if you expel some gas or air. This is perfectly normal. Small growths may be removed or tissue samples taken. As the scope is slowly withdrawn, the doctor carefully inspects the lining of the colon, rectum, and anus. The procedure takes from 30 to 60 minutes.

Will I have any side effects from my colonoscopy?

If you have had local anesthesia, you might feel groggy right after the test is finished. You will rest until the medications wear off. If you have had general anesthesia, you will remain until you recover from its effects. In either case, it's useful to take it easy for the rest of the day. Be sure to drink fluids after the test to replace those lost in cleansing your colon in preparation for your colonoscopy. You may see some blood in your stools for a few days. However, if you have heavy bleeding, severe stomach pain, or fever, call your doctor.

What is virtual colonoscopy?

Virtual colonoscopy is a new method, presently under study, that looks at the inside of the colon by taking a series of x-rays (spiral CT scans). You will prepare for this test the same as if you were having a regular colonoscopy. The doctor inserts some air into the colon. Using a high power computer, 2-D and 3-D pictures are reconstructed, letting the doctor see the inside of the colon on a computer monitor. The pictures can be turned for better views, saved, and looked at after the test, even years later. It is anticipated that the test can be done more quickly, without anesthesia, and probably at lower cost than the colonoscopy.

What is a cystoscopy?

The doctor inserts a pencil-thin, lighted instrument into your urethra, the tube that brings urine from your bladder, and is able to view the urethra, bladder, kidneys, and prostate. This examination is used to diagnose problems in these organs. Various instruments may be passed through the scope to obtain fluid or tissue samples.

How is a cystoscopy done?

For the procedure, you will lie on your back with your knees bent, legs apart, and feet or thighs supported. You will be asked to lie very still to prevent damage to the urinary tract. Your doctor will insert a thin, lubricated cystoscope into your urethra and bladder. A sterile solution is put through the scope to expand the bladder and give the doctor a clear view. This may give you a feeling of fullness and an urge to urinate, but it is a necessary part of the procedure to stretch bladder walls and to provide the doctor with a better view of the area. Urine specimens and tissue samples may be taken. Sometimes a catheter is put in to drain urine until the swelling in your urethra subsides. This test may be done with either local or general anesthesia. If local anesthesia is used, you will be free to leave after the test. After general or spinal anesthesia, you will be monitored until you recover from the effects of the anesthesia.

Are there any side effects to my having a cystoscopy?

For a day or two, you may need to urinate often and you may have a burning sensation during and after urination. Try to drink lots of liquids to prevent infection. You also may have pinkish urine for several days. If your urine is red with blood clots or if you cannot urinate within eight hours of the test, be sure to call your doctor. If you experience pain in your back, stomach, or side or if you have high fever or chills, notify your doctor.

What is a laparoscopy?

A laparoscopy is an examination that uses a lighted instrument to look at the outside surface of the intestines, liver, spleen, uterus, fallopian tubes and ovaries. It is used to evaluate pain or tumors of the stomach or pelvic area. Tissue may be removed through an endoscope to test for cancer. This procedure also makes it possible to determine whether or not cancer has spread in this area. It is a less invasive procedure than surgery. It may also be used after cancer has been treated to allow for "second-look" surgery to determine how successful treatment has been and to make sure that all cancer is gone from the site and the surrounding areas.

How is the laparoscopy done?

General anesthesia is usually used for this procedure. It may be necessary for the hair surrounding your navel to be shaved. In the operating room you will lie on your back on a tilted table, with your feet higher than your head. A small incision is made in your abdomen, below the navel. You also may have incisions near the pubic hairline. Gas (carbon dioxide or nitrous oxide) is pumped into your abdomen through a hollow needle to expand your abdomen. The laparoscope, a thin, lighted tube, is put through the cut so the doctor can look at the area in question. If the doctor needs other instruments, such as those used to take some tissue for biopsy, another small incision may be made further down in the pubic area. When the examination is finished, the scope is taken out and the gas is allowed to discharge. The doctor will use a few stitches or staples to close the incision.

Will I have any side effects from a laparoscopy?

You may have a few side effects from your laparoscopy. You will not be able to go home until the medications wear off, you have emptied your bladder and you can walk. Most patients experience cramping in the abdomen and referred pain in the shoulder as a result of the gas that was inserted which may irritate the diaphragm. You will be a little sore around the area of the incision, may have a dark coloration around your navel, some bloating in the stomach area and feel generally achy for a day or two. If you had a tube in your throat, you may have a sore throat. You may be able to get back to your regular routine in a day or so, depending on why you had the exam and what was found. Don't do any strenuous activity or exercise for about a week. If you have severe pain in your back or stomach area or if the incision is draining, call the doctor immediately.

Will I have scars from my laparoscopy?

Since the incisions are small, the scars usually disappear. Be sure to keep the area dry for about four days to allow the incision to heal properly.

What is a microlaparoscopy?

This is a new procedure that uses telescopes and instruments that are much smaller than normal. This means that smaller incisions are made and that you will heal more quickly.

What is a laryngoscopy?

This is an examination of areas of the mouth and throat used when you have problems such as blood-tinged sputum, difficulty in swallowing, a feeling of a lump in your throat, or a harsh whistling sound when you breathe. Your doctor may use one of two procedures: a flexible fiber-optic instrument that can be done in an office or a straight, hollow lighted laryngoscope that needs to be done in an operating room.

How is the examination done?

If it is being done in an office, the doctor will apply a numbing solution to your nostrils and the back of your throat. The lighted flexible instrument will be passed through the nostril, down the back of your throat. You will be asked to make several sounds to make your vocal cords move so the doctor can examine them. You will not be able to talk during the exam. You may feel several sensations during this exam. The anesthesia may taste bitter. Your throat may feel swollen, making you feel like you cannot swallow. You may feel like gagging. Try to relax as much as you can, taking panting breaths. The procedure usually takes 5 to 10 minutes. If the examination is being done in the operating room, you will be given a relaxant and general anesthesia. You will be asleep while the instrument is inserted through your mouth, and down your throat. Instruments may be passed through the scope to remove tissue samples or photographs may be taken. The procedure in the operating room usually takes 30 minutes to one hour.

Will there be any side effects from the laryngoscopy?

You may have a sore throat and some hoarseness for a few days. Try gargling with saltwater or using lozenges. If you had a biopsy taken, you may spit up small amounts of blood for several days after the examination. With general anesthesia, you may feel tired and achy for a few days. If you spit up a lot of blood, have a high fever, or if you have trouble breathing, call your doctor.

What is mediastinoscopy?

A mediastinoscopy is a surgical procedure in which a flexible or rigid viewing tube is inserted into the space between the breastbone and the lungs. The examination is done to detect cancer and to determine whether cancer has spread in the lung area.

How is a mediastinoscopy done?

This procedure is usually performed by a chest (thoracic) surgeon and a surgical team. You will be placed under general anesthesia, and a thin tube attached to a breathing machine may be passed into your windpipe to assure proper breathing. The doctor will make a two to three inch incision between the collarbones, just above your breastbone and will insert a long, thin scope behind your breastbone. You will not feel anything. The doctor will be able to look at the space, and take out lymph nodes or tissue. Then the scope will be taken out and a few stitches will be made to close the incision. The procedure takes about one hour.

Will I be able to go home right away after this examination?

You will need to stay in the hospital until you are fully awake and able to swallow. Depending on your condition, you may be allowed to go home later the same day or required to remain for one to two days. You may feel a little pain at the stitch site and you may have a sore throat from the tube. You may also have a general achy feeling for a few days. Your stitches will be taken out in about two weeks. You will probably have a small scar from this procedure. Call the doctor if your incision starts bleeding or if you have a fever, chest pain, shortness of breath, or difficulty swallowing.

What is a sigmoidoscopy?

A sigmoidoscopy is the primary test done to examine the inside of the lower part of the intestinal tract, which includes the sigmoid colon, rectum, and anus. The test is done on a routine basis, every three to five years, to screen for colon or rectal cancer. It is used in diagnosis when you have unexplained bleeding or pain in the rectum or a change in bowel habits. This test helps the doctor to detect tumors, polyps, inflammation, hemorrhoids, and other bowel disease.

Will I have to do anything special to prepare for my sigmoidoscope?

To prepare for this examination, the doctor will usually instruct you to have a tap-water enema the night before, or the morning of, the examination. Some doctors will ask you to have only a liquid diet for a couple of days before the examination along with the enemas. If bleeding, obstruction or diarrhea is present, you will be instructed not to do anything at all before the examination, and a local anesthetic jelly may be used before the procedure to ease discomfort. You will need to undress from the waist down and empty your bladder before the test begins. NOTE: Barium interferes with visual inspection of the colon, so be sure to wait at least a week after having a barium test (such as a barium enema) before scheduling a sigmoidoscopy.

How is the sigmoidoscopy done?
The test, often done in the doctor's office, makes most people apprehensive but it usually causes only mild discomfort. The test takes 15 to 30 minutes. You will be lying on your side with your knees drawn up. After inserting a gloved, lubricated finger into your rectum for a manual examination, the doctor will gently insert the lubricated instrument—a hollow tube called a sigmoidoscope or proctosigmoidoscope—into the anus. Most doctors use a flexible fiber-optic sigmoidoscope, an instrument with a two-foot long tube that can transmit light around the bends and allows viewing higher into the colon. Sometimes air is inserted through the scope to help clear the path. This will give you a feeling of being bloated and may cause you to pass gas. The doctor may insert other instruments, such as forceps or swabs, through the inside of the instrument to remove a small piece of tissue for examination or to take out small polyps. Most people say the thought of this examination is worse than the exam itself. You may be a bit uncomfortable and feel like you are going to have a bowel movement. You also may feel pressure or cramping, but in most instances, you will not feel any pain. Try to relax, taking slow, deep breaths through your mouth. If you need to pass air, don't be embarrassed or try to hold it in.

Will I be able to go right home after this examination?
The doctor will want to make sure you are not dizzy before you are allowed to leave. You may feel some pains in your abdominal area and may pass some gas. If you had a polyp removed or if you had a biopsy, you might have some blood on your stool for a few days. Call the doctor if you have heavy bleeding from the rectum, severe pain in your abdomen or a fever.

What kind of doctor should do the sigmoidoscopy?
This procedure is best done by a proctologist, a gastroenterologist, or a physician who is trained in the procedure. Complications from this examination are rare, but an inexperienced doctor could perforate the rectum or colon, causing serious problems.

What is a thoracoscopy?
A thoracoscopy looks at the surface of the lungs and the spaces between them through a flexible tube called a thoracoscope. You will usually be given general anesthesia. The doctor will make two or three small incisions in your side. A thin tube-like instrument containing a tiny camera is passed through one of the incisions, with surgical instruments passed through another. The doctor can see your lungs on a video camera. The doctor can take samples of tissue if needed. One lung is partially deflated during this test so that the doctor can see between the chest wall and your lung. You may have tubes

inserted in your chest to drain fluid and air. This procedure is sometimes done to see if a thoracotomy is needed. If you have a shortage of oxygen because you only have one lung, you will not be able to have this test.

What is a thoracotomy?

A thoracotomy is an exploratory chest operation used as a diagnostic tool. The chest wall is opened to see the internal organs, to get samples of tissue, or to treat disease. You will be brought to an operating room and given general anesthesia. A cut will be made in your chest wall and samples will be taken from the tissue in your lungs. Your breastbone may need to be split if the doctor needs to take tissues from both of your lungs. At the same time, the doctor can, if needed, take out a section of the lung, a lobe, or the entire lung. This is major surgery and is used as a diagnostic tool only when other procedures, such as thoracentesis, bronchoscopy, mediastinoscopy, or thoracoscopy do not give enough information to the doctor.

What examinations are used to view the upper gastrointestinal tract?

There are several examinations done to look at the interior lining of the upper gastrointestinal tract. When the doctor is looking at the esophagus, the tube that leads from the mouth to the stomach, an esophagoscope is used. For the stomach, a gastroscope is inserted. For the duodenum (the first portion of the small intestine), a duodenoscope is the instrument used. Often these three areas are checked during one combined examination, using a three-foot-long flexible tube that can transmit images around the bends in this area of the body. These tests are familiarly referred to as EGDs (esophagogastroduodenoscopy). The doctor can look for inflammation, tumors or bleeding and can take tissue specimens for a biopsy with flexible lighted instruments.

How are the scopes in the upper gastrointestinal tract done?

You will be given medication to relax you and to relieve pain. You will be drowsy but alert during the test. Your throat will be numbed to make it easier to pass the instrument. Lying on your left side with your head bent slightly forward, the doctor puts the tip of the thin instrument into your mouth and gently moves it down into the area to be examined, while looking through the eyepiece. You may be asked to swallow to help move it along, but you should not swallow during the examination unless you are asked to do so. The doctor may put air or water through the tube to help with the exam. Your saliva may be suctioned from your mouth. Sometimes a camera is used to take photographs. If needed, forceps or brushes may be inserted through the instrument to take tissue for biopsies.

Is this an uncomfortable test?

Some people find that the thought of this test is even more uncomfortable than the test itself. You will be drowsy from the medication and may not remember much about the examination. Your throat and tongue will feel numb and swollen. You will not be able to talk during the procedure. Some people say they feel like they cannot breathe with the tube in their throat, but this sensation is caused by the anesthetic. Just remember there is plenty of room for you to breathe. You can help by being as relaxed as possible. Try to breathe slowly as the tube is being inserted. When the tube is moved or as air is added, you may have some gagging, nausea, bloating, or cramping. These are normal reactions.

Will I have side effects from this test?

Very few. You may have the usual aftereffects related to the medication—drowsy feeling, dry mouth, blurred vision—for several hours after the test. Don't eat or drink for a couple of hours while your throat is still numb. The doctor will want to watch you for a couple of hours before you can go home. You should have someone drive you home. You may belch and feel bloated. Your throat may be sore, you may have a tickle or cough, and you may remain hoarse for several days. It may help to gargle with saltwater or use lozenges. You can go back to your normal schedule and diet. Call the doctor if you vomit blood, have black or bloody stools, have difficulty swallowing, are short of breath, or have chest pain, stomach pain, or a fever.

What is a barium swallow test?

This test, professionally known as an esophagography, requires you to swallow a liquid mixture containing barium sulfate, a chalky contrast dye that allows the physician to x-ray the area to see the inner lining of the esophagus. The test takes place in a radiology room where you are given a thick, milkshake-like liquid that contains the contrast dye. As you drink the liquid, you are moved into various positions while the radiologist views a florescent viewing screen. The test takes from 15 to 30 minutes to complete. Be sure to drink plenty of fluids after the test to help eliminate the barium from your system.

What is an endoscopic retrograde cholangiopancreatogram?

This test, referred to as ERCP, is a combination of two diagnostic procedures: an endoscope of the upper gastrointestinal area and x-rays of the ducts that drain the liver, gallbladder, and pancreas. An intravenous needle will be inserted in a vein in your arm and a mild sedative will be given to you. However, you will remain conscious during the procedure. The endoscope is passed into the duodenum, and a hollow tube is threaded into the opening of the ducts. An iodine-based contrast dye is injected through the endoscope and x-rays are taken. (Let your physician know if you are allergic to iodine or shellfish as the dye may cause an allergic reaction.) If needed, the doctor may insert instruments through the scope and remove tissue or perform other procedures. This is a test that must be done by an experienced gastroenterologist. The test takes one to two hours to complete. Depending on what procedures were performed, you will either return home after the sedatives have worn off, or you may need to stay at the hospital overnight.

Cytology

What is cytology?

Cytology relates to the formation, structure, and function of cells. When it is mentioned in connection with the diagnosis for cancer, it is sometimes called exfoliative cytology and refers to the technique of examining cells that have been normally shed or that have been scraped from living tissue. The cells, which cannot be seen by the naked eye, are examined under the microscope, usually by a pathologist or a technician trained to know whether the cells look normal or not.

What kinds of tests are cytological exams?

There are several different tests that use this technique. Among them are:

- Pap test to detect cancer of the cervix.
- Vaginal pool aspiration or endometrial aspiration to detect uterine cancer.
- Sputum tests to detect lung cancer.
- Urine-sediment tests to detect cancer of the urinary tract, especially bladder.
- Scrapings from the mouth to detect oral cancer.
- Cell samples from the esophagus, stomach, pancreas, or duodenum.
- Fluid tests from areas such as breasts, spinal cord, thyroid, prostate.
- Bone marrow tests.

How are cytological exams performed?

All of these tests are performed in a similar manner. A little fluid or tissue is taken from the area in question, either from cells that have been sloughed off, cells that have been scraped off, or cells that have been removed through a needle (aspirated). The material is spread on a glass slide, stained with dyes and examined under a microscope. This technique was first used in the Pap test. Today, fiber-optic instruments make it possible to obtain smears from less accessible organs, such as the stomach and pancreas.

How is the Pap test done?

The Pap smear is a simple, painless test that can be done in a doctor's office, a clinic, or a hospital. Its purpose is to detect abnormal cells in and around the cervix. While a woman lies on an examining table, the clinician inserts a speculum into her vagina to widen the opening. Living cells are collected in and around the cervix. The specimen is put either on a glass slide or into a vial of liquid and sent to a medical laboratory for evaluation. The test is usually done by a gynecologist or other specially trained health care professionals, such as physician assistants, nurse midwives, and nurse practitioners. The interpretation of the slide by the laboratory is an important factor in the diagnosis. The percentage of misinterpretations has been shown to be quite high, so it is important to have the test verified before any treatment is undertaken.

Can the Pap test detect cancers in the female tract?

A Pap test can accurately detect cancer of the cervix, but it is not a test for detecting cancer of the endometrium, fallopian tubes, or ovaries. In cases where these types of cancer are discovered through a Pap smear, it is because the cancer cells have passed down into the cavity of the uterus and continued through the cervix and into the vaginal discharge. (For information about Pap test results, see Chapter 20, Gynecological Cancers.)

How is a sputum test done?

You are asked to cough deeply to bring up some material, called sputum, from your lungs. The sputum is examined under the microscope to see if there are cancer cells present that have been shed from the inner lining of the breathing passages. The tumor is then located by such techniques as flexible fiber-optic bronchoscopy, because the sputum examination by itself does not tell the doctor where the tumor is located in the bronchial tree.

What is thoracentesis?

Thoracentesis—also called a pleural tap or pleural fluid analysis—is a test in which a needle is inserted through the chest wall to withdraw fluid that has accumulated between the lungs and the membrane that lines the chest cavity. Ultrasound or fluoroscopy is often used to guide the insertion of the needle. You need to be very still during the test, and cannot cough, move, or breathe deeply. The fluid will be sent to the laboratory to be tested for cancer cells. This is a relatively risky test, since the needle can accidentally puncture the lung or blood vessel.

What are pulmonary function tests?

Pulmonary function tests, also called lung function tests, are given to measure your breathing and evaluate your ability to get oxygen into your blood.

The tests measure the amount of air moving in and out of the lungs and indicate if there is an obstruction in the air passages. The tests, which are usually done in a pulmonary function laboratory or a respiratory therapy department, consist of various breathing exercises and can take up to two hours to complete. Pulmonary function tests are used in diagnosing lung cancer, as well as for evaluation purposes before chest or abdominal surgery.

What is a spinal tap?
A spinal tap, also called a lumbar puncture, spinal fluid tap, or cerebrospinal fluid (CSF) analysis, takes spinal fluid out of the spinal canal. The doctor, after numbing your lower back, inserts a small needle to get a sample. About two teaspoons of fluid are usually taken out to send to the lab. The test takes about 20 minutes. This is considered a safe procedure, although many people have a severe headache that lasts a day or two, after the test. Drink plenty of fluids to help replace the spinal fluid lost by your body. Be sure to call the doctor immediately if you develop a fever, stiff neck, a continuing headache, numbness, or weakness.

What is a bone marrow aspiration and biopsy?
This test is done to obtain a sample of the bone marrow—the soft tissue that fills the cavities inside the bone where the majority of blood cells are produced. Two techniques are used. A fine needle is used to withdraw liquid marrow, or a larger needle is used to obtain a small core of marrow tissue. Both techniques will often be used during the procedure. You may be given a mild sedative before the test. The doctor, after numbing your skin, inserts a long, hollow needle into the bone marrow, and a sample is drawn back through the needle. The samples are usually taken from your hip, although the breastbone or the shinbone may also be used. For a bone marrow biopsy, a special needle will cut out a tiny piece of marrow, called a core. The needle is pushed further and rotated until there is a piece of whole marrow in it. You will feel pressure as the needle enters the bone and a bit of pain as the needle is withdrawn. Bleeding rarely occurs after this procedure. The tests take about 15 minutes to a half hour. You will probably have to rest for 15 to 30 minutes after the test. If you have been given a sedative, you will need more time to recover. You should arrange to have someone drive you home after the test. For a few days, you may feel sore at the spot where the needle went in and have some swelling or bruising in that area. The area should be kept dry for 24 hours. Generally, the doctor can give you results of the test in 48 to 72 hours.

Imaging Techniques

What are the most common imaging techniques used in diagnosing cancer?

The most common are: ultrasound, nuclear scans, and x-rays, which include CT scans.

What is ultrasound?

Ultrasound is a noninvasive technique that produces an image, called a sonogram, of the inside of your body using high-frequency sound waves that bounce off tissues and create echoes. These are picked up and converted into electric signals. A computer analysis of the signals creates a two-dimensional image that is displayed on a screen like a TV. Ultrasound can differentiate the pattern of blood flow through the abnormal blood vessels that feed a tumor from that of normal blood vessels. Ultrasound is commonly used as a diagnostic test in many areas of the body. It also may be used during an operation to locate tumors in the brain or the abdomen.

Can ultrasound tell a solid tumor from one that is not solid?

A solid tumor looks solid on the screen because echoes are returning from all the particles inside it. A cyst filled with fluid looks hollow because fluid does not reflect ultrasound waves. The ultrasound test can tell the difference.

Can ultrasound tell the difference between a cancerous tumor and one that is not cancerous?

No. Ultrasound can confirm that there is a solid mass, but it cannot distinguish a malignant tumor from a benign one. The doctor, looking at the shape and consistency of the tumor as shown by ultrasound in combination with the medical history of the patient, may be able to say that the tumor is "highly suspicious" of being cancerous.

What are the advantages of ultrasound?

There are several. It is quick, does not hurt, and is relatively inexpensive. It does not use x-ray beams. You need little or no preparation and no needle or instrument will be put into your body. Ultrasound is considered safe—it is used to examine fetuses during pregnancy.

How is the test done?

You will be in a room especially set aside for ultrasound, either in a hospital or in a doctor's office. A radiologist and a technician will do the test that will take from 15 to 30 minutes. You will lie on an examining table. A gel that improves the transmission of the sound waves will be put on the area of the test. A small instrument that emits the high-frequency sounds will be passed back and forth across the area a number of times. The sound waves are converted to pictures on a monitor. You will be asked to hold your breath and be still while each scan is done. You may be asked to change positions so that additional pictures can be made. When you are finished, the gel will be wiped off.

What will I feel and hear?

The gel may feel cold and slippery. You will feel a light pressure when the instrument passes over the area of the test. You will not hear the high-frequency sounds.

What is MRI?

MRI stands for Magnetic Resonance Imaging. The scanner looks like a very large cylinder and contains a magnet weighing from five to one hundred tons. It resembles a CT scanner in that it takes sectional images of any part of the body, but rather than using an x-ray beam, it records water molecules within the body. MRI takes advantage of the body's magnetic properties such as the protons in the nucleus of hydrogen atoms. When exposed to a magnetic field, these protons line up in parallel rows, and after being knocked out of alignment by a burst of radio waves, give off radio signals as they fall back into place. A computer converts these signals into pictures. MRI can create sectional images of the body, similar to CT scans, but it does not expose you to any radiation.

What is MRI used for?

MRI is used to scan most areas of the body. There are several cancers for which MRI can be used in diagnosis. These include brain, spinal cord, breast, head and neck, lung, liver, bladder, bone, prostate, and endometrial areas. It has, in many centers, taken the place of CT scanning for some cancers.

Are there people who cannot have an MRI?

Yes. Since the MRI uses a strong magnet, you cannot have an MRI if you have an aneurysm, pacemaker, implanted pump, or any other metallic implant, inner ear implants, tattooed eyeliner, surgical clips, or metallic monitoring devices. The magnetic pull of the MRI might dislodge an implant, interfere with its operation, or even pull it out of your body. However, many implanted ports used by cancer patients are made out of material that may distort the MRI but will not cause them to be dislodged. You need to talk to your doctor and the radiologist to be sure you can undergo an MRI.

What do I do when I am having an MRI?

MRI is usually done in a special room that is part of the nuclear medicine or diagnostic radiology department. You will be asked to take off any metal

SELECTED TYPES OF ULTRASOUND TESTS

TYPE	PREPARATION	COMMENTS
Gallbladder	Eat a fat-free meal on the evening before the test and fast before test.	May be given an injection to make gallbladder contract during test; drug may produce cramping, nausea, dizziness, flushing, or sweating.
Kidneys	Lie on back for most of test.	Instrument passed over abdomen.
Liver	No special preparation.	Instrument passed over abdomen.
Ovary	No special preparation needed.	Probe inserted into vagina. Waves bounce off ovaries to create sonogram. Color doppler may be used with test.
Pancreas, spleen	Eat fat-free meal on evening before test and fast before test.	Instrument passed over abdomen.
Pelvic	Full bladder usually required. Drink several glasses of water about an hour before test and don't urinate till after test. Remove all clothing.	Instrument passed over abdomen. Tell doctor if you are pregnant, have an IUD, have had difficulty urinating, or have had barium enema or upper GI series within past two days, or proctoscopy or sigmoidoscopy within past day.
Thyroid	Remove jewelry from head and neck. Remove all clothing above waist.	Instrument passed over neck. Easier and less expensive than thyroid scan.
Intracavity ultrasound	No special preparation needed.	Inserted into the pelvic cavity to produce more detailed images than external ultrasound. Used for vaginal and prostate examinations.

(continued)

SELECTED TYPES OF ULTRASOUND TESTS *(continued)*

TYPE	PREPARATION	COMMENTS
Doppler and Duplex	No smoking for 30 minutes before test. Depending on area to be examined, clothing must be removed. Blood pressure cuff may be wrapped around one or both legs or arms.	Used to evaluate blood flow through major arteries and veins of arms, legs, and neck. If blood is flowing through vessel, reflected sound waves create swooshing sound. Sometimes used instead of arteriography and venography. Color Doppler ultrasound uses different colors to demonstrate speed and direction of blood flow.

objects that might be attracted to the magnet. In some cases you may be given a contrast dye, through a vein. You will either lie on a table, sit, or stand up to have the test taken. You will be secured by straps. The platform will move so that the part of your body to be examined is positioned in the center of the magnet. You will need to be very still while the test is being done.

How long does it take to do an MRI test?
The test takes anywhere from 20 minutes to two or more hours, depending on the test being done and on the facility.

Does it hurt to have an MRI?
No, it does not hurt. If the machine is the type that uses a tunnel-like cylinder, you may feel closed in. You might be uncomfortable, if the test takes a long time, because you must lie motionless. In addition, the machine makes loud, continuous, knocking sounds. If you think you may have problems, or if you have any feelings of claustrophobia, discuss this with your doctor before you make your appointment. Ask if there is a facility with an "open" MRI available in the area.

Will I be able to talk with the technician while the test is being done?
A microphone inside the machine makes it possible for you to talk to the technician during the procedure. To block out noise, you can request earplugs

or earphones to listen to music. In some medical centers, the MRIs are equipped with television with special earphones. It may be helpful to practice some relaxation exercises, or take a sedative before the test.

What is an MRA?
MRA (Magnetic Resonance Angiography) evolved from the MRI and is a noninvasive test used for imaging the coronary arteries and evaluating heart disease. It does not require the insertion of a catheter.

What is fMRI?
This term refers to functional Magnetic Resonance Imaging, a more recent discovery in this field, that is used primarily to track microscopic changes in blood flow to different areas within an organ as the organ performs its normal functions.

What is dynamic contrast-enhanced MRI?
Dynamic contrast-enhanced MRI, also called DCE-MRI, or three-time-point MRI (3TP MRI), uses high-resolution imaging, a contrast material (low molecular weight Gd-based extracellular contrast agent) and data from three strategically chosen time points (before contrast material is given, two minutes and six minutes after) to produce color maps of the tumor. 3TP MRI helps doctors pinpoint exactly where the cancer is, as well as helping to differentiate between benign and malignant disease. It is anticipated that this new method will offer a standardized, reproducible technique for using MRI to diagnose breast and prostate cancer. This procedure is now in clinical trials.

Is contrast-enhanced MRI being used in any other way?
Contrast-enhanced MRI, in combination with molecular tumor markers, is also being studied in clinical trials to see whether it can predict tumor response and disease-free survival in women with breast cancer who are getting adjuvant chemotherapy.

What is radiolocalization?
Radiolocalization, also called gamma-probe radiolocalization, uses a radioactive tracer that is injected around the tumor. The tracer is picked up by the lymphatics, which drain from the tumor and travel to the first draining lymph nodes. After the tracer accumulates in these lymph nodes, they create a radioactive "hot spot," which can be detected on the surface of the skin with a hand-held detector. If a hot spot is detected, a biopsy is performed through a small incision. This technique is being tested for use in melanoma and head and neck cancers.

What are nuclear scans?

Nuclear scans use a radioactive substance, called a radioactive tracer, to diagnose diseases. There are almost 100 different nuclear scanning procedures that provide information about nearly every major organ system in the body. These scans show the size, shape, and location of the internal organs in a way not possible with x-rays. Nuclear scans are used in the cancer field to detect cancers, to determine response to treatment, and to conclude whether or not cancers have spread to other organs such as the bone, liver, or brain. Nuclear scans can often tell the doctor many things that once required more complicated procedures, such as operations. However, the increased use of CT scans has replaced some of the nuclear scans.

How are nuclear scans done?

A small amount of the radioactive material is given, usually through an injection into the vein in your arm. The radioactive material accumulates in the organ that has been targeted. The doctor, using a special camera that measures the radiation in the radioisotope, scans your body. A picture or scan is made of the organ being studied. The doctor can see a tumor if there is one. The camera itself does not expose you to any radiation, since it is not an x-ray machine.

Are radio-labeled monoclonal antibodies ever used with nuclear scans?

These tests, presently being performed in investigational trials, are sometimes called immunoscintigraphy. A monoclonal antibody, targeted against a specific tumor, is combined with the radioactive material. When the material is injected into the vein, the antibody finds the tumor, which lights up on the scanner. This technique is being tested to see if it can detect cancers that cannot be found using other imaging methods or for the detection and staging of cancer.

What is a PET scan?

PET stands for positron emission tomography. PET scanning can provide valuable information not only about the structure of particular organs, but also about how they work. A radioactive substance is injected intravenously and you lie on a table as the scanner records a circular array of photos that are displayed on a computer. PET produces three-dimensional images of the body's metabolic and chemical activity by detecting positrons emitted by radio-labeled substances that are taken up by tissue. PET scans are used to detect and evaluate cancers and to check whether or not your treatment is working.

What is the advantage of a PET scan?

A series of studies in lung, breast, and colorectal cancer, and non-Hodgkin's lymphoma is underway to determine whether and when PET scans would be more valuable. The data coming from studies seem to show that PET scans are more accurate in detecting and staging cancer than are some other commonly used tests. This has led to more accurate treatment decisions and some changes in treatments, including avoiding major surgery or radiation. These are important data since PET scans are more expensive than other commonly used diagnostic tests.

What is meant by the term *hot spot*?

There are some radioisotopes that concentrate on the cancerous tissue, forming *hot spots* on the scan. Other radioisotopes accumulate in the normal tissue. In these scans, the areas that are abnormal have less radioactive labeling and are termed *cold spots.*

Are scans difficult to interpret?

You need someone who is skilled and has experience in reading scans. They must be trained in the specialty of nuclear medicine.

Are nuclear scans dangerous?

The amount of radioactive material that is used is very small. Most of it leaves your body within a few days, some within a few hours. Most nuclear scans have the same or less radiation exposure than do major x-rays. These diagnostic tests often give the doctors important information at less risk than other means of getting it. The main issue is whether or not the test is needed to decide on a specific treatment. However, if you are pregnant or breastfeeding, nuclear scans are not recommended. In addition, they usually are not ordered for babies.

Are nuclear scans painful?

Most nuclear scans are painless. If the radioactive material is injected, you will feel the pinprick as the needle is put into your vein. On rare occasions, there may be some soreness or swelling in the area where the needle was injected. If so, put a moist, warm cloth on the area every few hours. Depending on the test and how long it will take, you may feel uncomfortable lying for a long time on the hard table. You may want to ask for a pillow or blanket.

What will I need to do to prepare for this test?

It depends on what part of the body is being scanned. You will probably be asked to take off all your jewelry and metal objects. If the doctor is looking at organs such as the gallbladder, liver, or thyroid, you will be asked to fast for anywhere from two to 12 hours before the test. For some scans, you will need to take laxatives or an enema. You may be asked to drink several glasses of liquid. You will also be asked what medications you are taking and whether or not you have had other scans or tests recently.

Will I need to stay overnight in the hospital for these tests?

These tests are done without an overnight stay in the hospital. The testing usually takes place in the hospital radiology or nuclear medicine department and is done by a nuclear medicine physician with the aid of a technician.

Will I be able to go back to my regular routine after the test?

Yes. In most cases, you will be able to go back to your usual activities and diet after your nuclear scan.

When will I know the results of the scan?

It usually will take a couple of days before the doctor who ordered the scan will know the results. You need to ask to speak to the doctor who sent you for the test when you can call for the results.

Why is a bone scan done?

You may need a bone scan to find out whether or not cancer has spread from its original location, such as the breast, to the bone. The bone scan may also be done to see how the treatment being given to you for your cancer is working.

How long does it take to do a bone scan?

The scan itself takes about 30 to 60 minutes. However, you will have to wait about two to three hours after the radioactive material is injected, to give the material a chance to get through your body. You will need to drink four to six glasses of water during that time, to flush the material not being picked up by the bones out of your body. While you are waiting, you can read or go about your normal routine. Before the scan is taken, you will be asked to empty your bladder. You will lie down on an examining table and a large scanning camera will be passed over your body, recording the gamma rays emitted by the radioactive material in your bones.

What can a brain scan detect?

A brain scan may be done if, due to dizziness, numbness, or seizures, the doctor suspects that there may be a tumor in the brain. Sometimes, a brain scan may be used to see how well the treatment is working. In many cases, CT and MRI are used instead of brain scans.

Will I have more than one scan taken for my brain test?

Yes. Usually the first set is taken as the radioactive material travels up your neck arteries to the brain. Then, a couple of hours later, a second set of pictures is taken. You can expect that the doctor will take several different views of your head. You may have to move into different positions. Each scan takes

SCANS USED IN DIAGNOSING CANCER

TEST AND PROCEDURE	DISCUSSION
Bone Material injected in arm vein, travels through bloodstream to bone. Need to drink several glasses of fluid before scan. You lie on back or change positions as large camera scans back and forth above you.	If you have had barium for x-rays, you may need a laxative or enema. Empty bladder needed. Takes one hour plus three to four hours waiting time. Most material leaves body within a day.
Brain Material injected into arm vein. You sit up or lie on back while large camera scans as material goes through arteries in neck to brain.	Scan takes five to ten minutes; second set taken one to two hours later. Most material leaves body within a day. Not used as often now that CT and MRI are available.
Gallium Material injected into arm vein. After waiting period, lie on back while large camera moves over body. Need to be completely still during scan.	Gallium injection takes about five minutes. Return one to three days later for test. Takes one to two hours. Limited use.
Kidney Material injected into arm vein, travels through bloodstream to kidneys. You sit up or lie on back while large camera scans as material circulates through kidneys. Additional scan shows flow into collecting system, ureters and bladder.	More than one type of radioactive material may be injected, with additional scans taken. Test takes about one hour. May need to return in four hours or later for additional scans. Need to empty bladder after test.
Liver Material injected into arm vein. You sit up or lie on back while large camera scans as material circulates through liver and spleen. May be asked to hold breath or turn on side or stomach for more views.	No need to fast. Will wait about ten minutes after material injected before scan taken. Test takes about one hour. Most material leaves body within a day.

(continued)

SCANS USED IN DIAGNOSING CANCER *(continued)*

TEST AND PROCEDURE	DISCUSSION
Thyroid Liquid or capsule with radioactive material is swallowed about six hours before test. Need to hold head back while camera scans thyroid area. May sit or lie down. Two different tests may be needed—an uptake study and a scan.	Tell doctor if you are taking any medicine for your thyroid or other problems, including vitamin pills. Also if you have had any other scans or x-rays recently. One test takes about ten minutes for each measurement. Scan takes about half an hour. Both tests may be done again 24 hours after taking material.
Salivary gland Material injected into arm vein, travels through bloodstream to salivary glands then comes out through mouth. Camera gives picture of glands.	Examines parotid salivary glands located in cheeks and under jaw.
PET (Positron Emission Tomography)	Radioactive isotope injected into blood. Sophisticated equipment—PET machine and cyclotron—needed for test. Used in determining whether cancers have spread.

about five minutes. You will be asked to be absolutely still during that time, then you will be repositioned for the next one.

Why is a scan of the kidneys done?
A scan of your kidneys, also called a renal scan, renogram, renal scintigraphy, or renography, looks at how the kidneys and your urinary system are working. The doctor uses kidney scans, along with other diagnostic tests to find tumors. The scans are also used if you are allergic to the dyes used in another kidney test, intravenous pyelogram.

Is there more than one type of kidney scan?
Yes. Often two or more of the different types of kidney scans are performed, one after the other. Depending on what information is needed, the testing can take from one to four hours. You will receive an injection of the radioactive

tracer in the vein in your arm. The scan will be done. You will then receive a different type of radioactive material and further scans will be done, often several over a half-hour period.

Do I have to take any special precautions after the test?

The doctor will ask you to empty your bladder after the test. You can then go back to your normal routine and diet. However, for the next day, you should drink lots of fluids and take care to flush the toilet immediately after you urinate to reduce exposure to the tiny amounts of radioactive substance in your urine. Most of the radioactive material is flushed out within six to 24 hours.

What is a gallium scan?

A radioactive material (gallium citrate) is injected into your arm. One to three days later you come back for your body scans. The testing will take about one to two hours.

Why is a liver scan done?

This test, which focuses on the liver and the spleen, is most often done to find out if your cancer has spread to the liver from another part of the body, or to see how well chemotherapy or radiation treatment is working. A liver scan may also determine whether you have cancer of the liver.

How are thyroid scans done?

A small amount of radioactive material is introduced into your body either in beverage or pill form and you will be asked to return for the scan four to 24 hours later. Inform your doctor if you have an allergy to iodine or shellfish, and report any medications, herbs, or supplements you are taking. You will be instructed to avoid iodized salt and seafood for one week before the test. The scanning procedure is done as you lie on your back on an examination table and takes about 20 to 30 minutes.

X-Rays

What kinds of x-rays are used in diagnosing cancer?

It depends upon the part of your body that needs to be seen by the doctor. You may have a regular x-ray, such as a chest x-ray. You may have a contrast x-ray, where a substance—such as a chemical dye, air, or radioactive material— is put into the body in order to get more detail. A barium study is an example of a contrast x-ray. Or you may have a CT scan, which uses a scanner and a computer to make images. CT scans, ultrasound and nuclear scans have replaced some of the regular x-rays that were once performed in diagnosing cancer.

What is digital radiology?

Digital radiology records x-ray images in computer code instead of placing them on film. Using computer software, the radiologist enhances subtle variations in the image, making tumors easier to spot. Digital radiology images can be sent to other experts via computer so that information can be shared.

How much radiation will I get from my diagnostic x-rays?

You need to discuss this with your doctor. Some of these tests will give you a low dose of radiation, while others give quite a high dose. You also can ask the technician where you are having the test done what dosage the machine is giving, since machines in different offices and institutions can give different dosages, depending on the age of the machine and its calibration. When properly taken and read, x-rays are an important tool. However, the benefits must be weighed against the risks. What is most important is that you ask the right questions so that you can assure yourself you are in the hands of a skilled and competent practitioner.

When are lead shields used?

Shielding can help reduce the amount of scattered radiation absorbed, especially by the reproductive organs. There are several kinds of shields, such as lead aprons, lead-lined panels, and scrotal cups. Newer machines have built-in shields to avoid scattering.

What are CT scans?

CT stands for computerized tomography. Sometimes this test is referred to as a CAT scan (Computerized Axial Tomography). A scanner passes a pencil-thin beam of x-rays through a selected part of the body, creating a 360-degree picture of that slice in a few seconds. The information is processed in a computer, which shows the image on a TV screen. Information from several slices of the body can be combined to create views from different angles. The pictures are much more detailed than regular x-rays. CT scans can be taken of parts of the body that previously were difficult or impossible to see.

For what kinds of cancer are CT scans used?

CT scans can be used to detect abnormalities that cannot be seen with plain x-rays. It is used to examine cancer in the chest, in the space between the lungs (mediastinum), the upper abdomen, kidneys, liver, pancreas, adrenal area, bones, spine, and brain.

Can full-body CT scans detect cancer in people with no symptoms?

There is a difference in using CT scans to diagnose cancer in people who have symptoms and using them as a screening tool to detect cancer in people without symptoms. Although there are many radiology offices offering full-body scans as a preventive screening tool, there have been no long-term studies of benefits and risks of having them. At this time, there is no evidence that these scans can detect cancers of the breast, prostate, or any other particular disease early enough to make a difference in its management, treatment, or cure. The FDA has approved using a CT scan only as a diagnostic tool when a person has symptoms, or when there is some reason for further testing. It has warned that the use of full-body scans is unproven and possibly harmful. Full-body CT scans have high false-positive rates that can lead to more tests, usually unnecessary. The FDA has never approved, or cleared, or certified any CT system specifically for use in screening people without symptoms because no manufacturer has ever demonstrated to the FDA that its CT scanner is effective for screening for any disease or condition. The American College of Radiology also does not believe there is sufficient scientific evidence to justify recommending total body CT scans for people without symptoms, or a family history suggesting disease.

How is a CT scan done?

The test usually is done in the diagnostic radiology department of a hospital or an office. It needs to be performed by a qualified diagnostic radiologist, or an x-ray technician. You are asked to lie on your back on a narrow table that moves into the scanner. You will be alone in the room, but you will be able to talk to the technician who will be watching through a window in the room. You will be asked to lie very still while the pictures are being taken. The table will move a little bit every few seconds, as the machine takes a new slice of pictures. A large scanning machine moves around you. You may hear a buzzing or a clicking sound. When the test is finished you should be able to go back to your normal routine and diet.

Will I need to do anything to prepare for my CT scan?

Depending on what part of your body is being tested, you may need to fast for four hours before the test. You may need to swallow contrast dye, have it injected into your arm vein or get it through an enema. If you need to swallow the material, it may have an unpleasant taste. Some people say they get a flushed feeling when the dye is given. Others complain about a metallic taste in their mouths. All of these symptoms last only a few minutes. Usually, if you receive the contrast material, you will have one scan, receive the dye and then have a repeat scan. The day before the scan, you should drink large amounts of fluids to prevent dehydration. Tell your doctor if you suffer from

X-RAYS THAT MAY BE USED IN DIAGNOSING CANCER

TYPE	COMMENTS
Abdominal Can look at large and small intestine, stomach, spleen kidney, and diaphragm	You lie on back on table; may need to change positions for other views, with machine above you. Need to hold your breath and be still. Takes five to ten minutes. Ovaries cannot be shielded. Can shield testes.
Arteriogram Can look at arteries anywhere in body, including brain, lung.	You lie on back on table, with machine above you. Local anesthesia used. Contrast material injected through long, thin, flexible tube threaded through artery to area to be tested. Takes one to three hours plus four to six hours of rest after. Involves risk and can have complications. Major procedure. Make sure you understand what will be done before you have it.
Chest	Usually two views taken, one from the front and one from the side. You stand with hands on hips (for front view) or with arms forward or over head (for side view). You will be asked to take a deep breath and stand very still while the x-ray is being taken. Takes about ten minutes.
CT Scans Computerized tomography (CT) or computerized axial tomography (CAT). Can be used to detect cancer in the lungs, the space between the lungs (mediastinum), kidneys, liver, pancreas, adrenal area, spine, and brain.	If contrast material used, will need to fast for a few hours before test. You lie on table with part of your body to be tested in middle of a tunnel-like structure. Table moves every few seconds, as the machine takes a new slice of pictures. Large scanning machine moves around you. If in brain area, head is immobiilized in a brace. Need to lie very still while the pictures are being taken. Takes about an hour.
GI Series, Lower. Barium Enema X-ray of large intestine. Liquid barium enema used to make area tested visible on x-ray. Uncomfortable procedure.	Must clean intestine before test, usually using liquid diet, laxative, or enema, alone or in combination. You lie on table, x-ray film taken, enema tube inserted in anus and barium inserted. X-rays taken from various positions. You need to be completely still and hold breath while x-rays taken. You expel barium in bathroom. If air-contrast test done, air will be added through tube and additional x-rays taken. Takes 30 to 45 minutes.

X-RAYS THAT MAY BE USED IN DIAGNOSING CANCER (continued)

TYPE	COMMENTS
GI Series, Upper. Barium Swallow, Esophagram Can look at throat, esophagus, stomach, duodenum, jejunum, and ileum. Endoscopy has replaced this test in some cases.	If lower GI series also ordered, should be done before this test. Must fast and abstain from smoking and chewing gum for a period before exam. You lie on a table that will be tilted to various positions as x-rays are taken from different angles. You swallow barium several times during test. Depending on part of body being tested, can take from 30 minutes to several hours.
Intravenous Pyelogram (IVP). Can look at urinary tract, kidney, ureters, and bladder.	May need to fast and take laxatives before test. You will lie on back on x-ray table for preliminary film; then contrast material put in vein in arm. You will need to be still while x-rays taken, usually at five-minute intervals.
Lymphogram, also called lymphangiogram. Can look at lymph nodes, small lymph vessels and lymph glands. Used in diagnosis of lymphomas, and to evaluate treatment. CT scans may be used instead of, or in addition to, lymphograms.	May need to fast or have liquid diet before test. You will sit on specially constructed chair or lie on table. Blue dye will be injected into Webs between toes. Local anesthetic given and small cut made in each foot where contrast material slowly put in. X-rays taken after contrast material has spread, again 24 hours later, and maybe at 48 and 72 hours later. Test takes up to five hours first day and 30 minutes on successive days.
Mammography In diagnosis, used to evaluate breast lumps, calcifications, or other symptoms. Can also see early breast cancer before it can be felt.	No deodorant, perfume, powders, or ointment used under your arm or on your breasts. You will need to undress from waist up and remove any jewelry from your neck. Breast rests on flat surface. Compressor pressed firmly against breast to help flatten out breast tissue. You will be asked to hold your breath while x-ray is being taken. Several views many be taken of area in question. Takes about half an hour.

claustrophobia. A sedative can be prescribed to help you tolerate the proce-dure. Just before the test, you will need to remove your clothes and any metal objects, including hairclips, jewelry, and watches, and put on a gown.

Will there be any difference if the CT scan is of my brain?

There are a few differences. You will have to take off your dentures, hearing aids and any other objects, such as earrings or hairpins, that might come in the path of the x-ray beam. Your head will be placed in a headrest in the mid-dle of a doughnut shaped scanner ring. Your head may be secured with a spe-cial device to keep it still. Your face will not be covered.

Are there any after effects from the CT scan?

Usually there are none. Some people may have a reaction to the contrast material, such as itching or wheezing. Be sure to tell your doctor if you have any allergies of any kind or if you have been sensitive to iodine or shellfish.

What is an intravenous pyelogram?

An intravenous pyelogram can look at your kidneys, ureters, and bladder. First a preliminary x-ray will be taken. Then contrast material will be put in the vein in your arm. The doctor then will take several x-rays, usually five minutes apart.

When I have my intravenous pyelogram will I be alone in the room?

The doctor and technician will be with you while preparing you for the test and while the contrast dye is being injected. However, you will be lying on the table, alone in the room, while the x-rays are taken and probably for sev-eral five-minute periods between the x-rays. During this period, you probably also will not be able to move. Many times several x-rays are taken during the five minutes after the dye has been put in. Then an inflatable belt might be wrapped around on your stomach area to keep the dye in the kidneys. X-rays are again taken every five minutes for another 15 minutes.

Will I feel pain during my intravenous pyelogram?

Probably not. You may have a flushed feeling in your body or a burning sen-sation in your arm after the dye has been injected. You might feel some pres-sure from the belt, and be uncomfortable lying on the table waiting between x-rays. After the test you might be lightheaded.

What is a lymphogram?

A lymphogram may be used in the diagnosis of Hodgkin's disease and non-Hodgkin's lymphomas. It can look at lymph nodes, small lymph vessels, and lymph glands. In some institutions, CT scans are used in addition to, or instead of, lymphograms.

Is the lymphogram a painful test?

You will probably feel a little bit of pain from the injection given at the beginning of the test, but should not feel pain during the test itself. Your feet will be cleaned with an antiseptic solution. A small amount of blue dye, which is sometimes mixed with a local anesthesia, is injected into the webs of your feet. Within 15 minutes or so, you will be able to see the blue dye in the lymph vessels on the top of your feet. At that time, you will be given a local anesthesia so you will not feel the doctor making a small incision in each foot, where the contrast dye will, over the next hour or two, be injected into your feet. You might have a feeling of pressure when the dye is put in. You may find it hard to sit or lie for such a long time while waiting for the dye to go through your body. The doctor will be checking the spread of the dye through x-rays or a TV monitor. When all the dye is in your body, the incisions will be stitched up and covered. Then x-rays will be taken, usually of your chest, stomach area, and pelvis. The x-rays are repeated 24 hours later and sometimes at 48 and 72 hours later.

Will I have any side effects from my lymphogram?

You will probably have to stay on a liquid diet until all the x-rays have been taken. You may have some pain and swelling in your feet where the incisions were made. Keep your feet up for 12 to 24 hours after the test. Talk to the nurse about what you should do if swelling occurs. Sometimes icepacks are recommended to reduce the swelling, which may last up to a month after the test. Your urine and stool may have a bluish tinge for a couple of days. Your skin may look bluish and your eyes may see things with a bluish tone for about a week. The area where the cuts were made must be kept dry. The stitches will be taken out in a week or ten days. If you have a cough, fever, shortness of breath, or if the area around the cuts is tender, red, or has a discharge, call the doctor.

What is a barium swallow?

A barium swallow is used to get x-rays of the esophageal area. A barium swallow is given as a thick, milkshake-like liquid which has an unpleasant chalky taste, but is flavored to make it easier to take. As you sip the mixture, you will be moved to various positions so that the inner lining of the esophagus from the throat to the stomach is x-rayed. It is important to drink plenty of fluids to eliminate the barium, as barium can accumulate and block the intestines if it is not eliminated in one or two days.

What is an upper GI series?

Examination of the esophagus, the stomach, and the upper part of the small intestine (the duodenum) is referred to as an upper GI series. Sometimes the examination includes inspection of the entire 20-foot length of the small intestine. A barium swallow is included as part of this series.

How is the test done?

You will be given a liquid mixture containing barium sulfate. The mixture has a thick, chalky consistency and usually is sweetened with a flavoring. You will be secured to a tilting x-ray table that is moved to various positions so that the dye coats the GI tract. Your stomach may be massaged to make sure the barium is properly distributed. An inflatable belt may be used to compress the stomach. The radiologist observes the flow on a viewing screen and spot x-rays may be taken. The test is painless although you may feel nauseous or bloated. It usually takes about 30 to 60 minutes.

Will I be uncomfortable during the upper GI test?

You will probably feel uncomfortable when your stomach is compressed, either by the use of the technician's hand or the inflatable belt. In addition, you may feel uneasy when the table is tilted at different angles.

Will I have any aftereffects from the upper GI series?

Your stool will look whitish for a couple of days after the test. You need to eliminate the barium or it can harden. So if you don't see the whitish color on your bowel movements within three days or if your bowel habits change drastically, call your doctor.

Is a lower GI series the same as a barium enema?

The barium enema is part of the lower GI series. It is done in order to make it possible to take the x-rays of the lower gastrointestinal (GI) tract. For this test, a liquid called barium, that appears white on the x-ray film, is inserted as an enema into the colon. The barium coats the inside of the large intestine and x-rays reveal any polyps, growths, or constricted or displaced areas. Air may be pumped into the colon during the test to expand the bowel and make small tumors easier to see. This technique is called an air contrast or double contrast barium enema. The barium enema feels much like an ordinary enema, causing a feeling of fullness.

What preparations should be made before a barium enema?

Many people feel that preparation is the worst part of the test. Your bowels must be cleared as completely as possible. The doctor will provide you with exact instructions, which usually include a liquid diet and laxatives to help clear the colon of waste so that all areas of the colon can be inspected. You may be told to give yourself an enema on the morning of the procedure. The whole process can be tiring and debilitating. Your anal area may become sore. A warm bath can help with the soreness.

Will I be embarrassed or feel pain during the lower GI series?

Some people do feel embarrassed but the doctors and nurses who do this test often are aware of the problems and will help you get through them. You may be afraid you can't hold the barium in and that it might leak out on the table. To help keep the barium inside, a small balloon is sometimes inserted at the end of the enema tube. As the barium goes into your colon, you may feel like you need to have a bowel movement. Take slow, deep breaths through your mouth to help you relax. You probably will not feel pain, but you may feel uncomfortable. You may have some cramping or gas pains. To allow the doctor to better see the area, small amounts of air may be introduced through the enema tube. This may cause mild cramps or the make you feel as though you need to move your bowels. Breathe deeply and slowly through your mouth to help relax.

Will I have any side effects after the lower GI series?

You may have some soreness or irritation around your anal area. You should drink large amounts of fluid to keep the barium that remains in your system from getting hard and causing constipation. For a few days after the test, you may see some white or pink material from the barium on your bowel movement. If you have any bleeding from your rectum, pain in your stomach area, or fever, call your doctor.

Mammograms

How is a mammogram done?

Mammograms use x-ray beams that pass through the breasts, producing images of the internal tissue on a special type of film. You stand in front of the mammogram machine while a technician positions the breast between two compression plates. The breast is flattened and compacted, and you may be uncomfortable while the procedure is taking place. Two x-rays are usually taken, one from above and one from the side. The procedure is repeated on the other side. Sometimes after the film is developed, the procedure needs to be redone if the mammogram is unclear.

What is the difference between a diagnostic and a screening mammogram?

In a screening mammogram, two views of each breast are taken to see if any signs of early cancer are present. A diagnostic mammogram is taken when you have specific symptoms or when an irregularity is found on your screening mammogram. The technician will take different views, from several different angles. The area in question may be magnified to allow the doctor to see the details more clearly so that an accurate diagnosis can be made. The mamography facility and its staff should be certified by the Food and Drug Administration (FDA). This assures the quality of the equipment as well as the training of the technicians. There is information in Chapter 13, Breast Cancer, on checking to see that your mammography facilities are up to required standards.

What preparations are necessary before having a mammogram?
There are no special diets or other procedures. However, on the day of the examination, you will be asked not to use any deodorant, perfume, powders, ointment, or preparation of any sort in the underarm area or on your breasts, since these might obscure the results. Also, it is a good idea to wear a skirt or slacks with a blouse or sweater, since it is necessary to undress to the waist for the examination.

What is meant by the term *microcalcification*?
This means there are tiny specks of calcium in the breast. When these specks form a certain pattern, it is called a cluster. A cluster signifies to a doctor that the tissues surrounding the calcium specks may be cancerous. If the pattern is not clear, the doctor may advise you to have another mammogram in three to six months. If the pattern of calcifications looks suspicious to the doctor, you will have a biopsy. About half of the cancers detected by mammography are seen as these clusters on the mammogram.

What are macrocalcifications?
These are coarse deposits of calcium in the breast. They usually result from the aging of breast arteries, from old injuries or inflammations. Macrocalcifications are usually not cancer and do not need to be biopsied. About 50 percent of the women over 50 years of age have macrocalcifications.

Can a mammogram tell whether or not cancer is present?
Mammograms may indicate to a trained doctor a suspicion that cancer is or is not present. They can be used by surgeons to locate the site of the tumor and to check if there are additional tumors in the breast. However, they cannot be used alone to definitely tell whether there is cancer in the breast. Only the pathologist, looking at cells under a microscope, can tell whether they are cancerous. In addition, a negative mammogram **does not** guarantee that there is no cancer in the breast.

What is digital mammography?

Digital mammography, a technique that is still being studied, records x-ray images in computer code instead of placing them on film. Using computer software, the radiologist enhances subtle variations in the image, making tumors easier to spot. Digital mammograms also can be sent electronically (called *telemammography*), allowing consultation with experts. A study is presently being carried out, involving 49,500 women in the United States and Canada, comparing digital mammography with standard film mammography.

What is contour mammography?

Contour mammography is done with a special type of equipment that makes the exam more comfortable, photographs more breast tissue and uses lower doses of radiation.

Does having a mammogram hurt?

When you have a mammogram, your breast must be squeezed between two flat plates in order to get a good image. While most women feel that the squeezing of the breast is uncomfortable, it lasts only for a few seconds. A few women complain that the mammogram is painful. It is a good idea to schedule your mammogram between your periods, when your breasts are less likely to be tender. There is more information about mammograms in Chapter 13, Breast Cancer.

Biopsies

What is a biopsy?

A biopsy is the procedure in which a piece of tissue is obtained and examined under the microscope to determine whether cancer or other disease is present. This microscopic examination of the biopsy specimen is accepted by doctors in determining the nature of a tumor with complete accuracy. Therefore, whenever possible, a doctor insists on obtaining a sample of every tumor that could be cancer before treatment is attempted. The biopsy provides the most reliable basis for a diagnosis of cancer.

Who determines if the biopsy cells are cancerous?

The biopsy is "read" by a pathologist—a physician who specializes in the study of normal and diseased body tissues.

What kind of training does a pathologist have?

In order to be certified by the American Board of Pathology, the person must be a licensed doctor of medicine or osteopathy and have four years of training in both clinical and anatomic pathology, or three years of training in either specialty, or eight years of practical experience under circumstances acceptable to the board. The doctor must also successfully complete the examinations administered by the board. The pathologist is a vital member of the healthcare team, especially in the field of cancer. In these days of changing technology, with new instrumentation and new testing mechanisms, such as tumor markers, it is essential that the pathologist be well trained and expert in the cancer field.

Are all pathologists skilled in diagnosing cancer from these specimens?

As in all other specialties, the skill and competence of pathologists vary. A decision regarding whether cancer is the disease in the tissue being examined depends on the interpretation one individual pathologist makes of the cellular structure of the biopsy. Often, the specimens are sent to experts in larger institutions for consultation, especially by pathologists practicing alone in small communities. The Armed Forces Institute of Pathology in Washington, DC, is used by many pathologists for biopsy review (see Chapter 28, Where to Get Help). If your diagnosis of cancer is based on the single pathological report of a single pathologist in a small community, be sure to ask that a consultation with other pathologists be arranged. It is important that your doctor and the pathologist talk with each other and work together as a team.

How can the pathologist tell if cells are benign?

When looked at under the microscope, normal cells have an orderly appearance. They possess the distinctive features of the organ from which they came. The cells from the thyroid gland, for example, look very different from those of the skin. Normal cells from different organs carry genetic "messages" that determine their structure and function.

What does the pathologist look for when reading the biopsy?

The pathologist does many things. First is to look to see when the specimen is malignant or benign. If malignant, the next step is to identify the specific type of cancer cells present in the tumor and determine just how fast they reproduce themselves. With special stains and fixes, the pathologist can tell much from the tissue samples, such as whether the blood vessels or lymph channels have been invaded. With some kinds of tumors, the pathologist may test for dependency on hormones or other substances. All of this information will help your doctor determine the proper treatment for your cancer.

Can I get a copy of my own pathology report?
If you wish to have a copy, you need to ask your doctor for it, either right after surgery or when you go back for your visit. Most doctors are willing to go over the report with you and to give you a copy. Keep it with your medical records. Since it is written in medical language and mostly in medical shorthand, it might be difficult for you to read without help.

What should I expect the report to contain?
The report will tell you what kind of cancer was found, the grade of the cancer, the size of the tumor, how far the cancer has spread, and how aggressive the cancer is.

- Patient information: Name, birth date, identification number, type of surgery, tissue removed, and the date the biopsy was done. Make sure that you have the right report.

- Gross description: Color, weight, and size of the tissue taken out and received by the pathologist or laboratory.

- Microscopic description: What the sample looks like under the microscope and how it compares to cells next to it.

- Diagnosis: There may be two. If there are, the "clinical diagnosis," which is usually at the beginning of the report, is what the doctor expected before the tissue was tested. The "summary" or "final" diagnosis, normally found at the end of the report, tells you what was found in the tissue covered in the report itself. The type of tumor, cell of origin, histologic grade, and numerical grading system are usually covered.

- Tumor size: Measured in centimeters.

- Tumor stage: How advanced it is in the body. Were lymph nodes or blood vessels involved? Gives initialized description of tumor, nodes, and metastasis (TNM) as well as other staging information.

- Tumor margins: Was tumor found in edges of tissue removed? If the cancer cells come out right to the edge of the tumor, they are said to be "positive." If there are no cancer cells seen at the outer edge, they are described as negative, not involved, clear, or free from tumor. If "close" describes the tumor margins, it is neither negative nor positive. You need to ask the doctor for a definition of what these terms mean in a particular hospital or laboratory.

- Other information: Depending on the type of cancer you have, you may find information about hormone receptors, special markers, other tests or comments. If the pathologist sent the tissue somewhere for a second opinion, the words, "outside consultation" may be on it.

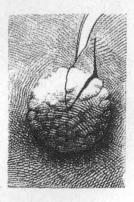 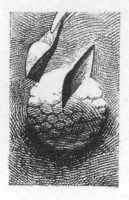 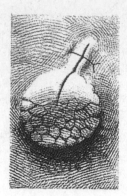

Incisional biopsy

- The report should be signed by the pathologist and have the name and address of the laboratory on it.

What is an incisional biopsy?

In an incisional biopsy, a part of the tumor is cut out and looked at microscopically. This method is usually favored if the suspicious mass is a large one. The object is to get as large a sample as possible, cutting down on the chances of getting a false reading from a bit of tissue that is not representative of the whole.

What is an excisional biopsy?

In an excisional biopsy, the tumor is removed totally. This method is selected when the tissue has been identified as cancerous, when strong suspicion exists that part of it may be, or may become, cancerous or when the tumor is small. When a punch is used to remove the tissue, this is called a punch biopsy. Many skin tumors, for example, are totally removed before the biopsy is performed.

What is a needle aspiration biopsy?

In a needle aspiration biopsy, also called a fine needle biopsy, a needle is used to extract either fluid or tissue from a suspicious mass. This fluid or tissue is then examined under the microscope. It can be used in diagnosing many kinds of cancers, such as breast, eye, lung, liver, gallbladder, and thyroid.

What is a core needle biopsy?

This is similar to a fine needle biopsy, but it uses a wide needle through which a tiny instrument can be inserted for cutting out the sample of tissue to be looked at under the microscope.

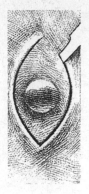 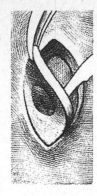 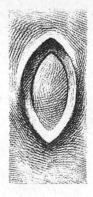 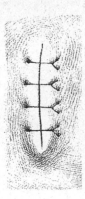

Excisional biopsy

What is a sentinel lymph node biopsy?

This is a relatively new procedure in which the surgeon finds and removes only the sentinel node—the first lymph node into which a tumor drains, and the one most likely to contain cancer cells. Studies continue to be carried out to verify that if no cancer cells are found in the sentinel node, there probably are no tumor cells in the remaining axillary nodes. Because sentinel lymph node biopsy involves removal of fewer lymph nodes than the standard lymph node dissection, the potential for side effects such as lymphedema is much lower. Sentinel node biopsy may be done on an outpatient basis or may require a one-day stay in the hospital.

What is the procedure for doing sentinel lymph node biopsy?

A blue dye and a low-level radioactive tracer are injected. After the dye and tracer have traveled from the tumor region to the lymph nodes (the wait may take from 45 minutes to 8 hours) the biopsy is performed. A gamma ray counter is used to locate the sentinel node or nodes. Once the area is pinpointed, the surgeon makes a small incision (usually one-half inch) and removes the suspected node. The node is then examined by the pathologist. If no cancer is found, further lymph node surgery is avoided. This surgery should be performed only by a team experienced in the procedure. **Be sure to ask beforehand how many sentinel node procedures your doctor has done.** (The answer should be at least 20.) Investigational trials are presently under way to determine if survival of patients with positive sentinel nodes who do not undergo node removal is different from survival for those who have a complete lymph node dissection.

What happens if cancer is found during sentinel lymph node surgery?

If the node is found to be cancerous during the surgery, the surgeon will usually remove additional lymph nodes. However, if the final pathology report is

TYPES OF BIOPSIES

TYPE	PROCEDURE
Incisional biopsy	Part of tumor is removed for examination. Used if suspicious mass is large.
Excisional or total biopsy	The entire tumor is removed for examination. Used when tumor is small, tissue has been identified as cancerous, or if there is strong suspicion that part of tumor is, or may become, cancerous.
Needle aspiration or core needle biopsy	Fluid or tissue is removed from lump, using a fine or a wide needle. The needle biopsy can be guided by touch or by an imaging technique, such as CT scan.
Endoscopic biopsy	Fluid or tissue is obtained by using long instruments, usually with a needle or knife; the optical instrument allows the doctor to see into the body cavity.
Punch biopsy	A punch is used to remove a sample of the tissue.
Ultrasound biopsy	This device is helpful in guiding needle aspirations or needle biopsies in many parts of the body.
Sentinel node biopsy	First lymph node into which the cancer drains is taken out. If no cancer found, no further lymph node surgery is done.
Stereotactic biopsy	Uses a scanning device to find the location of a tumor that is difficult to see. CT or MRI establish the perimeters of the tumor before the biopsy. Used for brain and breast tumors.

not available until after the surgery has been completed and cancer is found, follow-up surgery may be necessary to remove more nodes.

What is a stereotactic biopsy?
The stereotactic biopsy, sometimes called a stereotactic needle-guided biopsy, is a procedure that uses a scanning device to locate the site of a tumor that

cannot be seen. The radiologist will use imaging equipment to locate the area to be biopsied. The biopsy samples can be taken either with a fine needle or a core needle. Stereotactic biopsies can be used in diagnosing breast and brain cancer.

How is a stereotactic breast biopsy done?
It is used when something is found on the mammogram that cannot be felt. It can tell whether the cells are benign or malignant, without leaving a scar. The procedure is done in the radiology department. During the procedure, you may be sitting up or you may be lying on your stomach on an examining table that has an opening in the front end to accommodate the breast. You will be given local anesthesia to numb your breast. The radiologist will use imaging equipment to position the needle. Both aspiration and core biopsy samples can be taken.

What is a CT scan-guided biopsy?
A CT scan-guided needle biopsy, performed by an interventional radiologist, involves the insertion of a biopsy needle into the body to collect a tissue sample. It is usually done in area such as the chest where a shadow has been seen on an x-ray or CT scan. A CT scan is taken of the problem area and is used to guide the doctor in inserting the needle that will take the biopsy.

How is an ultrasound-guided needle biopsy done?
The ultrasound is used to guide the doctor. In diagnosing prostate cancer, for example, the probe is placed in the rectum and bounces high-frequency sound waves into the prostate. The different densities between normal prostate tissue and cancer show up as shadows on the ultrasound image. The ultrasound probes are often able to discover cancerous tissue that is missed by a digital examination. The biopsy is then done using the ultrasound to guide the probe. Ultrasound images allow the surgeon to guide a spring-loaded device that fires a needle through the wall of the rectum into the prostate to capture bits of possibly cancerous tissue. The needle is withdrawn so the sample can be analyzed. The device fires the needle so rapidly that it is virtually painless. Some five to ten percent of patients feel a little ache when the gun is fired. There is no anesthesia or catheter and you can usually return home when the procedure is completed.

What is a frozen section?
A frozen section refers to the procedure of preparing the tissue for the pathologist to read. There are two ways of preparing the tissue—via frozen

section, which is a quick procedure taking 15 to 20 minutes, or via a permanent section, which takes several days. The frozen section is a quick-reference method of determining whether or not cancer is present. The permanent section is a more accurate method.

When is a frozen-section biopsy used?
The frozen section is performed while the patient is in the operating room. Generally, it is used when a suspicious mass cannot be reached to obtain tissue by means other than an operation. It can also be used to determine whether the margins are adequate during surgery. The patient is prepared for the major surgery. The tissue is obtained, but the surgeon waits to proceed until the report is relayed from the pathologist.

How is the frozen section done?
The surgeon sends the section of tissue to the pathology laboratory, where it is quickly frozen and cut into razor-thin slices. The slices are placed on slides, fixed and stained. The slides are then looked at under a microscope. The frozen section slides are used to look quickly at the structure of the tissue. The entire procedure takes about ten to 15 minutes.

How does the permanent section differ from the frozen section?
The permanent-section biopsy takes considerably longer than a frozen-section biopsy. In this process, the tissue is put through a time-consuming multistage procedure that is highly complicated and that gives a high-quality slide. The tissue is put through a series of solutions to withdraw water and fatty substances. It is then saturated with warm liquid paraffin. When it has cooled and hardened, the tissue in paraffin is sliced into thin slices. The slices are placed on slides and stained so that the tissue can be studied under the microscope. Proper staining, which brings out cell formations and their nuclei, requires exact timing.

What are the advantages and disadvantages of the frozen and the permanent sections?
If the tumor is in an area where a permanent section cannot be done under local anesthesia, a frozen section eliminates a second operation. Although today's techniques have greatly improved the quality of frozen sections there can be some distortion of cells. For the permanent section, the tissue is fixed in the formaldehyde solution, the tissue shrinkage is more uniform and the slower process reduces tearing of the tissue and distortion of its structure.

The tissue cuts thinner and takes up the stain better than the frozen section. The pathologist has the whole tissue block available for cutting samples at a later date. The definition and character of a single cell is much clearer and more precise than in a frozen section. A permanent section is always done, even when a frozen section already has been completed.

Have there been advances in the kinds of microscopes being use by the pathologists?

Yes, there have been substantial advances. For instance, the electron microscope sorts out tumor cells by exposing fine structures visible only at magnifications at least ten times as high as a light microscope provides. It gives information that the standard microscope cannot give and permits the pathologist to tell the difference between primary and metastatic tumors and often to identify where in the body the cancer began.

Can the pathologist always tell where the tumor originated from the biopsy?

No, in about nine percent of the cases, the pathologist can confirm that the tissue contains cancer cells but is not able to tell where the primary tumor originated. The doctors call these "unknown primaries" or "tumors of unknown origin." Often the pathologist can identify the cell type, or uses tumor markers or hormone receptor analysis to try to determine the kind of cancer, so that treatment can start.

Staging and Grading

What is meant by staging a tumor?

Staging is the process doctors go through to tell how much cancer there is in the body and where it is located. It is necessary for the doctor to have this information to plan your treatment. Staging is also a "language" used to characterize your specific case.

Why is staging needed?

The doctor needs to determine the amount of cancer in your body and where it is located in order to give you the right treatment for your specific case. The treatment for breast cancer at one stage of the disease, for instance, is different from that at another stage. Your doctor also needs to anticipate the course your disease is likely to take. Staging makes it possible to compare the results of the different treatments being used by different doctors in different parts of the country and the world.

What is the doctor looking for when staging cancer?

The doctor wants to know basic information about the original tumor—or the primary tumor, as the medical professional refers to it. Information such as the size and cell type, whether it has spread to areas around the original site and whether it has spread to other organs of the body, away from the original site.

Are the answers to these questions important?

They are vital. Tumors must be staged at the beginning of the diagnosis to the fullest extent possible in order to give you the most effective treatment. For example, if the doctor finds that the cancer that began in your lung has already spread to other parts of your body, your treatment will differ from a lung cancer that has remained in the lung.

Are all kinds of cancer staged the same way?

No. There have been systems designed for specific kinds of cancer. Most staging has developed over time, as new knowledge has been acquired. Some staging systems are named after organizations, such as the FIGO classification for gynecologic tumors, or after persons who have developed them, such as Clark's and Breslow's classifications for melanoma. However, the most widely used system is the TNM method of the International Union Against Cancer and the American Joint Committee on Cancer.

What do the initials TNM stand for?

These initials are used in the staging system: T = tumor, N = nodes, and M = metastases.

T, plus a number one to four, is used to describe the size and the level of invasion. The higher the number, the larger the size of the tumor and the depth or amount of involvement in the local area of the tumor.

N, plus a number one through four, indicates whether or not there is evidence that the tumor has spread to the regional lymph nodes, the size of the nodes involved and the number of nodes involved.

M, plus a zero or a plus sign, indicates the absence or presence of distant metastases (cancer that has spread to other parts of the body). A letter is sometimes added to the M to show the other areas that are involved. P, for instance, could indicate "pulmonary," indicating that the cancer has spread to the lungs.

An X added to any of these letters indicates that staging cannot be assessed. Therefore, TX means the tumor cannot be assessed. A zero added to any T, N, or M means there is no evidence of cancer. Thus, N0 means lymph nodes are not demonstrably abnormal.

What is meant by Stage I disease?
Stage I means your cancer is the most curable. In lung cancer, for instance, Stage I is T1, N0 and M0 means the tumor is 3 cm or less in size and is not in the main bronchus, the regional lymph nodes are not involved and there are no metastases.

Do the letters and numbers mean the
same thing for every kind of cancer?
Each tumor type has its own classification system. However, A Stage I is always the most curable and a Stage IV is most difficult to cure. The definition of the size of the tumor varies from site to site, and of course the treatment will differ. The variation depends upon what the doctors know about each kind of tumor, how it spreads, what treatments are most effective at each stage, and what the prognosis is. Some cancers do not as yet have an agreed-upon classification. Others, such as the lymphomas, use a different system from the one just described.

What is meant by tumor grade?
Grading takes into account the structure of the cells and their growth patterns. Because of the differences in appearance and behavior in different tumors, the grading criteria vary. However, there are some basic principles that apply, describing the extent to which the cells conform to the normal tissue. There are two kinds of grading in cancer: histologic and nuclear.

What is meant by histologic tumor grade?
Histologic grading refers to how much the tumor cells resemble normal cells. This is also called *differentiation*. The lower the grade, the more the tumor cells resemble normal cells. Thus, Grade 1 refers to cells that are well differentiated, whose features and growth patterns nearly resemble normal cells. Grade 2 indicates that the cells are moderately well differentiated—there have been some changes in both the features of the cells and in their growth patterns. Grade 3 cells are poorly differentiated, with features and growth patterns that are abnormal. Grade 4 cells are undifferentiated and have very abnormal features and growth patterns. The doctor may refer to a tumor as being high grade or low grade.

What is meant by the nuclear grade of a tumor?
Nuclear grade refers to the rate at which the cancer cells in the tumor are dividing to form more cells (called *proliferation*). Cancer cells that divide more often are faster growing and more aggressive than those that divide less often. The nuclear grade is determined by the percentage of cells that are dividing.

A nuclear Grade 1 means that the cells are dividing slowly, with nearly normal nuclei. At the other end is a Grade 3 with fast-dividing cells and abnormal nuclei.

Why is it important for me to know the stage and grade of my cancer?
The only way you can get an accurate diagnosis is if you can supply the complete details on your cancer, giving stage and grade. It is important for you to have in your possession all the background information on your cancer diagnosis so that you will have it in your files to reference when you are seeking treatment and other opinions.

How long does it take to establish a diagnosis?
Ask your doctor about how long you will need to wait before you get a full diagnosis. The length of time will depend upon several factors—and the slightest delay will seem like an eternity because you will be living in fear of the unknown. A full evaluation can take from several days to two or three weeks—or may even have to be postponed because a decision cannot be made for any of a number of reasons. Don't be in a rush. Allow time for as many diagnostic procedures, additional consultations and reviews as you can. This is the point in your treatment that is most important to you—because what happens at this point sets the stage for determining much of the future course of your disease.

What should I be evaluating during the period while waiting for my diagnosis?
You should ask yourself the following questions:

- Do I have enough information and understand enough to make a judgment?
- Is this the right doctor for me? Do I feel comfortable with this doctor? Is the doctor giving me enough information? Am I happy with the hospital the doctor will send me to?
- Should I have a second opinion?
- Should I go to a major medical center for my treatment?

Web Pages to Check Out

www.cancer.gov: For general up-to-date information, and for clinical trials.

www.cancer.org: For general up-to-date information and community resources.

www.health.harvard.educ/fhg/diagnostics: More information on tests.

www.aidsmeds.com: CBC test results.

www.labtestsonline.org: Lab tests on line.

www.ahrq.gov/consumer/quicktips/tiptests.htm: Quick tips for medical tests.

Also see Chapter 2, Searching for Answers on the Web, for more information.

Seven

TREATMENT

A number of different methods—alone or in combination—are used in treating cancer. The goal is to find, remove, or destroy all of the cancer so that it cannot recur. Surgery, chemotherapy, and radiation are the most common treatments. Most cancer treatments include a combination, sometimes referred to as multimodality therapy. The treatments will vary depending upon the kind of cancer you have, your physical condition, the extent of your disease, how it is progressing, and how you respond to the treatment. In order to be certain that the treatment chosen is right for you, you should get as much information as possible about the treatment being recommended so that you can understand how the treatment will affect you and your lifestyle.

MOST TIMES A combination of treatments will be recommended to you. Among the treatments being used are:

- **Surgery:** taking out the tumor by operating on it.
- **Radiation:** the use of x-rays or radiation seeds.
- **Chemotherapy:** the use of drugs.
- **Hormonal:** the use of hormones.

- **Biologicals:** boosting the body's own defenses against cancer.
- **Investigational treatments**: new treatments or new ways of using older treatments being studied in a scientific manner.

Questions to Ask Your Doctor About Treatment

- **What treatments are available?**
- **What treatment do you recommend?**
- **Is this treatment necessary for me?**
- **Are there any other alternatives? What are they?**
- **Why do you think this treatment is preferable?**
- **What do you expect the results to be?**
- **How safe is the procedure?**
- **What are the side effects of the treatment and what can be done to relieve them?**
- **Can I be put on a program that doesn't interfere with my work schedule?**
- **How will we determine how well the treatment is working?**
- **When can I call you to ask further questions?**
- **Are there specific times when I can call and talk directly with you?**
- **Do I have a type of cancer that would be better treated at a major cancer center?**
- **Whom would you recommend for a second opinion?**

How will my specific treatment be determined?
Your doctor will consider many factors in determining the treatment for your cancer. Among them are:

- What kind of cancer you have and its pattern of growth and spread.
- Aggressiveness of the cancer.
- Predictability of the spread of cancer.
- The sensitivity of your cancer to specific drugs or other modes of treatment.
- Morbidity and mortality of the treatment procedure.
- Cure rate of the treatment procedure.
- The areas of your body affected by your cancer.
- Your physical state.
- Your lifestyle.

Are there standard treatments for the various types of cancer?
For most kinds of cancers, there are standard treatments that are used. These treatments are those considered most effective for the specific type and stage of cancer. Many times, there are several standard treatments for a particular type and stage of disease. If you look at the treatment tables in this book under each specific type of cancer, you will notice that a number of different treatments are listed.

If there is more than one standard treatment for a particular type and stage of cancer, how does the doctor decide which one I will get?
The doctor, in consultation with you, will choose the one that is determined to be best for you, depending on your general physical condition, your own preferences and concerns, and on other factors in your case. Sometimes, if the doctor feels that more than one kind of treatment is equally effective, you will be given all the treatment options and asked to make the choice you prefer. You need to ask questions about different kinds of treatment, so that you can be a partner in making these treatment decisions, particularly if there is a choice between two equally effective ones.

Is there a difference between standard treatment and state-of-the-art treatment?
In cancer treatment, the two terms mean the same thing, that is, the best treatment currently available for a specific type and stage of cancer.

What are the advantages of surgery?
Surgery, which is the most common treatment for cancer, allows the doctor to see the extent of the cancer and to define the cell type. Surgery removes the tumor by using a cutting instrument. The disadvantages of surgery are that both normal and cancerous tissues are taken out and that you may lose a portion of your body. In addition, surgery cannot cure cancers that have spread.

When is radiation used in cancer treatment?
Radiation can be used alone or before or after surgery and chemotherapy, for those tumors that are sensitive to it. Radiation can cure some localized tumors and control those that are more advanced. However, it can have side effects that develop over the length of the treatment. Radiation is divided into two basic kinds—external, where a machine is used, and internal, where the radiation is placed in or near the affected area. External radiation (also referred to as external beam, electron beam, or cobalt treatment) is the most common type. Internal radiation (also called radiation seeding, brachytherapy,

interstitial radiation, intracavitary radiation, or radium implant) may be used alone or in addition to external radiation.

What are the advantages of chemotherapy?

Chemotherapy, which uses drugs and hormones to destroy cancer cells, works on rapidly dividing cells. Usually used after surgery or radiation as a secondary or preventive treatment, it can cure some cancers that have spread. It can be taken intravenously or by mouth. There are known side effects to different kinds of chemotherapy.

When is hormonal treatment used?

Hormonal treatment is used in cancers that depend on hormones for their growth. The treatment either removes or adds hormones to the body. It may include the use of drugs to block the body's production of hormones or surgery to remove the hormone-producing organs.

What is biological treatment?

Biological treatment uses your body's own defenses against the cancer. It tries to boost, direct, or restore the body's normal defenses. Biologicals include both naturally occurring agents as well as those made in the laboratory. Most biological treatments are still considered experimental.

Are any of these treatments ever combined?

Yes. Often several types of treatment are given to the same patient in order to achieve better results than with one type of treatment alone.

Are the different kinds of treatment given one at a time or all together?

It depends on many factors, including the tumor and the extent of disease. Sometimes the different treatments are given one after the other. Other times, two or more treatment modes are intermixed. Sometimes, radiation therapy or chemotherapy is given first, before the operation. For other kinds of tumor, surgery is the first treatment used.

What are the newest types of treatments for cancer?

The newest treatments for cancer involve using biologicals to trigger the body's own defenses against cancer. These cancer-fighting methods, now in clinical trials across the country, are using substances called biological response modifiers. They include monoclonal antibodies, tumor growth factors, gene therapy, differentiation and maturation factors, colony-stimulating factors, tumor necrosis, and interleukins. Some of these substances occur naturally in the body, while others are made in the laboratory. Many of these

TYPES OF TREATMENT

TREATMENT	HOW AND WHEN USED	ADVANTAGES AND DISADVANTAGES
Surgery	Removes the tumor by cutting; most often used if tumor is small, if it is limited to a single area of the body, and if cancer has not spread to other parts of the body. It is the most frequently used method. There are a variety of surgical procedures that may be used besides the removal with conventional surgical instruments. Curettage means removing the cancer by scraping. Cryosurgery employs liquid nitrogen to freeze and kill abnormal cells. Mohs surgery is microscopically controlled. Laser surgery uses a beam of laser light to vaporize cancer cells.	*Advantages:* May cure localized tumors. Allows the doctor to assess the extent of the cancer and to define the cell type. *Disadvantages:* Normal and cancerous tissues are equally destroyed. You may lose body parts. Cannot cure cancers that have spread.
Radiation	External beam radiation or radiation seeds are often used—sometimes as a primary treatment and at other times before or after surgery or chemotherapy.	*Advantages:* May cure localized tumors and control more advanced disease. Minimal risk of visible deformity. *Disadvantages:* Both normal and cancerous tissue destroyed. May develop side effects over a period of time. Must be available to go for treatment every day for five or six weeks.
Chemotherapy	Uses drugs to destroy cancer cells. Can be used before or after surgery and radiation. Used when	*Advantages:* Works on rapidly dividing cells. Can cure some cancers that have

(continued)

TREATMENT	HOW AND WHEN USED	ADVANTAGES AND DISADVANTAGES
	cancer has spread within body system rather than localized in one spot. Used to control growthand for palliation. Many different drugs and dosages have been tested and many of the side effects have been lessened.	spread and can eliminate micrometastasis. *Disadvantages:* Resistance to tumor may develop. Affects good cells as well as cancer cells. Has side effects. Less effective for large tumors. Some tumors not sensitive to drugs.
Hormonal therapy	Uses or manipulates hormones. Hormones can be natural or synthetic. Can be given by injection or orally. In some cases, surgery is done before or after use of hormones.	*Advantages:* Can be used to block the hormones cancer needs to grow. *Disadvantages:* Can cause number of side effects, depending on specific drug or surgical procedure.
Biological	Uses the body's own defenses against cancer. Boost, direct, or restore normal defenses. Uses agents occurring naturally in body or made in laboratory. Usually used in combination with other treatments.	*Advantages:* Enhances the body's own immune system. Can make cells more sensitive to destruction by body's system. *Disadvantages:* Still primarily experimental. Often produces major side effects.
Investigational	Includes all kinds of treatments, combinations of different treatments along with new discoveries. Compares standard treatments with new ones.	*Advantages:* Patient gets latest available treatment. Payment for parts of treatment may be covered by study. *Disadvantages:* Can have unknown risks and side effects. May need to be done at major cancer centers, sometimes far away from home.

new treatments are still years away from being used for ordinary treatment. Doctors are experimenting with ways of combining various biologicals with each other and with standard treatments for more effective use. More information on these and other investigational treatments will be found in Chapter 11, New Advances and Investigational Treatments.

What are tumor markers?

A tumor marker is a substance that is found in higher amounts than normal in the blood, body fluids, or tissues of people who have cancer. Tumor markers can be used to monitor patients during treatment and to check for recurrence. For instance, a reduced amount of CEA (carcinoembryonic antigen) in the blood may indicate a favorable response to treatment, while an increase in CEA level may be an indication of a recurrence of colon or rectal cancer. Many tumor markers are being used in clinical trials in an investigational manner. For more information on tumor markers, see Chapter 4, What Is Cancer?

Where are these newest treatments being done?

Many of these treatments are available only at the comprehensive or clinical cancer centers designated by the National Cancer Institute. Some are available in local communities through clinical cooperative groups or through the community clinical oncology program. Some treatments are only being done at the National Institutes of Health Clinical Center. Chapter 28, Where to Get Help, gives information on these resources. The best information on clinical trials is found on the Web (www.cancer.gov) or by calling 1–800–4–CANCER.

With so much new information about cancer and its treatment, how does the ordinary doctor keep up with what is going on?

It is a serious concern to doctors, patients, and to the National Cancer Institute (NCI), the federal government's principal agency for research on cancer prevention, diagnosis, treatment, and rehabilitation. The NCI has created a computerized database to inform doctors, other health professionals, and the public of the latest and best treatments for cancer patients. Called PDQ for Protocol Data Query, it gives information on the state-of-the-art treatment for each type and stage of cancer, as well as information on more than 1,000 active investigational treatment studies under way in the United States. It is updated continuously to reflect the latest in treatment choices. You can get this information by accessing it on the Web or by calling the Cancer Information Service. Information on contacting these agencies is in Chapter 28, Where to Get Help.

How can I, an ordinary cancer patient, take advantage of the newest treatments?

It depends upon what kind of cancer you have and the stage of your cancer. Many of the newest treatments are still considered experimental and are available only to patients with advanced cancer for whom all other treatments have failed. Discuss the treatment in which you are interested with your doctor. You can call the National Cancer Institute's Cancer Information Service, a toll-free number (1–800–4–CANCER) for information on treatment. Trained information specialists can tell you the kinds of treatments available for your specific type and stage of cancer and, if appropriate, can conduct a PDQ search, or advise you on how to conduct a search, for those treatments being studied and where they are being conducted.

What is PDQ?

PDQ (Protocol Data Query) is a computerized service of the National Cancer Institute which lists the latest information on treatment for cancer patients. It has state-of-the-art treatment statements on more than 100 kinds of cancer. There are two versions of these statements—one written in simple language for patients and one written in medical language for health professionals. The information specialist can send you the state-of-the-art statement that gives you information on treatment. PDQ also gives information on the more than 1,000 clinical trials underway in the country. Or you can do your own search on the Web.

How can I get a PDQ search done for my kind of cancer?

You can call the Cancer Information Service or you can do your own search on the Internet. If you want a PDQ search, you will need to know the kind of cancer you have, the cell type, the stage of disease, and the kinds of treatments you have already had and when you had them. There is more information on clinical trials, their advantages and disadvantages in Chapter 11, New Advances and Investigational Treatments.

How can the doctor measure the effectiveness of the various kinds of treatment on the tumor?

Different people respond in different ways to treatment. Different kinds of cancers respond in different ways. The doctor uses several measurement tools: physical exams, x-rays, scans, and various laboratory tests to measure each person's response to the treatment. The doctor will do various tests, will check to see whether the signs and symptoms of the disease have disappeared, whether you feel better, have increased strength and decreased fatigue, whether your appetite has improved and gained weight, and whether your pain has gone away.

What if the treatment the doctor has chosen for me does not work?
There are many treatment programs that can be used. One may result in controlling your cancer even after another has failed to do so adequately.

Why are there so many different kinds of treatments?
Since no two cancers are truly alike and since people respond differently to treatments, two people with seemingly identical diseases may receive and respond to different treatments. Each type of cancer has its own way of growing and spreading. It also has its own way of responding to treatment. The treatments must be tailored to your individual cancer, to its size and its location in your body, to your physical condition, and to how you respond.

What is meant by adjuvant forms of treatment?
An adjuvant treatment is one that is being used **in addition to** a primary form of treatment. When radiation is used after surgery, the radiation is referred to as adjuvant treatment.

What is meant by palliative treatment?
A palliative treatment is a treatment that is intended to improve the condition of the patient. It might be used to relieve pain or to eliminate symptoms of the cancer. It is also used to prevent further complications or to give a psychological uplift.

Can I withdraw from a type of treatment once I have started it?
If you decide to stop the treatment, it is your choice. However, before you begin any kind of treatment you should make sure you understand what you are getting into. Your doctor should explain in detail the pros and cons of your recommended treatment as well as alternative forms of therapy that might be available to you. Of course, the final decision is yours, but you should understand that if you stop treatment, you may be losing valuable time that can never be regained.

What is meant by the term "informed consent"?
Informed consent is a legal standard that defines how much a person must know about the potential benefits and risks of treatment before being able to agree to undergo it knowledgeably with legal responsibility for the result. The question of informed consent is a very controversial and complex one, particularly if you are talking about surgery or other treatment procedures that carry some risks. Basically, you have the legal right to know everything you want to know about a treatment that is being proposed for you. If you should become involved in a clinical trial, informed consent is part of the process. You will be asked to sign a paper that explains the pros and cons of the treatments before

they are done. In most cancer treatment, however, it is up to you to ask about the major risks involved versus the benefits that are expected.

What is meant by the term "prognosis"?
Your prognosis is a prediction of what the outcome of your disease will be. A doctor bases the prognosis on your general physical condition plus the accumulated information about the disease and its treatment. A prognosis is only a prediction.

What is meant by the term "quality of life"?
This term is often used when talking about cancer treatment. It means how good the life is that you will be leading after treatment. Some people feel that they would rather live a shorter period of time than undergo disfiguring operations or long periods of painful treatment. Influencing your quality of life are such things as your general health, the side effects of your treatment, your ability to function normally, pain, your personal attitude, how you think about yourself (self-esteem), your spirituality, your family, work and social roles, sexuality, economic status, and your physical conditions. Each of these items needs to be examined as you assess your treatment for cancer.

Web Pages to Check Out

www.cancer.gov: For general up-to-date information, and for clinical trials.
www.cancer.org: For general up-to-date information and community resources.
www.cancer.gov: National Cancer Institute (PDQ treatment information).
www.consensus.nih.gov: National Institutes of Health Consensus Program.

Also see Chapter 2, Searching for Answers on the Web, for more information.

Eight

SURGERY

In most cases, surgery that is needed for cancer can wait while you get a second opinion. Make sure you understand all your biopsy and treatment choices before you agree to a scheduled time for surgery. Remember: once you have the operation, it's too late to change your decision.

SURGERY, REMOVING DISEASED tissue or an organ with some kind of cutting or other device, is the most often used treatment for cancer. You may need surgery for your biopsy, to take out a tumor that might be cancerous, to relieve pain, or to remove a tumor that is the result of spread of the cancer. It can also be used for diagnosis and prevention. Surgery is often the first step in your treatment plan when cancer is suspected. It is important to be certain that all the necessary diagnostic tests have been done before the operation is planned. Choose your surgeon carefully. It is important to ask questions before your surgery so that you know the reasons for the treatment, exactly what will be done, the expected results and any possible complications.

What You Need to Know About Cancer Surgery

▪ Many biopsies can be performed with means other than surgery. Be sure that the operation you are having is necessary. You can find more information on biopsies in Chapter 6, How Cancers Are Diagnosed.

▪ You are more likely to have a well-qualified surgeon if you choose one who is a fellow of the American College of Surgeons and is board-certified in the field of specialty. Doctors who specialize in cancer surgery are known as surgical oncologists.

▪ Many of the operations that, only a few years ago, required a stay in the hospital are now being done either in an outpatient area of the hospital or in a surgical center.

▪ You need to understand exactly what is going to be done, where the operation is going to take place, who will be doing the surgery, and how long the recovery will take before you agree to surgery.

Questions to Ask Your Surgeon Before Your Operation

▪ **What is this surgery for? Why do you feel I need it?**

▪ **Exactly what do you plan to do? Please explain it to me in simple terms, show me what parts of the body are involved and tell me how extensive the surgery will be.**

▪ **What are my chances for cure with the surgery?**

▪ **Will I have a scar from it? How long will it be and exactly where will it be? How disfiguring will it be?**

▪ **What other kind of treatment can be used instead of surgery?**

▪ **Is this surgery dangerous? What are the risks and what are the benefits?**

▪ **Do I have time to have a second opinion? If not, why do you feel this operation needs to be done on an urgent basis?**

▪ **Can I postpone having this surgery? What will happen if I do?**

▪ **Will I have a hospital stay or can the surgery be done as an outpatient procedure?**

▪ **How long will the operation take?**

▪ **After the operation, how will you let my family/friends know the outcome? Where will they meet you? (At this time, if there are specific instructions about how you want family/friends told, you should discuss this with your doctor.)**

▪ **How long will the recovery period be?**

- How disfiguring will the operation be?
- How disabling will the operation be? Temporarily? Permanently?
- Will I have drains, catheters, or intravenous lines?
- Will I need a blood transfusion? Can I bank my own blood?
- What are the possible aftereffects of the operation?
- How many times have you performed this operation?
- Whom do you recommend I see for a second opinion?
- How much will the surgery cost? Does that include all the costs?

Should I discuss fees with my surgeon?

Many surgeons volunteer this information. If yours does not, don't hesitate to ask. In addition to surgeons' fees and the costs of your hospital stay, you will probably be billed separately for the professional services of the assisting surgeon, anesthesiologist, and any medical consultants. You should familiarize yourself with the extent of your medical benefit plan beforehand. Your doctor's office staff may be able to help you find out how much your benefit plan will cover. If the plan will not pay all of the costs, discuss your situation frankly with your surgeon to see if you can work out a mutually acceptable solution. If you feel uneasy about talking with the surgeon about costs, remember that he or she knows it's important for you to be as relaxed and worry-free as possible in preparation for the surgery. (Part of the pledge of the American College of Surgeons says, "I promise to make my fees commensurate with the services rendered and with the patient's rights. Moreover, I promise to deal with each patient as I would wish to be dealt with were I in his position.")

Is surgery always the first treatment for cancer?

Surgery is often the initial treatment. However, there are some cases where chemotherapy or radiation therapy is done first, followed by surgery.

Is surgery ever used alone as a treatment?

Some cancers, such as basal or squamous cell skin cancers, are still treated by surgery alone. However, surgery is a local treatment, working only in one part of the body and thus is limited in what it can accomplish. Therefore, many kinds of cancer that in the past were treated with surgery alone, such as cancer of the breast, colon, and head and neck, now have additional treatments, such as chemotherapy or radiation, either before or after surgery.

Is surgery dangerous?

All surgery has some risk to it. How much risk is involved depends on many factors: the kind of operation being performed, the physical condition of the patient, the skill of the surgeon and the team performing the operation (including the skill of the anesthesiologist) and the caliber of the hospital and its facilities. You must weight the benefits against the risks. It is certainly a subject you should discuss with the doctor before going ahead with the operation.

Is there a special kind of surgeon who works with cancer patients?

There are doctors known as surgical oncologists who specialize in performing surgery on cancer patients. Before you have an operation, you should know whether or not your doctor has had special training in cancer treatment and experience in treating your kind of cancer. There are no easy guidelines, but one or two cases of treatment of a particular kind of cancer each year does **not** qualify as extensive experience. Each cancer has its own special history of how it grows and where it spreads. The choice of a surgeon is a very critical part of cancer treatment. It is very important that the doctor know how your cancer might spread so that the proper operation can be done. For more information on specialties of doctors and their training, see Chapter 3, Choosing a Doctor and a Hospital.

Are there any guidelines for choosing a surgeon?

Most of the time, your primary doctor will give you names of suggested surgeons. Moreover, whatever health plan you belong to might limit your choice. It is important that you take the time to check out the surgeon's credentials and check out the hospital where the operation will be done, as has been described in Chapter 3, Choosing Your Doctor and Hospital. Remember these basic points:

- It is best to have a surgeon who is board-certified and a Fellow of the American College of Surgeons. Although this professional accreditation is just a guide, it tells you that the doctor is well trained and that those qualifications have been verified.

- It is best to choose a doctor who has performed the operation many times. Although this does not prove the doctor is competent, as a general rule, the more experienced the surgeon is, the more competent.

- It is best to be in a hospital affiliated with a National Cancer Institute Cancer Center, or directly affiliated with a medical school or whose cancer program has been approved by the American College of Surgeons. At least, the hospital should be accredited by the Joint Commission on Hospitals (JCOH).

- It is important for you to understand that the surgeon is a new doctor to you who knows nothing about how much information you wish to have. If you wish to participate in the decision-making process, you need to take the lead by asking questions and talking to your surgeon about your wishes.

- It is best to choose a surgeon who is willing to answer your questions and to give you the time and attention you feel you need. Check your understanding of what the doctor has told you about the operation by repeating it in your own words.

- Ask the doctor to tell you the risks of the surgery based on your particular physical condition added to the statistical evidence (both national and local) compiled over the years for the particular operation you will have. You should also ask what the risks are if you do **not** have the surgery.

- It is best to have a surgeon who knows and can work with your general practitioner or internist. Remember it is the surgeon who will be in charge of your care while you are in the hospital.

- It is best to choose a surgeon who is part of a group or who is hospital-based, since this will probably offer you the best total care both before and after the surgery.

- If you are getting a second opinion, it is best to get it outside of the particular group practice where your primary physician is located or where the first surgeon is located.

- The time to get a second opinion is before making arrangements to have the surgery done.

What determines whether the doctor will operate or whether another type of treatment will be used?

There are several factors that the doctor considers before the decision to operate is made. Among them are the following:

- Is surgery the treatment of choice for this site and this cell type of the cancer?

- Can similar results be obtained from a different kind of treatment?

- What is the risk of the operation? Are the potential results worth the risk?

- Is it technically feasible to remove the primary tumor and a reasonable margin of surrounding healthy tissue?

- Is there any indication that the cancer may have spread outside the primary site?

- Is the person's physical condition good enough to withstand the operation?

When is preventive surgery done?

There are several factors the doctor takes into consideration when deciding whether or not to do preventive surgery—such as if you are at high risk for cancer or you have a condition that is known to be precancerous; whether

TYPES OF SURGERY

TYPE	DESCRIPTION
Preventive	Removal of tissue or an organ not presently malignant. Used when person is known to be at high risk, the tissue or organ is not vital, and removal lessens possibility of cancer.
Diagnostic; also may be called biopsy or staging	Removal of tissue to determine whether it contains cancer cells. Used when symptoms or tests are suspicious for cancer.
Exploratory	Looking at the organ or area suspected to determine the cause of the problem.
Treatment	Taking out the tumor, organ, or tissue to cure or control the cancer or improve the person's quality of life. May be used alone or as part of a sequence with other therapies.
Ambulatory or Outpatient	Done in an outpatient area of the hospital or in a surgical clinic. Person does not need to stay in hospital overnight. Tests are done a day or so before the operation.
Emergency	Must be done immediately. Essential to save person's life, preserve function of organ or limb, to stop hemorrhage or remove damaged organ.
Urgent	Must be done as soon as possible, usually within twenty-four hours.
Planned	Surgery can take place within a few weeks. Many operations for cancer fall into this category.
Elective	Not absolutely necessary, but better off if done or if patient desires it to be done.
Reconstructive	Correcting functional or cosmetic defects that result from the original surgery. May be done immediately or many years after original surgery.
Palliative	Treating complications incidental to cancer. Used to relieve problems or pain.

the tissue or organ to be taken out is vitally needed; the seriousness of the operation; and whether doing the surgery will put you at a much lower risk for developing cancer or a recurrence. For example, removing a polyp in your colon or a mole on your skin is a relatively simple procedure that can reduce your risk of cancer. On the other hand, removing a breast as a preventive measure is a much more difficult decision. You need to be sure you understand the risks involved, the type of procedure that will be done, the anticipated results, and the success rate before you have any surgery.

What kind of surgery is used for diagnosis?
There are several types of procedures—such as endoscopies and biopsies— that are used in diagnosis and staging of cancer. Depending on the site, the doctor may do several procedures to determine how extensive the cancer is before taking out a tumor, especially if the surgery will be radical or alter the way you look or the way your body functions. The diagnostic and staging surgeries are described in Chapter 6, How Cancers Are Diagnosed.

What is exploratory surgery?
Exploratory surgery is done so that the doctor can see the organ or area suspected of causing the problem which cannot be resolved through the use of diagnostic tests.

Are most cancer operations urgent surgery?
Most operations for cancer are not urgent. Rather they fall into the planned or elective categories. You normally have time to arrange for a second opinion and to think through the procedures you will be having before the operation needs to be scheduled.

When is reconstructive surgery done?
Reconstructive surgery tries to restore a person to as near normal as possible following surgery for cancer. The use of surgery for rehabilitation is fairly recent. It can achieve not only cosmetic improvement but also increase function and self-esteem. In order to achieve the best results, it is wise to consider and prepare for reconstructive surgery before the primary surgery is done so the plastic surgeon will be part of the planning team.

What kinds of palliative surgery are performed on cancer patients?
Palliative surgery is done to relieve suffering, or minimize the symptoms of the disease, improving the person's quality of life even if a cure is not possible. Palliative surgery can be used to treat complications incidental to cancer or to treat side effects such as pain.

Does it make any difference what day of the week I go into the hospital for surgery?

You may not have a choice. Normally you are scheduled to go when there is an empty bed. However, you should be aware that it is better not to go into the hospital before a weekend or a holiday, when the hospital may not be as fully staffed as during a normal week.

What kinds of tests will I have before my operation?

You will need to have the routine tests, such as a chest x-ray and an EKG to test lung and heart functions. Your blood also will be tested. You will be asked questions about your medical history. Make sure you discuss any chronic health problems or allergies you have, any medicines you are taking for any reason—no matter how unrelated to your surgery they may seem. Any of these items could interfere with your anesthesia. Usually, all of this is done on an outpatient basis a few days before the operation.

Will I need to sign a consent form for my surgery?

Before an operation can take place, you will need to sign a consent form. Make sure you take the time to read it over and that you understand what is going to be done and what alternate procedures your doctor has in mind should the intended one not work out.

What kinds of things should I know in order to make an informed choice about the operation?

There are several things you should know if you are to make an informed choice. Among them are:

- The likelihood of being cured, or having your condition improved by the operation.
- The benefits and risks of *not* having the operation.
- The alternative kinds of treatment that are available.
- How disabling and disfiguring the operation is going to be.
- The risk of death or serious disability from the operation or from its complications.

Will I need to bank my blood for my operation?

This is an important question. You need to ask the doctor whether or not there is a possibility that you will need to have any blood transfusions during your cancer operations. If your doctor thinks you will need blood transfusions during your operation, it would be wise to make plans to bank your own blood. Depending on how much blood you need to bank, you may need a few weeks before your operation to do it.

How long will I need to fast before I have surgery?

It depends upon the kind of surgery that you are having done and the place where you are having it. Be sure to discuss the timetable with your doctor. The American Society of Anesthesiologists in 2002 put out guidelines for fasting, based on improved anesthesia techniques. These guidelines recommend permitting clear liquids up to two hours before surgery, a light meal up to six hours before and a heavier meal eight hours before. However a survey has found that most patients are still being told to take nothing after midnight. And, according to the type of surgery, the patients exceed even this time period, with some people not having liquids for up to 20 hours and solids for 37 hours before the operation. This kind of fasting can result in patients suffering from thirst, with headaches, hypoglycemia, discomfort, and other side effects. It is important that you understand how long you need to fast and that you not exceed the timetable.

Will I have drains, catheters, and intravenous lines after my operation?

What will be needed will depend on the location and the extent of your operation. Many times, these procedures are routinely done as part of surgery. If you are informed, you and your family will not be alarmed after surgery.

If I have outpatient or ambulatory surgery, will I be able to go home right after my surgery?

According to the results of a large, long-term study on the aftermath of outpatient surgery, more than one-third of serious post-operative complications occur more than 48 hours after the procedure. It's a good idea to have someone with you when you leave the outpatient area and at home for 24 hours or longer. Refrain from driving, drinking alcohol, or making important decisions for at least a day. Be sure you have the telephone number of the doctor who performed the procedure, the anesthesiologist (if one was involved) and the center where the procedure was done. You should also have written instructions about medications to take or avoid, what to eat and drink, activity level, bathing instructions, wound care and what to do in case of an emergency. Don't forget to ask which postoperative symptoms are normal and which warrant medical attention.

Are there different ways diseased tissue is removed?

There are a number of different techniques. See the chart below.

What is cryosurgery?

Cryosurgery, or cryoablation as it is sometimes called, uses cold liquid gas to freeze and kill cancer cells. A small cut is made so that a thin catheter tube can be put into the tumor. The doctor inserts a device, called a cryoprobe, into the catheter tube and pumps liquid nitrogen into the tip of the probe. The liquid nitrogen freezes and kills any abnormal tissue. Ultrasound, CT scans, and MRIs are used to guide the probe to make sure it reaches the exact tumor site and to monitor and record the tumor cells that are killed. Depending upon the location of the tumor and the type of cryosurgery used, the procedure is done either in an operating room, using local or general anesthesia or in a doctor's office. The treated area sloughs off the dead cells and leaves a sore that eventually heals. Cryosurgery is being used for cancers of the skin, bone, brain, spine, liver, cervix, kidney, and prostate.

What is laser treatment?

Laser (light amplification by simulated emission of radiation) treatment uses a narrow, intense beam of light to shrink or destroy tumors. Lasers are more

SURGICAL TECHNIQUES

TYPE	DESCRIPTION
Cryosurgery, cryoablation	Use of cold liquid gas to destroy a tumor by freezing.
Laser	Use of intense, narrow light beam to shrink or destroy a tumor.
Mohs surgery	Shaves off tumor a thin layer at a time. Usually used for skin cancer.
Laparoscopic	Makes small cuts in skin. Small instruments and video cameras used to perform surgery.
Bloodless	Loss of blood lessened by use of lasers, harmonic scalpels, argon beam coagulators.
Electrosurgery	Use of high-frequency current.
Chemosurgery	Use of chemotherapy drugs on tumor before, or instead of, surgery.
Stereotactic surgery	Uses computer-assisted techniques to allow the surgeon to remove tumors in areas that are normally difficult to reach.
Intraoperative chemotherapy or radiotherapy	Use of chemotherapy or radiation treatment during the operation.

precise than scalpels, shorten operating times, and allow surgeons to reduce the use of anesthesia. Since laser heat seals blood vessels, there is less bleeding, swelling, or scarring and healing time is often shortened. They also bring fast and effective treatment to previously inaccessible areas. Lasers are used in treating many kinds of cancer such as cervical, skin, lung, vaginal, vulvar, penile, and vocal cord. It may also be used to help relieve symptoms caused by cancer.

Is laser surgery being used in treating cancer?

There are several different kinds of lasers. The three most often used are:

- carbon dioxide laser: removes thick layers from the skin's surface without penetrating the deeper layers; often used for skin cancer.

- Nd: YAG laser: penetrates deeper into tissue than other kinds of lasers; sometimes used to treat throat cancer.

- argon laser: can pass through only superficial layers of tissue; also used in photodynamic therapy.

What is the Free-Electron Laser?

A "Star Wars" type laser, known as the Free-Electron Laser, is being used in selected hospitals for brain surgery, with hopes that in the future it will find other applications. The FEL laser, originally developed for the missile defense program, is capable of generating laser beams of incredible delicacy. To date, it has been used only on tumors on the outside surface of the brain, so that surgery can be done without cutting through normal tissue. (For information on facilities operating with FEL lasers, go to www.sbfel3.ucsb.edu. There is more information on the use of lasers in cancer treatment in Chapter 11, New and Investigational Treatments.)

What is laser-induced interstitial thermotherapy?

Lasers are directed to areas between organs in the body. The laser light raises the temperature of the tumor, which damages or destroys cancer cells. This treatment uses the same idea as hyperthermia—heating the cells to help shrink tumors by damaging cells or depriving them of what they need to live.

What is Mohs surgery?

Mohs micrographic surgery is a surgical technique usually used for skin tumor removal. The advantage of Mohs surgery is that only the tissue which has been invaded by the tumor is removed, preserving healthy skin and allowing for the best possible cosmetic effect. A thin layer of skin at the tumor site is removed and examined under the microscope using a special instrument. If evidence of tumor cells is found at the edges of the sample, the doctor will remove and examine another skin sample. These steps are repeated until no tumor is detected under the microscope. Depending on the extent of the tumor, this process may be repeated several times. The process may take more than an hour per sample.

What will I do to prepare for Mohs surgery?

When preparing to have Mohs surgery, you will probably be advised to set aside a day for the necessary number of procedures. Small or superficial wounds may be left to heal by themselves. Some wounds may need to be stitched closed. Very large wounds may require a flap or a graft from elsewhere on your body to repair the surgical procedure. Mohs surgery has a high cure rate because the tumor is seen microscopically and can be completely removed.

What is laparoscopic surgery?

Laparoscopic surgery, also known as minimally invasive or keyhole surgery, uses cameras and video monitors to aid in performing surgery. A small cut is made in the skin and a harmless gas, such as carbon dioxide, is used to expand the body cavity and enlarge the working area. Through additional small cuts (each about 1/2 inch long), a rod shaped telescope, attached to a camera, and other long and narrow surgical tools are placed into the space. The video camera lets the doctors "see" inside the body while doing the surgery. Depending on the site, other small incisions may be needed. For instance, when using this method for colon cancer, another incision is made to bring the intestine out so that the doctor can take out the part with cancer and sew the two ends back together.

What are the advantages of laparoscopic surgery?

Instead of making a large cut into the skin and the underlying muscles, surgeons are able to make small entry cuts and perform all the major surgery previously done with a large opening. That means that you will feel less pain after the operation, will be in less danger of infection, and will recover faster. Only small scars—one or two inches long instead of the usual eight or 12 inches—are left after surgery. Not all hospitals have the equipment necessary to perform laparoscopic surgery, since the equipment is expensive and surgeons need special training. Even surgeons who are very skilled in regular techniques must be specially trained to perform surgery using the video monitor and display—since they are performing in a two-dimensional field instead of the three-dimensional operating field to which many are accustomed. Some patients with many prior operations have a great deal of scar tissue so they are not good candidates for this type of surgery. These procedures are still under study.

What is bloodless surgery?

Bloodless surgery means that no blood transfusions are given during the operation. It is being used for removal of some cancers. The doctors use lasers and harmonic scalpels, argon beam coagulators and drugs to lessen the loss of blood. This kind of surgery results in a shorter stay in the hospital.

What is a harmonic scalpel?

A harmonic scalpel uses ultrasound vibrations to cut tissues and seal blood vessels. The scalpel vibrates at more than 55,000 times per second. Hysterectomy, colon surgery, and conization of the cervix are among the uses of an harmonic scalpel.

What is electrosurgery?

Electrosurgery, or electrocautery, uses an electric probe or needle to burn and destroy tissue.

What is chemosurgery?

Chemosurgery is the use of anticancer drugs to shrink the tumor before surgery or to remove the tumor instead of operating.

What is intraoperative chemotherapy?

Intraoperative chemotherapy is an investigational treatment. A single, high dose of chemotherapy drug is given directly to the tumor or the area of the tumor during the operation.

How is radiation used during an operation?

The surgery is begun and after the tumor is exposed or taken out, the patient is given radiation therapy directly to the area. The operation is then completed. This is called intraoperative radiation therapy. Intraoperative radiation can deliver a single high dose directly to the tumor, because surrounding organs sensitive to radiation, such as the skin, intestines and liver can be held aside or shielded. The exposed tumor can also be felt or seen directly, rather than viewed on a scan or x-ray. This treatment is still being studied through clinical studies.

Is stereotactic surgery used in treating tumors?

Stereotactic surgery uses computer-assisted techniques to allow the surgeon to locate and remove tumors that are deep or difficult to reach. CT scanning and MRI, attached to special computer-assisted stereotactic instruments allow a tumor to be viewed in three dimensions.

Questions to Ask the Anesthesiologist

- **What kind of medication will I be given before I am taken into the operating room?**
- **Who will be administering the medication and anesthesia?**
- **How will they be given to me?**
- **Are you an anesthesiologist or an anesthetist?**
- **Will my allergies be a problem?**
- **What kind of anesthetic are you going to give to me?**
- **What are the side effects?**
- **What are the risks?**
- **How long will the operation take?**
- **How long will it take before I regain consciousness?**
- **Will I go to a recovery room after the operation?**
- **What are the fees for your service?**
- **If you do not want to be fully unconscious during surgery, are elderly, or have lung problems, ask: Is general anesthesia absolutely necessary or is there another choice?**

Who gives the anesthesia?
Anesthesia should be given either by an anesthesiologist or under the direction of an anesthesiologist. An anesthesiologist is a doctor specializing in anesthesia—the physician who can choose the most appropriate type of anesthesia to be used—and during surgery is responsible for maintaining all the body's vital functions.

What is an anesthetist?
Anesthetists are not medical doctors. Usually they are specially trained nurses who give anesthesia under the direction of a doctor. A hospital's department of anesthesiology, besides being responsible for the administration of anesthesia during surgery, usually sets the standards for the way in which the operating room and the recovery room are run.

Will I meet the anesthesiologist?
Most times, you will meet the anesthesiologist before surgery. Make sure you talk about any chronic health problems, allergies or drug sensitivities you have, any medicines you are taking for any reason no matter how unrelated to your surgery it may seem. Any of these items could interfere with your anesthesia. Of course,

the information is also available to the anesthesiologist from your medical history and other available medical records as well as by consulting with your surgeon.

Can I decide what kind of anesthesia I would like?
The decision on the kind of anesthesia to be used is usually made by your anesthesiologist and surgeon. However, if you have preferences, you should discuss any feelings and needs you have with the doctors. If you prefer to be asleep instead of awake during the surgery (even though you will not experience any pain in either case) you should talk to the doctor.

How long can a person stay under anesthesia?
It varies depending upon the kind of drugs used and the condition of the patient. Surgeons are not under the same pressure to hurry through operations as they once were, mainly because of advances in methods of anesthesia and better monitoring of patients during surgery.

How does the anesthesiologist decide what kind of anesthesia to use?
It depends upon the kind of operation, what the surgeon needs during the procedure and the physical needs of the patient.

What will the anesthesiologist do during the operation?
The anesthesiologist will be present during the operation and after it, monitoring your condition, watching your blood pressure, pulse rate, temperature, and the electrocardiographic recording of the action of your heart. The anesthesiologist can administer glucose, plasma, whole blood, and various other drugs as needed.

Does the anesthesiologist work only in the operating room?
The anesthesiologist works in the operating room and in the recovery room. It is the responsibility of the anesthesiologist to alleviate pain, relieve anxieties before the operation, increase the safety in the operating room, provide the best conditions for the surgeon during the actual operation, and help ensure complete and comfortable recovery afterward. Advances in anesthesiology have made it possible to operate on patients who not long ago would have been considered poor surgical risks because they were too young, too old, or too feeble.

Is anesthesia painful?
Not with today's procedures. Probably an hour or so before the operation, you will be given something to make you drowsy and relaxed. You may also be given medication to dry up mucous and salivary-gland secretions, which will help the effectiveness of the anesthesia. The anesthesia will be given in the operating room.

What is topical anesthesia?

An anesthetic is sprayed or painted onto the surface of the area. Topical anesthesia can be used for eye, nose, and throat procedures. Sometimes it is followed by injections of local anesthetics. It can also be used when tubes are being put into the trachea (windpipe) or esophagus (food passage).

When is local anesthesia used?

Local anesthesia is used for minor operations when a small area needs to be numbed or temporarily deadened. It is injected directly into the tissues at the site to be operated on. Only a small area is made insensitive.

What is regional anesthesia?

Regional anesthesia is injected into the nerves that transmit pain sensations from a particular area. A larger area can be made insensitive than with a local. If regional anesthesia is used, you will be aware during the entire procedure, although you may be given a sedative injection or intravenous medication to help you relax. The affected area may continue to be numb for sometime after the operation. The advantage of regional anesthesia is that your heart, lungs, blood pressure, and general condition are not greatly affected because only specific nerves are blocked. This means that some poor-risk patients can be operated on who could not withstand general anesthesia.

How is general anesthesia used?

With general anesthesia you are put into a drug-induced sleep. The anesthesiologist aims at producing a sleep of just enough depth to permit safe surgery. The anesthesia may be light for a superficial procedure. Or you may be given a deep anesthesia so that an operation on the heart, lungs, or abdomen can be carried out.

TYPES OF ANESTHESIA

KIND	DESCRIPTION
Topical	Sprayed or painted directly on the area involved.
Local	Limited to a certain part of the body. Used in most minor operations. Patient awake during procedure.
Regional	Affecting a larger part of the body than local anesthesia. Patient awake during procedure.
General	Affecting the whole body. Patient asleep during procedure. Used for most major operations.

Is general anesthesia dangerous?
Although anesthesia entails some risks, it is necessary for surgery. In the case of many cancers, general anesthesia is used so that you will be asleep and relaxed during the operation.

How is general anesthesia given?
After you reach the operating room, the anesthesiologist will probably insert an intravenous (IV) needle into your arm so that any drugs needed during the operation can easily be injected. If you are to be asleep during the operation, a drug will be injected and within seconds you will be sleeping. If a mask is to be used, or an endotracheal tube is to be inserted, it will be done after you are asleep so you will not be aware of it. Sometimes, you will be given a short-acting muscle relaxant to make it easier to pass a tube. Muscle relaxants may also be given during surgery to decrease the amount of general anesthetic needed. If you are having spinal anesthesia, a needle is inserted into the spinal canal, the area surrounding your spinal cord, either in the middle (just below the waist) lower down (saddle block) or at the base (caudal).

Questions to Ask in the Hospital or Surgical Center

- Why is this blood test/x-ray being taken? What will this test determine?
- Why am I being given this drug? What will it accomplish?
- What drugs have been prescribed for me and what is their purpose?
- How long do I need to stay here?
- Can I get out of bed and walk around?
- When can I go home?
- Will I need to stay in bed at home? For how long?
- Will I need help? Will I be able to take care of myself?
- When will I be able to go back to my normal activities? (Ask specific questions based on your case: When can I drive a car? When can I play tennis? When can I do my household chores? When can I resume sexual activities?)
- What symptoms, if any, should I report to you? If I have a problem when can I reach you on the phone? Who else should I call if I cannot reach you?
- What symptoms can I ignore?
- When can I safely go back to work?
- What medications should I continue to take?
- What exercises will I be permitted to do? When?

Are there any special procedures that need to be done the night before an operation?

It depends on what operation you are having done, where it is being done, and the particular procedures that your doctor follows. Any of the following may be needed:

- **Fasting:** You will usually not be allowed to eat or drink for a period of time before an operation so it can be done on an empty stomach. Your doctor or nurse will tell you what the fasting rules are. If you fast for a longer time than recommended by your doctor, you run the risk of suffering from headaches, hypoglycemia, or other side effects.

- **Enema:** You may need an enema before some operations because there may be temporary interference with normal functioning of the intestines and the bowels may not move for several days.

- **Sedative:** You may be given a sleeping pill to take so that you will have a good night's sleep before the operation. An hour or two before you go to the operating room, an injection is usually given so that you will be in a calm, semiconscious state.

- **Shaving:** Depending on the location of the operation, you may have a wide area shaved and cleansed before the operation. It's a good idea to ask whether extensive shaving is really necessary. Often, if you ask, the extent of the shave can be limited.

- **Stomach tube:** If you are having an operation in the area of the stomach you may need to have a thin tube inserted so that the stomach and bowels will be empty and free of fluids and gas. The tube is inserted in the nostril and slid down the throat to the stomach. You may be given some anesthetic to numb the area. The tube is usually put in the night before, or the morning of, the surgery and left in place throughout the operation and for a number of days after it to help suction off fluid and gas.

- **Urinary catheter:** For some operations, especially those in the pelvic and bladder area, a catheter (a flexible, narrow tube) is inserted so that the bladder will be empty. This may be done in your room or in the operating room.

Who will be in the operating room during the surgery?

Several people help with the operation, no matter how minor. The size of the team depends upon the extent of the operation. It may include the surgeon, one to three assistant surgeons, anesthesiologist or anesthetist, chief operating room nurse, nurse in charge of surgical supplies, scrub nurse who handles the instruments, circulating nurse who gets additional supplies, and any additional required personnel.

How can the doctor determine during the operation if the tissue is cancerous?

If the type of cancer and the degree of malignancy are not known definitely before the operation, the doctor takes out a piece of the tumor (or the whole tumor if it is small) and sends it to the pathologist. The pathologist does a frozen-section biopsy. The results come back from the pathology laboratory in 15 to 20 minutes, allowing the doctor to know the results and continue with the operation as necessary.

What determines how radical the surgery will be?

Different kinds of cancer have different tendencies to spread. The surgeon must understand the history of the kind of cancer being operated on, the growth rate and how the tumor spreads. The doctor must also take into consideration whether or not the lymph nodes are involved and whether there is any indication that the cancer has spread to other parts of the body. The physical condition of the patient is also a determining factor. The surgeon gathers as much information as is possible about the cancer before the operation. But in most cases, all the questions cannot be answered until the doctor actually looks at and examines the diseased area. Doctors usually try to remove the visible cancer tissue plus some of the surrounding tissue, even if it seems normal. This is done in case the nearby tissue contains cancer cells that could later lead to the recurrence of the cancer.

What is meant by the term *clear margins*?

This means that in the area around the tumor, no cancer cells are present and all the cancer has been removed from the area.

What is tumor debulking?

This term, used in cancer surgery, means removing as much of the tumor as possible.

What is lymph node dissection?

A lymph node is a small bean-shaped organ that is part of the lymph system, the part of the body responsible for fighting infections. Lymph nodes are found throughout the body—under the arms, behind the ears, in the groin, in the stomach area, behind the knee and in many other areas. A lymph node dissection takes out some of the lymph nodes in the area of the cancer, so that they can be looked at under the microscope to evaluate whether or not the cancer has spread. This procedure, which can be done separately or during a cancer operation, is called a lymph node biopsy or a lymphandectomy. When you are told this is part of your surgery plan, you should be sure to ask the doctor exactly what this means in terms of scars and how the loss of the lymph nodes will affect the lymph drainage in that part of your body.

What is sentinel node dissection?

With sentinel node dissection, a surgeon may only have to remove one lymph node, or a small cluster of two or three nodes, to know if cancer has spread, leaving the noninvolved lymph nodes that perform important functions intact. Lymph node surgery can lead to uncomfortable side effects, such as lymph backup, which causes swelling, mild discomfort, and numbness. Usually, both a dye and a radioactive tracer are used. Results are more reliable if both dye and tracer are used, rather than if only one is used. The blue dye used will stay in the body for a few months to a year. You will be able to see it under your skin. The blue also may show up in your urine immediately after surgery. You should understand that even with an experienced medical team, about five percent of the time, no particular sentinel node will take up the dye or tracer, so that more extensive dissection will need to be done. Many studies are underway involving sentinel lymph node dissection to determine how effective this procedure is in different kinds of cancer.

What if the doctor finds the tumor has spread too far to remove it all?

The doctor's decision will depend on the kind of operation being done, the condition of the patient, and the history of the disease. For some cancers, like lung cancer, the lung itself may not be removed. Radiation and chemotherapy will then be used. In other kinds of cancer, the doctor may remove as much cancer as possible and then treat the patient with radiation or chemotherapy.

How long do operations generally take to perform?

The location and complexity of the tumor, the procedure being used and the surgeon's dexterity all have a bearing on the length of time involved. Some operations are complete within an hour or two. Others may take many more hours. Ask your doctor this question when you are being scheduled for surgery.

Should I make arrangements for the doctor to talk with someone I designate as soon as the surgery is completed?

If you want someone to be able talk to the doctor after your operation, be involved with any decisions that might be necessary, or to be there when you come back to your room, make sure you tell your doctor who that person is, ask where the person should wait and how long the procedure will take. Some hospitals and surgicenters have a special waiting room, while others will tell you to have family and friends wait in your room. Also, if you feel strongly that someone should not be told anything until you are alert, be sure to explain this to your doctor beforehand. These are all things you want to discuss before the operation.

Does the length of time I spend in the operating room indicate the seriousness of the operation?
It depends on the individual case. There are several situations that can make your time in the operating room longer, but have no bearing on your own operation. For instance:

- You were taken from your room some time in advance of the actual operation.
- The anesthesiologist may make some additional preparations that last 30 minutes or even an hour.
- The surgeon takes longer than expected on the operation before yours, thus starting on your operation later than scheduled.
- You could spend more time than anticipated in the recovery room.

Those people who are waiting for you should understand that they should not judge the length or seriousness of the operation by the amount of time you spend in the operating room.

Will I need to go to a recovery room after my operation?
It depends upon the kind of anesthesia given and the length and seriousness of your operation. If you had topical anesthetic and a simple skin cancer removed, you probably will not need to go into the recovery room. However, for most other procedures, you will be watched and checked by the medical team until you are stable enough to move. The recovery room has equipment for monitoring your heart action and respirators for assisting you in breathing if you need them. You can get intravenous fluids and blood in the recovery room. Normally the recovery room is run by a physician anesthesiologist so that you can be monitored when you wake up from the anesthesia. Respiration therapists will probably help you cough and inflate your lungs as soon as you wake up. If you have had general anesthesia, you may spend several hours in the recovery room.

Will things seem hazy as I come out of general anesthesia?
Sometimes they do. Voices may seem very loud or they may seem like they are coming from a long way off. People may seem to be moving differently from the way you think they should. You will probably feel groggy, your arms and

legs may feel like lead, and you may feel cold. Vision, hearing, and sense of balance can all be affected by anesthesia and it takes time for the effects to wear off. You will be half asleep, and until your vital signs are stable and there is no apparent problem, you will be kept in the recovery room.

How long does it take for the anesthesia to wear off after an operation?

Once the operation is finished, it can take anywhere from minutes to hours before you wake up, depending upon the kind of anesthesia you are given and the dose. Some people find that after general anesthesia, they are light-headed for as long as a few days. Don't worry, it will pass and there should be no permanent effect from it.

Is it wise to have someone waiting in my room to stay with me when I get out of the recovery room?

It is a good idea, because someone who knows you may be able to spot problems more quickly. It will also be a comfort for you to know that someone is there even if you are drowsy or sleeping most of the time.

Will I be able to get painkilling drugs after the operation if I need them?

You will probably experience some pain immediately after surgery and for a few days following. How much pain you have and how severe it will be depends on what was done and where in the body your operation was done. There are many painkilling drugs that can be used with perfect safety. In some hospitals and surgicenters, patient-controlled units are available so that you can have pain medicine whenever you need it. If you are having pain, be sure to inform the nurse so that you can get pain medication. If you have any problems, talk with your doctor, telling where the pain is, how long the painkillers are lasting, what kind of pain it is, how often it comes back, and what relieves it. There is considerable detail about pain and pain medication in Chapter 27, Living with Cancer.

Will I be staying overnight in the hospital after my operation?

You need to ask this question when you are setting up the operation with your doctor. It will depend on the operation being done, on the health plan you are under, and the facility where the operation is being done. These days, many operations that used to require an overnight in the hospital are being done as one-day surgery. The tests are done ahead of time, you come to the hospital or surgicenter early in the morning, the operation is completed, you spend time in a recovery room and you go home. If you are not going to stay overnight, make arrangements for someone to stay with you for at least the

first 24 to 48 hours after surgery. You also should think about getting a referral for a visit from the local Visiting Nurses organization.

What are the general procedures that are followed after an operation?
It depends on your doctor, the hospital, the operation performed, and your
own physical condition. There are some common procedures that will probably be followed:

- If you are going to be staying overnight, when you return to your room
  from the recovery room, you will probably spend some time lying flat in
  bed. You will be encouraged, after you recover from the anesthesia, to
  change your position and move your legs often, to stimulate your circulation. You may be given a little machine to blow into to make you breathe
  deeply so you will not get pneumonia.

- Your dressings will be checked often and changed if necessary. If you have
  a drain coming out of your incision, it will be checked and removed as
  soon as possible.

- Unless you had surgery of the stomach or intestinal tract, you will usually
  be given sips of water within a few hours after your operation and a bland
  diet the next day.

- The next day, you will probably be allowed to get out of bed and walk a little.
  This speeds your recovery and minimizes the complications from surgery.

- If you are having trouble with stomach gas, you will be encouraged to
  move about and walk as much as you are able. A record will also be kept
  of how much fluid you get and how much you urinate.

- Depending on the operation, you may need intravenous fluids and medications, antibiotic drugs, blood transfusions, and enemas.

**What will the nurses be checking on during my
first day after surgery?**
They will be checking your general color and appearance, your blood pressure, pulse, temperature, and rate of breathing. They will observe if your
reflexes are getting back to normal and if you are swallowing properly. They'll
come in to give you your medicine and help you with other things you may
need. They will make you move in your bed, sit up, dangle your legs over the
side of the bed, and help you to walk. They will be checking for proper elimination of both urine and stool.

Why is deep breathing important?
It is important that you begin deep breathing early after an operation to prevent pneumonia and other complications. If your breathing is shallow, the air

sacs around the edges of your lungs don't fill out. You may be asked to blow into a special machine to help you with your breathing.

Will I have soreness around my incision?

You will have some soreness around the incision but if it is unusually painful, let your doctor or nurse know at once.

What happens to the stitches in my incision?

This depends on the kind of sutures used during your surgery. In many cases, doctors use sutures that dissolve over time. But occasionally, the end of a suture will poke out of an incision like a whisker. If this happens, your surgeon can easily remove it. Surgical staples, sometimes used to close the incision, removed during the first office visit.

When will the stitches be taken out?

The stitches made out of a material that will dissolve do not need to be taken out. Ordinarily stitches are usually removed between the fifth and tenth day after the operation. If there is an area that has tension on it or is not healing firmly, the stitches may be left in for a longer time. You will feel only a slight tugging, but usually no pain when the stitches come out. If staples are used instead of stitches, they are usually taken out on the fourth to sixth day.

How can I take care of the drains that have been inserted?

If drains were inserted, they will be emptied by nurses while you are in the hospital. One of the bothersome results of surgery is caring for drains. If drains are left in when you go home, you must learn to drain them yourself. They will often be left in place for a week or two until the wound is no longer draining fluid or the wound shows signs of becoming infected. Though drains are inconvenient, they don't hurt. Be certain you have good instructions on how to care for drains before leaving the hospital and notify the doctor's office if you have any of the problems listed below.

How long will I be in the hospital?

Most people go home from the hospital very quickly these days. You may be in overnight or for a few days. Many times you will be sent home with your drain in and instructions on how to monitor it. You need to be sure that you discuss with the doctor and nurse what kind of support you have at home, and what needs you may have for help, before you are discharged from the hospital. If you need assistance, ask for appointments with the social worker and the discharge planner. They are employees of the hospital who are there to try to aid you in getting assistance if you cannot take care of yourself when you go home.

What problems can occur after surgery?

There are a number of complications that can occur after surgery, though most people recover quickly and resume their normal activities without problems. Soreness near the incision, especially when twisting or stretching; a mild sore throat (if a breathing tube was used) or discomfort in the abdomen, upper chest, shoulders and neck area can result from the surgery, but these symptoms usually disappear quickly. More serious complications such as lower urinary tract infections, pneumonia, the formation of blood clots, and pulmonary congestion or other lung-related problems sometimes occur following surgery.

What kinds of problems following surgery should I be aware of that require me to contact the doctor?

You should contact the doctor immediately if:

- your incision begins to bleed or leak fluid.
- your incision becomes red, swollen, or feels warm.
- you develop a fever.
- there is increased pain in your abdomen or pelvic area.
- you develop chest pain, shortness of breath, or leg pain.
- you become light-headed or dizzy.

Is it common to have sexual problems following cancer surgery?

After surgery, many people find that it is some time before they are able to resume their normal sexual activities. The whole process of hospitalization, surgery, scars, and tenderness of the areas that have been disturbed may make sex uncomfortable. Worry and concern about the future do not make for a happy atmosphere for sexual pleasures. But as time goes on, most people find that sexual desire returns and sexual activity is again a satisfying part of life. In some cases, accommodations must be made for the changes made in the body by surgery. Losing a body part may make you feel embarrassed. Naturally, the changes vary depending on where surgery was performed. Each type of surgery in each area of the body can affect your sexual being in a different way. Women who have had breast cancer and women and men who have had surgery in the reproductive area have very specific problems. Those who have had to have a colostomy or urostomy face a whole other set of circumstances. Facial cancer, limb amputations, and laryngectomy, all make it necessary to adjust to changes in appearance, which have a bearing on how you feel about yourself. Pain can be a common problem, often related to changes made by the surgery or by pain in some other part of the body. Some of these problems are discussed in the chapters relating to operations in the specific areas involved. Other information about dealing with sexual problems, feelings, and pain can be found in Chapter 27, Living With Cancer.

What is lymphedema?

Lymphedema is an accumulation of lymph fluid in the arms or legs and causes swelling. Not being able to drain, the lymph fluid remains in the soft tissue where infections can develop. People who have had lymph node dissection, the removal of lymph nodes during cancer surgery, are at greatest risk. Lymphedema is most commonly seen in women who have had axillary nodes removed during breast cancer surgery. However, lymphedema also occurs when the pelvic and inguinal groups of nodes in the legs are removed. Those with melanomas in the arms, thigh, or leg may be subjected to lymphedema as well. Men who have had surgery (or radiation) for prostate cancer, women who have had radical surgery and node dissection for gynecologic cancers, or those who have ovarian, testicular, colon-rectal, pancreatic, or liver cancer which has spread to the lower area of the abdomen are all at risk for lymphedema. Curiously enough, not everyone who has lymph node surgery has lymphedema. Lymphedema, however, can occur soon after surgery or even as many as 15 years after surgery.

Does lymphedema mean my cancer has spread?

Many people fear that lymphedema means that the cancer has spread or returned. Another fear is that the swollen, nonfunctional limb may be permanently disfigured. It is important to discuss your fears with the health care professionals in your life, so that they can help you to learn the necessary measures you need to take to keep lymphedema under control. Positioning, massage, exercise, special garments, and pumps are all used in treating lymphedema.

How can you tell if you have lymphedema?

About half of patients who have lymphedema report a feeling of heaviness or fullness in the affected arm or leg. A slight indentation may be visible when the skin on the arm or leg is pressed. Depending on how extensive the problem is, a deeper fingerprint may take anywhere from five to 30 seconds to return to normal. At the extreme, the arm or leg may swell to one and a half to two times its normal size. You should always be aware of any signs of infection in the involved area—redness, pain, heat, chills, swelling, or fever. Infections can move quickly and become serious very rapidly.

How important is it to get immediate care?

Immediate care is essential. Untreated, the condition can result in a permanently swollen arm or leg. Awareness of the possibility of lymphedema and the need for immediate medical attention may help keep the problem from becoming chronic. Obesity, immobility, poor nutrition, prior radiation or surgery, concurrent medical problems such as diabetes, hypertension, kidney disease, cardiac disease, or phlebitis can all be contributing factors to the onset of lymphedema. Those who have any of those problems should be extremely aware of the symptoms and the need for lifelong adherence to the dos and don'ts for prevention and control of lymphedema. (See Chapter 13, Breast Cancer, for further discussion of lymphedema. The same information pertains, regardless of whether your arm or your leg is affected.)

Web Pages to Check Out

www.cancer.gov: For general up-to-date information, and for clinical trials.

www.cancer.org: For general up-to-date information and community resources.

www.sbfel13.ucsb.edu: For facilities with FEL lasers.

www.yoursurgery.com: Searchable site that provides information on surgical procedures, complications, and post-operative care.

Also see Chapter 2, Searching for Answers on the Web, for more information.

RADIATION TREATMENT

More than half of all people who have cancer will receive some type of radiation treatment, either as the primary treatment or in combination with other treatments. Radiation therapy uses x-ray waves or a stream of energy particles to destroy cancer cells or to damage them so they cannot continue to multiply.

RADIATION TREATMENT HAD its beginnings in the late 1800s, when x-rays and radium were discovered. Within a few years, scientists found that x-rays were capable of damaging body tissues. Subsequently researchers uncovered the curious fact that x-rays and radium did more damage to cancerous tissue than to normal, healthy tissue. Although radiation therapy is not a new field, research and improved technology, especially in the past 25 years, have made it a major treatment for cancer. It is an area that is rapidly growing and changing, thanks to new, improved equipment, advances in the use of computers, and new uses for radiolabeled antibodies, and radiosensitizers. The intricate details of the effects of these powerful types of radiation on living cells, especially cancer cells, are still being studied.

What You Need to Know About Radiation Treatment

- Radiation is used to kill cancer cells, which are growing and dividing more rapidly than most of the normal cells around them. Sometimes radiation is used to shrink tumors before or after other treatments or to relieve symptoms.

- You may have radiation before you have an operation, during it, or after the operation. Sometimes, your radiation will be combined with chemotherapy treatments and biologic response modifiers.

- Electron beams, high-energy x-rays, radioactive isotopes, protons, and neutrons are all forms of radiation used to treat cancer. There are many advances in the manner in which radiation therapy is given, along with sophisticated instruments that are now being used in defining the area of treatment.

- If you are having external beam radiation treatment, you will probably have a treatment every weekday for about six weeks.

- When undergoing radiation, you will need to take special care of your skin in the treatment area.

- Newer high-dose internal radiation (brachytherapy) treatments have shortened the treatment time for internal radiation from several hours to several minutes and allow many patients to go home the same day.

- You may have some side effects from the treatment, depending on the area of your cancer and the method being used. Talk with your radiation oncologist and nurse about steps you need to take to minimize side effects.

Questions to Ask Your Radiation Oncologist Before You Have Radiation Treatments

- **Exactly what type of radiation treatment will I be getting?**

- **Who will be responsible for coordinating my radiation treatment? For giving my treatment?**

- **If I have questions about my radiation treatment who should I ask?**

- **Can I continue to work during these treatments?**

- **Where is the best place to have the treatments?**

- **How long will it take for each treatment? For the whole series?**

- **Will I be able to drive myself to and from my treatments?**

- **What side effects can I expect? How long will they last? Can these side effects become chronic? Are there possible long-term side effects?**

- **How do I handle side effects if they occur?**

- **What side effects should I report to the radiation oncologist?**

- How much will this treatment cost? Is it covered by insurance?

- How much of a risk is involved? Will the radiation affect the sur-rounding areas?

- Will I be having other kinds of treatment in addition to the radiation?

- Are there any alternatives to radiation treatment?

What is radiation treatment?

Radiation treatment consists of using high-level x-rays or a stream of energy particles, tens of thousands of times the amount used to produce a chest x-ray, to destroy the ability of cells to grow and divide. Both your normal cells and the cancer cells will be affected, but most normal cells are able to recover quickly. Radiation oncologists carefully limit the amount of normal tissue being treated to lessen the effects on these cells.

What does radiation treatment actually do to malignant cells?

Radiation damages DNA so that the life cycle of the malignant cell is dis-rupted and is unable to reproduce its DNA and form new cells. Radiation does not distinguish between tumor cells and healthy cells, but normal tissue is able to recover with little or no permanent damage. Cancer cells are also sometimes able to repair their DNA damage. That is why radiation must be given repeatedly on a continuing basis.

Are there different kinds of radiation treatments?

You may hear several different terms. External beam radiation (also called radiotherapy, x-ray therapy, or cobalt therapy) directs radiation from an out-side source into the body. Internal therapy (also called brachytherapy or interstitial therapy) uses a radioactive source inserted into the body near the cancer. Gamma knife (also called stereotactic radiation) delivers intense doses of radiation to small local tumors in targeted areas, such as the brain, largely sparing surrounding tissues. Intraoperative radiation is radiation given during an operation. Radiolabeled antibodies that can attach to the tumor are also being used.

When is radiation treatment used?

Radiation is used to cure or control your cancer. It is often used to preserve normal organs, to keep the body functioning fully and to avoid disfiguring surgery. It may be used along with surgery or it may be preferred to surgery if there is a pre-existing condition that makes surgery impossible or if surgery would be too disfiguring or debilitating. Radiation can be used before an operation to shrink a tumor. It may be used after the operation to stop any cancer cells that remain from growing. Sometimes, instead of having an operation, you may be given radiation along with chemotherapy drugs to destroy the cancer. Radiation is also used to treat symptoms of cancer, such as to reduce pressure, bleeding, or pain.

Is radiation treatment ever used alone?

It can be used alone in some kinds of cancer. However, many treatments for cancer include more than one form of therapy and radiation is often used in combination with surgery or chemotherapy.

Is radiation more successful with some cancers than with others?

Yes. There are many cancers where radiation has been very successful. Hodgkin's disease, breast cancer, and some lymphomas respond well to radiation, especially when the disease is diagnosed and treated in the early stages. Certain cancers of the head and neck, and cancer of the cervix have had good cure rates with radiation. Early cancers of the bladder, prostate, and skin, and certain brain and eye tumors respond well to radiation. For some cancers, radiation is better than surgery because it gives a high potential for cure with little or no loss of function. Psychologically, radiation may be a better choice in cases where surgery might change appearance.

Are there cancers that cannot be treated with radiation?

Yes. Sometimes because of the location of the tumor, previous treatment, or radiosensitivity, radiation therapy would not be the best treatment. Every kind of tissue, each kind of cancer and each patient has a different sensitivity to the effects of radiation. Different cancers spread and grow in different ways. Some kinds of radiation treatment work better for some cancers than others. The general theory in using radiation is that the radiation dose must be large enough to destroy the cancer cells but not so great as to seriously damage surrounding normal tissues. Sometimes the dose required to kill the cancer would also do permanent damage to the surrounding normal tissue. This is the major limitation in the use of radiation in the treatment of cancer and an important consideration when treatment is recommended.

Why does radiation treatment work for some people and not for others?

There are many different reasons. Sometimes the tumor is too large for the radiation to have any real effect. Or the tumor may be resistant to radiation. In some cases, the cancer may have already spread too far for the radiation treatment to be effective.

Does a tumor ever continue to grow while radiation treatment is being given?

Not usually, but it depends on what kind of cancer the person has, the exact area being treated and whether the treatment is given to cure that disease or to relieve other symptoms. Some kinds of cancer continue to grow for a short time during radiation, but then shrink or disappear altogether. Sometimes the cancer will continue to grow outside the area being treated (known as the field of treatment) even while it is shrinking where the treatment is being given. Sometimes the radiation is given because of symptoms such as pain. The treatment makes the person feel better, even though the cancer may continue to grow elsewhere. There are cases where a particular tumor in a particular person proves not to respond to radiation treatment. Unfortunately, this cannot be predicted before the treatment starts. In these instances, other forms of cancer treatment, such as chemotherapy, may be used.

What does the term *radiosensitive* mean?

This term refers to how sensitive a cell is to radiation treatment. Some kinds of cancer cells are more susceptible to destruction by radiation than others. The radiation oncologist takes this fact into consideration when planning your treatment.

What is meant by the term *radioresistant*?

This term refers to cells that are not affected by radiation treatment. Tumors are not likely to shrink when treated with it. Some kinds of cancer are more resistant to radiation treatment than others.

Are children's radiation treatments different from adults?

Yes, as is true for all radiation treatment planning, the dose of radiation is planned particularly for the person receiving it. The radiation oncologists and physicists also take into consideration the fact the child is still growing. Particular areas of concern are the bones, and organs such as the breast, thyroid, testes, or ovary, which need to be carefully shielded. Accurate markings and treatment for children are particularly important to prevent unnecessary long-term complications.

Will I have a choice as to the location where I have my radiation treatments?

Have a frank discussion with your doctor about why a specific radiation oncologist or radiotherapy department is being recommended. You may want to explore whether or not it would be advantageous for you to use a larger medical center, rather than a small hospital or private office closer to home.

A large radiation center will have several types of equipment and beams to use for treatment, whereas a smaller general hospital or private office may have less sophisticated equipment. You must weigh for yourself the advantages of convenience versus the technology and expertise a larger medical center may have to offer. Of course, your type of health insurance may limit where you receive your treatment. Radiation treatment is a science in which many advances have been made, both in technology and in application. The radiation team and their equipment will be playing an important part in your treatment. **Look for a center near you using computers to achieve three-dimensional planning and treatment.**

Will I be able to drive myself to and from my treatments?

Some people are able to drive themselves to their treatments. Others prefer to have their family and friends drive them. Often it depends on where on the body you receive the treatment, how well you feel in general and the side effects of the treatment for your specific cancer. You may decide to drive yourself for the first few weeks and then have someone else drive you towards the end of your treatment. You need to discuss these issues with your nurse and radiation oncologist before you decide on your transportation needs. If you need help with transportation, discuss it with the nurse at the radiation facility or with the discharge planner where you had your original treatment. Many times you can get rides through services in your own community, such as the American Cancer Society, the American Red Cross, or community groups like FISH, senior citizen transportation services, or civic organizations.

What kind of doctor will I go to for my radiation treatments?

Radiation is a very specialized field, requiring treatment from a team especially trained in therapeutic radiology. The radiation oncologist, sometimes called a therapeutic radiologist, heads the team and plans the treatment.

What does the radiation oncologist do?

The radiation oncologist will examine you, take your medical history and study all the pertinent information about your case to evaluate whether or not radiation treatment would be of benefit to you. The radiation oncologist is experienced in the natural history of cancers, when radiation can be used for treating cancer and how much to use to produce the best results while causing the least amount of damage to normal tissues. If you are to have radiation treatment, the radiation oncologist will decide what treatment should be used, supervise its administration and evaluate you at intervals during the course of the treatment to see whether it is working.

Who are the other members of the team?

This will vary from place to place, but there are usually several other people who work with the radiation oncologist. The *radiation physicist* and the *dosimetrist* help in calculating the dose, planning the exact treatment field, creating special blocks or shields and devising other treatment setup aids. They use a computer to plan the treatment and to calculate the distribution of the radiation dose. The *radiation therapist* (sometimes called a radiation technologist) is the person who is responsible for following the plan, getting you ready for your treatment and giving your daily treatment under the direction of the radiation oncologist. The *radiation therapy nurse* has specialized training in radiation and in helping to manage any side effects, both emotional and physical. The nurse may also coordinate complex treatment schedules and protocols. A dietitian, a physical therapist, a social worker or other health care professionals may also be part of the team's services. Before you agree to go to a facility for treatment, be sure you understand what kind of team will be treating you.

What will determine what kind of radiation treatments I will receive?

The radiation oncologist will take many factors into consideration in planning your treatment, including the cell type of your cancer, where it is located, what stage it is in, how it might spread, your age and general health, what side effects the treatment may give you, and the kind of equipment needed to carry out the treatment.

What is the difference between a rad and a gray?

Both are terms for describing radiation dosage, the amount of radiation that is absorbed by the tissues in the body. Rad stands for radiation absorbed dose and had been used for many years by radiation oncologists to describe doses of radiation. In 1985, the International Commission on Radiation Units and Measurements officially adopted the term gray as the unit of radiation dose to replace the term rad. One gray equals 100 rads or 100 centigrays (cGy). One rad equals 1 centigray.

External Radiation

What is external radiation?

When external radiation is being given, a machine directs high-energy rays or particles at the cancer and at normal tissue near the cancer.

What kind of radiation beams are used in treatment?

There are several kinds of beams used: x-rays (produced by specially designed equipment), gamma rays (emitted by radioactive materials), electrons (produced

TYPES OF RADIATION

TYPE	WHAT IT IS	WHEN USED
External radiation	Machine, such as a linear accelerator, delivers x-rays or gamma rays to tumor on or in your body. Machine is usually some distance from your body. Three-dimensional conformal radiation aims radiation in multiple directions. Intensity-modulated radiation can deliver radiation while sparing surrounding healthy tissues. Proton and neutron beam radiation uses protons and neutrons that can pass through healthy tissues with little damage but destroy tumor cells at end of their path.	Linear accelerator is most commonly used type of radiation treatment. Used for many different tumors. Low-energy beams used to treat surface tumors; high-energy or megavoltage used to treat most other cancers. Proton therapy and neutron therapy are still being investigated in clinical trials.
Brachytherapy or **internal radiation.** Also called **radium** or **cessium implant, interstitial radiation, intracavitary, intraluminal.**	Radioactive material (such as the commonly used iodine or palladium as well as gold, cessium, iridium, phosphorus) is placed on the affected tissue, or in the body near the tumor. It is either sealed in a container and inserted into a body cavity, given orally, or injected into the bloodstream or the affected area. Interstitial places implant directly into tumor. Intracavitary places it into body cavity. Intraluminal is inserted into hollow organs.	Can be used for several cancers such as uterine and prostate. Gives radiation closer to cancer cells. Can be given at higher doses than external radiation. Palladium seeds can deliver a higher dose of radiation than iodine. However, there are more side effects with palladium seeds.

TYPES OF RADIATION *(continued)*

TYPE	WHAT IT IS	WHEN USED
Gamma knife or **rotogen knife. Cyber knife.** Also called **strereotactic radiation**	Delivers intense dosages of radiation to targeted areas, largely sparing surrounding tissues.	Used for cancers in the head, mostly inside the brain.
Conformal. Also called **three-dimensional conformal radiation therapy, intensity modulated radiation therapy**	Radiation beams target cancer from several directions, after computer has mapped location.	Being used for prostate and other cancers.
Intraoperative radiation	External radiation given during an operation. Investigational treatment done at major centers and hospitals.	Being used for cancers of the breast, colon, rectum, stomach, brain, pancreas, and gynecologic organs.

by an x-ray tube), neutrons (produced by radioactive elements), protons, heavy ions (such as carbon and neon) and negative pi-meson (small, negatively charged particles). X-rays, gamma rays, and electrons are known as low-LET (linear energy transfer) radiation. Neutron beams, heavy ions, and negative pi-mesons (pions) are known as high-LET radiation. Facilities for high-LET radiation are limited.

What machines are used to give radiation treatments?

Several machines, with different characteristics, are used for giving radiation externally. They are usually defined by the amount of energy they emit. Kilovoltage and orthovoltage machines give out low-energy rays, less than one megavolt. This type of equipment has limited use today, usually only for surface skin cancers. Megavoltage equipment, such as linear accelerators and cobalt units, emits energy greater than one megavolt and directs a more precise, intense beam to a tiny target area in the body with less scattering of radiation to surrounding normal tissue. These machines, which give the maximum dose beneath the skin rather than on it, allow much higher doses of radiation to be given to deep-lying tumors. Linear accelerators are the most widely used machines, found in most hospitals as well as in some private radiotherapy offices. Cobalt units, once the most common equipment, are easier to operate and maintain than the linear accelerators, but take longer to give the treatment.

What is conformal radiation therapy?

In conformal radiation therapy, or 3-D conformal beam radiation therapy, a computer is used to make a precise map of your tumor. The radiation beams are then aimed from several directions. This will give more radiation to the tumor while reducing the damage to the normal cells. Intensity modulated radiation therapy not only aims the beams in several directions but also adjusts the strength of the beams. These treatments are being studied in clinical trials.

What is neutron therapy?

Neutron beam radiation is a highly effective form of radiation treatment that is used for treating inoperable, radioresistant tumors anywhere in the body. Because of the effectiveness of neutrons in killing tumor cells, the required dose is about one-third the dose used with other types of radiation. Usually the treatment is completed in ten to 12 treatments instead of the 30 to 40 treatments needed with other types of radiation. Side effects are similar to other forms of radiation treatment. Careful computerized treatment planning is necessary to avoid the effects on normal tissues. Boron neutron therapy delivers boron molecules into the nucleus of the cell. It selectively targets cancer cells, leaving healthy tissue unharmed.

What is proton beam radiation?

Proton beam radiation therapy, instead of using x-rays, focuses *proton beams* on the cancer. Protons are parts of atoms that cause little damage to tissues they pass through but are effective in killing cells at the end of their path. This means that proton beam radiation may be able to deliver more radiation to the cancer while reducing side effects on nearby normal tissues. Conformal proton beam radiation therapy is similar to conformal radiation but uses proton beams instead of x-rays. Proton beam radiation is expensive, and there are very few proton beam facilities in the United States at this time.

What is a gamma knife?

A gamma knife is not a knife at all—it is stereotactic radiosurgery. High-energy x-rays are used to destroy deep-seated tumors and other lesions, primarily in the brain. It can be performed with a roentgen knife or with a gamma knife, a delicate, costly device, available at a limited number of hospitals. Several advanced mechanical technologies can be combined with the roentgen knife, including CT scan, angiography and linear accelerator. Other types of similar stereotactic surgery tools are known as Cyberknife, X-knife, and Clinac. They were designed originally for whole-body use but have been modified to treat other parts of the body.

When is a gamma knife used?

The gamma knife, along with computerized treatment software, enables physicians to locate and radiate relatively small targets, such as inside the brain, with great precision.

What are hypoxic cells?

Hypoxic cells (also called anoxic cells), which can be identified by using a tool known as a hypoxic marker, are cells that have a reduced oxygen supply. Cells sensitivity to radiation depends on the amount of oxygen in their environment. The greater their oxygen supply, the more susceptible they are to radiation. If there is little oxygen (hypoxic), they are less sensitive. When cells become hypoxic, tumors become very large and their blood supply is diminished.

What is a radiosensitizer?

A radiosensitizer is a substance or a procedure that makes cancer cells more susceptible to the effects of radiation treatment. Several chemotherapy drugs are used as effective radiosensitizers.

Are radiolabeled antibodies used to treat cancer?

Yes, they are. Radioactive isotopes are attached in the laboratory to antibodies, which may be produced from cells taken from a patient's tumor. The antibodies, reinjected into the patient and carrying the radioactive isotopes, travel through the bloodstream to the tumor. The isotopes attach to the tumor and attack and kill cells.

What is a radioprotector?

Radioprotectors are chemical compounds that may be able to protect normal cells against short-term radiation damage. They allow the normal cells to repair themselves while the tumor cells are still being treated. Radioprotectors allow radiation oncologists to give higher doses of radiation than would normally be safe for the surrounding tissues. They also may eliminate the problem of second cancers sometimes induced by radiation treatment. There are radioprotective substances presently being tested in clinical trials.

Is radiation ever used before an operation?

Sometimes radiation is done before an operation to shrink the tumor. In some special cases, radiation is used both before and after an operation, with a large single dose given 24 to 48 hours before surgery, followed by radiation sometime after the operation. This is sometimes referred to as a "sandwich" technique.

Is external beam radiation ever used during an operation?

Yes. This is called intraoperative radiation therapy. The surgery is begun and after the tumor is exposed or taken out, the patient is given radiation therapy directly to the area. The operation is then completed. Intraoperative radiation can deliver a single high dose directly to the tumor, because surrounding organs sensitive to radiation, such as the skin, intestines and liver can be held aside or shielded. The exposed tumor can also be felt or seen directly, rather than viewed on a scan or x-ray. Sometimes, the intraoperative radiation is given in addition to external radiation. Intraoperative radiation therapy is being used with cancers of the breast, colon, rectum, stomach, brain, pancreas, and gynecologic organs. This treatment is being studied in clinical trials at selected institutions.

Will the radiation treatment be done right in the operating room if I am having intraoperative therapy?

It depends on the hospital. Some have an operating room in the radiation department. In others, you are moved to the radiation therapy area and then returned to the operating room. These issues are also being studied in clinical trials at selected institutions.

Is hyperthermia ever used with external radiation treatment?

Some centers are using hyperthermia—raising the temperature of the area of the tumor—before radiation treatment. Hyperthermia can be applied locally (only to the site of the tumor), regionally (to the tumor site and the surrounding tissue), or to the whole body (elevating the core temperature of the body). There is more information about hyperthermia in Chapter 11, New Advances and Investigational Treatment.

What is meant by the terms *boost* and *conedown*?

Once the regular radiation treatment is finished, an additional high dose may be given to a smaller area where the tumor was found. This is referred to as a "boost" dose in a "conedown" or reduced area. It may also be called "shrinking field technique." It is used to help avoid excess radiation to radiosensitive organs that are in the area of the tumor.

PLANNING YOUR TREATMENT

How long do external radiation treatments last?

External beam therapy is given on an outpatient basis, although sometimes it is started in the hospital and completed at a clinic or given at a radiation center. Usually the treatments are given daily, except on weekends, for two to eight weeks, depending on the reason for the treatments. For some types of cancer, you might have some time off between treatment cycles. Your radiologist will discuss your treatment plan with you.

What steps will the radiation oncologist take in planning my external radiation treatments?

The radiation oncologist will thoroughly examine you and study your x-rays, CT scans, pathology slides, hospital records, and any other pertinent information about your case. Then the radiation oncologist will discuss the recommendations on the type and duration of radiation treatment. The next step probably will be a treatment planning session.

Will I have my first treatment at my first appointment with the radiation oncologist?

Probably not, although it depends on how complex your case is. It is highly unlikely that you will have your first treatment during your first appointment, because your treatment plan needs to be set up. Treatment plans are different for each patient, so it may take several visits before your treatment actually begins. Timing of your first treatment depends on the kind of cancer you have, the kind of treatments you have already had, the stage of your particular disease, your physical condition, and how complicated your treatment plan will be.

How is the dose of radiation decided upon?

The dose varies with the size of the tumor, the extent of the tumor, the tumor type and grade and its response to radiation. Computers are used to determine the treatment volume and the distribution of the dose within that volume. Several plans may be generated from which the radiation oncologist will select the one that provides the desired distribution of the dose.

Will my normal cells be affected by radiation?

All cells are affected by the radiation, whether they are normal or malignant. The normal tissues have a greater capacity to recover from the damage induced by the radiation than do the cancer cells. The radiation oncologist plans the treatment so that normal tissues are irradiated as little as possible. In addition, some areas will be shielded and protected from the radiation.

Why is the radiation treatment sometimes given from different angles?

One way of giving the maximum amount of radiation to the tumor—and the minimum amount to normal tissue—is by aiming radiation beams at the tumor from two or more directions. The patient, or the machine, is rotated. The patient and the machine are placed so that the beams meet each other where the tumor is located. The tumor thus gets a high enough dose of radiation to be destroyed but normal tissues escape with minimum radiation effects since the beams take different pathways to reach the tumor.

Why is the radiation given over a period of time instead of all at once?

The radiation must be strong enough to kill the tumor and still allow the normal tissues to heal. The radiation oncologist determines the total radiation dose necessary and divides it into the number of single-treatment doses that will add up to the total dose by the time of the last treatment. This process, dividing the doses of radiation, is known as *fractionation*. Fractionation is a very important part of planning and delivering radiation since it affects both the tumor and the normal tissues.

What is hyperfractionation?

When a radiation oncologist gives you the regular dose of radiation in a shorter time, it is known as *hyperfractionation*, or accelerated fractionation. Hyperfractionation uses the same amount of time but increases the total dose by giving it two or three times a day, usually separated by several hours. Hypofractionation gives fewer than five doses a week. There are several studies looking at the use of these methods to plan radiation treatment to get the best results with the least damage to normal cells.

What is meant by simulation?

Simulation is another term for the session that determines your treatment plan. This is the process in which the radiation oncologist, working with the physicist, determines the area to be treated, the methods to be used, and the positions the machines will use. You will be asked to lie very still on a table below a special x-ray machine, called a simulator, which outlines the area to be treated, called the treatment field. This x-ray will be used to define the precise areas where the treatment will be directed, called the treatment port. Some simulators give three-dimensional views of the tumor and surrounding areas. Others include ultrasound devices that produce images of internal structures. Sometimes information on the contour of your body is fed into a computer to help guide the planning process. During this planning session, those areas that need to be shielded will also be pinpointed.

How long does the simulation session last?

Depending on where your radiation is going to be given and how complex the planning is, the session may last from 15 minutes up to two hours, with one hour being an average. You may find this procedure long and exhausting. If you have just had an operation, you also may find that the simulation session is uncomfortable. If you are taking pain medicine, you may wish to bring it with you for comfort. Once the simulation is completed, you will be given an appointment to start the treatment.

Will I need to remain in the same position for my treatments?
Usually, you will be lying in exactly the same position each day so that you will get the precise amount of radiation to the target site, but it will be for a much shorter time than the simulation. During the simulation process, retaining or positioning devices, such as bite blocks, casts, or molds may be designed especially for you. Headrests, armboards or handgrips may also be used to assure accurate positioning. Sometimes, especially for children, a custom-made body-cast may be used. Some of these supports actually help you to be more comfortable while you are in the correct position for the treatment. Some newer machines do not need these blocks.

How are the casts, forms, or molds made?
You are put in the position you will assume during treatment. The mold or the cast is made right on your body, using whatever material has been chosen, such as plaster, plastic, or foam. Small windows are cut into the mold to allow the beam to be directed to the precise area to be treated. The radiation oncologist can use the mold over and over again to be sure the beam is always directed to the correct area.

What is a bite block?
A bite block is a specially made dental impression that you bite into for positioning during radiation treatment. The bite block is attached to a stabilizing device to hold your head in the right place. It will be used throughout the course of your treatment to make sure you are in the same position each time the treatment is done. In addition, other devices such as plastic or plaster forms may be made to help you stay in exactly the right place.

How will I be shielded from, unnecessary radiation?
There are many safeguards to protect you from unnecessary radiation to the parts of your body that do not need treatment. All the machines are shielded so that the large amounts of radiation are given only to a specific area. The treatment field is usually lit with a light that outlines the surface through which the radiation will pass. A series of safeguards in the machine limits the radiation to this lighted area of your body. Shields, usually made out of lead blocks, are used to protect the areas of your body not needing treatment.

What parts of the body are covered with these shields?
That depends upon where the radiation is being given. Lead cases and blocks, based on your own anatomy, will be used throughout the course of your treatment to protect your vital organs and to keep you in the proper position for radiation. For example, in giving radiation to the ovary, your kidneys would be shielded. The ovaries may be shielded or moved, for instance, in women of childbearing age who are getting radiation for Hodgkin's disease. Moving the ovaries requires surgery (oophoropexy). Medicine can also be used to turn off the ovaries temporarily and keep a woman's eggs from being damaged.

What are portal films?
Portal films, sometimes also called port or beam films, are taken through the treatment machine to confirm that the treatment field and the placement of blocks are in the correct position.

How will the spot be marked where the radiation is to be given?
Once the location has been decided, the radiation oncologist or the radiation therapist will draw marks on your skin. Marking pens, indelible ink, or silver nitrate may be used. You will be asked not to wash away these markings. After your first week of treatment, you may have permanent markings put on your skin. Usually a small pinpoint tattoo is placed on the corners of the treatment field.

How is the permanent tattoo done?
Usually it is a very simple process, which substitutes for the ink markings used for your original treatments. A drop of ink is placed on your skin, and with a needle, a tiny, permanent, black dot is made on the skin itself. For sites that are most visible, such as on the face, a mask or head holder may be made of plastic and the markings placed on it rather than on the skin itself.

Is the treatment plan ever changed?
Your original radiation treatment plan may be added to, subtracted from, or changed, as the radiation oncologist feels is appropriate. Interruptions to allow for rest periods are common. There are a number of reasons for making changes as the treatment goes along. The initial estimate of the length of treatment should not be regarded as rigid. Do not be alarmed if the plan is changed. It does not mean that the disease is getting worse or that the disease has progressed.

GETTING YOUR RADIATION TREATMENT

Can I wear my own clothes while I am having a radiation treatment?
It depends upon where on your body the treatment is being given. You will probably have to undress, so wear clothing that is easy to get on and off. You might even want to bring your own robe.

What will happen during my treatment?
Depending upon where on your body the treatment is given, you may need to undress and put on a robe or a hospital gown. Then you will go into the treatment room and sit in a special chair or lie on the treatment table. The marks on your skin will be used to locate the treatment area. Special shields will be placed between the machine and the parts of your body to help protect your normal tissues and organs. The casts will be put in place to help you keep your position and to make you comfortable during treatment.

Will I be alone in the room during treatment?
The radiation therapist will leave the room and will direct the machine from the control room. You will be watched on a television screen or through a window. The machine, which is very large, will make a steady buzzing noise when the beam is on. Some treatment machines rotate around you, making noises as they move. You might hear clicking or whirring sounds. If you are concerned about what will happen in the treatment room, make sure you discuss it with the radiation therapist or the radiation oncology nurse before you begin your treatments.

What is the actual treatment like?
You will usually be in the treatment room for ten to 25 minutes. The radiation beam is turned on for one to five minutes depending upon the treatment schedule, and the tumor usually is irradiated from two or more directions. Most people say that they feel nothing while the treatment is being given. A few say that they feel warmth or a mild tingling sensation. You will feel no pain or discomfort and it will be unusual if you have any kind of sensation. If, by any chance, you do feel ill or very uncomfortable during the treatment, tell the radiation therapist. The machine can be stopped at any time. You need to remain very still during treatment, but you can breathe normally. Try to relax. Some people bring their headsets so they can listen to music in the treatment room. You may feel cold in the treatment room, since the temperature is kept cool for the proper operation of the machine.

Will the radiation I am getting make me radioactive?
No. External beam radiation does not cause your body to become radioactive. There is no need to avoid being with other people because of your treatment. You can hug, kiss, and have sexual relations with others, without any worry.

Is it safe for a pregnant woman to accompany me to my daily radiation treatments?
Basically, the levels in the radiation department waiting room should be safe for all.

Why can't the radiation therapist stay in the room with me while I am having my radiation treatment?
The machine, although it pinpoints the beam at a specific part of the body, does scatter some of the radiation. Although the amount of radiation outside the beam is tiny during any one radiation treatment session, over months and years, it could add up to a dangerous amount for the treatment personnel. It is important for the staff who is working with radiation all day long not to be exposed to these scattered beams. All personnel who are working with radiation must be carefully monitored with badges that measure their accumulated doses, so that they will be able to tell when the maximum amounts, set by the Food and Drug Administration, have been reached.

How many radiation treatments will I get?
The number of radiation treatments depends upon the kind of tumor, the extent of the disease, the type of equipment being used, the dose involved and your physical condition. The most usual schedule is to have a treatment each day for five days, with weekends off. Usually you do not have treatments on holidays since most radiation departments are not fully manned on weekends and holidays. For some kinds of cancer, a few treatments are needed over a few weeks. For other kinds, the treatments may last longer. Sometimes the radiation is given over several days. Sometimes there will be a treatment followed by several days or weeks with no treatment.

What will happen if I miss one of my treatments?
It is better if you do not miss your treatments because the treatment program is precisely planned. If you have important events that you need to attend or a vacation scheduled, you need to discuss changes with your radiation oncologist to see if it is possible to modify your appointments.

Will I have tests each time when I go for my radiation treatments?
There may be some tests during the course of the treatment, but not each time. It will depend on your treatment plan. Usually tests such as blood

counts are taken so the radiation oncologist can determine if the radiation is doing damage to other structures. Sometimes x-rays and other tests are needed to determine if the radiation oncologist should change the treatment plan.

How can the radiation oncologist tell if the radiation treatment is working?

After you have had several treatments, your radiation oncologist will begin checking you to find out how well the treatment is working. For some cancers, the radiation oncologist can use regular x-rays to see whether the tumor is shrinking and can do other tests to find out whether the radiation is causing any damage to normal cells. For instance, you may have blood tests to check the level of white blood cells and platelets, which may be reduced during treatment. Your own reports of how you feel may be one of the best indicators of the treatment's progress. You may not be aware of changes in your cancer, but you will be able to notice any decrease in pain, bleeding, or other discomforts you may have had.

What is total body radiation?

This means that the whole body is treated with radiation. It is used in preparation for bone marrow transplantation.

What is hemibody radiation?

In hemibody radiation, a large single dose of radiation is given in a single treatment to about half of the body, either the upper or lower half. It is usually used if there is large amount of local disease in the gynecologic area or the abdomen. It may also be used in cancers of the lung, esophagus, prostate, and digestive system.

Can radiation be used to treat pain?

Radiation can be used to treat cancer pain, especially in the bone. It has been shown to be useful in treating pain due to pressure on nerves, or lymphedema associated with several types of cancers including colon, rectum, kidney, ovary and other gynecologic organs, lung, and metastases in the liver, and bone. Often treatments that last two to three weeks give rapid and sustained pain relief without any major disruptions in quality of life.

Managing Side Effects from External Radiation

Does everyone have side effects from radiation?

Although the radiation beam travels directly to the area being treated, there is no way for the beam to get there without other normal tissues being affected.

Most side effects are the result of the damage done to normal surrounding cells. These normal cells will usually recover and many side effects disappear after a period of time. The extent of side effects from radiation varies greatly. The side effects range from slight in some people to severe in a few instances. They depend on the intensity of the treatment, the location of it, and your tolerance and physical condition. Some people go through their radiation treatments with very little suffering from side effects. Others do have serious problems. Most side effects begin after the second or third week of treatment. On the following chart, we have listed the most common side effects experienced by people receiving radiation treatment. It is important to understand that no one experiences all of them and that your radiation oncologists and nurses can help you minimize some of them. There is no relationship between the severity of the side effects you experience and the effectiveness of the treatment. Some people are just better able to tolerate the radiation than others.

Will I be very sick from radiation?

Most people do not get very sick from radiation treatment, although many people do complain about being tired. Most people are able to work, keep house and enjoy some leisure activities while having radiation treatment. Some people prefer to take a few weeks off from work near the end and after radiation treatments. Others work fewer hours. This is a subject you need to discuss with your doctor and your employer. You may also want to ask family and friends to help you with daily chores.

Are there any specific problems I should report to my radiation oncologist or nurse during radiation treatment?

Your radiation oncologist will tell you what problems, if any, you need to watch for and how you should deal with them. As a rule, you should contact the radiation oncologist or nurse if you have any cough, sweating, fever, or unusual pain over the course of your treatment. As soon as any of the side effects discussed in this chapter begin, you should tell your radiation oncologist, radiation therapist, or nurse so they can help you to control the problems.

Will I get sick enough from side effects to stop treatment?

Very few people are unable to complete their entire treatments because of side effects. Of course, this depends on your own physical condition, the reason for the radiation treatment, how long they are going to last and where they are being given. Sometimes the radiation oncologist will give you a rest from treatment if your blood counts are down or if you are having a severe reaction. It is very important that you discuss side effects with your healthcare team.

POSSIBLE SIDE EFFECTS OF EXTERNAL RADIATION TREATMENT

POSSIBLE SIDE EFFECT	THINGS YOU SHOULD KNOW
All Sites:	
Dry or itchy skin; redness, tanning, sunburned look; skin may become darker than normal.	■ When taking a bath or shower, use lukewarm water only, no soap, gently sponge your skin and pat it dry.
	■ Don't put salves, deodorants, powders, perfumes, bandages, medications, cosmetics, suntan lotion, or other self-remedies on your skin in the treated areas during treatment or for three weeks after treatment, unless ordered by the radiation oncologist giving you radiation. Stay away from talcum powder because it contains an abrasive; use cornstarch instead. Ask the nurse or radiation therapist to suggest what you should use during and after treatment.
	■ Keep the treated areas out of the sun. Be sure to prevent sunburn during treatment and after completion of treatment. After treatment, the use of a sun block is recommended for the skin that has been radiated to prevent further damage. You will always have to be careful about protecting the treated area from the sun. If treatment is to head and neck area, wear a wide-brimmed hat when outdoors.
	■ Heat or cold may further shock your sensitive skin. Do not apply hot or cold objects to the skin without radiation oncologist's permission. Do not use hot-water bottles, ice packs, hot-water compresses, electric heating pads, hot packs, or heating lights on treatment areas.
	■ Try not to rub, scrub or scratch the treatment area. Do not wear tight-fitting or irritating clothes over the treated areas—no corsets, girdles, belts, or other articles of clothing that leave a mark on your skin. Check with the radiation oncologist or nurse about shaving in the treatment area. Use soft shirts and loose collars if radiation is in the head and neck area.

(continued)

POSSIBLE SIDE EFFECTS OF EXTERNAL
RADIATION TREATMENT *(continued)*

POSSIBLE SIDE EFFECT	THINGS YOU SHOULD KNOW
All Sites:	
Dry or itchy skin; redness, tanning, sunburned look; skin may become darker than normal.	■ If skin blisters or cracks or become moist be sure to tell the radiation oncologist and nurse. Ask them what to do for treatment. Remember these skin reactions are temporary and should disappear within a few weeks after treatment is completed.
Changes in blood counts	Bone marrow cells are sensitive to radiation and treatment may depress their ability to function normally, especially if you've had chemotherapy or previous radiation. In some cases, if red or white cells or platelets become low, treatment may be temporarily discontinued to allow blood count to return to normal. Low white blood counts mean greater susceptibility to infection. Lowered red blood cell count may cause dizziness and fatigue. Low platelet counts can cause areas of hemorrhage, which usually appear as blotchy, bruised spots on skin.
Hair loss	Depends on the site of radiation. If hair is present within the area being treated, loss may occur. Areas affected are scalp, beard, sideburns, eyebrows, armpits, pubic area, chest, and body hair. Use an electric shaver instead of a blade razor for shaving. Hair usually grows back; starting about two months after treatment has ended. Hair may grow back a little thinner.
Feeling weak and tired; extreme fatigue	A natural reaction to radiation treatment, fatigue is one of the most common complaints. Get extra rest. Don't try to force yourself to do things if you feel tired. Limit activity. Rest for an hour or so a day; go to bed early. Get help with daily chores. Fatigue will usually begin to disappear two to three weeks after completion of radiation treatments.
Loss of appetite	See eating hints in Chapter 27, Living With Cancer.
Sluggish bowels	See hints in Chapter 27, Living With Cancer.

POSSIBLE SIDE EFFECTS OF EXTERNAL
RADIATION TREATMENT (continued)

POSSIBLE SIDE EFFECT	THINGS YOU SHOULD KNOW
All Sites:	
Sexual	Potential infertility and sexual dysfunction should be thoroughly discussed before beginning treatment. Some side effects such as being tired or feeling sick may make it difficult to have intercourse. Depending on location of treatment, may have problems having erection or orgasm, or may not enjoy sex or desire to have it. Women and men in reproductive years may become sterile. Fertility counseling before treatment is recommended. Women may have decreased lubrication or shrinking of vaginal tissues.
Head, neck, upper chest, mouth, and throat: Thick saliva	Saliva problems may begin during third or fourth week of treatment. Rinse with club soda or Peridex to refresh your mouth and thin out the saliva. Check your local pharmacy for Xerolube (put two or three drops on your tongue and work it through your mouth). Use it as often as you need it.
Dry mouth	Usually occurs near end of treatment and lasts from several months to several years. May result in serious dental problems. See a dentist experienced in this area. See hints in Chapter 27, Living with Cancer.
Sore throat, red tongue, white spots in mouth, sore mouth, unable to wear dentures, lumplike feeling when swallowing (rare)	Usually begins two to three weeks after treatment starts. Symptoms should lessen after fifth week of treatment and end four to six weeks after treatments stop. Make sure you report it to your radiation oncologist. See hints in Chapter 27, Living With Cancer.
Loss of taste or change in taste	Usually occurs during third or fourth week of treatment and may return to normal from three weeks to three months after treatment is completed. The x-rays may have destroyed some of the tiny taste buds on your tongue. Many patients prefer egg and dairy dishes instead of meat.

(continued)

POSSIBLE SIDE EFFECTS OF EXTERNAL
RADIATION TREATMENT (continued)

POSSIBLE SIDE EFFECT	THINGS YOU SHOULD KNOW
Problems with teeth	Have a complete dental examination before radiation treatment begins. Brush your teeth after every meal or snack with a soft toothbrush. Use fluoride toothpaste with no abrasives and a gentle mouthwash. Floss once or twice a day. Apply fluoride every day. If you have dentures, expect to take them out before each treatment.
Earaches	Ear and throat are closely related—sometimes ears can be affected by treatment. If your ears bother you, tell the radiation oncologist. Sometimes ear drops will be ordered. Sometimes radiation to the brain results in hardening of earwax, which can damage hearing.
Drooping or swelling skin under chin	Fatty tissue under the chin sometimes shrinks after treatment, leaving loose skin that droops or swells. If you notice lumps or small knots on side of neck or in shoulder, tell the radiation oncologist.
Breast: Dry, tender, moist, or itchy skin in armpit (axilla), under breast, or breast area.	Can occur during third or fourth week of radiation treatment. If itchiness continues, ask the radiation oncologist or nurse for something to put on it. If area is moist, be sure to talk with the radiation oncologist or nurse, who can give you something to put on it. You will probably also need to let the air get at the area several times a day. Sometimes the side effects of radiation continue for four to six weeks. Do not be alarmed, but do discuss them with your radiation oncologist or nurse. You might have a sore breast or swelling in the treatment area. Make sure you contact the radiation oncologist to report these effects. Breast swelling can continue for up to one year. Breast may become hard gradually, softening after one to two years. Skin may darken and become thick. Can last from one month to two years. If you have had a breast removed, it is best not to wear an artificial breast (prosthesis) until a month or so after radiation treatment has ended.

POSSIBLE SIDE EFFECTS OF EXTERNAL
RADIATION TREATMENT *(continued)*

POSSIBLE SIDE EFFECT	THINGS YOU SHOULD KNOW
Upper Abdomen: Nausea, vomiting, feeling of fullness	Nausea and indigestion can cause loss of appetite. Nausea can be controlled with various medications. See Chapter 27, Living With Cancer.
Lower Abdomen: Diarrhea, feeling sick to your stomach, cramps, rectal burning with bowel movement (rare), inflamed bladder (rare)	Usually occurs during third or fourth week of treatment. Varies from one to two soft stools a day to as many as ten watery stools a day. It is best to start diet with foods that are low in fiber early in treatment and not wait until you have this problem. Radiation to the rectal area may result in irritation to the anal opening. Cortisone creams will help. Cortisone suppositiories may be used for rectal spasms. Medications are available to calm bladder spasms (feeling the constant need to urinate). See Chapter 27, Living With Cancer, for further information.
Brain	Temporary swelling can cause headaches and tiredness. If severe, tell the radiation oncologist. Can be relieved with steroid-type medication. Disorientation may be experienced immediately following treatment, but a nap can usually dispel this feeling.
Long-Term Side Effects	**Bladder and Prostate Cancer:** Urgency and frequency of urination; possible bleeding; bladder that may require cauterization.
	Breast and Chest: Scarring of lung; damage to heart and its blood vessels. Breast tissue may be scarred and feel hard to the touch. Some Hodgkin's patients may be at increased risk for breast cancer.
	Head and neck: Saliva production and taste sensations altered; persistent tooth decay and gum and bone infections. Rarely, decreased range of motion in opening and closing mouth.
	Breast: Prolonged fatigue, slight deterioration of mental ability.
	Rectal: Frequent diarrhea or occasional constipation with urgency of urination.
	Esophagus: Swallowing difficulties, reflux, heartburn.

Are there some general dos and don'ts for people getting radiation treatment?

Yes, there are some general guidelines. Nearly all cancer patients having radiation treatment need to take a few extra steps to protect their overall good health and to help the treatment succeed. Later in this chapter there are comments on specific areas of radiation. But if you are getting radiation to any part of your body, here are some general recommendations:

- Be sure to get plenty of rest. Sleep as often as you feel the need. Your body will use a lot of extra energy over the course of the treatment.

- Eating well is important. If you are losing weight, tell the doctor.

- Tell the radiation oncologist about any medicine you are taking before you start treatment. If you need to take medicine, even aspirin, let your radiation oncologist know before you start. You also need to tell the radiation oncologist if your medicines are changed during your treatment. If you are a diabetic and you are eating less while you are having treatment, your insulin dose may need to be changed.

- Do not bare treatment areas to the sun during treatment. Wear sunscreen at all times.

- Expect your skin to turn a shade darker than its normal color. This is usually a temporary condition.

- Hair loss is not normally a side effect of radiation treatment unless hair is present within the area being treated. Areas that may be affected are the scalp, beard, eyebrows, armpits, and pubic and body hair.

- If you are having problems with nausea and vomiting, ask your radiation oncologist about anti-vomiting medicine and about how often you should be taking it. Read the information in Chapter 27, Living With Cancer, for more eating hints.

- If your throat or mouth is sore or you have pain when swallowing, tell your radiation oncologist. You can get a mouthwash medication that, when swallowed or gargled, can numb your mouth so you can eat more normally.

What kind of clothing should I wear?

Loose fitting clothing is the best. You need to stay away from clothes that increase friction in the treated area. Watch out for belts, girdles, high shirt collars, bras (especially underwire), heavy seams in denim or corduroy pants and shirts, and groin bands on men's briefs. Use cotton underwear because it encourages the exchange of air and decreases moisture. Women who are having radiation in the pelvic region also should not wear nylon pantyhose. It is best if you wash your clothes with soaps formulated for baby's clothes, since they have fewer chemicals in them.

What should I do if my skin gets irritated?
Because the skin in the treatment area is more sensitive, you need to take steps to try not to irritate it. Don't scrub it with a washcloth or a brush. Don't use soaps, creams, lotions, or powders on it without first checking with the nurse or radiation therapist. Don't apply anything hot or cold to it. Don't scratch or rub the skin in that area. Do not use adhesive tape, because your skin is sensitive and may come off with the tape. Don't expose it to the sun. Wear loose-fitting clothes. However, if you do see an irritation, or if your skin looks like it's going to blister or crack, be sure you report it to your radiation oncologist immediately.

Does it make any difference what kind of soap I use?
Your nurse can give you advice. Many soaps irritate sensitive skin. Wash with warm water or warm water and mild soap. If you use soap, make sure it is thoroughly rinsed from your skin. Pat your skin dry with a soft, clean towel.

Will my skin get dry or itchy?
Again, it depends on many factors. Some people will have dry skin or itchiness during treatment. Do not scratch. Trim your fingernails to prevent damaging your skin unconsciously while you sleep. If you have allergies, try to stay away from substances that normally cause itching. Use tepid water when bathing to reduce the loss of oils from the skin. Pat your skin dry. Do not rub skin with a towel or have massages. Stay away from soaps that dry the skin or have perfume or detergent in them. Do not use talcum powder because it contains an abrasive. You may use cornstarch for itchy skin, but do not use it if you have a moist reaction on your skin. If you have dry skin, it may help to drink more water and juices. Talk with your technician and nurse about medicine you might take to reduce the itchiness.

Why can't I use lotions on my dry or itchy skin?
Many products you can buy in the store, such as lotions or petroleum jelly, leave a coating that can interfere with your radiation treatment or healing. If your skin does become dry, ask the nurse or technician to suggest what you should use during and after treatment.

Why should I be careful about using hot compresses or ice packs?
Do not apply anything—hot or cold—to your skin without checking with your radiation oncologist. Skin that has undergone radiation is less resiliant to extreme temperatures. Do not use ice packs, hot-water bottles or compresses,

heating pads, heat lamps or sun lamps on your treatment areas. If you are in a cold climate, make sure you wear warm clothing. Heat or cold may further irritate your already sensitive skin.

Will my skin get darker or redder?

It depends on the condition and color of your skin, the area and kind of radiation, your age and physical condition, medicine you might be taking and the other types of treatment you may be getting. Most people do not see any changes during the first two weeks of treatment. Some people get little reaction at all. Others find their skin looks light pink or red, sunburned or tanned. Sometimes it turns a bit rough and might even peel slightly. You may find that your skin has thickened, is more leathery, or is not as flexible or as movable as before. Tell your radiation oncologist or nurse when you first note reddening of your skin. If you are taking any medications, make sure you tell the radiation oncologist and nurse what they are, so that they may decide whether they need to watch your skin more closely during treatment.

What happens if my skin feels wet?

You should report this immediately to your radiation oncologist. The area may be painful, bright red, and moist. This can happen, especially after many radiation treatments and in areas where the skin creases. This is called "weeping" of the skin, because the upper layers have shed. It is not a burn. Your radiation oncologist may stop the treatment for a while, block the affected area, or treat a different area. You will get medicine to prevent infection and to reduce the pain. The nurse will teach you how to do soaks (there are several kinds that can be used) or to apply moist dressings to the area, and how to keep the area clean. The goal will be to minimize the loss of fluids, prevent infection, and make you as comfortable as possible while the skin heals. Depending on the size of the area, it can take from one to three weeks for the skin to heal.

Do most people get severe skin reactions?

Most people do not get severe skin reactions from the radiation because of skin-sparing effects of modern equipment but people with light complexions and sensitive skin may have problems. Some patients may have severe reactions due to the need for high doses of radiation for a particular situation.

Will the skin reactions go away after my treatment ends?

Most of the skin reactions will disappear a few weeks after treatment is finished. In many cases, however, your skin in the treated areas may remain dark and thicker with less feeling. Call your radiation oncologist immediately if your skin cracks, blisters, or becomes moist after your treatment ends.

Will I be able to shave or use deodorants?
You should not use razors or deodorants in the treatment area during treatment. Shaving can result in small cuts that can become infected and can also lead to moist skin reaction. If you must shave, use an electric razor but check with the radiation oncologist, nurse, or radiation therapist. Deodorants can affect the radiation treatment. Cornstarch may be used instead of deodorant. You should wait several weeks after your treatment has ended to use roll-on deodorants or to shave skin in the treatment area because these activities may pull on the skin and cause damage.

May I go swimming while I am having my radiation treatments?
You probably can, as long as it does not cause your skin to become too dry. You need to rinse your skin well with fresh water if you have been swimming in saltwater or in a chlorinated pool.

Will I need to do anything to take care of my skin after the radiation treatments have ended?
Yes. You should use some kind of lotion or moisturizer on your skin in the treated area two to three times a day. Use a product that is not perfumed and that will wash away with water (petroleum jelly is not recommended, for instance).

Will I be able to go out in the sun after my treatment is finished?
Do not expose the treatment area to direct sunlight for at least a month after you have finished radiation. If you expect to be in the sun for more than a few minutes during that time you will need to be careful, making sure the area is covered. After that you will need to be cautious when you go out in the sun—at the beach, on a boat, working in your garden, riding in a car, at a picnic, or skiing. Protect your treated skin with a cover-up or a shirt, and a broad brimmed hat. Don't use thin, gauzy materials for your cover-up fabric. If you sit in the sun, use a sunscreen, and stay in the direct sun only for a few minutes each time. If you see any reaction, such as redness or irritation, stay out of the sun until it goes away. Do not take foolish chances. Ask your radiation oncologist or nurse about using sunblock.

Will radiation affect my blood counts?
Sometimes it may, especially if you've had chemotherapy or radiation before. The radiation oncologist may find you have low white blood cell counts or low levels of platelets, which can affect your body's ability to fight infection and to prevent bleeding. If your blood tests show these problems, you may have to go off treatment for a week or so to allow your blood counts to come back up.

Will I feel tired from the radiation?

Probably, but it depends on the individual, the dose and the area of radiation, what treatments you have had before or during your radiation, and your general physical condition. It is the most common side effect. Most people, after a few radiation treatments, find they tire easily. Some people complain of feeling tired a few hours after treatment. Some who take their treatments every day say they feel tired all the time. The stress related to the treatment plus your trips to the treatment center also can add to your fatigue. If you feel tired, you should rest and take naps if you can. The feeling may begin after three or four weeks and should gradually start to wear off within a few weeks after your treatment ends, but may last up to a year. The following should help:

- Eat when you feel tired. Sometimes a small amount of food will give you the extra energy you need.

- Rest when you feel tired. Some people get tired more quickly and need more rest during this time. Try to get more sleep at night. Rest during the day if you can. Don't feel you must keep up your normal schedule of activities if you feel tired. Don't feel guilty for resting.

- Exercise. It has been found that exercising can help to reduce your fatigue.

- Reduce your activities. You may wish to take some time off from work, or work a reduced schedule for a while.

- Don't be afraid to ask others for help. Family, friends, and neighbors can help you in shopping, childcare, housework, or driving.

Does my diet have to change during treatment?

No, your diet does not need to change, unless you are having treatments in the area of your stomach and your intestines. However, it is important for you to eat well to speed tissue repair. You should try to maintain your normal weight through a well-balanced, nutritious diet and have sufficient rest. Your appetite may be affected, but it is important that you eat properly. Good nutrition is essential also for several months after treatment. You should be careful to have both good nutrition and plenty of rest to help your body repair and replace the normal cells. Radiation oncologists have found that patients who eat well can better withstand both their cancer and the side effects of treatment. Try also to keep emotional stress to a minimum. There is further information and diet tips in Chapter 27, Living with Cancer.

Can I continue my usual activities during treatment?

Continue as much of your normal activity as you can without feeling tired and strained. Many people find they can continue to work during the treatment period. Others find they can continue some activity, but less than the normal amount. This is a time to listen to your body and to take good care of yourself. In addition, your radiation oncologist may suggest that you limit some activities, such as sports, that might irritate the area being treated.

Does radiation treatment put patients at risk for lymphedema?
Radiation treatment may increase your risk for lymphedema, or swelling in your arms and legs, especially if you have had surgery or chemotherapy. This is true in some types of cancer, including breast cancer, malignant melanoma of the arms or legs, prostate cancer (if whole pelvic radiation is given), soft tissue and bone sarcomas, and some gynecologic cancers. There is more information on lymphedema in Chapter 8, Surgery.

Will radiation treatment affect my emotions?
It is common for people who are having treatment for cancer to feel upset, depressed, afraid, angry, frustrated, alone, or helpless. These feelings are due to many things, including the changes in their everyday living, their fear about cancer, or the fact that they can't do everything they could before. Radiation treatment may add to these emotions, either because of fatigue or from the strain of traveling to radiation treatments every day. However, the treatment itself does not cause mental distress. Some people tell us they feel depressed or nervous during their treatments. You may want to ask your radiation oncologist or nurse about meditation or relaxation exercises that you can use during treatment. For example, some people find it soothing to listen to audiocassettes. If you are having some problems with coping, it may be useful for you to talk about them to someone—a nurse, a social worker, a good friend, or a chaplain. Or check with your radiation oncologist's office about support groups that might be run in the facility where you are having your treatment or by an organization such as the American Cancer Society or Cancer Care.

Other Side Effects in Head and Neck Area

Is there anything special I should know about getting radiation in the head and neck area?
There are several things you should know about the changes in your system if you are getting radiation to any area of the head and neck—including the brain, mouth, throat, neck, and upper chest.

- Be sure you check with a dentist experienced in treating cancer patients before you begin radiation treatment, so that any dental work needed can be taken care of.
- You may experience some soreness in the area of the mouth and throat.

- You may notice that your tongue is red and that there are white spots in your mouth. You might have a hard time swallowing, feel pain or a lump in your throat, or feel your food sticking in your throat due to irritation of the tissues in the area of the throat and swallowing tube (esophagus). You might not be able to eat with your dentures. All of these are temporary side effects that usually begin two to three weeks after treatment starts and usually begin to decrease after the fifth week of treatment. They usually end some four to six weeks after treatments finish. Of course, you should report any of these problems to your radiation oncologist.

What can I do to minimize symptoms?

- Smoking and drinking irritate your mouth and throat, especially during treatment. Don't use tobacco, alcoholic beverages, or hot, spicy, rough, or coarse foods like pepper, chili powder, nutmeg, and vinegar, since they can irritate your mouth.

- Stay away from coarse foods such as raw vegetables, dry crackers, chewy meat, and nuts.

- Have liquid rather than solid foods.

- Don't eat sugary snacks. With the production of less saliva, sugar promotes more tooth decay than usual.

- Don't breathe in strong fumes, such as paints and cleaning solutions.

- Brush your teeth and tongue with a soft, narrow toothbrush within 30 minutes after you eat and at bedtime. Dip the brush bristles into hot water to make them softer. If you regularly use dental floss to clean between your teeth, be gentle so that you do not damage the gums. Massaging your gums can help to improve circulation, clean the teeth and stimulate saliva.

- Use a fluoride toothpaste with no abrasives. You may need to use a solution or tablet after brushing to show whether you have missed any plaque. Rinse your mouth well with a solution of salt and baking soda after you brush (2 tablespoons of salt and/or baking soda in a pint of water). Do not use commercial mouthwashes, since they contain alcohol and may cause burning. If you wear dentures, soak them in diluted hydrogen peroxide (and rinse with water) at least weekly to clean. Apply fluoride every day. Moisturize your lips with petroleum jelly, or aloe gel.

- Don't shave with razor blades in the areas being treated. You may shave with an electric razor. You may find that whiskers, sideburns, eyebrows, head hair, hair in your armpits, or chest hair fall out temporarily, depending on the dose of radiation and the area being treated. Some men with a great deal of hair on their chests who have chest radiation will find that the hair in the treated area falls out within a few weeks. It may grow back in two months after the treatment is ended, sometimes a little thinner than originally.

- Stay out of the sun, wear a cap, wide-brimmed hat or scarf when you are outside if you are having radiation in the area of your head. Don't use any sunblocking or suntanning products on your skin during the course of your treatments, without discussing it with your radiation oncologist or nurse.

- Don't use starch in your collars if you are having radiation in the head and neck area. Wear soft shirts and loose collars to prevent irritation to the treated area.

- You may have earaches caused by hardening of the wax in your ears.

- You may have swelling or drooping of the skin under your chin. There may also be changes in your skin texture.

- See Chapter 27, Living With Cancer, for hints about eating during this period.

Why do I need to see a dentist before I begin radiation treatments to the head and neck area?

You need to take special care of your teeth and mouth before, during, and after radiation because the treatments can affect your teeth. You should visit your dentist, or a dentist who has had experience treating persons who have had head and neck radiation before your treatment starts. The dentist will probably take x-rays, examine your mouth, and try to do any major work that is necessary or will become necessary within the next year. Ask your dentist to discuss with your radiation oncologist any dental work you need before treatments begin. If your dental work includes taking out teeth, it must be done at least ten days before you start your radiation treatment. The dentist will also explain the special care you should take to protect your teeth and mouth. Your dentist will probably want to see you often during the time you are having treatment. Young people, especially, need to be closely watched to ensure that the radiation does not lead to abnormal development of teeth that are still in the formative stages.

Will I be able to wear my dentures?

You may notice that your dentures do not fit as well. This may be due to swelling of your gums caused by the radiation. You may need to stop wearing them until the radiation treatments are finished. Discuss this with your radiation oncologist, nurse, and dentist. It is important not to let your dentures cause gum sores that might become infected.

Is there anything I can do for my dry mouth?

Dry mouth is a difficult side effect for people who are having radiation to the head and neck area. Your glands will be producing much less saliva than usual, making your mouth feel dry. It may be helpful to suck on ice chips and sip drinks, such as water or carbonated beverages, often, throughout the day. Sugar-free candy, sucking lemon drops, or chewing gum may also help. You will probably need to increase the amount of liquids you drink and perhaps use a humidifier. You may wish to carry a water bottle so you can rinse frequently. There are also a number of artificial saliva products that may help. These products have different properties, are semiliquid or gel, come in spray or liquid forms, and are usually used after rinsing, brushing, flossing, and at bedtime. There are also moisture-stimulating toothpastes, and chewing gum that can be used to stimulate saliva. Talk to the nurse or radiation oncologist about these products. The radiation oncologist also can prescribe drugs that help stimulate the flow of saliva.

Will my loss of saliva be permanent?
If you had a low flow of saliva before you began radiation treatment, you may be left with permanent dryness. Younger people are more likely to recover some of their saliva flow than are older people. Loss of saliva flow makes it even more important to take special care of your teeth, both during and after treatment.

Will my taste buds change?
You may find that you have a loss of taste or change in the way foods taste as a result of radiation to the head and neck area. This usually happens during the third or fourth week of treatment. It may return to normal by three months after treatment. You might not recover all your taste sense. The radiation may harm some of the tiny taste buds on your tongue. Salty and bitter are usually most severely affected.

What can I do for a sore mouth?
Some people who have radiation treatments to the head and neck area suffer from painful sores or swelling of the membranes in their mouths. The soreness may appear in the second or third week of radiation therapy, and decrease from the fifth week on. It will probably end a month or so after your treatment ends. It may make eating, speaking or swallowing difficult. Ask your radiation oncologist or nurse about rinsing with baking soda and water to keep the area clean and to prevent infection. Also ask about relief measures such as medicines that will numb the area so that you will be able to eat and swallow. You may need to take antibiotics for infections resulting from mouth sores or pain pills to relieve the discomfort.

Will I lose my hair as a result of my radiation treatment?
It depends on where the radiation treatment is being given. For instance, if your scalp area is being treated, you will lose your hair on your head. You can

also lose your beard or eyebrows if you are being treated in those areas. Usually hair begins to grow back two months after you have finished treatment, but it might grow in thinner. If you are going to lose the hair on your head, you might wish to buy a hairpiece before you begin treatment. See Chapter 10, Chemotherapy, for information on wigs.

What do I need to do to protect my skin if I lose my hair?

The area may be somewhat tender. If your scalp is affected, you may want to cover your head with a hat, turban, or scarf while you are in treatment. Of course, when you are outside you should wear a protective cap or scarf. If you plan to buy a toupee or a wig, try to do it before your hair falls out so you can match your color and style. You should use a mild shampoo (baby shampoo is the mildest) and use a cool setting on your hair dryer. For more information on selecting wigs and hairpieces, see Chapter 10, Chemotherapy.

Will my hair grow back?

Usually your hair will grow back. The amount of hair loss will depend on how much radiation you received and the type of radiation treatment you had. Your hair may not start to regrow for a few months following the end of your treatment. It may have a different texture, or color and may be thinner than before.

Other Side Effects in Breast and Chest Area

Is there anything special I should report if I am getting radiation in the breast and chest area?

You should watch for dry, tender, moist or itchy skin in the area of your armpit and under your breast or breast area. If your skin becomes inflamed or weepy, if you run a fever, notice a change in the color or amount of mucus when you cough, or feel short of breath, be sure to tell the radiation oncologist immediately.

Will I have soreness in my breast from radiation treatments in that area?

Some patients who get radiation treatment after a lumpectomy or mastectomy have sore breasts or swelling in the treated area. These side effects should disappear in four to six weeks, but sometimes swelling may persist for a year or more. It is a good idea to go without a bra or wear a very soft one during the time you are having radiation treatment in this area. It will help reduce the irritation to your skin. Your skin may stay slightly darker, and the pores may continue to be enlarged and more noticeable.

Will I have the same feelings in my breast as before the treatment?
Some women say the skin on their breast is more sensitive after radiation treatment while others say it is less sensitive. The skin and fatty tissue on your breast may feel thicker and leathery. Your breast may be firmer or harder than before. Although many women have little change in size, some women's breasts may be larger or smaller after radiation treatments.

What is radiation pneumonitis?
Radiation pneumonitis is an inflammation of lung tissue, usually resulting from radiation to the lung. It normally occurs several months after treatment is finished. People who have had a lung problem, such as bronchitis, are more apt to get it. It can be painful and may cause coughing or shortness of breath. It usually lessens in time, although for some people, there may be permanent scarring.

Other Side Effects in the Abdominal Area

Will I have any other side effects from radiation in my abdominal area?
You may have some problems with an upset stomach, a feeling of fullness, vomiting, or nausea. Depending on where the radiation is being given, you may also have diarrhea, or cramps. Rarer side effects include rectal burning with your bowel movements or an inflamed bladder. If you are going to have treatment in your digestive area, it is best to start a diet with foods that are low in fiber early in your treatment cycle and not wait until you have diarrhea. You need to discuss these side effects with your radiation oncologist or nurse. You also may need medicines prescribed to help you relieve these problems. See Chapter 27, Living with Cancer, for more information on managing these side effects.

Is there anything special I should do if I am getting radiation in the pelvic area?
If you are getting radiation therapy to any part of the area between your hips, known as the pelvic area, you may experience some of the problems discussed in the question directly above. You may also find that you need to urinate often or that it might be uncomfortable to urinate. Increasing the amount of fluids you drink may help you. Talk to your radiation oncologist about medication that might help you with this problem.

Sexual Side Effects

Will I have problems having sex after my radiation treatments?
It depends on where the radiation was given, the dose, and the duration. Both men and women who have had radiation treatments can have problems—some

temporary, some permanent. For instance, they may not enjoy sex as much, may not desire to have sex, or have some problems in having an erection or an orgasm. Other side effects, such as being tired or feeling sick may make it difficult to have sexual intercourse. Women who receive radiation treatments in the pelvic area also may have decreased lubrication and some shrinking of vaginal tissues. Men who have radiation in the pelvic area can have reduced sperm production or become sterile.

Male Sexual Problems

Can I father a child while having radiation treatments?
It depends on the area being treated and the dose of radiation being given. If the radiation area includes the testes, your sperm will be reduced both in number and in strength and may have genetic damage. Since you can still father a child, make sure you discuss the use of birth control methods with your radiation oncologist.

Will I become sterile from radiation treatment?
This will depend on the dose of radiation and the location of treatment. If your sexual organs are in or close to the field of radiation, the treatment may cause sterility. Radiation therapy for cancers of the prostate, testicle, and penis can affect sterility since the body often stops producing sperm. Sperm production can begin again within six months to several years after treatment, although radiation therapy close to sexual organs can sometimes cause permanent sterility and possible genetic damage. Be sure to check with your doctor about whether sterility is a possible side effect so that you can make decisions about how you wish to deal with that possibility.

What can be done if the doctor says I may become sterile?
You may want to explore the possibility of having semen frozen and stored at a sperm-banking facility so that you may be able to have children later on.

Does radiation therapy cause erection problems?
It can, especially if you had erection problems before having radiation. Some men find there is no change in their ability to have erections. The one-third of men who do have a change, find that it develops gradually over the year or two following radiation. Radiation can affect erection by damaging the arteries that carry blood to the penis. As the area heals, internal tissues can become scarred, and the walls of the arteries may lose some elasticity, causing the erection to be less firm. Radiation may also hasten hardening of the arteries, which may narrow the pelvic arteries. Men who have high blood

pressure or have been heavy smokers may be at higher risk for erection problems because of prior damage to the arteries.

Should I have my testosterone level checked?

If you notice that you have problems with erection or lose the desire for intercourse, discuss with your doctor the possibility of having a blood test to check your testosterone level. You may need to take replacement testosterone. (However, if you have prostate cancer, you will not be able to take replacement testosterone.)

Is painful ejaculation caused by radiation?

After radiation to the pelvic area, some men ejaculate only a few drops of semen. Toward the end of radiation treatments, you may feel a sharp pain as you ejaculate. The pain results from irritation in the urethra; it should fade within several months after treatment. If it does not, see your radiation oncologist.

Will my erection problems be permanent?

Many of the sexual problems that men experience after cancer treatment are temporary. Pain that occurs with erection after radiation usually lessens or disappears. One way of judging whether the change is permanent or temporary is to test if your reactions vary depending upon circumstances. Do you have trouble getting or keeping an erection every time you have sex? Are you able to do better when you stimulate yourself? Yes answers indicate that the problem may be temporary. If your sleep erections are firm and long lasting, you will know that physically you function well and the problem probably lies with stress or psychological pressures. There is more information on sexuality in Chapter 14, Prostate Cancer and Other Male Cancers, and Chapter 27, Living with Cancer.

Female Sexual Problems

Will I continue to get menstrual periods during radiation treatment to the pelvic area?

It depends upon the dose of radiation, where in the pelvic area it is given, length of the treatment, and how close you are to menopause. Your periods may stop temporarily, especially if you have a lower dose of radiation or your ovaries are moved and shielded. Often, however, your loss of periods will be permanent.

POTENTIAL SEXUAL SIDE EFFECTS OF RADIATION TREATMENT

SIDE EFFECT	WHO AFFECTED, FREQUENCY AND TREATMENT
Infertility or sterility	Often in men and women if treatment is in pelvic area. Fertility counseling, sperm banking, blocking, or moving and shielding of ovaries.
Dryness in vagina	Often in women with treatment in pelvic area. Use of vaginal lubricant.
Reduced size of vagina	Often in women with treatment in pelvic area. Stretching walls of vagina three times each week through intercourse or by using a dilator.
Painful intercourse	Often in women with treatment in pelvic area. Use of lubricant, changing positions, relaxing vaginal muscles.
Weak orgasm or trouble reaching orgasm	Often. Practice teasing techniques; delaying orgasm until excited.
Erection problems	Often. Check for hormone imbalance; use of medications or implants.
Low sexual desire	Often. Check for depression, anxiety, pain, or other causes. Sexual counseling.

What changes will I notice if my periods stop?

The changes will probably be more abrupt and intense than those of people who have natural menopause. You may have hot flashes, dryness or irritation of your vagina, among other possible symptoms. If you have already gone through menopause, you may notice little or no change.

Will my vagina be swollen?

If you have radiation in the pelvic area, the sensitive tissues in the area of the vagina may become pink and swollen. Your vagina may feel tender. After treatment is finished, there may be less elasticity in the vaginal area. The tissues of the vagina may develop scar tissue, narrowing the passage and making it difficult for you to have a vaginal exam or intercourse. Your radiation oncologist or nurse will discuss vaginal stimulation, which usually begins about two weeks after treatment is completed to help prevent the narrowing of the muscles and tissues that form the walls of the vagina.

How is vaginal stimulation done?

It can be done either with intercourse or with the use of a dilator. Intercourse and the physical movement associated with lovemaking will stretch the vaginal tissues and muscles and help prevent scar tissue formation. If you are sexually active and have intercourse at least three times per week, you will probably not need to use a dilator.

What is a dilator?

A dilator is a tube, usually made out of plastic that is used to keep the vagina open. It comes in different sizes and you may need to change sizes as your vagina relaxes. Your radiation oncologist or nurse may supply you with a dilator, or give you a prescription for one. You will probably be told to use the dilator three times a week unless you have sexual intercourse at least three times a week.

How do I use a vaginal dilator?

You apply a water-soluble lubricant to the rounded end of the dilator, lie on your back in bed with your knees bent or by standing with one foot up on a step or the toilet. Insert the rounded end of the dilator into the vagina gently and as deeply as you can without causing discomfort. Let it stay in place for 10 to 15 minutes. Withdraw and clean the dilator with hot, soapy water, rinsing it well. Do not be alarmed if slight bleeding or spotting occurs following dilator use, especially the first few times you insert it. If you are unable to insert the dilator easily, have pain or increased bleeding, check with your radiation oncologist or nurse.

What can be done to prevent pain during intercourse?

There may be several causes of pain—the sexual activity itself, the shortening or narrowing of the vagina, or the lack of lubrication. Spread a generous amount of water-based lubricating gel around and inside the entrance of your vagina before having intercourse or use a lubrication suppository that melts during foreplay. There are also vaginal moisturizers that you can use to keep your vagina from becoming dry and irritated. Make sure you are fully aroused before you have intercourse. It is only when you are highly excited that your vagina expands to its fullest length and width and the walls produce lubricating fluid. Let your partner know if any kind of touching causes pain. Show your partner the positions that are not painful. Try different positions, such as kneeling over your partner with your legs on either side of the body or facing each other while lying on your side.

Is there a way to teach myself to relax my vaginal muscles?
Once you have felt pain during intercourse, without realizing it, you may tighten the muscles that ring the entrance to the vagina each time you have intercourse, making it more painful. If you become aware of these muscles, you can learn to control them by doing Kegel exercises. These are the same muscles that control your flow of urine. Try starting to urinate, then shutting off the flow for a few seconds, and starting again. Notice that when you relax the muscles, the urine starts to flow again. Practice tightening and relaxing these muscles when you are not urinating. To exercise the muscle, tighten to the count of three and then relax. You should practice this tightening and relaxing action ten times, one or two times a day. Then during lovemaking, when you are both aroused and ready for intercourse, take a few seconds to tense your vaginal muscles and then let them relax as much as possible before penetration. If you feel any pain, you can signal your partner so you can stop a moment to tighten up and then relax your vaginal muscles.

Are there any medications that would be helpful in making me relax my vaginal area?
Medications, including antispasmodics and analgesics, are sometimes used to help relax the body before intercourse and prevent the tightening of the pelvic muscles. You should consult your doctor or a sex therapist to determine if medication might be helpful to you.

Is it unusual to have bleeding after intercourse?
Radiation to your vagina can make the lining more fragile. You may find some light bleeding after intercourse. It may be several months after your radiation treatments are completed before full healing takes place.

Can I have sexual relations if I am having radiation treatment in the pelvic area?
It depends. Some radiation oncologists advise women not to have intercourse during the treatment period. Other women find that intercourse is painful. However, some radiation oncologists encourage sexual activities to prevent the narrowing of the walls of the vagina. You need to discuss this with your doctor.

Can I get pregnant during radiation treatment?
If you are of childbearing age, you need to be aware that there are serious risks to becoming pregnant while you are having radiation treatments. Most radiation oncologists feel you should take precautions not to become pregnant because there is a high risk of fetal death, malfunction, or retardation.

If you are already pregnant, you need to discuss this with the radiation oncologist before starting treatments.

Will I be able to have children after having had radiation treatments?
It depends on where the radiation has been given, the dose of the radiation, how long the ovaries were exposed to it, and your age. Some women are sterile temporarily. For others, it is a permanent condition. It may be possible to use surgery to move the ovaries out of the radiation field (this is called *oophoropexy*), thus shielding them, or to use drugs to temporarily turn off the ovaries. Women may be able to have children after these procedures. There is more information about pregnancy after cancer treatment in Chapter 27, Living with Cancer.

Internal Radiation or Brachytherapy

What is internal radiation?
The radiation oncologist places a radioactive material, such as iridium, directly into or on the area to be treated. The material can be implanted in tissues or inserted into body cavities, administered orally, or intravenously. The materials are absorbed or metabolized by the body. Internal radiation, or brachytherapy as it is often called, allows the radiation oncologist to give a higher dose of radiation to the area, while not harming most of the normal tissue around it. Because the radiation is concentrated in the tumor, it is possible to expose cancer cells to a higher dose during a shorter period of time than would be possible with conventional radiation sources. It can also be called a radium implant, interstitial, or intracavitary radiation.

What kinds of materials are used in internal radiation?
Most commonly, the substances include iridium, cesium, gold, cobalt, iodine, and phosphorus. The devices containing the radioactive materials come in several different forms, such as wires, ribbons, tubes, capsules, and needles. Sometimes a seed gun is used to inject grains or seeds into the area of the tumor. The radiation oncologist chooses the best source according to the site to be treated, the size of the tumor, and whether the implant is temporary or permanent.

Questions to Ask Your Radiation Oncologist about Internal Radiation

- **Why is internal radiation being recommended?**
- **What kind of radioactive material will you be using?**
- **How will the radioactive material be put in my body?**
- **Will I need surgery to have radiation implanted?**
- **Will I need anesthesia? Will it be local or general?**

- **Will I need to be in the hospital for this procedure? For how long?**
- **Will I have to stay in bed during this time?**
- **Will I be able to have visitors? Will there be any restrictions on the visitors?**
- **Will the implant be permanent or temporary? Will I need anesthesia when the implant is removed?**
- **Will I be radioactive while the implant is inside me? For how long?**
- **What side effects should I expect?**
- **When will it be safe to have intercourse?**
- **When will I be able to get back to my normal routine?**

How is interstitial radiation done?

Using a computer to define the area and calculate the dose needed, and a CT scan, MRI, or ultrasound to help guide the placement, the oncologist implants a container that will hold the radioactive materials within or near the cancerous tissue. The container is then filled with radiation seeds. After the required radiation dose has been given, usually in one to six days, the implant usually is removed, although some implants stay in permanently.

What is high-dose-rate brachytherapy?

High-dose-rate brachytherapy uses the same procedure as interstitial radiation but higher dose implant materials. It may also be referred to as high-dose-rate remote brachytherapy or remote brachytherapy. The radioactive materials stay in usually for five to 15 minutes, for each of three to ten treatments. You are usually able to go home after each treatment, which are usually given a week apart.

What is ultrasound seeding?

Many times, the implant is positioned with the help of ultrasound along with the computer. For instance in prostate cancer, the doctor implants radioactive material directly into the tumor with long needles. Ultrasound scans are first used to create a map of the prostate, to calculate the exact number of seeds needed for complete coverage and to ensure accurate placement. A treatment-planning computer constructs the implant model so that the seeds will be distributed properly. When the seeds are being placed, images on the ultrasound screen allow the doctor to see the needle's exact position in the prostate.

What is intracavitary radiation?

A container is put into a cavity of the body, such as your uterus or vagina, as close to the tumor as possible. The radioactive material is placed in the container, which is usually removed after the dose of radiation has been given (within 48 to 72 hours). Intracavitary radiation is most often used in the treatment of gynecologic cancers.

Is the radioactive material ever swallowed?
Some radioactive material comes in liquid form and may be swallowed or injected into the bloodstream or into a body cavity. When the radioactive substance is injected, it is not sealed in a container.

What is intraluminal radiation therapy?
The radiation is delivered to a hollow organ, such as the esophagus. A specially designed tube or container is placed in the inner open space (or lumen) of the organ. Radioactive seeds are placed in the tube near the cancer.

Will I need to have anesthesia for my internal radiation treatment?
It depends upon which type you have. For most of the implants, you will need to be in a hospital or a major radiation center and will get either local or general anesthesia, so that the radiation oncologist can place the substance into your body.

What is meant by the term *afterloading*?
If the container for the radioactive substance is positioned in your body through an operation, the radioactive material is inserted into the container at a later time, after the proper position has been checked. That is known as afterloading. In some institutions, specialized equipment allows for remote afterloading (high-dose-rate brachytherapy). A catheter may be placed in the body. The radiation is delivered through the catheter that is connected to the treatment machine. A computer is used to direct the radiation source through the tubing to the area of the cancer.

Will I need to be in a hospital if I am having the treatment using afterloading?
It depends on the type of treatment you are having. For some kinds of cancer, you will need to stay in the hospital for a few days. If you are in a center that is using the high-dose remote afterloading technique, you will probably be able to go home after you have spent an hour or two in the recovery room.

How long is the implant left in the body?
It depends upon the kind of cancer, where it is located, the amount of radiation that the radiation oncologist needs to treat you and the type of implant being used. Some implants with a low dose rate may be left in for from one

to seven days. Others with a high dose rate may be removed after 15 minutes. Still others remain in the body permanently.

Are the high-dose implants done in a different way?
Hollow tubes, called catheters, are placed in or near the tumor. The catheters are connected to the delivery system and the radioactive material is given via catheter for the prescribed period of time. This allows the radiation oncologist to give a high dose of radiation over a short period of time to an exact tumor site within the body.

Are some implants left in permanently?
There are some implants, such as prostate seeds, that are left in permanently. Usually these are put into the body through a hollow needle, hollow tube, or a seed gun. They lose some energy each day. You usually have to take some precautions for a few days after you have had the treatment.

Will the implant spread radiation to others?
It depends on the implant. Usually if the implant is in a sealed source, such as a needle or a hollow applicator, neither you nor any of your body excretions, such as blood, urine, or stool, become radioactive. Items you touch, such as bed linens, also do not become radioactive. However, if your treatment uses radioactive material that is unsealed, your urine and stool may contain some radioactive materials and extra care will be taken.

Will I get regular hospital care when I have a radioactive implant?
It depends on what kind of implant and where it is. If it is not in a sealed source, your hospital care may be a bit different than usual. There may be a lead shield close to your bed to protect hospital personnel. Nurses and other hospital personnel may be limited as to how long they can remain in your room and how close they can come to you and your bed. You might notice that they come into your room more often but for shorter periods of time. Your bed may be close to the window wall. The nurses will probably not come close to the side of your bed, but will talk with you from the foot of the bed or from the doorway. They will probably be wearing film badges to measure radiation. Housekeeping personnel may be changing your linens less often or only when soiled. Naturally, the restrictions for hospital personnel depend upon what part of your body the implant is in, the kind or radioactive material used, and the dose. Pregnant nurses may not be allowed to take care of you. Most times, you will be assigned to a single room. Although personal contact is limited because of the radiation implant, you should not hesitate to call a nurse if you need one for any reason.

What if I need help?

Your bedside table, call bell, and television controls will be put within easy reach so that you can be as self-sufficient as possible. If you need help, you should ask for it. But you will notice that the nurse will work quickly, concentrating on doing what needs to be done in the shortest period of time possible.

Will I be allowed to have visitors?

It depends on what hospital you are in. Most will restrict visitors to persons over 18 years old and persons who are not pregnant. Visitors are usually asked to sit at least six feet from your bed. They will probably have to limit their visits to less than 30 minutes each day.

Will I be in pain as a result of my implant?

Most of the time you will not have severe pain. However, you might be uncomfortable, especially if you have an applicator containing the radioactive material. If you have an applicator in the gynecologic area, you may have some low back pain. Depending on the location of your implant, you may have to stay in bed and restrict your movements so that the radiation source will not become dislodged and harm sensitive organs. You may be given sleeping pills or other medication to relax you. If you feel you need medicine for pain, be sure to let your nurse and radiation oncologist know.

Is it dangerous for me to touch the implant while it is in me?

It is important that you do not touch the implant while it is in your body. Although the container is sealed, touching it could cause radiation damage to your skin.

Will I have any side effects from this treatment?

If you have had general anesthesia, you may feel drowsy, weak, or nauseated for a short time after your operation. Be sure to tell your nurse if you have any burning, sweating, or other unusual symptoms. Depending on what kind of implant you have had and where it is located in the body, there may be some other side effects.

Will I be able to eat while the radiation implant is in my body?

Yes, you will usually be given a special diet with lots of fluids. The nurses will place the food where you can manage it without having to move your body. If your implant is in the vaginal area, you will be given pills to discourage bowel movements while the applicator is in your body. If you have an implant in the head and neck area you may have difficulty eating and talking.

How is the implant removed?

This is usually done right in your room. You will be given some pain medication about half an hour before the radiation oncologist comes in to take out the applicator. Once the implant is removed, you will then be allowed to get out of bed. Usually the nurse will help you move around until you are steady on your feet.

Is internal radiation used alone?

Sometimes internal radiation is used alone. Other times it is used in addition to external-beam radiation, either before or after the internal radiation treatment.

COSTS OF RADIATION TREATMENTS

How expensive is radiation treatment?

Radiation treatment, with its complex equipment and sophisticated staff, can be very expensive. The cost will depend on the type, the complexity, and the number of treatments that you will have. Although most health insurance policies pay for radiation treatments, you need to talk with the staff of the radiation department to find out how much of the cost will be covered under your specific policy.

What items are included in the cost?

You will probably see costs for a variety of items, such as initial consultation, treatment planning, simulation, dosimetry calculations, and weekly treatment fees.

Do Medicare and Medicaid pay for radiation treatments?

Both Medicare and Medicaid cover the major portion of the cost. For Medicare, if the radiation oncologist is a participating physician (one who has agreed to accept the charges established by Medicare), the physician will be paid 80 percent of the recognized charge. You will pay the other 20 percent. If you have a Medigap insurance policy, it will usually cover the 20 percent copayment. Be sure you are not confused by the "billing balance" that some radiation oncologists add to your copayment bill. For instance, if Medicare pays $100 as the "reasonable" charge, a nonparticipating radiation oncologist may charge $120 for the procedure. Medicare would pay the patient or physician $80. If you pay the $20 copayment, $20 will remain as the billing balance. You should be aware that some states have legislated against the practice of balance billing.

Web Pages to Check Out

www.cancer.gov: For general up-to-date information, and for clinical trials.

www.cancer.org: For general up-to-date information and community resources.

www.radiologyinfo.org: Explanations of all types of radiation, how procedures work, how to prepare for procedures.

www.youngwomenshealth.org: Information for young women on fertility and cancer treatment.

Also see Chapter 2, Searching for Answers on the Web, for more information.

Ten

CHEMOTHERAPY

Most people are afraid of chemotherapy, and especially of its side effects, fearful that the cure is worse than the disease. But chemotherapy has changed and so has the treatment for its side effects. Not all who have chemotherapy get nauseated or lose their hair. Although it's a difficult treatment to get through, most will tell you that it is worth the effort. By knowing what to expect and what to do if you have a problem, you will be able to deal better as you proceed through treatment.

CHEMOTHERAPY MEANS THE use of drugs to treat cancer. To most people, chemotherapy is frightening because of the possible side effects caused by the use of the potent drugs needed to disrupt the cancer cells' ability to grow and multiply. Over the past several years, great progress has been made, both in preventing some of chemotherapy's most serious side effects and in lessening and minimizing those that do occur. Chemotherapy treatment also has proven itself to be very effective—more than 50,000 cancer patients are being cured each year with cancer drugs, used alone or combined with other kinds of treatment.

What You Need to Know About Chemotherapy

- Your chemotherapy may be given in several ways—in pill, capsule, or liquid form, by applying it to the skin, by injecting it into a muscle, in a vein, or through an internal or external pump.

- Often a variety of drugs are given. Each drug acts on the cell in its own way and at different times in the cell cycle.

- How fast your cancer cells will be destroyed by the drugs varies with the medication and the type of cancer.

- You will be given your chemotherapy drugs one at a time, in sequence or in combination. Your treatment may be weekly, monthly, or even daily. You normally have some rest time between treatments, to give your normal cells a chance to rebuild and regrow.

- Sometimes the treatment lasts for long periods of time—up to one or two years. Some people may be on and off chemotherapy for several years.

- Most people worry about the side effects of chemotherapy treatment. Side effects vary greatly from drug to drug and from person to person. Every person doesn't get every side effect and some people get few, if any at all. If you do have side effects, there is much you and the health care team can do to help lessen and relieve them.

- Chemotherapy is a serious treatment that must be given carefully by experienced medical professionals. Medical oncologists are the physicians who most often prescribe and supervise the treatment. Nurses play a major role in the administration of the drugs and in treating and dealing with side effects.

What is new in the chemotherapy field?

There are many new advances in chemotherapy now being studied. They include new drugs, new combinations of drugs, and new ways of administering them. Here are several developments.

- Attaching drugs to monoclonal antibodies that can find and kill the tumor cells without destroying normal cells.

- Packaging drugs inside a fat module (called a liposome) to selectively kill cancer cells while producing fewer side effects.

- Adding growth factors to stimulate the patient's own system for cell regrowth.

- Using colony-stimulating factors and chemopreventive drugs to lessen side effects.

- Searching for new drugs to use when the body becomes resistant to the chemotherapy drugs being given.

- Using monoclonal antibodies to strengthen the immune system's ability to destroy cancer cells.
- Discovering new chemotherapy drugs.

Questions to Ask Your Doctor Before You Have Chemotherapy

- **Is this the standard treatment for my kind of cancer?**
- **Am I eligible for any clinical trials?**
- **What is the purpose of using chemotherapy for my cancer?**
- **What are the names of the chemotherapy drugs that will be used? Why a combination of drugs? What is each drug supposed to do?**
- **Who will be responsible for giving me my treatment?**
- **Where will I get my treatment? Will it be in the hospital or in the doctor's office?**
- **What is the treatment schedule?**
- **How many treatments will I have?**
- **How will the drugs be given to me at each treatment? Will a port or pump be used? What are the advantages and disadvantages of getting my treatments in this way?**
- **How long will it take for each treatment?**
- **What are the possible side effects? What should I do if these side effects occur? Which ones should I report immediately? To whom?**
- **Will the chemotherapy cause premature menopause? Will I become infertile? How will it affect me sexually?**
- **May I continue to take my other medications while I am on chemo? What should I do about birth control?**
- **Will my diet be restricted?**
- **May I drink alcohol?**
- **Is there any special nutritional advice I should follow?**
- **Are there any special precautions I should take while I am on chemotherapy?**
- **Can I have an immunization shot while I am taking this drug?**
- **If I have questions about my chemotherapy whom should I ask?**
- **Can I continue to work during these treatments?**
- **Will I be able to drive myself to my treatments?**
- **How much will it cost? Will my health care plan cover all of these costs?**

- How much of a risk is involved?
- Will I be having other kinds of treatment in addition to the chemotherapy?
- Are there any alternatives to chemotherapy?
- What if I don't have this treatment at all?

What is chemotherapy?

Chemo means chemical and *therapy* means treatment. Thus, chemotherapy is simply the treatment of cancer using chemicals (drugs).

What does chemotherapy do?

In simple terms, the chemicals destroy the cancer cells, either by interfering with their growth or by preventing them from reproducing. Most times, chemotherapy uses a variety of drugs. They may be given during the same treatment or on different days. The various drugs work in different ways to interrupt the cell life cycle. Some affect the cycle during one or more of its phases of growth but have no effect on the cell during the other phases. Others affect the cell throughout the whole cycle.

When is chemotherapy used?

Chemotherapy is used for many different reasons:

- It can cure some kinds of cancer.
- It can be used to keep cancer from spreading.
- It can be used to achieve long-term remissions in some kinds of cancer.
- It can be used before surgery to reduce a large tumor.
- It can be used after surgery to kill the cells that may have been left behind or are in another part of the body.
- It can be used with radiation therapy, either before, during, or after the radiation treatments.

Is chemotherapy ever used alone as a treatment?

Like other treatments for cancer, chemotherapy is sometimes used alone. Many times, however, chemotherapy is used in combination with another kind of treatment—usually surgery or radiation therapy.

What does chemotherapy do that is different from other kinds of treatments?

Chemotherapy is known as a systemic treatment, which means that it goes through your whole body system, unlike surgery or radiation, which concentrate on one specific body part. It's used when there is the possibility that cancer cells may be deposited in a different place from the primary tumor or may be circulating throughout the body via the bloodstream. Drugs used in chemotherapy enter the bloodstream either by being injected directly into it or by being absorbed through the tissues. Therefore, the drugs reach wherever tumor cells may be growing.

What effects does chemotherapy have on cancer?
Chemotherapy can cure some cancers. In others, chemotherapy makes the tumor shrink. When this does not happen, the drugs at least stop the tumor from growing or make it grow more slowly. Sometimes, the drugs stop the growth for a period of time. There are times when chemotherapy is used to relieve pain and other symptoms, which allows the person to live a longer, more comfortable life. There are some types of cancer, however, for which chemotherapy has little or no effect on the growth of the cancer.

What are the different kinds of chemotherapy?
Chemotherapy drugs are classified by their structure and function. They fall mainly into the following five classifications:

- **Alkyating agents** are called non-cell-cycle-specific agents because they attack all cells in a tumor whether the cells are resting or dividing. They work in any phase of the cell cycle by stopping or slowing down cell growth.

- **Antimetabolites** are drugs that interfere with the cells' ability to reproduce themselves. These drugs are designed to starve cancer cells by interfering with vital life processes. They fool the cell by introducing the wrong building elements or blocking synthesis of the right ones.

- **Natural products** include plant alkaloids and antibiotics. Plant alkaloids stop cell division at one of its phases. Antibiotics are made from molds like penicillin but are stronger and do not act in the same way as regular antibiotics. Rather, they interfere with cell division and damage more cancer cells than normal cells.

- **Hormones** are naturally occurring substances that stimulate or turn off the growth or activity of specific cells or organs. In cancer treatment, the environment is changed either by adding or removing the hormones, thus antagonizing the growth-stimulating hormones that promote growth of cancer cells in certain tissues.

- **Miscellaneous agents** don't fit into any of these other categories but act against cancer cells in a variety of ways.

How many different kinds of chemotherapy drugs are now in use?

There are about 100 different chemotherapy drugs that are presently in use in the treatment of cancer, some of which are still under investigation. The National Cancer Institute sponsors an international cooperative chemotherapy program, involving many research laboratories of the federal government, the universities and medical schools and the pharmaceutical industry. This program encourages scientists of all kinds to search for drugs to cure cancer. Chemotherapy is one of the most heavily studied areas in cancer treatment. Scientists are creating new chemical compounds, studying plant specimens, and extracting antibiotics from natural fermentation products and soil samples. At the same time, many of the world's top chemists are searching for ways to improve the activity of known drugs. There is more information about new chemotherapy agents and the clinical trials that test them in Chapter 11, New Advances and Investigational Treatments.

Who prescribes chemotherapy?

We cannot stress strongly enough that chemotherapy should be prescribed by a doctor who has been trained in the use of drugs and drug combinations for the treatment of cancer. This may be a medical oncologist, who is a specialist in internal medicine with specific training in the overall care of the cancer patient, or a hematologist, who is a physician who deals with blood diseases. Some chemotherapuetic drugs may be prescribed by other doctors, but it is important that the doctor have special training in treating cancer patients. Most chemotherapy drugs are too risky to be prescribed by general physicians who have not been specially trained.

Do nurses play a role in administering the chemotherapy drugs?

Nurses play a major role in actually giving you the drugs. They are specially trained and know what side effects to look for and how to cope with them. In most places, the nurses must be certified in giving chemotherapy, usually using national standards of the Oncology Nursing Society. Most state boards of nursing also have rules based on these standards.

Why is it important to have specially trained personnel dealing with chemotherapy drugs?

Every chemotherapy plan must be individually tailored. The doctor chooses the drug or combination of drugs, determines the dosage, the best way to give the drugs, how often to give them, and how long the treatment will last. Chemotherapy, and especially combination chemotherapy, in which more than one drug is used, may be dangerous if the proper dosage is not prescribed. In addition, it is a field of medicine that is continuously changing. New forms of treatment may not always reach the doctors who are not specializing in this field. If you are living in a community that does not have a specialist to give you the drugs, make sure you have a consultation with a cancer center, a medical school, or a large medical center to confirm your treatment plan.

Where will I get my chemotherapy?
You may get it in one of several places—in your doctor's office, your hospital's outpatient department, a clinic, a hospital, or even in your home. It depends on the drugs you are being given, their potential side effects, your physical condition, and your doctor's preference. For some drugs that have serious side effects, the first doses of the drugs may be given in the hospital so that the health care team can closely watch you and make minor changes if needed.

How does the doctor decide on what kind of drug to use?
The doctor takes many things into consideration, such as the type of tumor you have, the extent of its growth, how it is affecting you, and your general condition. Also considered are the responses of chemotherapy in similar patients and what kind of drugs are most likely to damage or kill the cancer. However, individual differences among patients and the effects of the anti-cancer drugs on various kinds of tumors make this an inexact science. The medical oncologist cannot always specifically predict how the drug will affect the tumor of any given patient, although the major side effects of any particular drug can be anticipated.

Does each patient get the same dose of drug?
The doses are most often calculated according to your body surface area (per meter squared) and occasionally by your weight (in kilograms). The body surface area is determined by a formula using height and weight. When more than one drug is used, the dose for each drug is usually lower than when each drug is used alone. What the doctor is trying to do for each person is to give the "maximum tolerated dose"—that is, the amount of the drug which will give the greatest anticancer effect with the least amount of damage to normal cells.

How often will I get chemotherapy, and for how long?
This will depend on the kind of cancer you have, the drugs being used, how long it takes your body to respond to the drugs, and how well you tolerate them. Treatment schedules vary widely. Chemotherapy may be given daily, weekly, or monthly. Some drugs are given every four to six weeks, with other drugs given weekly in between. There are also drugs that may be given every day for a short time or drugs that may be taken in pill form once or twice a day over a long period of time. Many times, you are given a rest period in between treatments to allow your body to build healthy new cells and regain strength.

How is chemotherapy given?

Chemotherapy can be given in several ways:

- It can be put on your skin (topical).

- You can swallow it just like any other medicine, either in a pill, a capsule, or in liquid (PO) form.

- You can have it injected into your vein through a thin needle, usually in your arm or on your hand (intravenous or IV) or into your artery (intraarterial or IA); it can also be given IV through catheters, ports, and pumps.

- You can have it injected through a thin needle into a muscle in your arm, buttocks, or thigh (intramuscular or IM), beneath the skin (subcutaneous or SQ), directly into a tumor (intralesionally or IL), into the spine (intrathecally), directly into the stomach area (intraperitoneally), or into the bladder (intravesically).

- It can be delivered to specific areas of the body, such as your liver, using a catheter (long thin tube) that is put into a large vein and stays there as long as is needed.

How will the doctor decide what method to use?

Some drugs can be given only in one way. For instance, most drugs are given IV (injection into the vein) because they are better able to reach the cancer cells everywhere in the body. If the drug can be given in different ways, the decision will hinge on the necessary dose, preferences of the patient and doctor, what kind of cancer is being treated, and the location of the cancer.

How is topical chemotherapy used?

The drug, usually in a cream base, is applied to the area once or twice a day, with cotton swabs or a special applicator. The area will become red and tender, the skin will die and shed, and healthy skin will regrow. You need to be careful to apply the drug only to the area affected and to treat the area gently while the treatment is progressing. Fluorouracil is one of the topical chemotherapy treatments used for some skin cancers.

Are there any precautions when taking chemotherapy pills or tablets orally?

Taking chemotherapy orally is convenient—but it is important that you take great care in taking the drugs on time and as instructed. Take only the amount that has been ordered, nothing more and nothing less. It's a good idea to have a pill box to store the pills you will take each day or to use a calendar with the doses marked on it and space for you to record when you have taken the drugs. Most of the drugs are taken on an empty stomach with water, although a few need to be taken with food. Discuss with the nurse and doctor what to do if you miss a dose. Also be sure to tell them what other medicines you are taking, including over-the-counter drugs and vitamins. Do not take any new medications without checking with your doctor and nurse.

Are there any drugs that I can inject myself?
You can give yourself some drugs that are injected under the skin, or as the health professionals say, subcutaneously. The process is similar to what diabetics do when giving themselves insulin. If you are to do the injections yourself, the nurse will instruct you how to do this properly.

Does it hurt to get a chemotherapy drug?
Taking your drug in a pill, capsule, topical, or liquid form is no different from taking any other medicine. If you are getting a drug injected into your muscle, you usually just feel a pinprick, similar to an antibiotic shot. If you are taking a drug that needs to be injected into the vein, the process takes longer, but usually does not involve pain. Depending on the drugs being used, it may take anywhere from a few moments to several hours when given intravenously. Some people say they feel a temporary burning sensation in the area of the injection. Others feel warmth throughout the body. Some people say the needle insertion hurts. If you have any pain, burning, or discomfort that occurs during or after an IV treatment, be sure you report it to your nurse.

How is the drug injected IV?
IV stands for intravenous. It is the most common method for giving chemotherapy because it is the quickest way to get the medication into the bloodstream to all parts of the body. The drug or drugs will be injected into your vein. It can be done through a thin needle, usually placed in your arm or on your hand. Or the doctor may use a device with catheter that is put into a large vein in the chest, neck or arm. You might hear that called a central venus access or a vascular access device.

Do some people have a hard time getting repeated IV treatments?
Sometimes, after repeated IV treatments, veins become difficult or impossible to access. The nurse will attempt to use veins in the hands, which are easier to see, or veins in the lower arm which have more fatty tissue. However, sometimes after several chemotherapy sessions, some veins become scarred or collapse. When this happens, a vascular access device can be put in place so that treatments can continue.

Are there different kinds of vascular access devices?

There are several different kinds of vascular access devices, which can remain painlessly in place in the skin to provide easy access to a large vein in the chest, neck, or arm. These devices include peripherally inserted central catheters, midline catheters, tunneled venus catheters, implanted ports, and implanted pumps. These devices are usually used if you are getting continuous infusion chemotherapy or several drugs at one time, if your treatment is going to last a long period of time, or if the drugs can cause damage if they leak onto the skin.

What is a peripherally inserted central catheter?

This is a device, usually referred to as a PICC, that can be put into a vein by a specially trained nurse or a doctor, without surgery, can be removed easily and can remain in place for 12 to 30 days, until the treatment is completed. Keeping it clean at the point where it exits your body is important.

What is a midline catheter?

A midline catheter, used when it is not possible to use a regular IV, is put in less deeply than the PICC.

What is a tunneled central venus catheter?

A tunneled central venus catheter has more than one tube. It is put into one of the central veins and comes out either at the chest or abdomen. It can stay in for months or years. Keeping it clean at the point where it exits your body is important.

What is a port?

A port is a small disc made out of steel, titanium, or plastic. It is placed under the skin surface, usually in the chest or arm, by a surgeon. Since it is completely under the skin, it requires no special care. Drugs are injected into the port through a needle. The port can be used as needed and can remain in place for a long period of time. Another surgery is done when treatments are completed to remove the port. You should know that although it is a rare occurrence, a clot might develop in the large vein at the port site. If your arms or face begin to swell, you should contact your doctor immediately.

What is meant by continuous infusion?

Continuous infusion means that chemotherapy drugs are given over a longer period of time, such as those that take two or more hours. Usually continuous infusion drugs are given using a tunneled central venus catheter, such as a Hickman catheter or an implanted port.

What does a pump do?

The catheter may be attached to a pump that will control how fast the drug is given. There are two kinds of pumps—external and internal. The external pump, usually portable, connects to the catheter. You will be able to move around while it is being used. The internal pump, on the other hand, will be placed inside your body. It might be right under the skin or it could be put in the abdomen.

Are there any new developments in chemotherapy drugs and the way they are given?

The following techniques and developments are currently under investigation:

- Attaching a drug to monoclonal antibodies or other structures that will find and kill cancer cells, leaving normal cells alone.

- Cutting off the tumor's blood supplies, or anti-angiogenesis, by using drugs that slow or stop new blood vessels from growing.

- Targeting specific proteins, such as using signal transduction inhibitors (STIs.)

- Using implanted, refillable pumps to deliver anticancer drugs directly to affected organs.

- Isolating cancer cells from a patient's tumor in the laboratory and testing different drugs against those cells before chemotherapy has begun on the patient to match drugs more closely with an individual's disease.

- Using biological drugs—that is, those made by the body itself.

- Prescribing more intensive drug treatments, in sequence, for shorter periods of time, ensuring patients get full doses of each drug as quickly as possible, and adding growth factors to help overcome the side effects of the more intense doses.

More information on new developments in cancer treatment is discussed in Chapter 11, New Advances and Investigational Trials.

Will it make a difference if I have to miss a treatment?

If you are unable to make a treatment, call the doctor and discuss how you can reschedule it so that it doesn't interfere with the effectiveness of the treatment.

Will I be able to drink wine and cocktails while I am on chemotherapy?

It depends on the drugs you are taking. Usually you can drink small amounts. Talk with your doctor about how much beer, wine, or other alcoholic beverage you can have while you are in treatment.

Can I take other pills or drugs during treatment?

There are some medicines that may interfere with how your chemotherapy works in the body. To be safe, you should tell your doctor about any medicine that you are taking, regardless of whether it is prescription or over the counter. Make a list with the names of the medication, how often you are taking them, and the dosage. Discuss the list with your doctor before you start treatment so he can make sure nothing will interfere with your chemotherapy drugs. If you begin to take a new medicine while you are on chemotherapy, be sure to tell the doctor.

What are some of the drugs that can alter how chemotherapy drugs work in the body?

Such drugs include antibiotics, anticoagulants, anti-seizure pills, aspirin, barbiturates, blood-pressure pills, cough medicine, diabetic pills, hormone pills, sleeping pills, some vitamins and herbals, and tranquilizers and diuretics (water pills).

Will I be able to have dental work done while on treatment?

You usually will. Again, it depends on the drugs you are taking. Regular cleaning and cavity repairs are usually not a problem. However, be sure to tell your dentist that you are on chemotherapy. If the dentist is going to perform oral surgery, take out a tooth, or give you an injection, tell your doctor so that blood counts can be taken a few days before the dental work is going to be done. If your blood counts are normal, you can have minor dental surgery.

Will I be able to continue working while I am having chemotherapy drugs?

Most people find they are able to continue working while they are being treated. Some feel very tired when they are going through treatment and find they need to alter their normal schedules. It depends on your general health, the type and extent of cancer you have, and what drugs you are getting. If you wish, you may be able to schedule your treatments so that they cause the least disruption with your work schedule or your children's schedules.

How will the doctor know whether or not the drug is working?

There are several ways of measuring how well your treatments are working. You will have physical exams, laboratory tests, scans, x-rays, blood counts, and blood chemistry tests. Don't be surprised by the number of tests that will be done while you are having treatments. Some, like blood counts, will be used by the doctor to help adjust the doses of drugs. Your nurse can explain why the various tests are being done. Do not hesitate to ask your doctor about test results.

Do chemotherapy drugs ever stop being effective?

Sometimes drugs lose their effectiveness against a particular cancer. Scientists believe that in some cases, cancer cells are multiplying more quickly than the drug can kill them. Other times, cancer cells undergo change and are able to survive and even grow rapidly in the presence of drug that previously was effective. When this happens, the cells are said to "mutate" and are called "drug resistant."

How do cells become drug resistant?

Some cancer cells make genetic changes that allow them to produce a large amount of an enzyme that overrides a drug's usefulness. In other cases, the cell membrane changes in a way that allows it to block the entry of the drug into the cell or reduces the time the active drug remains in the cell. Scientists are currently working on ways to overcome drug resistance, including different ways of administering drugs or testing other drugs that could prove effective over the mutated cancer.

What is meant by combination chemotherapy?

When more than one drug is being used for treatment, it is called combination chemotherapy. Many times two to five drugs are used in combination in an attempt to kill cells in different phases of their reproductive cycle and to delay or prevent resistance to the drugs from occurring. Sometimes, several drugs are given during the same treatment. Sometimes the drugs are given sequentially; one drug is given for several weeks, followed by the next drug. There are hundreds of different combinations of drugs, many of which are known by the initials of the drugs that will be given. For instance, the combination chemotherapy regimen MOPP, used in lymphoma, stands for mechlorethamine, oncovin (vincristine), procarbazine, and prednisone. ABVD, another combination used in lymphoma stands for adriamycin (doxorubicin), bleomycin, vinblastine, and dacarbazine.

Why are female hormones used to treat prostate cancer and male hormones used to treat breast cancer?

Cancers that start in breast tissue in women and in the prostate gland in men depend on the presence of the hormones for their growth. Scientists feel that treatment with opposing hormones may affect these cancers by changing their normal environment. Thus male hormones are sometimes used to treat breast cancer, and female hormones are used to help suppress the growth of cancer of the prostate. Other hormones used in cancer treatment include corticosteroids, such as cortisone and prednisone for certain types of leukemia and lymphomas. Doctors also sometimes remove glands that secrete hormones, such as the ovaries or testicles, to help slow down malignant growth.

MAJOR CHEMOTHERAPY DRUGS AND HORMONES, THEIR USES AND MOST COMMON SIDE EFFECTS (For Biological Response Modifiers, see Chapter 11, New Advances and Investigational Treatments)

NAMES AND USES	COMMON SIDE EFFECTS (All patients do not have all side effects)	OCCASIONAL SIDE EFFECTS (Some patients may have other side effects not listed)
Altretamine (Hexalen, hexamethyl-melamine) Alkylating agent. Used in ovarian, lung, endometrial, cervical cancers and non-Hodgkin's lymphoma. Taken as a pill.	Nausea and vomiting (may worsen with continued treatment; taking drug with food at bedtime may help), fever, chills and sore throat, low blood counts, decreased sperm count, problems with fetus. Pregnancy prevention essential.	Confusion, hallucinations, diarrhea, cramps, bloody urine, skin rash, hair loss, weight loss, loss of feeling in fingers, difficulty walking and moving, difficulty sleeping, depression, second cancers (leukemia).
Amifostine (Ethyol) Reduces side effects of chemotherapy and radiation. Given IV.	Nausea, vomiting (may be prevented by taking antinausea medicine), and low blood pressure.	Drowsiness, sneezing, hiccups, chills, muscle and stomach cramps, flushing of face and neck.
Aminoglutethimide (Cytadren, Elitpen) An aromatase inhibitor used in breast, adrenal, and prostate cancers. Taken as a pill.	Skin rash with fever, sluggishness and tiredness (usually goes away slowly four to six weeks after treatment is finished).	Swelling of face, weight gain, leg cramps, fever, chills, sore throat, loss of appetite, drowsiness, mild nausea and vomiting, leg cramps, blurred vision dizziness when getting up from lying down or sitting.

Amsacrine
(AMSA, m-AMSA, acridinylanisidide NSC–24992) Leukemia, lymphoma, melanoma, colon, and breast cancer. Given IV.

Orange urine, fever, chills, sore throat, mouth sores, loss of fertility.

Nausea and vomiting, seizures, headaches, dizziness, heart and liver problems, anemia, pain at injection site, skin rash, numbness in fingers or toes, diarrhea.

Anastrozole
(Arimidex) Hormone or hormone inhibitor: Used in breast cancer. Taken as pill.

Tiredness, lack of energy, weakness, hot flashes, vaginal dryness, sweating.

Headache, diarrhea, nausea, appetite problems (increased or decreased), pain in legs, shortness of breath, difficulty in breathing, swelling of arms or legs.

Asparaginase
(Elspar, l-Asparaginase, Oncaspar) An enzyme used mostly in leukemias, lymphomas, and soft tissue sarcoma. Usually given IV or in muscle.

Nausea and vomiting, loss of appetite. May have allergic reaction; tell doctor or nurse if lightheaded or short of breath, have pain in your back, or feel queasy.

You may need to drink extra liquids to prevent kidney problems.

Difficulty in breathing, fever, chills, sore throat, joint pain or inability to move arm or leg, puffy face, skin rash or itching, stomach pain, unusual bleeding or bruising, drowsiness, confusion, seizures, or hallucinations, severe headaches, mouth sores, swelling of feet or lower legs, unusual thirst, yellow skin or eyes, low blood counts.

Azacytidine
(5–Azacytidine, ladakamycin, NSC–102806) Antimetabolite. Leukemia, melanoma, colon, and rectal cancers. Given IV.

Nausea and vomiting, diarrhea, hair loss, liver damage, muscle weakness, restlessness, sleeplessness, tiredness, low blood counts.

Fever, chills, sore throat, anemia, drowsiness and sluggishness, confusion, skin rash, mouth sores.

(continued)

MAJOR CHEMOTHERAPY DRUGS AND HORMONES, THEIR USES AND MOST COMMON SIDE EFFECTS (continued)

NAMES AND USES	COMMON SIDE EFFECTS (All patients do not have all side effects)	OCCASIONAL SIDE EFFECTS (Some patients may have other side effects not listed)
Bicalutamide (Casodex, ICI 176,334) Nonsteroidal antiandrogen (hormone). Cancer of the prostate. Taken as a pill.	Breast tenderness, pain, swelling, hot flashes, general, back or pelvic pain.	Constipation, diarrhea, headache, nausea, anxiety, insomnia, urinary tract infection.
Bleomycin (Blenoxane, BLM) Antibiotic used in several cancers such as squamous cell, Hodgkin's disease, sarcomas, melanoma, thyroid, testicle, kidney, esophagus, endometrium, and ovary. Given IV, in muscle or under skin.	Darkening or thickening of skin, changes in fingernails or toenails, skin rash, peeling redness or tenderness, fever.	Fever and chills, nausea, vomiting and loss of appetite, sores in mouth, headache, swelling and pain in joints, unusual taste sensation, coughing, shortness of breath, or other chronic lung problems.
Buserelin (Buserelin acetate, HOE 766, Suprefact) A luteinizing hormone-releasing hormone (LH-RH) analogue used in prostate cancer. Injected under skin or inhaled through nose.	Pain at injection site, hot flashes, impotence and breast enlargement (males), irregular or lack of menstrual periods and spotting, bone pain, difficulty urinating.	Infrequent nausea, vomiting, diarrhea, and constipation, headache, muscle weakness, depression.

Busulfan
(Myleran, BSF)

An alkylating agent used for chronic myelogenous and acute lymphocytic leukemia, polycythemia vera, and bone marrow transplant. Given as a pill or, for bone marrow transplant, IV.

Low blood counts. When given at high dose for bone marrow transplant: nausea and vomiting, mouth sores, dizziness, blurred vision, confusion, seizures.

If you miss a dose, do not double the next dose; check with your doctor.

Fever, chills, sore throat, hair loss, unusual bleeding or bruising, darkening of skin, pain in joints, side, or stomach, swelling of feet or lower legs, diarrhea, missing periods, breast enlargement, impotence, sterility, eye problems.

Capecitabine
(Xeloda)

Antimetabolite used for breast and other types of cancer. Taken as a pill.

Sores in mouth, fever, chills or sore throat, diarrhea, tiredness, nausea and vomiting, low blood counts, tingling of hands and feet, skin rash.

Constipation, pain in stomach, heartburn, headache, dizziness, eye pain, headache, swelling of ankles.

Carboplatin
(Paraplatin, CBDCA, carboplatinum, JM–8, NSC–24120)

An alkylating-like agent. Used for cancer of the ovaries. May also be used for neuroblastoma, leukemias, cancers of the bladder, brain, breast, testes, head and neck, endometrium, cervix, and lung. Given IV.

Nausea and vomiting (may be preventable by taking antinausea medicine), low blood counts, fever, chills and sore throat, kidney problems, weakness.

Skin rash, hair loss, tingling of hands and feet, blood in urine, pain injection site, hearing loss, eye problems, constipation, diarrhea.

(continued)

MAJOR CHEMOTHERAPY DRUGS AND HORMONES, THEIR USES AND MOST COMMON SIDE EFFECTS (continued)

NAMES AND USES	COMMON SIDE EFFECTS (All patients do not have all side effects)	OCCASIONAL SIDE EFFECTS (Some patients may have other side effects not listed)
Carmustine (BCNU, BiCNU) An alkylating agent used for multiple myeloma, Hodgkin's disease and non-Hodgkin's lymphomas, melanoma, cancers of the brain, colon, rectum, stomach, and liver. Given IV.	Nausea and vomiting (may be prevented by taking antinausea medicine), hair loss and darkening of skin, redness, burning, pain or swelling where injection is given, lung problems, low blood counts.	Fever, chills, cough and sore throat, unusual bleeding or bruising, shortness of breath and flushing or face, mouth sores, diarrhea, difficulty in swallowing, dizziness, eye problems.
Chlorambucil (Leukeran) An alkylating agent used in leukemias and lymphomas, multiple myeloma, cancers of the breast, ovary, and testicle. Given as a pill.		Nausea and vomiting, diarrhea, loss of appetite, loss of hair, fever, chills, sore throat, mouth sores, seizures, cough, shortness of breath, joint, stomach or side pain, skin rash, changes in period, sterility, itchiness, eye problems, second cancer (leukemia).
Cisplatin (Platinol-AQ, Platinol, Platinol-Q, platinum, cis-platinum) An alkylating agent used in lymphoma,	Nausea and vomiting may last up to three days (may be prevented by taking antinausea medicine). Loss of appetite, diarrhea, metallic taste.	Hair loss, seizures, dizziness, loss of taste, blurred vision, change in ability to see colors, difficulty in hearing, ringing in ears, sores in mouth, fast

sarcoma, cancers of the testicle, ovary, bladder, brain, adrenal glands, breast, cervix, uterus, endometrium, head and neck, esophagus, lung, skin, prostate, and stomach. Given IV with intravenous fluids.	numbness and tingling in finger, toes or face. kidney damage. IMPORTANT: drink extra liquids to prevent kidney problems.	heartbeat or wheezing, fever, chills, sore throat, decreased urination, swelling of feet or lower legs, unusual bleeding or bruising chest pain, heart attack.
Clarabine (Leutatin, chlordeoxyadenoise, 2–CdA, CldAno) An antimetabolite used for leukemias and lymphomas.	Lower blood counts, headache, fever and chills, cough, nausea, vomiting, loss of appetite, nausea (antinausea medicine can be prescribed), skin rash.	Diarrhea, constipation, pain in stomach, dizziness, trouble sleeping.
Cyclophosphamide (Cytoxan, Neosar, Endoxan, Procytox) An alkylating agent used in lymphomas and Hodgkin's disease, myeloma, neuroblastoma, retinoblastoma, sarcomas, Wilms' tumor, cancers of the ovary, breast, prostate, head and neck, lung, bladder, cervix, stomach, and uterus. Given IV or taken as a pill.	Nausea, vomiting, loss of appetite, loss of hair, low blood counts. IMPORTANT: drink extra liquids to prevent bladder problems. If you miss a dose, do not double the next dose; talk to your doctor.	Blood in urine, pain when urinating, black tarry stools, fever, chills, nasal stuffiness and sore throat, cough and shortness of breath, dizziness, confusion, fast heartbeat, sterility (may be temporary), skin darkening, metallic taste during injection, blurred vision, cataract, second cancers (leukemia, bladder).

(continued)

MAJOR CHEMOTHERAPY DRUGS AND HORMONES, THEIR USES AND MOST COMMON SIDE EFFECTS *(continued)*

NAMES AND USES	COMMON SIDE EFFECTS (All patients do not have all side effects)	OCCASIONAL SIDE EFFECTS (Some patients may have other side effects not listed)
Cyclosporine (Cyclosporin A, CsA, Sandimmune, Neoral) An immunosuppressant agent used in bone marrow transplant. Given with other drugs to reverse multidrug resistance. Given IV.	Headache, tremor, hypertension, hairiness (women), kidney problems.	Diarrhea, loss of appetite, nausea and vomiting, hiccups, constipation, confusion, depression, facial flushing, shortness of breath, wheezing, enlargement of breasts, hearing loss.
Cytarabine (Ara-C, Cytosar-U, arabinosyl, Tarabine) An antimetabolite used in the leukemias and the lymphomas. Given IV or less commonly, under the skin or in the spinal cord.	Nausea, vomiting, diarrhea, lowered blood counts, anemia, metallic taste.	Mouth sores, loss of appetite, black tarry stools, ulcers, dizziness, headache, lung problems, tiredness, bone, joint or muscle pain, heartburn, irregular heartbeat, fever, chills, sore throat, numbness or tingling in fingers, toes or face, reddened eyes.
Dacarbazine (DTIC, DTIC-Dome, imidazole carboxamide) An alkylating agent used in melanoma, Hodgkin's disease, soft-tissue sarcomas, neuroblastoma and cancers of the bladder and islet cell. Given IV.	Nausea and vomiting (antinausea medicine prescribed; may be severe but lessens with each additional daily dose), redness, pain or swelling at injection site, lowered blood counts, anemia.	Fever, chills, sore throat, mouth sores, metallic taste, sensitivity to sun, flushing of face, skin rash, diarrhea, hair loss, confusion, blurred vision, liver problems.

Drug	Effects	Side Effects
Dactinomycin (Actinomycin-D, ACT-D, Actinomycin-C, Cosmegen) An antitumor antibiotic used for Wilm's tumor, sarcomas, choriocarcinoma, leukemias, melanoma, cancers of the testicle, uterus, endometrium, and ovary. Given IV.	Nausea and vomiting (may happen about one hour after a dose and may last several hours; may get worse as treatment continues; antinausea medicine may be used), hair loss, low blood counts.	Mouth sores, skin rash, acne, loss of appetite, hair loss, diarrhea, fever, chills, sore throat, redness, pain or swelling at place or injection, tiredness, anemia, hair loss, black tarry stools, mouth sores, stomach pain, liver problems, darkening of skin, may activate skin reactions from past radiation.
Daunorubicin (Cerubidine, Daunomycin, Rubidomycin, DNR) An antitumor antibiotic used for acute nonlymphocytic leukemia lymphomas, neuroblastoma, and Wilms' tumor. Given IV.	Nausea and vomiting (may be prevented by taking antinausea medicine; may happen about one hour after a dose and last for several hours), red urine (usually lasts one or two days after each dose), redness, burning or pain at injection site, hair loss, low blood counts, back pain, flushing, chest tightness.	Fever, chills, sore throat, shortness of breath, joint or stomach pain, skin rash or itching, mouth sores, darkening or redness of skin, especially in areas where radiation was given, irregular heart beat, liver problems.
Dexamethasone (Decadron, Hexadrol, Dexone, DXM) Adrenal corticostroid used for brain metastases, breast cancer, leukemias, myeloma, lymphomas. Also used as antinausea before chemotherapy. Given as tablet, ointment, syrup, inhaler, or IV.	Loss of or increased appetite, weight gain, aggravation of, or bringing on of, diabetes, swelling of arms, ankles and legs, higher blood pressure, depression.	Nausea and vomiting, aggravation of peptic ulcers, skin rash or dryness, growth of facial hair, acne, poor wound healing, mouth sores, irregular or lack of menstrual periods, sleeplessness, headache, dizziness, muscle weakness, cataracts, back pain, infections, bone loss.

(continued)

MAJOR CHEMOTHERAPY DRUGS AND HORMONES, THEIR USES AND MOST COMMON SIDE EFFECTS (continued)

NAMES AND USES	COMMON SIDE EFFECTS (All patients do not have all side effects)	OCCASIONAL SIDE EFFECTS (Some patients may have other side effects not listed)
Dexrazoxane (Zinecard, ADR–529, ICRF–187, NSC–169780) Given to patients with breast cancer to protect heart while on chemotherapy. Given as IV.	Lower blood counts, mild nausea and vomiting, loss of appetite, hair loss.	Mouth sores, tiredness, fever, seizure, shortness of breath.
Docetaxcel (Taxotere, RP 56976, NSC–628503) Antimicrotubule used in cancer of the breast, ovary, lung, and head and neck. Given IV.		Nausea and vomiting, diarrhea, taste changes, tiredness.
Doxorubicin (Ardiamycin, Rubex, Adriamycin RDF or MDV, Adria, hydroxydaunorubicin, hydroxydaunomycin, Doxil) An antitumor antibiotic used in leukemias, lymphomas, Wilm's tumor, neuroblastoma, multiple myelomas, sarcomas, cancers of the breast,	Nausea and vomiting (may be prevented by taking antinausea medicine), red urine (usually lasts one or two days after each dose), hair loss, loss of appetite, heart problems, low blood counts.	Mouth sores, darkening, of soles, palms or nails, may reactivate skin reactions from past radiation, fever, chills, sore throat, diarrhea, eye problems, fast or irregular heartbeat, shortness of breath, pain in joint, side or stomach, redness, burning or pain at injection site.

Drug	Side effects	
ovary, bladder, thyroid, stomach, cervix, endometrium, liver, esophagus, head and neck, pancreas, prostate, testes, and lung. Given IV.	Diarrhea, nausea and vomiting, mild hair loss, tiredness.	
Edatrexate (10–EDAM, 10–ethyl-10-deaza-aminopterin, NSC–626715) Antimetabolite used for cancers of lung, head and neck. Given as IV.	Mouth sores, lower blood counts, skin rash.	
Epirubin (4'–epidoxorubicin, 4'–epi-adriamycin, NSC–256942) An antitumor antibiotic used for leukemias, lymphomas, sarcomas, cancer of the breast, ovary, and lung. Given IV.	Low blood counts, red urine, nausea and vomiting (may be prevented by taking antinausea medicine), loss of appetite, hair loss, darkening of nail beds, skin rash, may reactivate skin reactions from past radiation.	Flushing of face, irregular heart beat, fever, tiredness, headache.
Estramustine (Emcyt, Estracyt, estramustne phosphate) A hormone used in prostate cancer. Taken as a capsule.	Nausea and vomiting loss of appetite, diarrhea, impotence, loss of libido. Do not take more or less than your doctor ordered or more often than ordered. If you miss a dose, do not double the next dose; talk to your doctor. Do not take within an hour before, or two hours after, you have had milk, milk formulas, or other daily products.	Shortness of breath, slurred speech, vision changes, breast tenderness or enlargement, skin rashes, fever, chills, sore throat, severe or sudden headache, dry skin, sudden loss of coordination, pains in calves of legs.

(continued)

MAJOR CHEMOTHERAPY DRUGS AND HORMONES, THEIR USES AND MOST COMMON SIDE EFFECTS (continued)

NAMES AND USES	COMMON SIDE EFFECTS (All patients do not have all side effects)	OCCASIONAL SIDE EFFECTS (Some patients may have other side effects not listed)
Etoposide (VePesid, Toposar, VP–16, VP–16–213, EPEG, NSC 141540 Etoposide phosphate) A plant alkaloid used in cancers of the breast, testes, lung prostate, brain, bladder, adrenal cortex, stomach, uterus, lymphomas, leukemias, trophoblastic tumors, neuroblastoma, and sarcomas. Given as IV or taken as capsule.	Nausea and vomiting (mild and more common when taken as capsule), hair loss, loss of appetite, low blood counts.	Lung problems, fever, chills, sore throat, mouth sores, stomach pain, diarrhea, unpleasant taste in mouth, constipation, local pain at site of injection, sleeplessness, tiredness, headache, eye problems, muscle cramps, second cancer (acute myeloid leukemia).
Exemestane Armatase inhibitor used in breast cancer.	Hair loss, hoarseness, nausea, vomiting, loss of appetite.	
Floxuridine (FUDR, 5–FUDR, fluorodeoxyuridine) An antimetabolite used in gastrointestinal adenocarcinoma metastatic to the liver and cancers of the breast, ovary, cervix, bladder, kidney, and prostate. Usually given IV or pumped directly into the liver.	Loss of appetite. If pumped directly into liver; problems with catheter, infections.	Nausea and vomiting, diarrhea, mouth sores, stomach pain and cramps, hair loss or thinning itching, swelling or soreness of tongue, ulcers, fever, chills, sore throat, scaling or redness of hands or feet, low blood counts.

Fludarabine (Fludarabine phosphate, Fludara, 2–fluoro–ARA, AMP, FAMP, NSC–312887) An antimetabolite used in leukemias and lymphomas. Given as IV.

Nausea and vomiting (can be prevented by taking antinausea drugs), fever, chills, cough, pneumonia, sore throat, nose-bleeds, skin rash, low blood counts, tiredness, swelling of hands and ankles.

Anemia, loss of appetite, constipation, stomach cramps, mild hair loss, sleeplessness, tiredness, blurred vision, muscle pain, problems walking.

Fluorouracil (Adrucil, Efudex, Fluoroplex, 5–FU, 5–Fluorouracil) An antimetabolite used in cancers of the stomach, colon, rectum, breast, pancreas, bladder, cervix, endometrium, esophagus, head and neck, islet cells, liver, lung, ovary, prostate, and skin. Usually given IV. Can be taken mixed with water. For skin, a cream is used.

Nausea, mouth, tongue and lip sores, diarrhea, skin darkening (sensitive to sun), low blood counts, eye tearing.

Loss of appetite, hair loss, skin rash or dryness, vomiting, poor muscle coordination, swelling of palms and soles, nail loss or brittle nails, eye irritation, increase of tears, blurred vision, headache, confusion.

Fluoxymesterone (Halotestin, Ora–Testryl) An androgen used in breast cancer. Taken as a tablet.

Acne, yellowing of eyes and skin, swelling of arms and legs; voice deepening, hoarseness, menopause, and vaginal dryness.

Patchy hair loss, breast swelling, acne, swollen hands and feet.

(continued)

MAJOR CHEMOTHERAPY DRUGS AND HORMONES, THEIR USES AND MOST COMMON SIDE EFFECTS *(continued)*

NAMES AND USES	COMMON SIDE EFFECTS (All patients do not have all side effects)	OCCASIONAL SIDE EFFECTS (Some patients may have other side effects not listed)
Flutamide (Eulexin, Euflex) An antiandrogen used in prostate cancer. Given as a capsule.	Nausea and vomiting, diarrhea, breast enlargement, breast tenderness, loss of sexual interest, impotence, hot flashes.	Anemia, pain, skin rash, muscle aches.
	If you cannot swallow capsule, open it and mix the contents with apple-sauce, pudding, or other soft foods. Do not mix in liquid because it does not dissolve well in water.	
Fulvestrant (Faslodex, ICI 182, 780) Antiestrogen used in breast cancer. Given intramuscularly.	Nausea, vomiting, constipation, diarrhea and stomach pain, headache, back pain, hot flashes.	
Gefitinib (Iressa, ZD1839) Growth factor inhibitor used for non-small cell lung cancer.	Rash, acne, dry skin, diarrhea.	
Gemcitabine (Genzar, gemcitabine hydrochloride, dFdC)	Low blood counts, nausea and vomiting (may be prevented by taking antinausea	Hair loss, drowsiness, unable to sleep, facial swelling, uneven heart

Antimetabolite used in cancers of the breast and pancreas. Given IV.	medicine); diarrhea, constipation, mouth sores, skin rash, liver problems, swelling of hands and ankles, fever, headache, back pain, chills, muscle aches.	beat, difficulty breathing, heart attack, depression.
Goserelin (Zoladex, ZDX, ICI 118,630, NSC–606864) Leutinizing hormone-releasing hormone (LH-RH) used in prostate, endometrial and breast cancer. Given by depot (pellet of drug is injected beneath skin of abdomen where it is slowly released) or implanted.	Hot flashes, impotence, decreased sex drive, breast enlargement in men, spotting, irregular or lack of menstrual periods, vaginal dryness, bone pain, retention of urine, acne, scaly skin, sweating, headaches, depression, bone pain.	Nausea and vomiting, diarrhea, constipation, loss of appetite, discomfort where pellet is implanted, headache, difficulty sleeping, kidney damage.
Hydroxyurea (Hydrea) An antimetabolite used in leukemia, melanoma, head and neck, prostate, cervix, and ovary. Taken as a capsule.	Low blood counts. Do not take more or less than your doctor ordered or more often than ordered. If you miss a dose, do not double the next dose; talk to your doctor. If you cannot swallow capsule, open it and dissolve the drug in water. Discard the white powder that does not dissolve and is floating on top of the water. You may need to drink extra liquids to prevent kidney problems.	Mild nausea, vomiting, skin rash and itching, mouth sores, diarrhea or constipation, hair loss, loss of appetite, drowsiness, tiredness, confusion, redness of face.

(continued)

MAJOR CHEMOTHERAPY DRUGS AND HORMONES, THEIR USES AND MOST COMMON SIDE EFFECTS *(continued)*

NAMES AND USES	COMMON SIDE EFFECTS (All patients do not have all side effects)	OCCASIONAL SIDE EFFECTS (Some patients may have other side effects not listed)
Idarubicin (Idamycin, Zavedos, Idarubicin hydochloride, NSC–256439) An antitumor antibiotic used for leukemia. Given IV.	Nausea and vomiting (may be prevented by taking antinausea medicine), diarrhea, low blood counts, fever, chills, sore throat, red urine, hair loss, heart and liver problems, loss of appetite, mouth sores, skin rash.	Anemia, tingling or numbness of hands and feet, seizures.
Ifosfamide (Ifex, Mitoxana, Holoxan, Naxamide, Isophosphamide, NSC–109724) An alkylating agent used in lymphoma, sarcoma, melanoma, leukemia, cancer of breast, ovary, pancreas, stomach, testes, and lung. Given IV. **Mesna** (Mesnum, Mesnex, Uromitexan, NSC–11389l) is given with this drug to protect bladder.	Nausea and vomiting (may be prevented by taking antinausea medicine), loss of appetite, bladder infection, blood in urine.	Fever, chills, sore throat, lower blood counts, hair loss, constipation, diarrhea, confusion, disorientation, seizures, drowsiness, tiredness, burning pain where drug was injected, stuffy nose, sterility, mouth sores, darkening of skin, skin rash, lung and heart problems, anemia.

Drug	Side Effects
Imatinib mesylate (Gleevec) Used in lymphoma, soft tissue sarcoma, brain, lung and gastrointestinal tumors. Given as IV.	Nausea and vomiting, retaining fluids, stomach pain, bleeding, muscle cramps, swelling around eyes and lower legs, diarrhea, skin rash, headache, bleeding, tiredness, joint pain.	Liver problems, low blood count, indigestion.
Irinotecan (camptosar, CTP–11, camptothecin–11) Used in cancers of the colon, rectum, lung, cervix, and ovary. Given IV.	Low blood counts, anemia, diarrhea, nausea and vomiting (may be prevented with antinausea medicine), loss of appetite, stomach pain, constipation, flushing, cramping, diarrhea, hair loss, tiredness, eye tearing.	Mouth sores, heartburn, skin rash and darkening, fever, chills.
Letrozole (Femara) Hormone or hormone antagonist Used in breast cancer. Taken as a pill.	Bone, joint and muscle pain, headache, tiredness, nausea.	Hot flashes, vomiting, loss of appetite, chest pain, constipation, diarrhea.
Leuprolide acetate (Lupron, Lurpon Depot, Leuprorelin acetate) A gonodrotropin-releasing hormone (GnRH) analogue used in prostate, breast and islet cell cancers and endometriosis. Injected under skin or in muscle; pellets inserted into skin.	Loss of appetite, nausea, constipation, taste change, diarrhea, dry mouth, itchy or dry skin, acne, hair loss or growth, hot flashes, impotence, breast tenderness or enlargement, loss of sexual desire, decrease in size of testicle, irregular or lack of periods, vaginal dryness, decreased bone density.	High blood pressure, swelling of arms and legs, sleeplessness, headache, dizziness, depression, anxiety, blurred vision, tiredness, sluggishness, mood swings, pain at site of tumor.

(continued)

MAJOR CHEMOTHERAPY DRUGS AND HORMONES, THEIR USES AND MOST COMMON SIDE EFFECTS *(continued)*

NAMES AND USES	COMMON SIDE EFFECTS (All patients do not have all side effects)	OCCASIONAL SIDE EFFECTS (Some patients may have other side effects not listed)
Lomustine (CCNU, CeeNU) An alkylating agent used in lymphoma, melanoma, multiple myeloma, cancers of the brain, breast, lung, colon, rectum and kidney. Taken as a capsule.	Nausea and vomiting (may happen but usually does not last more than 24 to 48 hours), loss of appetite, low blood counts. You may need to take two or more different types of capsules to get the right dose. If you take on an empty stomach at bedtime, you may have less stomach upset.	Mouth sores, hair loss, anemia, shortness of breath, tiredness, diarrhea, chills and fever, irregular menstrual periods, darkening of skin, skin rash or itching, awkwardness in walking, confusion, slurred speech, kidney problems, second cancers (leukemia).
Mechlorethamine (Mustargen, nitrogen mustard) An alkylating agent used in lymphomas, sarcomas, leukemias, lung cancer, and brain tumors. Given IV or used topically prepared in an ointment for mycosis fungoides.	Low blood cell counts, nausea and vomiting (may be severe; usually begins one hour after IV given—anti-nausea medicine must be taken), irritation of veins, hair loss, burning pain at incision site. Skin rashes, itching and other skin problems when used as ointment.	Metallic taste, loss of appetite, fever, chills, sore throat, shortness of breath, wheezing, vein discoloration (where drug administered), mouth sores, confusion, diarrhea, drowsiness, headache, ringing in ears, loss of hearing.

Drug	Notes	Side effects
Megestrol acetate (Megace) A hormone or hormone inhibitor used in breast cancer. Taken as a pill.	Vaginal bleeding, retention of fluid, weight gain.	Blood clots, nausea.
Melphalan (Alkeran, Alkeran IV, L-PAM, L-phenylalanine mustard, L-sarcolysin) An alkylating agent used in multiple myeloma, melanoma, cancers of the ovary, breast, thyroid, testes, and bone marrow transplants. Given as a pill usually, higher doses IV.	Nausea and vomiting (especially if given IV in larger doses; antinausea medicine may be given), low blood counts. Do not take more or less than your doctor orders or more often than ordered. If you miss a dose, do not double the next dose; talk to your doctor.	Mouth sores, diarrhea, skin rash or itching, fever, chills, sore throat, missed or irregular menstrual periods, cataracts, second cancers.
Mercaptopurine (Purinethol, 6–MP, 6–mercaptopurine) An antimetabolite used in leukemia and non-Hodgkin's lymphoma. Given as a tablet. IV is being investigated.	Occasional nausea and vomiting. Do not drink alcohol without discussing it with your doctor. You may need to drink extra liquids to prevent kidney problems.	Skin rash and itching, mouth sores, diarrhea, fever, chills, sore throat, joint, side or stomach pain, darkening of skin, headache, yellowing of eyes and skin, anemia.

(continued)

MAJOR CHEMOTHERAPY DRUGS AND HORMONES, THEIR USES AND MOST COMMON SIDE EFFECTS (continued)

NAMES AND USES	COMMON SIDE EFFECTS (All patients do not have all side effects)	OCCASIONAL SIDE EFFECTS (Some patients may have other side effects not listed)
Methotrexate (Folex, Folex PFS, Mexate, Mexate-AQ, Abitrexate, Rheumatrex amethoptrin) An antimetabolite used in choriocarcinoma, hydatiform mole, multiple myeloma, leukemia, lymphomas, sarcomas, cancers of the breast, head and neck, lung, bladder, brain, cervix, esophagus, kidney, ovary, prostate, stomach, and testes. Most commonly given IV, also injected in the muscle, or taken as a tablet.	Mild nausea and vomiting, diarrhea, mouth sores. Do not take more or less than your doctor ordered or more often than ordered. If you miss a dose, do not double the next dose; talk to your doctor. You may need to drink extra liquids to prevent kidney problems. Do not take aspirin or other medicine for swelling or pain without first checking with your doctor. When very high doses are given, it is followed by the drug leucovorin calcium to counteract life-threatening side effects (called leucovorin rescue).	Loss of appetite, stomach pain, yellowing of eyes or skin, low blood counts, fever, chills, sore throat, cough, shortness of breath, blood in urine or dark urine, hair thinning, headache, dizziness, blurred vision, drowsiness, or confusion, joint pain, skin rash, reddening of skin (sensitive to sun), anemia, flank pain, blurred vision, confusion, seizures.

Mitomycin (Mutamycin, Mytomycin C) An antitumor antibiotic used for leukemia, cancers of the stomach, pancreas, bladder, breast, cervix, esophagus, gallbladder, head and neck, rectum, and lung. Given IV or directly into an organ.	Nausea and vomiting (may be prevented by taking antinausea medicine), loss of appetite, burning pain at injection site, fever, chills sore throat, fatigue and tiredness, low blood counts.	Hair loss, diarrhea, mouth sores, blurred vision, blood in urine, numbness or tingling in fingers and toes, purple-colored bands on nails, skin rash, cough, difficulty breathing, kidney or lung problems.
Mitotane (Lysodren, o,p'DDD) An adrenal cytotoxic agent used in adrenal cancer. Taken as a tablet.	Nausea and vomiting, loss of appetite, depression, dizziness or vertigo, diarrhea, skin rash. You may get dizzy, drowsy, or less alert than normal. Make sure you know how you react to this medicine before you drive, use machines or do other jobs that need an alert mind. Do not take more or less than your doctor orders or more often than ordered. If you miss a dose, take the missed dose as soon as you remember. If it is almost time for the next dose, skip the missed dose, go back to your regular schedule and do not double the next dose, talk to your doctor. Do not stop taking this medicine without first checking with your doctor.	Tremors, blurred or double vision, lightheadedness, shortness of breath, wheezing, flushing, muscle twitching, lethargy, drowsiness, headache, hypertension, fever, chills, sore throat, loss of appetite, brain damage.

(continued)

MAJOR CHEMOTHERAPY DRUGS AND HORMONES, THEIR USES AND MOST COMMON SIDE EFFECTS (continued)

NAMES AND USES	COMMON SIDE EFFECTS (All patients do not have all side effects)	OCCASIONAL SIDE EFFECTS (Some patients may have other side effects not listed)
Mitoxantrone (Novantrone, mitoxantrone hydrochloride, DHAD, DHAQ, NSC–301739) An antibiotic used for leukemia, lymphoma, breast, prostate, and liver cancers. Given IV.	Nausea and vomiting (usually can be prevented with antinausea medicine), mouth sores, hair loss (usually mild), blue-green urine (may last for 24 to 48 hours) low blood counts.	Diarrhea, abdominal pain, skin rash, dry skin, chest pain, anemia, problems with breathing, cough, heart damage, headache, liver problems, blue streaking in or around the vein.
Nilutamide (Anadron) Antiangrogen used in prostate cancer.	Hot flashes, back pain, weakness, constipation, pelvic pain, nausea, diarrhea, swelling, and fluid accumulation in limbs.	
Octreotide (Sandostain, l-cysteinamide, SMS) A hormone analogue used for VIPomas, cancers of the pancreas, and breast. Given IV.	Stomach pain, loose stools, loss of appetite, vomiting, low blood counts, tiredness, dry mouth.	Heartburn, swollen stomach, pain at site of injection, jaundice, hair loss, skin problems, dizziness, lightheadedness, depression, problems with breathing, cough, heart damage.
Oxiplatin (Eloxatin, Sanofi-Synthelobo) An alkylating agent used for cancers of the colon, rectum, breast and ovary. Given IV.	Nausea and vomiting, numbness or tingling in hands, feet, or lips.	Low blood counts, difficulty walking.

Drug		
Paclitaxel (Taxol, NSC–125973) A plant alkaloid used in cancer of the ovary, breast, and lung, head and neck, prostate and stomach, esophagus, bladder, endometrium, cervix, and lymphoma. Given IV.	Fever, anemia, low blood counts, hair loss (usually 14 to 21 days after treatment starts; sudden and complete); flushing, shoulder, muscle and joint pain, numbness, burning, tingling, loss of feeling in feet and hands; mouth sores (occur three to seven days after first dose gets better five to seven days after).	Chest, stomach or leg pain, fever, chills or sore throat, mild nausea and vomiting, diarrhea, fatigue, headache, alterations in taste, pain at injection site, wheezing, trouble breathing.
Pamidronate (Aredia, pamidronate disodium, APD) Used in multiple myeloma; for bone mets in breast cancer and Paget's disease. Given IV.	Nausea and vomiting, fatigue, fever, burning at site where drug was injected, bone pain, general pain.	Anemia, stomach pain, loss of appetite, tiredness, fever, chills and sore throat, sleeplessness, vision problems, heart palpitations.
Pentostatin (Nipent, 2′–deoxycoformycin, dCF, covidarabine, NSC–218321) Used for leukemia and lymphoma. Given IV.	Low blood counts, infections, anemia, fever, chills, sore throat, nausea and vomiting, mouth sores, diarrhea, loss of appetite, skin rashes, dry skin, liver problems, cough, sore muscles	Taste changes, muscle pain, headache, tiredness, sleeplessness, confusion, sluggishness, slurred speech, depression, seizures, coma, shortness of breath.
Pipobroman (Vercyte, NSC–25154) Chronic granulocytic leukemia, polycythemia vera. Taken as tablet.	Low blood count, anemia, nausea, vomiting.	Abdominal cramps, diarrhea, skin rash.

(continued)

MAJOR CHEMOTHERAPY DRUGS AND HORMONES, THEIR USES AND MOST COMMON SIDE EFFECTS *(continued)*

NAMES AND USES	COMMON SIDE EFFECTS (All patients do not have all side effects)	OCCASIONAL SIDE EFFECTS (Some patients may have other side effects not listed)
Plicamycin (Mitracin, Mithramycin) An anti-tumor antibiotic used for leukemia and cancer of the testes. Given IV.	Severe nausea and vomiting, mouth sores, diarrhea, loss of appetite, burning pain at injection site.	Bloody or black tarry stools, nosebleed, liver or kidney damage, mouth sores, fever, chills and sore throat, headaches, depression, nervousness, drowsiness, flushing, redness or swelling of face, skin rash or small red spots on skin, dark nails, anemia.
Prednimustine (Sterecyt, Mostarinia, Leo 1031, NSC—134087) Used in leukemia, lymphoma, cancers of ovary, breast and prostate. Taken as a tablet.	Low blood counts.	Mild nausea and vomiting, diarrhea, confusion, lightheadedness, fever, swelling, hives, hair loss, skin rashes, fever, swelling of arms and legs.
Procarbazine (Matulane, Nutulanar, Ibenzmethyzin) An alkylating agent used in Hodgkin's disease, non-Hodgkin's lymphoma, multiple myeloma,	Nausea and vomiting, constipation, low blood counts, tiredness, trouble sleeping, nightmares. When taken with certain foods and drinks can cause very dangerous reac-	Anemia, diarrhea, weakness, dizziness, depression, headache, muscle pain or twitching, sweating, visual disturbances, hallucinations, seizures, frequent urination, blood in urine,

melanoma, brain and lung cancers. Taken as a capsule.	tions. Do not eat foods containing tyramine, such as ripe cheeses (especially cheddar), spicy sausages, chicken livers, pickled herring, foods that are aged or overripe. Do not drink alcohol, including beer and wine. Do not take any other medicine unless prescribed by your doctor, including over-the-counter medicine. You may also be drowsy. Make sure you know how you react to this medicine before you drive, use machines or do other jobs that need an alert mind.	sterility, breast enlargement, irregular menstrual periods, loss of appetite.
Raloxifene (Evista) Antiestrogen. Investigational. Used for breast cancer. Taken as a pill.	Hot flashes, vaginal discharge, dryness or itching, blood clots.	Leg cramps, constipation, pain with intercourse, sinus irritation or infection, bladder control.
Streptozocin (Zanosar, strepozotocin) An alkylating agent used in cancer of the pancreas, carcinoid tumors, and Hodgkin's disease. Given IV.	Nausea and vomiting (usually occurs within one to four hours after receiving a dose and may be severe—may be prevented by taking antinausea medicine), low blood counts, liver, and kidney problems, second cancers.	Diarrhea, mild anemia, stomach cramps, bone marrow depression, confusion, depression, anxiety, nervousness, shakiness, redness or pain at place of injection, diabetes.

(continued)

MAJOR CHEMOTHERAPY DRUGS AND HORMONES, THEIR USES AND MOST COMMON SIDE EFFECTS *(continued)*

NAMES AND USES	COMMON SIDE EFFECTS (All patients do not have all side effects)	OCCASIONAL SIDE EFFECTS (Some patients may have other side effects not listed)
Tamoxifen (Nolvadex, Nolvadexalpha-tamoxifen, Med Tamoxifen, Novo-Tamoxifen, Tamofen, Tamone, Tamoplex, taxomifen citrate) An antigestrogen used in breast cancer. Taken as a tablet.	Hot flashes, burning at site where drug was injected, vaginal discharge, nausea, irregular menstrual period, weight gain, blood clots. Women more susceptible to cancer of the endometrium and uterine sarcoma as well as to strokes. Do not take more or less than your doctor ordered or more often than ordered. If you miss a dose, do not take the missed dose at all and do not double the next dose; talk to your doctor. You should use birth control measures while you are taking this medicine, but do not take birth control pills since they may change the effects of the tamoxifen. Tell your doctor right away if you do get pregnant while on the medicine.	Vaginal bleeding, nausea and vomiting, loss of appetite, endometriosis, bone and tumor pain, visual changes, skin rash and itchiness, dizziness, loss of hair, depression, light-headedness, confusion, fluid retention, headache, anemia, swelling of legs, low blood counts.

Teniposide (VM–26, Vumon, PTG, thenylidene-lignan-P, NSC–122819) A plant alkaloid used in lymphoma, leukemia, cancer of lung. Given IV.	Low blood counts, mild hair loss, fever, chills, sore throat, nausea and vomiting (usually can be prevented with antinausea medicine), diarrhea, mouth sores.	Loss of appetite, flushing of face, dizziness, loss of muscle coordination, diarrhea, sluggishness, confusion, tiredness, seizures.
Thioguanine (Tabloid, 6–Thioguanine, 6–TG, Lanvis Thioguanine Tabloid, aminopurine-6-thiol-hemihydrate, NSC–752) An antimetabolite used in leukemia. Taken as tablet. IV is investigational.	Low blood counts, diarrhea, mouth sores, fever, chills, sore throat, skin rash, unsteady gait.	Nausea and vomiting, jaundice, loss of appetite, unsteadiness.
Thiotepa (Thioplex, TESPA, TSPA, Triethylenethio-phosphoramide, NSC–6396) An alkylating agent used in lymphoma, cancer of the breast, ovary, bladder, and lung. High dose used with bone marrow transplant. Given IV. May also be given in artery, in muscle, or put into specific areas of body.	At high doses: low blood count, mouth sores, infections, nausea and vomiting, hair loss, fever, chills, sore throat, hives, skin rash, dry skin.	Headache, allergic reaction, dizziness, burning at injection site, stomach pain, blood in urine, frequent urination, weak legs, loss of appetite, diarrhea impaired fertility, second cancer (leukemia).
Topotecan (Hycamptamine, NSC–609699) Used in ovarian cancer. Given IV.	Low blood counts, anemia, nausea and vomiting, diarrhea, hair loss, headache.	Dizziness, lightheadedness, fever, chills, sore throat, weight loss, general tiredness, blood in urine, loss of appetite, constipation, stomach pain, mouth sores, skin rash, dry skin, acne, fever blisters.

(continued)

MAJOR CHEMOTHERAPY DRUGS AND HORMONES, THEIR USES AND MOST COMMON SIDE EFFECTS (continued)

NAMES AND USES	COMMON SIDE EFFECTS (All patients do not have all side effects)	OCCASIONAL SIDE EFFECTS (Some patients may have other side effects not listed)
Toremifene (FC–1157A, Fareston, toremifene citrate, toremifenum) Used in breast cancer. Taken as a tablet.	Low blood counts, nausea, vomiting, dizziness, pain in stomach, bleeding or discharge from vagina, hot flashes, sweating.	Loss of or increased appetite, diarrhea, constipation, dry eyes, cataracts, dizziness, vertigo, tiredness, lack of energy, headache, sleeplessness, tumor flare.
Traztuzumab (Herceptin) Used in breast cancer. Given IV.	Fever and chills, heart failure, anemia, low blood counts, diarrhea.	Lung problems, nausea, vomiting, pain.
Uracil Mustard (Uramustine, NSC–34462) Used for leukemias, lymphomas, and cancer of ovary. Taken as tablet.	Low blood counts, nausea, vomiting, lack of appetite, diarrhea.	Greater risk for infection, bleeding, anemia, loss of hair, skin rash, nervousness, irritability, depression, confusion, lack of menstrual periods. If you are sensitive to aspirin, you may develop reactions, including bronchial asthma.
Vinblastine (Velban, Velsar, Alkaban AQ, Velbe, vinblastine sulfate, vincaleukoblastine, VLB) Plant alkaloid used in leukemia, lymphomas, neuroblastoma, melanoma, cancer of the testis, breast, kidney, bladder, cervix, head and neck, ovary and lung. Given IV.	Low blood counts.	Nausea and vomiting, stomach cramps, loss of appetite, diarrhea, mouth sores, hair loss, burning pain, redness or swelling at injection site, constipation, skin rash and itching, sensitive to sun, pain in jaw, joints, bones, muscle, back, or limbs.

Drug		
Vincristine (Oncovin, Vincasar PFS, leurocristine) A plant alkaloid used in leukemias, lymphomas, sarcomas, neurblastoma, Wilm's tumor, melanoma, multiple myeloma, cancers of the colon, rectum, brain, breast, cervix, ovary, lung, and thyroid. Given IV.	Hair loss, numbness or tingling in hands or feet.	Pain in arms, legs, jaw or stomach, pain in testicles, mouth sores, fever, chills, sore throat, severe constipation, metallic taste, hoarseness, agitation, confusion, lightheadedness, dizziness, drooping eyelids, jaw or joint pain, blurred or double vision, anemia, stomach cramps.
Vinorelbine (Navelbine, vinorelbine tartrate, 5'noranhydro-vinblanstine, NVB) Vinca alkaloid used in breast and lung cancer. Given IV or taken as a capsule.	Low blood count, nausea and vomiting, tiredness, stomach pain, chest pain, difficulty breathing.	Tenderness over length of vein where drug injected, constipation, pain in jaw or tumor.
Zoledronic acid (Zometa, zolendrondate) Biophosphanate used to treat bone metastases in multiple myeloma, breast, prostate, lung, and other solid tumors. Given IV.	Fever, joint pain, lack of appetite, anemia, bone pain, spinal cord compression.	Bone fractures.

What hormones are used for breast cancer?

Today the hormones usually given for breast cancer are in three classifications: Antiestrogen selective ER modulators (SERM), aromatase inhibitors, and progestins. Since the development of new hormone types, the older hormones, such as estrogens, and androgens are rarely used.

What is a selective ER modulator?

An antiestrogen selective ER modulator, or SERM as it is often referred to, is a drug that blocks estrogen at the estrogen receptor (ER). At the same time it can act like estrogen in some other tissues. Tamoxifen is the most commonly used SERM. Toremifene (Fareston) and raloxifene (Evista) are also used.

What does an aromatase inhibitor do?

An aromatase inhibitor blocks the formation of estradiol, a female hormone, by interfering with an aromatase enzyme. It is a type of hormone therapy used in postmenopausal women who have hormone-dependent breast cancer. Anastrazole (Armidex), letrozole, and exemestane are the hormones most often used. They target only the aromatase and are being studied for use in women with ER-positive breast cancer. Aminoglutethimide therapy, which was once the major aromatase inhibitor used, is only used today for women without ovarian function.

What progestins are being used?

Megestrol acetate (Megace) is a synthetic form of the hormone progesterone. It is sometimes used to treat advanced breast cancer, especially in women for whom tamoxifen is not working well. It may also be used to treat advanced endometrial cancer.

What hormones are being used for prostate cancer?

Leutinizing hormone-releasing hormone (LH-RH) and oral nonsteroidal antiandrogen are the two types of hormones being used for prostate cancer. In the past estrogens were also used but are not often used because the newer hormones produce fewer side effects.

What leutinizing hormone-release homones (LH-RH) are used?

Leuprolide (Lupron) and goserelin acetate (Zoladex) are most often used. LH-RH agonists are often given with an antiandrogen hormone such as flutamide (Eulexin).

What antiandrogens are used?

Most commonly, flutamine (Eulexin), bicalutamide (Casodex), or nitlutamide (Anadron) are used in prostate cancer to block male hormones.

What biologic response modifiers are being used in cancer treatment?

There are several types that are being used, including interferons, inter-leukins, tumor necrosis factors, and colony stimulating factors to stimulate or restore the ability of the immune system to fight infections and other diseases. Sometimes these biologic response modifiers are combined with chemotherapy. There is more information on the use of these substances in Chapter 11, New Advances and Investigational Trials.

SIDE EFFECTS

Do all chemotherapy drugs produce some side effects?

The extent of side effects varies greatly from patient to patient and from drug to drug. The side effects range from slight in some people to severe in a few instances. Some drugs have more noticeable side effects than others. Some people go through their entire chemotherapy treatment without suffering side effects. Others have serious problems. We have listed the side effects as known for each drug. It is important to remember that no one experiences all of them. Remember, too, that the doctors and nurses can help you minimize many adverse effects. Sometimes your own attitude can play a role in how severe your side effects will be. Research shows that techniques such as relaxation can help you experience milder side effects. (See Chapter 27, Living With Cancer.)

Why do you get side effects from chemotherapy?

Many drugs kill the fast growing cancer cells. They also can harm the normal ones, especially those cells that grow fast or are not fully developed. Your mouth, stomach, and intestines, the roots of your hair (hair follicles) and the bone marrow are areas of the body that normally have fast-growing cells. Thus, they may be affected by the chemotherapy. When they are, side effects may result. But normal cells repair themselves faster than the cancerous ones and give the normal tissues a chance to do this, drugs are generally given in cycles, with rest periods in between.

What are the most common side effects?

The most common side effects of chemotherapy are nausea and vomiting, hair loss, fatigue, and the decreased ability of the body to make red and white blood cells and platelets (bone marrow suppression).

Are the side effects of all the drugs the same?

Each drug has its own potential side effects. When drugs are combined, the side effects can change. You should talk to your doctor and nurse about what side effects to expect for the kind of chemotherapy drugs you will be getting.

What can be done to minimize side effects?

Great progress is being made in preventing some of the most serious side effects of chemotherapy. Many new drugs and techniques can increase the powerful effects of chemotherapy on the cancer while decreasing its harmful effects on healthy cells in the body. In addition, many things can be done to help minimize or lessen side effects, if you get them. There is, for instance, a wide range of drugs that can help curb nausea and vomiting. Do not hesitate to discuss any side effects with your healthcare team. If the side effects are severe, your drugs or treatment schedule may need to be changed. There are many suggestions on ways of treating side effects in Chapter 27, Living With Cancer.

How long do the side effects last?

Some of the side effects, such as nausea and vomiting, can occur with each treatment and last for a relatively short time. Others, like tiredness, come on gradually and go away in the same manner. Some cause permanent changes, such as damage to the heart, lungs, nerves, kidneys, or other organs.

How can I describe my side effects to my healthcare team?

It is useful if you are able to give your healthcare team exact details about the side effects. Keeping a written log has helped many patients remember details that can be useful to the health care team. Keep track of when you had your last treatment, when the side effect started in relation to the treatment, how long it lasted, how many times a day it happened, when happened (morning, mealtime, nighttime), exactly what the side effect was (nausea alone, vomiting alone, both together, retching), what you had eaten/drunk before it started, what else accompanied it (diarrhea, constipation, feeling weak, dizzy), whether it kept you from your normal daily activities, what you were doing when it happened (eating food, drinking, taking medicine), how often it happened, and what helped to alleviate the problem. The more information you can give, the more help you will receive.

How long does it take to recover from the side effects of chemotherapy?

When your chemotherapy treatments are completed, most normal cells recover quickly and the side effects start to disappear as the healthy cells have a chance to grow normally. However, the time it takes to get over all the side effects and regain your former energy varies from one person to another, and depends on the kinds of drugs you have been getting, the side effect itself as well as on your own physical condition.

Do the side effects mean that the drugs are working?

There does not seem to be any relationship between the side effects and what is happening to the tumor. Neither the appearance of side effects nor their absence seems to have any relation to the effectiveness of the drug. One person may have no side effects and yet the drug may be making the tumor shrink greatly. Another person's tumor may also be shrinking with the person experiencing considerable side effects. It depends upon the body's tolerance to the drugs being given and the responsiveness of the cancer cells to them. The doctor will do tests to see if your treatments are working.

Are there any serious side effects I should report to the doctor immediately?

You should promptly report the following symptoms to your doctor:

- Fever over 100°
- Any kind of bleeding or bruising
- Development of any rash or allergic reaction such as swelling of eyelids, hands, or feet
- Shaking, chills
- Marked pain or soreness at the area where the drug was injected
- Any pain of unusual intensity or duration, including headaches
- Increasing "pins and needles" tingling sensations in your hands and/or feet
- Shortness of breath or inability to catch your breath
- Severe diarrhea
- Bloody urine

Any other new, unexpected symptoms that arise should be reported promptly to the doctor.

Will I have nausea and vomiting?

It depends on the dose and the drug being used. Some drugs are much more likely to cause this side effect while others rarely do. Thanks to new chemotherapy drugs and to new drugs called antiemetic agents, that control nausea and vomiting, these symptoms are not as common as they once were. These antiemetic agents are usually given before the chemotherapy treatments begin and are given as long as the drug is likely to cause vomiting. They are usually taken regularly around the clock. Among the brand names you might hear are Reglan, Zofran, Kytil, Ativan, Decadron, Compazine, Torecan, Marinol, Xanax, Benadryl, Anzemet, Inapsine, and Haldol. They can be given intravenously (IV), orally, intramuscularly, under the skin (subcuntaneously) rectally, under the tongue, or as a skin patch. You may take more than one since the different medicines affect different pathways.

When does the nausea and vomiting usually happen?

It depends on the dose, the drug used, and the physical makeup of the patient. Nausea and vomiting can begin as early as an hour after the treatment is given or as late as eight to twelve hours later. It may last for just a few hours or as long as three or four days. Some people feel mildly nauseated most of the time. Others become severely nauseated for a limited time after the treatment. Some even begin to feel nauseated before the treatment starts (called anticipatory nausea). Be sure you tell your nurse and doctor if the nausea or vomiting has lasted more than a day or has been so bad you cannot even keep liquids down.

Can relaxation techniques be used to help relieve my nausea and vomiting?

Studies have found that some people's nausea and vomiting can be helped with methods that are used to cope with stress. There are several methods that you might wish to try, including rhythmic breathing, biofeedback, imagery, and visualization. Others have found that hypnosis and acupuncture are helpful. There are additional details about these methods in Chapter 27, Living with Cancer.

Is marijuana being used to reduce nausea and vomiting?

There has been much interest in the use of marijuana to treat chemotherapy-induced nausea and vomiting in cancer patients. Some patients use marijuana itself. Dronobinol, a synthetic form of the active marijuana constituent THC (delat-9-tetrahydrocannabinol), is currently available by prescription under the trade name Marinol for use as an antiemetic for mild nausea and vomiting.

Is there something I can do about my lack of appetite when I feel nauseated?

First of all, most people find that they can eat a light meal or snack before they have a chemotherapy treatment. Don't be too hard on yourself if side effects make it difficult to eat. Try small amounts of food and eat more often. On the days you are feeling well, eat regular meals. You need a balanced, high-protein diet in order to maintain your strength, to prevent body tissues from breaking down, and to rebuild the normal tissues that have been affected by the drugs. There is additional nutritional help in Chapter 27, Living with Cancer.

Will I lose my hair?

Not all drugs cause hair loss, but it is a common side effect. The rapidly growing cells that make up the hair roots (follicles) are sensitive to chemotherapuetic drugs. If you do have hair loss, your hair may become thinner or it may fall out altogether.

Will I lose my hair in places other than on my head?

The hair follicles of the beard, mustache, eyelashes, eyebrows, armpits, chest, legs, and pubic area are all rapidly growing cells and are sensitive to some of the drugs used in chemotherapy. Sometimes the loss is partial. Many times, while there is a complete loss of scalp hair, hair loss in other body areas is much less common.

Will my hair fall out gradually or all at once?

Hair loss differs from patient to patient and from drug to drug. It may fall out gradually or in clumps. Your scalp may become sensitive, flaky or irritated. Use a soft bristle brush to lessen pulling on the hair. If you have long hair, cut it short before it begins to thin—the weight of long hair may hasten the loss. Don't use rollers, or a curling iron and don't tease your hair. Use a mild or moisturizing shampoo.

What should I do to prepare for losing my hair?

You need to think about what would make you most comfortable—wearing a wig or a hairpiece, a turban, scarf, cap, leaving your head uncovered or a combination of any or all of these alternatives. Try some hats and scarves to see how they might look. You also need to think about ways to conceal lost eyebrows. Some people find that horn rimmed glasses or other glasses that are fitted with the rim coming just in front of the eyebrows can help. You may need to practice using eyebrow pencil and false eyelashes.

Are there any general hints about buying wigs and hairpieces?

- Buy the wig before you start losing your hair. If you can, get the wig before you start having chemotherapy treatments. Get your first wig the same color as your natural hair so you can start wearing it as your hair begins to thin.

- Buy the wig yourself—don't send someone else to do it for you. Bring a friend along for moral support. It is essential that the wig or hairpiece fits you well, is comfortable to wear, is flattering on you, and pleases you. Many people find it useful to buy more than one wig, especially if they need to wear it for more than six months. (Some people choose to experiment with wigs of different colors.)

- You might want to consider borrowing a wig or hairpiece. Some hospitals and some American Cancer Society offices have wig banks where you can get them free.

- Wigs are tax-deductible medical expenses and may be covered by some medial insurance policies. You'll need to get a prescription from your doctor.

- A good synthetic wig washes better, is less expensive to maintain, is cooler and costs less than a real-hair wig.

Will my hair grow back the same as it was before?

When your hair begins to regrow, it will be thick and soft and sometimes even better than before. It usually begins to grow back once the chemotherapy is stopped. Occasionally, it will begin to regrow while you are still under treatment.

What can cause my urine to change color while I am on chemotherapy?

Some drugs can temporarily change the color of your urine. Some may turn it red, orange, bright yellow, or blue-green, or cause it to take on a strong or medicine-like odor. Your doctor or nurse can tell you if the drug you are taking can cause this side effect.

Why does the doctor tell me to drink more fluids?

Some of the drugs can affect your kidney and bladder. You will be advised to increase the amount of liquids in your diet—water, juice, coffee, tea, soup, soft drinks, broth, ice cream, soup, popsicles, and gelatin—to ensure good urine flow and help prevent problems.

Are there any signs I should watch for if the drugs I am taking are known to affect my kidney and bladder?

If you see any of these changes, you need to inform your doctor:

- Pain or burning when you urinate

- Frequent urination

- A feeling that you must urinate right away

- Reddish or bloody urine

- Fever or chills

Will the drugs damage my bone marrow?

Many types of chemotherapy, while stopping the growth of the tumor cells, also stop the growth of cells in the bone marrow that is responsible for producing most of your blood cells. Since bone marrow cells duplicate rapidly in order to maintain normal blood counts, these cells are particularly sensitive to the drugs. Among the cells involved are white blood cells that help fight fungal and bacterial infections, red blood cells that help carry oxygen to various parts of the body and platelets that help blood to clot. Three types of drugs usually have this side effect: alkylating agents, antimetabolites and antitumor antibiotics. When your bone marrow is not producing enough red and white blood cells, the condition is referred to as bone marrow depression.

What is a drop in blood count called?

If the drop is in the white blood cell count, it is called leukopenia. In the red blood cells it is called anemia. In the platelets it is called thrombocytopenia. If all of them drop, it is called pancytopenia.

When is my blood count checked?

If you are taking drugs in these categories, your blood count usually will be checked before you are given each chemotherapy treatment. If your counts are slightly low, your treatment may be held up for a few days until your count comes back up again.

What if my blood count is very low?

If your blood count falls very low, you will be carefully monitored. A serious drop in white blood count makes your susceptible to infections. A serious drop in your platelet count puts you at risk for bleeding. In some cases, you may need to have a transfusion of blood cells, either red cells or platelets.

What can be done if I have anemia?

Anemia can make you feel very tired, short of breath, dizzy, and unable to concentrate. You may need a blood transfusion. The doctor may give you erythropoietin, a natural hormone that stimulates your bone marrow to make more red blood cells.

What flu-like symptoms do some people have?

Some people report that they feel as if they have the flu a few hours to a few days after they have had their chemotherapy—muscle aches, headache, tiredness, nausea, slight fever, chills, sore throat, and little or no appetite. Usually, these symptoms last for a few days. However, since these symptoms also can be caused by an infection or by the cancer itself, be sure to report them to your doctor.

Will I get tired?

Many people do get tired during treatments, which is often caused by the lack of red blood cells. You may feel tired, weak, dizzy, chilled, and sometimes short of breath. The feeling of fatigue usually begins to wear off a few weeks after your treatment ends and will gradually go away. The following also should help:

- Eat well, including plenty of iron-rich foods, such as green leafy vegetables and red meat. Sometimes a small amount of food will give you the extra energy you need.

- Rest when you feel tired. Some people get tired more quickly and need more rest during this time. Try to get more sleep at night. Rest during the day when you feel you need it.

- Don't feel you must keep up your normal schedule of activities if you don't feel like it. Use your leisure time in a restful way.

- Reduce your activities. You may wish to take some time off from work, or work a reduced schedule for a while.

- Don't be afraid to ask others for help. Family, friends, and neighbors can help you in shopping, childcare, housework or driving.

- To prevent dizziness, get up slowly from a seated or lying position.

What are the side effects of a low platelet count?

Too few platelets can affect the blood cells that help stop bleeding. You may bruise and bleed more easily than usual, even with a small cut. It is best to avoid situations that might result in an injury, such as contact sports. Be careful when you use sharp tools or knives. Use heavy gloves when you reach in the oven or work in your garden or workshop. Blow your nose gently and avoid forceful sneezing. Use an electric razor for shaving.

Are there any signs I should report to the doctor that signal low platelet counts?

There are several things you need to report to your doctor:

- Unexpected bruises
- Small red spots under your skin
- Pink or reddish urine, or black or bloody bowel movements
- Any bleeding from your gums or nose

What precautions should I take if my white blood count is too low?

A low white blood count makes it difficult for your body to fight infection. Many parts of your body, including your mouth, skin, lungs, urinary tracts, rectum, and reproductive tract can get an infection. You should take several precautions:

- Try to stay away from crowds and people who have colds, flu, or any other disease you can catch such as the measles or chickenpox. This is particularly important the first ten days after starting chemotherapy because your white blood count will automatically drop, making you susceptible to infections.

- Clean cuts and scratches with warm water and an antiseptic, and keep them clean until the sore heals. Don't scratch or squeeze sores, such as pimples. Brush your teeth with a soft brush.

- Be careful not to cut or nick yourself when working with knives and scissors. Don't cut or tear the cuticles of your nails. Use an electric razor when shaving. Protect your hands with gloves when doing heavy work.

- Make sure all food is washed well and thoroughly cooked. Don't eat raw seafood or share utensils.

- Let somebody else clean the litterbox and take care of the pets.

- Wash your hands often during the day, especially before you eat and before and after you go to the bathroom. Clean your rectal area gently but thoroughly after each bowel movement. Don't use tampons, enemas, or rectal suppositories.

- Take warm (not hot) showers and baths. Use lotion on your skin to prevent dryness and cracking.

- Do not get immunization shots without first checking with the doctor.

- Inspect your body for signs of infection in your nose, on your lips, in your eyes or in the genital or rectal area. If an infection should develop, tell the doctor about it right away.

- If you get a cold or the flu, call your doctor. Do not take any medicine that has not been prescribed by the doctor, including aspirin, cough medicine, vitamins, antibiotics, painkillers, or any other types of medicine.

What are the signs of an infection?

You need to call the doctor if any of the following occur:

- Fever
- Chills, cough, sore throat
- Sweating
- Loose bowels (may be due to the drugs) burning feeling when you urinate
- Unusual vaginal discharge or itching
- Redness or swelling, especially around a sore, pimple, or boil

What kind of eye problems might I get from chemotherapy drugs?

Some of the drugs can cause serious problems with your eyes. You might have blurred vision. Your eyes might tear a lot or they may be very dry.

Cataracts, problems with your retina, and glaucoma are other eye problems that may be caused by the drugs.

What should I do if I have eye problems?

Before you get chemotherapy, you should have an eye exam so that you and your ophthalmologist know where you are starting from. If you see any changes, such as blurry vision, or tearing or burning while you are taking the chemotherapy, have your eyes checked against your first exam. The doctor also may give you eye drops if your eyes are dry.

What can I do about the sore spots inside my mouth?

Some drugs can cause sores in the mouth and throat, they make the tissues dry and irritated and cause them to bleed. It is important to take steps to prevent these sores from becoming infected by taking good care of your mouth and teeth. Brush your teeth after each meal, using a soft toothbrush. If your gums are extremely sensitive, use a cotton swab or gauze. Make sure that your toothpaste does not contain abrasives. Or you can use a paste of baking soda and water. Rinse your toothbrush well after each use and store it in a dry place. Do not use a commercial mouthwash that contains a large amount of salt or alcohol. Ask the nurse about using a saltwater or baking soda rinse. You might want to use a numbing medication, such as those used for teething babies, to soothe your mouth pain. If you are having trouble eating, ask the doctor to prescribe a numbing medication that you can use before meals. See Chapter 27, Living with Cancer, for more information on dealing with mouth sores.

Is the metallic taste in my mouth a common side effect?

It is not common but it can happen to some people who are getting chemotherapy drugs. Try sucking on sugar-free hard candy (peppermint seems to work especially well) or rinsing your mouth frequently to mask the taste.

Will chemotherapy affect my teeth?

Certain chemotherapy drugs cause a reduction in saliva in your mouth. Saliva protects your teeth against tooth decay. It is important, if possible, to have your dentist do any dental work that may be needed before you start chemotherapy. You should also ask the dentist to show you the best ways to brush and clean your mouth while you are having treatment. The dentist might prescribe the daily use of a fluoride gel in a small tray that fits over your teeth. Fluoride mouthrinse may also be recommended. It is important to be under the care of a dentist who has experience in treating people undergoing chemotherapy.

Will I experience diarrhea?

Some chemotherapy drugs, the antimetabolites or antitumor antibiotics, affect the cells lining your intestines and may cause you to have soft stools, or diarrhea. If it lasts more than 24 hours or if you have pain and cramps along with the loose stools, you need to talk with your nurse or doctor. You should try a diet that is low in roughage (avoid foods such as raw vegetables, bran, beans, fresh fruit) and high in low-fiber foods (such as yogurt, mashed potatoes, chicken, turkey, white rice, and noodles). Diarrhea can easily cause you to lose fluids and become dehydrated. Make sure you drink plenty of clear liquids (apple juice, clear broth, water, ginger ale) and that you eat foods that are high in potassium (bananas, oranges, potatoes). If you are lactose intolerant, you should avoid anything that contains dairy products. You should not take any medicine for your diarrhea without discussing it with your doctor. There is additional information on dealing with diarrhea in Chapter 27, Living with Cancer.

Will constipation be a problem for me?

It may be, since some of the chemotherapy drugs can cause constipation. In addition, you may be eating differently or be less active than you were before. Try to prevent constipation by drinking lots of fluids (at least eight glasses a day), such as water, juices, or broth. Warm drinks work especially well to help loosen the bowels. Eat fruits and vegetables if your diet allows. A glass of prune juice or a few tablespoons of bran in the morning may help. Keep active with light exercise such as walking. If you do become constipated, discuss how your normal bowel pattern has changed with your doctor or nurse. You may need to take a laxative or a stool softener but only with the approval of your doctor or nurse. There is additional information for dealing with constipation in Chapter 27, Living with Cancer.

Do people on chemotherapy have problems with retaining fluids?

The drugs themselves, hormonal changes due to the drugs, or the cancer itself may cause your body to retain fluids. If you notice any swelling or puffiness in your face, hands, feet or stomach area, tell your doctor or nurse about it. You may need to cut down on the amount of salt you are using in your foods or cut out salt altogether from your diet. In addition, you may need medication to help your body get rid of the excess fluids.

Is the tingling in my fingers and feet a result of my chemotherapy?

Because some chemotherapy drugs affect the cells of the peripheral nervous system, damage to the nerve endings of the hands and/or feet may result. You may feel numbness, burning, and tingling. You may have problems with walking, picking up objects, buttoning your clothes and keeping your balance. Your muscles may feel weak, tired, or sore. Sometimes the nerves in other parts of your body are affected and you may feel pain in your jaw, or stomach, lose some of your hearing, or become constipated. You should discuss any of these symptoms with your doctor. Many times, these effects start after you have had several chemotherapy treatments and are only temporary. However, sometimes they can signal serious problems that can become permanent.

What can be done if I have these side effects?

Massage, physical therapy, and acupuncture may be used to help circulation. There are several treatments that can be used including glutamine, vitamin B supplements, nonsteroidal anti-inflammatory drugs (NSAIDS), anticonsulsants, antidepressants, and amifostine. Reducing the dose of your drug or changing to another drug may also be necessary. If your balance is affected, you should take precautions to help keep you from falling or burning yourself.

Are skin rashes common during chemotherapy?

You may have some minor skin problems while you are on the drugs, including itching, peeling, dryness, redness, and acne. Most of these are easily taken care of. Use cornstarch like a dusting powder to ease the itching. Take quick showers or sponge baths and apply cream and lotion to your moist skin to help prevent dryness. Do not use cologne, perfume, or aftershave lotion that contains alcohol. Keeping your face clean and dry and using over-the-counter medicated creams can help your acne. Make sure you tell your nurse and doctor right away if you have sudden itching, a rash or hives, or if you begin wheezing, or have any trouble breathing.

Do patients sometimes suffer from irritation at the point where the drug is injected?

This may happen. If the rash is a reaction from the drug, it normally disappears in 30 to 90 minutes. However, if it is caused by the drug leaking out at the site of the injection, it can produce serious, permanent tissue damage. If you feel any burning or pain when you are getting drugs intravenously, report it immediately to the person giving the drugs. Cold compresses and pain medication may be used to help alleviate the discomfort.

Is it unusual for dark circles to form on my fingernails?

Some drugs cause darkening of the beds of your fingernails. This is a harmless side effect and will usually disappear when chemotherapy has ended. You may also find that your nails become brittle or cracked or develop vertical lines or bands. Try nail strengtheners to help keep the problem to a minimum and protect your nails by wearing gloves when washing dishes, gardening, or doing other work around the house. If they get worse, be sure to tell your nurse or doctor.

Do veins ever get darker when a person is on chemotherapy drugs?
Some drugs can irritate your veins and some discoloration may develop along the pathway. It may look as if someone has marked it with a felt-tipped pen. The darker your skin, the darker the vein becomes. Exposure to the sun makes the veins look even more prominent. Don't be alarmed. The coloring usually fades on its own a few months after treatment is finished.

Will I be more sensitive to the sun during my treatment?
Some drugs can increase the effects of the sun on your skin. Check with your doctor or nurse. You may need to be careful when going outside, even if you are just taking a walk. Wear a hat and use sunblock. Be extremely careful if you go to the beach: wear a sunscreen with protection factor of at least 15. The doctor may advise you to stay out of the sun or use a product to block out the sun's rays entirely.

What is radiation recall?
You may experience certain side effects if you have had radiation treatments before your chemotherapy. The skin where you had your radiation treatments may get patchy and red—anywhere from light to very bright in color—and you may have an itchy or burning sensation. A few people get blisters or wet, oozing areas of skin that peel. If you have radiation recall, clean the affected skin gently using mild soap and lukewarm water, and use cool, wet compresses to soothe the itching and burning. Tell your doctor or nurse about these reactions.

Do people on chemotherapy have personality changes?
This is not a common side effect. However, chemotherapy brings major changes into a person's life and causes people to feel fearful, anxious, angry, or depressed at some times during their treatments. These are perfectly normal feelings that can be dealt with, many times, by talking with friends and family members, by attending support groups made up of people going through the same kind of experiences, or by discussing them with your healthcare team, your clergy, social worker, or psychologist.

How expensive is chemotherapy?
The costs vary depending on the drugs being used, how often they are given, the dosage, and whether you get them at home, in an office, or in a hospital. Added costs include the cost of the visit, the tests involved, and the charge to administer the drug.

Will my insurance cover chemotherapy?

Most health insurance policies, including Medicare Part B (that helps pay for doctors' bills and many other medical services) cover at least part of the cost of many of the drugs. You need to discuss these costs with the healthcare team at the place where you are getting your treatment. There is more information on insurance in Chapter 27, Living with Cancer.

Are cancer patients on chemotherapy at a higher risk for getting shingles?

Shingles (or herpes zoster) is a painful viral infection of certain nerves that causes a skin rash along the course of the affected nerve. People with lymphoma are more susceptible to shingles. Others who are receiving chemotherapy drugs that suppress the immune system are also at a higher risk.

Are chemotherapy drugs available free of charge to patients who are unable to pay for them?

Many prescription drug manufacturers make their medications available free-of-charge to patients who do not have the means to pay for them. Call the Cancer Information Service, 1–800–4–CANCER, for further information. Usually the physician must certify that you are unable to afford the cost of the drug and are unable to obtain assistance elsewhere.

Is there anyone who can give me help with my hair, makeup, and nails while I am undergoing chemotherapy?

There is a nationwide program, called Look Good . . . Feel Better, that has been developed by the Cosmetic, Toiletry, and Fragrance Association in cooperation with the American Cancer Society (ACS) and the National Cosmetology Association. It helps women deal with the changes in their appearances that may result from chemotherapy or radiation treatments or from the illness itself, such as loss of hair, eyebrows and lashes, changes in skin tone and texture, or brittleness of nails. Cosmetologists give practical, one-on-one advice on appearance changes, including specific recommendations for skin care, hair styles, wigs and accessories, eyebrow and eye makeup, and nail care, taking into consideration the changes you may have in your skin and nails. You can learn how to put on scarves and turbans and the different styles of wigs that are available. The American Cancer Society, along with cancer centers and hospitals around the country, runs the program locally with members of the National Cosmetology Association offering their services on a voluntary basis to help women with cancer learn the beauty techniques. Call the American Cancer Society at 1–800–ACS–2345 or 1–800–395–LOOK to find programs located near you.

Sexual Side Effects

Will being on chemotherapy affect my sexual relations?
Chemotherapy may, but does not always, affect sexual organs and functioning in both men and women. The side effects depend on the drugs being used, as well as your age and your general health. In general, men and women on chemotherapy may have less desire for sex than usual. This may be due to the physical effects of the drugs, or may result from feeling unattractive due to hair and weight loss, or other side effects. In addition, several drugs used alone may cause infertility and sterility. Combinations of drugs appear to prolong infertility. Drugs used to manage side effects of the treatment can also alter your sexual functions.

FEMALE SEXUAL SIDE EFFECTS

Are irregular menstrual periods a side effect of chemotherapy?
Some drugs can affect the ovaries, reducing the amount of hormones they produce. Depending on the drugs you are taking, your menstrual cycle may come earlier or later, or it may last longer than usual. Sometimes it will stop temporarily or last as long as you are on chemotherapy. Women taking androgens may find that their voices deepen, hair growth increases, and sexual desire increases. Women who are menopausal may have bleeding. These changes usually disappear when you stop taking the drugs. You may have the symptoms of menopause—hot flashes, itching, burning, or dryness of the tissues of your vagina. These symptoms may be much more intense than they would be if you were having menopause naturally.

Can chemotherapy cause premature menopause?
Chemotherapy can cause periods to stop temporarily or permanently. In younger women, this loss of estrogen puts extra stress on the body because it happens before you have had the full benefit of estrogen for such tasks as building bone mass. For any woman of childbearing age, premature menopause means the temporary or permanent loss of the ability to bear children. Many women under age 35 may recover their menstrual periods but begin menopause sooner than they would have without chemotherapy. The damage to the ovaries depends on the type of drugs and the size of the doses. It is important that you discuss the possible effects of chemotherapy on your reproductive capacity with your doctor before undergoing treatment.

What can I do about the vaginal dryness?
You usually can relieve the dryness by using a water-based vaginal lubricant. There are many on the market, such as Astroglide, K-Y Jelly, Lubrin, Condom

Mate, Ortho Personal Lubricant, Replens, Surgilube, and Today Personal Lubricant. There are also lubricating vaginal suppositories (Lubrin, Condom Mate). If there is some pain during intercourse, try using a gel lubricant during intercourse for lubrication. Vaseline is **not** recommended because it is not water-based and can increase the chance of infection. You also should have your doctor check your estrogen level, which gives information on how well your ovaries are functioning and whether the dryness is due to a physical change in your vagina. Light bleeding after intercourse is not unusual because the lining of the vagina thins when you are on chemotherapy.

Am I more at risk for vaginal infections?
The changes in the tissues can make you more likely to get vaginal infections. It may be helpful to wear cotton underwear and panty hose with a ventilated cotton lining. Do not wear tight pants or shorts. The doctor may also prescribe a vaginal cream or suppository to reduce the chance of infection. If you have any symptoms of infections—itching, burning, or redness—check with your doctor so the problem can be diagnosed and proper treatment begun.

Can I get pregnant while I am on chemotherapy?
Even if your period stops, it is possible for you to get pregnant. And while it may be possible for you to get pregnant while on chemotherapy, it is not advisable because some of the drugs used may cause birth defects. Once treatment is finished your menstrual periods may return and you may be able to have a normal pregnancy. Many women have become pregnant and have had perfectly healthy children after being treated with chemotherapy. If you are of childbearing age, it is important to discuss the subject of birth control and childbearing thoroughly with your doctor before you start the treatment.

**If I am pregnant before I start my chemotherapy,
can I still have the baby?**
If you are pregnant, it may be possible to put off starting the chemotherapy until after the baby is born. If you need the chemotherapy before then, the doctor will usually wait until after the twelfth week of pregnancy. Women are no longer being advised to terminate their pregnancies as they sometimes were in the past. There is more information on pregnancy and cancer in Chapter 13, Breast Cancer.

Will a woman become infertile as a result of the treatment?
Sometimes the drug will cause damage to the ovaries that may result in infertility, making a woman unable to become pregnant. This may be a temporary condition or it may be permanent, depending on the type of drug given, the

dose used, and the woman's age. In addition, some chemotherapy drugs can damage your heart or lungs, making it difficult to go through pregnancy. If you wish to have children after you finish your treatments, you need to discuss this with the doctor before you start on chemotherapy.

Will I be able to preserve my eggs and use them to have a baby after treatment ends?

It is more difficult for women to freeze their eggs than for men to freeze their sperm. However, some women have their unfertilized eggs frozen; others freeze fertilized eggs.

Will I be able to have in vitro fertilization after my treatment ends?

Yes. Doctors agree that even if your ovaries are no longer functioning because of the chemotherapy drugs, you should be able to sustain a pregnancy.

MALE SEXUAL SIDE EFFECTS

What are the effects of chemotherapy on the male sex organs?

Often men who are undergoing chemotherapy have fewer sperm cells. The sperm may also have some abnormalities. These sometimes result in infertility, affecting a man's ability to father a child, either temporarily or permanently. This, of course, does not mean that erection or intercourse is affected. Production of sperm may return to normal when chemotherapy is completed, although some drugs cases permanent sterility. Since the effect of chemotherapy on the sperm and unborn child is not fully known, it is advisable to use birth control during this period.

Can sperm be stored for future use?

For men desiring children, freezing or storing sperm for future use prior to chemotherapy treatments may be an option. This alternative needs to be discussed with the medical team before treatment.

Will I have sexual side effects from hormonal treatment?

Men taking estrogens sometimes get enlarged breasts and have decreased sexual desires.

Web Pages to Check Out

www.cancer.gov: For general up-to-date information and for clinical trials.

www.cancer.org: For general up-to-date information and community resources.

New drugs are being developed and tested every day. If you do not find the drug you are taking listed in the book, check the following Internet sites:

www.cancer.org: Drug section gives mechanisms of action, side effects.

www.cancersource.com: Good section on drugs and their side effects.

www.nlm.nih.gov/medicineplus/druginfo: Drug information, both prescription and over-the-counter medications.

www.cancer.gov: Good information on chemotherapy and on how to deal with side effects from their booklets "Chemotherapy and You" and "Eating Hints." Put name of booklet in the search window on this site to view online and to print.

www.fda.gov/oder/cancer: U.S. Food and Drug Administration. Product Approvals by Cancer Indications—Cancer type or alphabetical listing.

Manufacturers of drugs also have patient information on their Web sites. Over 50 companies research and produce chemotherapy drugs; several also produce drugs to counter side effects. Among them:

www.amgen.com: Amgen.

www.bayerpharma-na.com: Bayer Pharmaceutical Division, U.S..

www.bms.com: Bristol-Myers Squibb Company.

www.gsk.com: GlaxoSmithKline.

www.pfizer.com: Pfizer, Incorporated.

www.novartis.com: Novartis Pharmaceuticals Corporation.

You can also search for information on a particular drug by putting its name into your search engine.

Also see Chapter 2, Searching for Answers on the Web, for more information.

Eleven

NEW ADVANCES AND INVESTIGATIONAL TREATMENTS

An exciting array of medical advances—from cyberknives that allow doctors to operate without cutting to "smart bombs" that target cancer cells—are being used in medical settings across the country. The scientific advances include new substances that might prevent cancer, new methods for detecting cancer cells for diagnosis, new treatments and improvements on old treatments, and using genetics in treatment and to help identify cancer risks. Clinical trials continue to be the link between research and progress. Before you have any treatment, check to see if there is a clinical trial for your type and stage of disease. If you are interested in joining a clinical trial, talk with your doctor, call the Cancer Information Service and ask specifically for information on clinical trials, or check out clinical trials on the Web (www.cancer.gov).

MANY OF THE promising breakthroughs are happening in the field of molecular medicine—a science whose name was hardly in any vocabulary a few years ago. Views from this window of molecular research have dramatically changed the ways scientists think about diseases. Some of the terminology is unfamiliar. Some of the techniques are complicated and hard to understand. But this is where much of the exciting new research is happening, with brilliant scientific minds using high-tech instruments to find future treatments and cures. This chapter covers some of the new exciting developments in this field, new research in genetics and what it means for cancer treatment in the future, how you can take part in clinical trials, and what stem cell and bone marrow transplants are all about.

WHAT YOU NEED TO KNOW ABOUT NEW ADVANCES AND INVESTIGATIONAL TRIALS

The most exciting advances are taking place in the new and growing area of molecular science, which is transforming the theory and practice of medicine. You may already have heard about new specialists called molecular biologists, molecular oncologists, and molecular geneticists. Some of the latest developments include:

- **Nanotechnology**—the development of miniature tools that can enter the cells and interact with DNA and proteins—is in the early phases of discovery. These tools may be able to detect disease at the earliest molecular change, in a very small amount of cells or tissue. They may also be able to enter and monitor cells within a living body.

- **Proteonics** uses computer software to perform a sophisticated analysis on a single drop of blood. This technique produces a printout that will indicate if cancer is present. Clinical trials are now testing this analysis in cases of ovarian and prostate cancer.

- **New chemotherapy agents** including molecularly targeted drugs, zero in on animal proteins that are fundamental to the cancer itself. These drugs target special cancer-causing molecules, eliminating cancer cells while avoiding serious damage to other noncancer cells.

- **Biological substances** trigger the body's own defense against cancer. Scientists are finding hundreds of substances that boost, direct, or restore many of the normal defenses in the body. You will hear many different names, such as colony stimulating factors, tumor necrosis factor, interleukins, interferons, cytokines, and gene therapy.

- **Genes** responsible for illnesses, even those that have complicated genetic patterns, are being found at a dizzying rate. This advance is transforming the way that cancer is detected, diagnosed, treated, even predicting who is at risk for developing certain cancers. This gene–cancer connection is opening a new, exciting field of exploration. However, this genetic resource also presents many difficult decisions for families in the future.

- **New tools** are allowing pathologists to be more precise and more sensitive in determining whether a tumor is malignant, how far it has spread, and how much the tumor has shrunk.

- **Surgery** can now be done using robotic scalpels and microcameras that allow doctors to see inside the body where they could never see before.

- **New treatments** and new ways of using treatments with radiation, drugs, hormones, or biological agents, often used in combination with molecular approaches and computerized delivery systems, are being tested in clinical trials.

- As in the past, the clinical trial remains the critical link between researchers with microscopes and test tubes and the transfer of new techniques to patients. Each clinical trial is designed to answer a set of research questions. You need to fit into the guidelines for a trial—usually a certain type and stage of cancer and certain health status—to be eligible to take part.

- The basis for a new treatment is often the standard treatment, that is, the state-of-the-art treatment presently in use. Most new treatments are designed on the basis of what has worked in the past and how it can be improved upon and are tested against the state-of-the-art standard treatments.

- More than 50 prevention trials are underway, scientifically studying how various substances, such as vitamins, minerals, hormones, or drugs, can prevent cancer from ever forming or stop or reverse its development.

How will nanotechnology work?

Nanotechnology is the use of miniature tools to detect and treat disease. In its early phase of development, it works by looking at and interacting with DNA and proteins in the cells.

How big is a nanometer?

A nanometer is a billionth of a meter or 1/80,000 the width of a human hair.

What are some of the nanodevices being tested?

There are several that have potential to be effective in the cancer field, both in the area of diagnosis and of treatment. You will probably begin to hear the word nanopores, nanotubes, quantum dots, and nanoshells. They work with molecules that represent some of the changes associated with cancer, such as damaged DNA sequences or a protein found in a specific cancer. The molecules binding to the cantilevers cause the cantilevers to bend. In diagnosis, nanotools should help to detect cancer in its early stages by identifying changes within DNA. Nanotechnology may also be useful for developing ways to eradicate cancer cells without harming healthy, neighboring cells.

Researchers can already link nanoshells to antibodies that recognize cancer cells. Scientists envision letting these nanoshells seek out the cancer cells and deliver treatments to tumor cells while leaving neighboring cells intact. The researchers' goal is to create a single nanodevice that will do many things: assist in imaging inside the body, recognize precancerous or cancerous cells, release a drug that targets only those cells, and report back on the effectiveness of the treatment. It will take from five to 15 years before this kind of treatment will be generally available.

DIAGNOSIS

New high-technology imaging techniques have replaced exploratory surgery in the diagnosis of cancer for some patients. Spiral CT scans trace a spiral path, making cross-sectional images of the body. Virtual endoscopy and colonoscopy allow doctors to see inside organs without doing surgery. Magnetic resonance imaging (MRI) is being used to detect hidden tumors by mapping the variations of the various atoms in the body on a computer screen. Positron emission tomography (PET), which produces 3-dimensional images of the body's metabolic and chemical activity, is in use for diagnostic purposes. Here are some of the advances in the diagnosis of cancer:

- A spiral CT scan, where an x-ray machine rotates continuously around the body, tracing a spiral path to make cross-sectional images of the body. This technique, being used as a screening method for lung cancer, makes 3-dimentional pictures, can detect small abnormal areas better than conventional CT scans and is faster, exposing people to less radiation.

- A virtual endoscopy, using spiral CT scans, allows the doctor to see inside organs and other structures without surgery or special instruments. One type of virtual endoscopy, known as CT colonography or virtual colonoscopy, is under study as a screening technique for colon cancer.

- A combined PET and CT scanning procedure may provide a more complete picture of the tumor's location and growth or spread than either test alone. A PET scan creates colored pictures of chemical changes (metabolic activity) in the tissues. Since cancer tumors are more active than normal tissue, they show up differently on a PET scan.

- A contrast-enhanced MRI helps doctors, with the use of color maps, pinpoint exactly where the cancer is, differentiate between benign and malignant disease, and predict tumor response.

- A thin, flexible fiberoptic instrument, called an endoscope, equipped with a light, a video camera, and electronic instruments allows the physician to obtain tissue and remove small growths in one procedure. One of the most rapidly advancing fields in medicine, this microchip technology allows the doctor to fast-forward diagnosis. Small amounts of tissue can easily be removed for biopsy, to determine diagnosis, to stage tumors, and to decide whether or not an operation is needed.

- High-resolution video technology equipment allows the entire operation team to observe the endoscopic procedures, permitting surgeons to perform more complex procedures.

- New mammography techniques improve the quality of mammograms and detect and distinguish different kinds of breast tumors. Among some techniques that are being used are: digital mammography, which uses computers to increase the ability to view breast tissue that is more dense; telemammography, which transmits images electronically; MRI to screen woman at high risk, and stereotactic needle biopsies which investigate lumps that cannot be felt.

- Thin hollow needles guided by x-rays for *biopsies called skinny* or thin needle aspiration biopsies. These needles allow access to both superficial and deep areas of the body without causing tissue damage. They can be used with great precision to reach tissues in the deepest recesses of the body, such as the liver, pancreas, and prostate and lymph nodes in the pelvis. A syringe attached to the needle allows cells to be withdrawn. These new advances are playing an increasingly important role in diagnosis and in cutting costs by eliminating major surgery and hospital stays.

- A computerized, laser-powered instrument measuring the amount of DNA in cells helps evaluate the risk of the recurrence of some cancers, including breast, prostate, and bladder cancer. Called flow cytometry, the procedure is performed on cancer cells that have been removed from the patient. It can determine whether some patients would benefit from less aggressive treatment or detect whether the person is resistant to certain drugs.

- Radiolabeled monoclonal antibodies find tumors undetectable by present technology and pinpoint the spread of metastatic tumors. The antibodies collect wherever the cancer has spread but will pass through the body if no cancer is present. Ultrasound equipment can differentiate between cysts and solid masses.

- Research continues to find ways to identify gene alterations or rearrangements to help predict whether a tumor will be aggressive or if it has metastasized.

SOME TUMOR MARKERS THAT MAY INDICATE CANCER

TEST NAME	HOW MAY BE USED IN CANCER
Alphafetoprotein (AFP)	Higher levels may indicate primary liver or germ cell cancer. Higher levels also found in cirrhosis, hepatitis, and pregnancy.
Calcitonin	May be used in diagnosis of cancer of thyroid. Higher levels also found in cancer of the breast, liver, lung, and kidney.
CA 15–3 (Cancer Antigen 15–3)	May be used to monitor response to breast cancer treatment. Higher levels also found in cancers of ovary, lung, and prostate as well as noncancerous conditions of breast, ovary, endometriosis, pelvic inflammatory disease, and hepatitis. Pregnancy and breast feeding may also cause levels to rise.
CA 19–9 (Cancer Antigen 19–9)	May be found in patients with cancers of colon, rectum, stomach, bile duct, and pancreas. Gallstone, pancreatitis, cirrhosis of liver, cholecystitis may also have higher levels.
CA 27–29 (Cancer Antigen 27–29)	Found in blood of most breast cancer patients. Can be used to monitor recurrence. Higher levels also found in cancers of colon, stomach, kidney, lung, ovary, pancreas, uterus, and liver. Pregnancy, endometriosis, benign ovarian and breast conditions, kidney and liver disease can also cause higher levels.
CA–125 (Cancer Antigen 125)	Protein found in blood. Higher levels found in women with ovarian cancer. Used to assess prognosis, monitor treatment, and determine recurrence in ovarian cancer. Also found in women with cancers of uterus, cervix, pancreas, liver, colon, lung and digestive tract, endometriosis, pelvic inflammatory disease, and peritonitis. NOTE: Menstruation and pregnancy also can cause increase.

SOME TUMOR MARKERS THAT MAY INDICATE CANCER *(continued)*

TEST NAME	HOW MAY BE USED IN CANCER
CEA (Carcinoembryonic Antigen)	Used to monitor colorectal cancer, especially if it has spread. Also to monitor its recurrence. Elevated levels found in cancers of breast, lung, prostate, pancreas, stomach, cervix, bladder, kidney, thyroid, liver, ovary, melanoma, and lymphoma. NOTE: May be found in higher levels in smokers, people with lung and bowel diseases and others who do not have cancer.
Estrogen or Progesterone Receptor (FR) or (PR)	Used to determine whether breast cancer will respond to hormone treatment and whether person is at (ER) increased risk for recurrence.
HER1 EGFR (Epidermal Growth Factor Receptor)	Protein found on surface of some cells to which epidermal growth factor binds, causing cells to divide. Found in high levels on surface of many types of cancer cells.
HER2/neu (Human epithelial growth factor 2) c-erbB-2	Protein involved in growth of cancer cells. Higher levels found in breast, ovary, and other cancer. Produced by HER2/neu gene.
HCG (Human Chorionic Gonadotrophin)	May be used to screen for choriocarcinoma, or to monitor treatment of gestational trophoblastic tumors. Higher levels also found in cancers of testes, ovary, liver, stomach, pancreas, and lung. NOTE: Pregnancy and marijuana use can also cause elevated HCG levels.
LDH (Lactate Dehydrogenase)	Can be used to monitor treatment of cancer of testes, Ewing's sarcoma, non-Hodgkin's lymphoma, and some leukemias. NOTE: Since protein found throughout body and almost all cancers and other diseases can cause it to rise, cannot be used for diagnosis.
NSE (Neuron Specific Enolase)	Used to provide information about extent of disease, prognosis, and treatment response in small cell lung cancer and neuroblastoma. Has also been found in cancers of pancreas, thyroid, kidney, testes, Wilms' tumor, and melanoma.

(continued)

SOME TUMOR MARKERS THAT MAY INDICATE CANCER (continued)

TEST NAME	HOW MAY BE USED IN CANCER
PSA (Prostate Specific Antigen)	Rising levels may indicate prostate cancer. Used in combination with other tests to detect prostate cancer. Useful in monitoring effectiveness of treatment or for recurrence. NOTE: Also higher in men with prostatitis, or nodular prostatic hyperplasia.
PAP (Prostatic Acid Phosphatase)	Present in small amounts in blood but may be found in higher levels in some prostate cancer patients. Also higher in other prostate conditions. Elevated levels also found in cancers of testes, leukemia and non-Hodgkin's lymphoma, and in noncancerous conditions.

What is proteomics?

Proteomics is the study of the patterns of serum proteins found in a person's blood. A new test combines proteomics with an artificial intelligence computer program that "trains" the computer to tell the difference between patterns of small proteins found in the blood of cancer patients from those who do not have cancer. It is presently being tested for prostate and ovarian cancer, but it may be able to be used in other diseases.

How is the test done?

A drop of blood is taken by sticking a needle in a person's finger, called a needle stick. Computer software detects key patterns of small proteins in the blood. Using mass spectroscopy, a technique that sorts proteins and other molecules based on their weight and electrical charge, the scientists analyze the blood protein. The test and the analysis take about 30 minutes.

How well does the test perform in prostate cancer?

Although this test is still being evaluated, scientists are very encouraged. It has been effective not only in men with normal PSA levels, but also men whose PSA levels were a little elevated (four to ten nanograms of antigen per milliliter of fluid), and who would otherwise have needed a biopsy to determine whether cancer was present. This is an especially significant advance, since 70 to 75 percent of men biopsied because of an abnormal PSA level do *not* have prostate cancer.

How has the test been used in ovarian cancer?
The test for ovarian cancer works in a similar manner. The artificial intelligence program has found a pattern of a handful of proteins among thousands that can be used to tell the difference between women with ovarian cancer and women with problems that are not cancer.

Are tumor markers and biomarkers the same thing?
A tumor marker, sometimes called a biomarker, is a general medical term for the substance that is found in higher amounts than normal in the blood and other body fluids or tissues of people who have cancer. There are a several different kinds of tumor markers presently being used in the cancer field, such as the PSA test for prostate cancer and the CA 125 test for ovarian cancer. They are used to diagnose disease, to monitor patients during treatment, and to look for recurrence. Most tumor markers cannot be used alone in diagnosing cancer. For instance, when adults have a higher than normal amount of carcinoembryonic antigen (CEA) in their blood it may indicate cancer of the colon or rectum. However, since this protein is also found in the blood of people who do not have cancer, such as smokers, it cannot be used as a definite diagnostic tool. Presently many new tumor markers are being researched in clinical trials.

What might be the future use of these tumor biomarkers?
Scientists believe that in the future tumor markers will be used for many other kinds of cancer and will be used in combination with other tests to determine whether cancer is present or not.

TREATMENT

New Surgical Techniques

Are there new techniques being used in surgery?
Several new tools and methods make surgery easier and less invasive. Among them:

- Performing "minimally invasive surgery," making small incisions and using new technology, video cameras, and surgical robots.

- Sentinel node biopsy that looks at the node closest or "sentinel" to the tumor to see if cancer has spread. This one node is removed, rather than the 15 to 35 nodes that are normally taken out. Clinical trials are underway to study the impact of this biopsy.

- Using harmonic scalpels (that cut and seal blood vessels), argon beam coagulators, and drugs that allow the doctors to do "bloodless" surgery.

- Laser surgery, using a carbon dioxide, argon or Nd:YAG (neodymium: yttrium-aluminum-garnet) laser, to remove colon polyps and tumors blocking the esophagus and colon, to treat abnormal tissue and some cancers of the skin, lung, colon, penis, cervix, vagina, vulva, head and neck, vocal cords, and breast. Lasers are more precise than scalpels, shorten operating and healing time, and usually can be utilized in an outpatient setting.

New Radiation Techniques

Are there any new advances in treating people with radiation?
There are several areas of research, including:

- Using a new device called a cyberknife, a 3-D computer with a robotic arm, to give large doses of radiation from several directions to attack damaged tissue while sparing healthy cells. It makes adjustments as it goes along and maintains its precise radiation beam. It can be used for patients who are too weak to have surgery or chemotherapy.

- Combining radiation with monoclonal antibodies and chemotherapy to boost the response rates in several kinds of cancer.

- Linking a radiosensitizer, a substance or a procedure that makes cancer cells more sensitive to the radiation treatment. Some chemotherapy drugs are being used, making tumor cells that were previously resistant to radiation more susceptible.

- Attaching radioactive isotopes in the laboratory to antibodies produced from cells taken from a patient's tumor. The antibodies, reinjected into the patient and carrying the radioactive isotopes, travel through the bloodstream to the tumor, where the antibody-carrying isotopes attach to the tumor and kill the cells. This treatment, called radiolabeled antibody therapy is being tested in Hodgkin's disease, non-Hodgkin's lymphoma, lung, and liver cancer.

- Using particle radiation, such as fast neutrons, protons, helium ions, deutrons, heavy ions (carbon, neon, argon) and negative pi-mesons, to give greater doses or distribute doses with less harm to surrounding tissues than the substances now being used. Studies include use in sarcomas, gliomas, melanomas, cancer of the sinuses, salivary gland, lung, prostate, and head and neck cancer.

- Using high-energy photons to destroy minute regions of the brain with minimal damage to surrounding tissues. Called stereotactic radiosurgery, it allows patients to arrive early the day of the treatment, undergo radio-surgery that is focused on the site, and go home the next day.

- Giving a large single dose of radiation directly to the tumor during an operation with minimum effects to nearby normal tissue. Called intraoperative radiation, this is being tested with cancers of the breast, colon, rectum, stomach, brain, and gynecologic organs.

- Trying new ways to kill most of the tumor with the least damage to normal cells by changing treatment schedules, such as giving smaller daily doses of radiation more frequently—often twice a day (called hyperfractionation) or the regular dose of radiation in a shorter time (accelerated fractionation).

- Using radioprotectors, chemical compounds that protect normal cells against short-term radiation damage. These allow the normal cells to repair themselves while the tumor cells are still being treated and permit higher doses of radiation than would normally be safe for the surrounding tissues.

New Chemotherapy Treatments

What new methods are being used in chemotherapy treatment?
There are several new methods under investigation in clinical trials for different kinds of cancers. Among them are:

- Linking chemotherapy drugs to monoclonal antibodies to make a "smart bomb"—a treatment that is able to find its way to specific cells and deliver a higher dose directly to the tumors while sparing healthy tissues. The antibodies work in stopping tumor growth either by acting on the tumor itself, by using the immune system, or by delivering a drug or radioactive compound to the cancer.

- Giving dose-dense chemotherapy—reducing the time between doses of chemotherapy, thereby condensing the schedule. Drugs that can reduce side effects of the treatment are making this treatment possible.

- Using drugs, such as STI571 (Gleevec) that can turn off the signal of a protein known to cause cancer.

- Giving drugs called taxanes to prevent the growth of cancer cells by affecting cell structures called microtubules. Taxanes include paclitaxes (Taxol) and docetaxel (Taxotere).

- Giving drugs directly to a limited area of the body, such as the liver, to prolong the time that the tumor is exposed to chemotherapy, while doing little damage to normal tissues.

- Adding an agent that causes the blood to slow down, making the cancer cells more vulnerable to the drugs.

- Finding drugs that can overcome the resistance sometimes developed by cancer cells to chemotherapy agents. Chemosensitizers are being tested that may reverse resistance in some patients.

- Giving drugs at carefully selected times of day, based on the rhythmic biologic cycle of an individual, using portable pumps to deliver single or several drugs. This area of research, called circadian chemotherapy, is also testing whether some anticancer drugs may be more effective if given based on circadian rhythm.

- Several new chemotherapy agents are in Phase I trials or will soon be entering those trials. Over 100 drugs are presently being tested in Phase III trials.

What clinical studies are being conducted using angiogenesis?

There is considerable research in the field of blood vessel formation (angiogenesis), in which doctors can evaluate the level of oxygen found in tumors to help identify those people whose cancers are more likely to recur and those who might benefit from more aggressive treatment. The trials are studying both sides of the issue—how to get more oxygen into tumors to enhance the effect of treatment as well as how to use drugs (angiogenesis inhibitors) to choke off the oxygen supply to tumors, thus starving them.

Hyperthermia

Is hyperthermia being used in treatment?

Heat therapy (hyperthermia) is a potential treatment that has been studied for many years and continues to be investigated in clinical trials, either alone or with radiation, chemotherapy, and biological therapy. Scientists think that exposing tissue to high temperatures may shrink tumors by damaging cells or depriving them of substances they need to live. Local (applying heat to a small area such as a tumor), regional (heating an organ or a limb), and whole-body hyperthermia are being studied.

How is the area under treatment heated?

There are a number of clinical trials of this treatment method being conducted. External and internal heating devices can be used. For local hyperthermia, the area may be heated externally with high-frequency waves. Or it may be heated internally with a sterile probe, such as thin, heated wires or hollow tubes filled with warm water, implanted microwave antennae, or radiofrequency electrodes. In regional hyperthermia, magnets and devices that produce high energy are placed over the region to be heated or the area is treated with perfusion—the patient's blood is removed, heated, and then pumped into the region that is to be heated internally. Whole body heating uses warm-water blankets, hot wax, inductive coils (like those in electric blankets), or thermal chambers.

Photodynamic Therapy

What is photodynamic therapy?
Photodynamic therapy, also known as phototherapy, photochemotherapy, or photoradiation therapy, uses three elements: a light-sensitizing drug, light (usually from a laser), and oxygen. The drug is a photosensitizing substance that makes cells more sensitive to light. The substance is injected into the body and is absorbed by all cells. The agent remains in or around tumor cells for a longer time than it does in normal tissue. When the treated cancer cells are exposed to a light (usually red) from a laser the light is absorbed by the photosensitizing agent. This light absorption causes a chemical reaction that destroys the tumor cells. The light exposure must be carefully timed to coincide with the period when most of the agent is no longer in the healthy cells but still remains in the cancer cells. Advancements in photosensitizers, fiberoptic probes, and two new types of lasers (argon-pumped dye and pulsed gold vapor) have created a new interest in photodynamic therapy because they have enabled doctors to use the treatment on tissue that was once unreachable by other treatment. For instance, the fiberoptic probe can be directed through a brochoscope into the lungs to treat lung cancer, or though an endoscope into the esophagus to treat esophageal cancer.

What are the advantages and disadvantages of photodynamic therapy?
There are several advantages. Cancer cells can be selectively destroyed while most normal cells are spared. The damaging effect of the photosensitizing agent occurs only when the substance is exposed to light and the side effects are relatively mild. A *disadvantage* is that the laser light cannot pass through more than about *one-third of an inch of tissue* (1 centimeter).

What kind of cancer has been treated with photodynamic therapy?
This treatment has been used in clinical trials in cancers of the esophagus, lung, bladder, brain, larynx, mouth, skin, lymphoma, gynecological cancers, and cancers of the stomach, head, and neck.

Are there any side effects from photodynamic therapy?
The most common side effects are skin and eye sensitivity for six or more weeks. Other side effects may include some pain in the treatment area, coughing, trouble swallowing, pain in the stomach, and shortness of breath or pain when breathing. These side effects are usually temporary.

Must patients take any precautions when being treated with photodynamic therapy?

The light-sensitizing substance remains active for six or more weeks after the injection. You need to protect yourself from direct and indirect sunlight and from bright indoor light. When outdoors, nontransparent clothing that covers the body from head to toe must be worn, including a wide-brimmed hat, gloves, socks, and shoes. The eyes must also be protected with sunglasses that have a 100 percent ultraviolet block to prevent eye injury.

Enhancing the Immune System with Biologic Therapy

One of the relatively new developments in cancer involves the increased use of biological therapy to trigger the body's own defenses against cancer. This treatment, sometimes called immunotherapy or biological response modifier therapy, uses the immune system, either directly or indirectly, to fight cancer and lessen the side effects caused by other treatments. It is believed that cancer cells probably are present at some time in everyone, but that the immune system is usually able to stop the cells before they have a chance to become cancers. Scientists are finding hundreds of substances that boost, direct, or restore many of the normal defenses of the body. Many occur naturally in the body while others are made in the laboratory. Many are still years away from being used in ordinary medical practice. Doctors are just beginning to experiment with ways of combining various biologicals with each other and with standard treatments for more effective use.

What substances are being used in biological therapy?

The substances are called biological response modifiers and include monoclonal antibodies, colony-stimulating factors, interleukins, interferons, vaccines, and gene therapy.

What are monoclonal antibodies?

A monoclonal antibody is a substance that can find and attach to a specific protein on cancer cells. Monoclonal antibodies are produced in the body in small quantities. However, they can be produced in a laboratory in great quantity and designed to hone in on target cancer cells. They have potential in the prevention, detection, and treatment of cancer. Transtuzumab (Herceptin) and rituximab (Rituxan) are examples of monoclonal antibodies approved for cancer use.

How can monoclonal antibodies be used in treating cancer?

They may be used in several ways:

- To interfere with the growth of cancer cells by programming them to act against cell growth factors.

- To enhance the immune system's response.

- To deliver substances directly to the tumors by linking them with chemotherapy drugs, radioisotopes, other biologic response modifiers, or other toxins.

- To help destroy cancer cells in bone marrow removed from a patient in preparation for a bone marrow transplant.

Monoclonal antibodies are being studied for use in diagnosing cancer of the colon, ovary, and prostate.

What are radiolabeled monoclonal antibodies?

They are monoclonal antibodies that have been made radioactive and can be used to detect minute cancer that has spread in the body. After being injected into the bloodstream, the radiolabeled antibodies attach to cancer cells and are detected by special sensing devices. Investigations using radiolabeled monoclonal antibodies in the detection of many different cancers are ongoing.

What are some of the agents linked to the monoclonal antibodies?

The agents include radioisotopes, plant and bacterial toxins, chemotherapy drugs and biologic agents. One of the toxins, ricin, is being tested in clinical trials for leukemia, lymphoma, melanoma, and cancers of the colon, rectum, lung, and breast.

What are colony-stimulating factors?

Colony-stimulating factors (also called tumor growth factors or hematopoietic growth factors) are naturally occurring substances that stimulate the bone marrow to produce white and red blood cells and platelets.

What are colony-stimulating factors used for in treating cancer?

Investigations are underway in many areas:

- To produce more red blood cells and lessen bleeding problems, enabling patients to tolerate larger doses of chemotherapy.

- To boost white blood cells that fight infection, allowing greater amounts of chemotherapy to be given.

- To enhance chemotherapy drugs, increasing their effectiveness.

- To separate cancer cells from bone marrow that has been removed from a patient.

What are some of the colony-stimulating factors being investigated?

There are several that are being tested, such as:

- Sargramostin (GM-CSF) to stimulate the growth of early bone marrow cells.
- Filgrastin (GM-CSF) to stimulate the growth of granulocytes.
- Erythropoietin to stimulate the production of red blood cells.
- Oprelvekin to reduce the need for platelet transfusions.

Researchers are also studying colony-stimulating factors in clinical trials for use in treating colorectal cancer, lung cancer, and melanoma.

How are growth factors given to patients?

Growth factors are usually given either intravenously or subcutanteously (under the skin). Sometimes patients are able to give them to themselves, after instruction by a nurse.

What is interferon?

Interferon, discovered in 1975, is a cytokine, a protein that helps to regulate the immune system. Interferons used in cancer treatment are made naturally by the body when cells are stimulated by an agent such as a virus, or produced synthetically in a laboratory by putting some interferons into bacteria and cultivating a large quantity of them.

Are there different kinds of interferons?

There are three groups of interferons: alpha, beta, and gamma. Alpha interferon is most widely used in cancer treatments. Interferons can improve the way the immune system acts against cancer cells, slowing growth or promoting them into cells that act more normally. Scientists also think that some interferons stimulate natural killer cells, T cells, and macrophages, boosting the way the immune system fights cancer.

What is interleukin?

Interleukin is a group of natural, hormone-like substances that are made in the body by lymphocytes, a type of white blood cell. Interleukins are a type of cytokine that carry signals between the blood-forming cells that are part of the immune system. There are several interleukins, but interleukin-2 (IL–2) is the one most often used in cancer treatment. It stimulates many immune cells to grow and become more active.

What cancer vaccines are being studied?

Scientists are developing vaccines that may encourage the patient's immune system to recognize cancer cells, help the body reject tumors, and prevent cancer from coming back. The vaccines are designed to be given after the cancer has developed but when the tumor is still small, so that they can kill the tumor. Vaccines are being studied in treating melanoma, cancers of the breast, ovary, prostate, colon, rectum, and kidney.

GENES, GENETIC TESTING, AND GENE THERAPY

One of the areas of research that has the greatest potential for cancer is that involving genes. As discussed in Chapter 4, What Is Cancer?, genes are the biological units of heredity. It is estimated that each human has from 30,000 to 100,000 genes. Each gene is a blueprint for making a specific enzyme or other protein. A flaw in a gene causes the body to work in an abnormal manner, such as allowing cancers to grow.

How are genes arranged?

The genes are arranged on chromosomes—rod-like structures composed of DNA and protein. Each cell, in humans, contains 46 chromosomes (23 pairs) located within a central structure known as the nucleus. Genes that normally direct how often a cell divides are called proto-oncogenes. Today, the Human Genome Project has completed the sequencing of the DNA of all cells. This major step will allow researchers to continue their search to understand how a cell is transformed into a cancer cell and why its offsprings no longer follow the rules of dividing when they should, maturing when they are supposed to, and dying on schedule.

What is an oncogene?

When there is a defect (mutation) in the gene, it is called an oncogene. The defect is transmitted on the chromosome. The cells, instead of slowing down and dying, are turned on all the time, dividing quickly, thus forming tumors.

What progress is being made in the treatment of the cancer in these oncogenes?

Scientists have found some ways of turning off the oncogenes and stopping them from producing abnormal cells. For instance, defects in the HER2/neu gene cause breast cancer to grow quickly and spread. Chemotherapy is not effective in these cases. But women with breast cancer who test positive for the HER2/neu gene have been found to respond to the anticancer drug,

SELECTED GENE ABNORMALITIES IN CANCER

GENE	DESCRIPTION
Bcr-abl	Breaks on chromosomes 22 and 9, genetic rearrangement that leads to Philadelphia chromosome. Produce abnormal *bcr-abl* gene that prevents leukemic cells from dying in a normal fashion.
HER2/neu c-erbB-2	Gene that makes human epidermal growth factor 2. Abnormalities in this gene in breast, ovary and some other cancers. Tumors grow rapidly, more likely to spread, less likely to respond to chemotherapy.
Lynch Syndrome 1	Family syndrome. Family that has many members with colon cancers without developing polyps or other cancers.
Lynch Syndrome 2	Family syndrome. Family with two or more generations of cancer of the colon and endometrium, and sometimes ovary and breast. Also called hereditary nonpolypotic colonic cancer, type 2, or the family syndrome of Lynch.
Li-Fraumeni syndrome (SBLA syndrome)	Family syndrome. Family that has three or more members who has one or more cancers and is at risk for developing sarcomas, breast, bone and brain tumors; lung, laryngeal cancer and leukemia, and adrenal cortical neoplasia. It is believed that changes in one gene, p53, may account for the Li-Fraumeni syndrome.
myc	Family of oncogenes (c-*myc*, N-*myc*, L-*myc*). Seen in cancers of the breast, lung, stomach, colon, and in leukemia and neuroblastoma.
p53 gene	Alteration of a gene p53, located on chromosome 17p; may indicate predisposition for cancers of the colon, lung, breast, bladder, liver, leukemias, or melanoma. Also see Li-Fraumeni syndrome.
Philadelphia Chromosome (Ph¹)	Abnormal chromosome that indicates chronic myelogenous leukemia.
ras family of oncogenes	Includes N-*ras*, H-*ras*, K-*ras*. Has been detected in cancers of the bladder, lung, colon, rectum, breast, and in some leukemias.

USES OF SELECTED BIOLOGIC THERAPY

NAME	USE
Alpha interferon	Treatment of leukemia, melanoma, chronic myeloid leukemia, AIDS-related Kaposi's sarcoma. Also may be useful in metastatic kidney cancer and non-Hodgkin's lymphoma.
Bacillus Calmette-Guerin (BCG, TheraCys, TICE BCG)	Treatment of superficial bladder cancer following surgery. Stimulates inflammatory, possibly immune response. Instilled in bladder for about two hours; treatment usually once a week for six weeks.
Filgrastim (G-CSF) Sargramostim (G-CSF)	Increase number of white blood cells and stimulate production of stem cells. Decreasing infection for bone marrow transplants, stem cell support and other high dose treatments.
Erythropoietin	Increase red blood cells. Reduce need for red blood cell transfusions in chemotherapy patients.
Interleukin 2 (IL–2, Aldesleukin)	Melanoma, cancer of the kidney. Also being studied in cancers of colorectal, ovarian, lung, brain, breast, some leukemias and some lymphomas.
Levamisole (Ergamisole)	Used in combination with fluorouracil (5–FU) after surgery to stimulate macrophages and T lymphocytes in Stage III colon cancer (Duke's C).
Monoclonal antibodies transtuzumab (Herceptin), rituximab (Rituxan)	Substance that can find and attach to a specific protein on cancer cells to deliver treatment or aid in diagnosis.
Oprelvekin	Reduces need for platelet transfusions in chemotherapy patients.
Vaccines	Being studied in melanoma, cancers of the breast, ovary, prostate, colon, rectum, and kidney.

trasuzamab (Herceptin). This is a monocolonal antibody, a substance produced in a laboratory that can locate and bind to a cancer cell. It blocks the effects of the HER2/neu growth factor that sends signals to the breast cancer cell to grow. Another example is STI517 (Gleevec), which turns off the signal of the *bcr-abl* protein in chronic myeloid leukemia cells. Other treatments are underway in clinical trials for other cancers where gene abnormalities have been identified.

What is a tumor supressor gene?

This is a gene that protects or limits cells from dividing and repairs DNA. When this gene is damaged, it is turned off and cells divide rapidly and grow out of control. Some genes, such as the APC gene, the one for familial adenomatous polyposis are so powerful that the carriers are almost certain to get the disease. Others, such as BRCA1 and BRCA2, that put a person at a greater risk for breast cancer, may be related to a combination of factors. Scientists have found more and more of these genes, including BRCA1, BRCA2, p53, and the one that causes retinoblastoma (RB). There are some ongoing clinical trials using gene therapy to replace these defective genes.

What is a genetic screening test?

A test to determine whether a person has an inherited gene, like the p53 gene, that predisposes a person to some kinds of cancer.

What is Lynch syndrome 2?

Lynch syndrome 2, sometimes known as the hereditary nonpolypotic colonic cancer, type 2, or the family syndrome of Lynch, is one of the cancer family syndromes. It is used to describe a family with two or more generations diagnosed at an early age with cancer of the colon and endometrium, and sometimes of the ovary and breast. Many members of the family are found to have multiple primary cancers. Lynch 1 is the term used for a family that has many members with colon cancers without polyps or other cancers.

What is the Li-Fraumeni cancer family syndrome?

The Li-Fraumeni cancer syndrome, also called SBLA syndrome, describes a family that has three or more members who have one or more cancers and are at risk for developing sarcomas; breast, bone, and brain tumors; lung, laryngeal cancer, and leukemia; and adrenal cortical neoplasia. It is believed that changes in one gene, p53, may account for the Li-Fraumeni syndrome.

What kind of counseling is available for families who may have an inherited genetic tendency?

Some of the major medical centers have genetic counselors with expertise in discussing the issues with families. They have specialized training in presenting information in an unbiased manner, so that you can make your own decision as to what you wish to do. They can talk with you about the way in which families inherit cancers, the types of cancers in your family, who might need to be tested, the benefits and costs of testing. There are many issues that need to be explored before the decision is made to have the tests. If you need this kind of counseling, be sure to seek out the experts in this emerging field.

Is it wise to be tested for any of these genetic tendencies?
It depends on which one it is. For some kinds of cancer, people who are found to inherit a trait will be able to take preventive action. For instance, people who test positive for the inherited gene for familial adenomatous polyposis (a rare condition in which the lining of the colon sprouts hundred of tiny wart-like polyps that left untreated almost always leads to colon cancer), might choose to have more frequent exams to find new polyps. They may decide to have preventive surgery. They may, in the future, be encouraged to enter trials to test chemopreventive agents that might prevent colon cancer. There are, however, many ethical questions and issues that need to be discussed and resolved before you decide to have the testing.

Questions to Discuss with a Genetic Counselor Before Having Any Tests

- Why do I want to have this test?

- What will I do with the information from it? How will it affect my life, my work, my insurance benefits?

- Am I prepared to hear the results?

- What are the advantages of having it? The disadvantages?

- Who will be notified if I have the test? Will the information be put on my medical records? Is there any way it can be kept confidential?

- If I test positive, what are the next steps? Will I need further testing? Is there anything that can be done to make any difference in my risk?

- What will the test cost? Who will be doing the test?

- How will the test affect my family? My relationships with my children, my brothers and sisters?

What is the Cancer Genetics Network?
It is a national network, sponsored by the National Cancer Institute, of eight centers that are studying the inherited predisposition to cancer. It seeks people who have a personal or family history of cancer or who are interested in participating in studies about inherited susceptibility to cancer. Information about the Network is on the Web (www.epi.grants.center.gov/CGN/) and in Chapter 28, Where to Get Help.

PARTICIPATING IN A TREATMENT CLINICAL TRIAL

New cancer treatments, such as biologic therapy, gene therapy, or new combinations of chemotherapy, radiation and surgery, start in the basic research laboratories with careful studies in test tubes and on animals. The research points out the new methods most likely to succeed, and how they can be used safely and effectively. If the investigational treatment shows promise of being better than the standard one, it is tested in a clinical trial. The trial helps find out if a promising new treatment is safe and effective for patients. During a trial more and more information is gained about a new treatment, its risks and how well it may or may not work. Most investigational (or experimental) drugs or agents being used are available only through doctors and scientists working closely with the National Cancer Institute or pharmaceutical companies, under strict U.S. Food and Drug Administration regulations. These regulations govern the use of investigational agents. If your physician is using a Phase II drug, for instance, it has already gone through extensive evaluation to determine its safe dosage.

Questions to Ask Before Participating in a Clinical Trial for Treatment

- What is the purpose of the clinical trial?
- What are the possible benefits?
- Who is sponsoring it? (NCI? A major cancer center? A pharmaceutical firm?)
- Who has reviewed it?
- Why do the doctors who designed the study believe that the treatment being studied may be better than the one now being used?
- What are the disadvantages compared to the standard treatment?
- Who will be giving the treatment?
- How long will I be in the study?
- What kinds of tests are involved? Are they in addition to the tests that would normally be done?
- What will the treatment consist of? How does it differ from the standard treatment?
- Will I be hospitalized?
- What are the possible side effects or risks of the new treatment? How do they compare with the standard treatment?
- What are my other choices?

- How does the treatment I would receive in this study compare with the other choices in terms of possible outcomes, side effects, time involved, cost to me and quality of life?

- What will happen in my case if I don't have this treatment?

- What will happen in my case if I do have it?

- How could the study affect my daily life?

- Can I stop my participation at any time? What happens if I do?

- Will I have to pay for the tests or the treatment?

- Will my overall charges be more than if I received standard treatment? Will insurance routinely pay for them? How often have you been successful in getting all costs reimbursed by insurance for this treatment?

- Does the study include long-term follow-up care? How often will that be and what will it consist of?

What does the word *protocol* mean?

Protocol is the term used to describe the treatment program. It is the outline or plan for use of an investigational procedure or treatment. A protocol gives the rationale for the study, and its goals. If drugs or radiation are involved, it describes the type, method of administration, dose, and duration. In addition, the protocol gives the criteria for participation.

What does the term *randomization* mean?

Randomization refers to the manner of choosing people who have similar traits, such as type and extent of disease, by chance (randomly) placed into groups that are comparing different treatments. The groups are considered comparable. Results of the different treatments used in different groups can be compared because irrelevant factors or preferences do not influence the distribution of people. Neither the doctor nor the persons receiving the treatment can choose the group to which they are assigned. Randomization is important because bias can alter the results of a trial.

What is meant by an experimental drug?

The words investigational and experimental are used when new anticancer drugs are in the research stages. The Food and Drug Administration (FDA) is the agency that regulates the introduction and clinical testing of the new drugs. (While the National Cancer Institute, along with drug companies, may be involved in conducting the tests, they are not regulatory agencies.) The FDA has established and administers strict regulations governing the introduction and clinical testing of new drugs. These regulations require that certain standards of safety and effectiveness be met and that a carefully planned clinical study be undertaken.

Why should I consider participating in a cancer treatment clinical trial?
There are many reasons for participating.

- The studies offer the most sophisticated, up-to-date, high-quality cancer care available when a new treatment is tested.

- You will be carefully monitored throughout the trial.

- There are safeguards built into the trial to protect you. For example, a special review board looks at the study to see that it is well designed and that potential risks to patients are reasonable in relation to the potential benefits.

- You usually will be tested more often and will be monitored more frequently.

- Exploring all the options for treatment may help you feel more in control and more a part of a vital decision affecting your life.

- If a new treatment is successful, you would be the first to benefit.

- You are actively trying to help yourself and future cancer patients.

What are the disadvantages in my being treated through a clinical trial?
You need to think carefully about the downside to make sure you are making the right decision for yourself.

- You may not receive the new treatment. Some people will be in the group that receives standard care for comparison to the new approach. You will be randomly assigned to receive either the new or the standard treatment. You need to remember that the standard care means the best treatment generally available. However, some people are uncomfortable with the fact that they may not receive the new treatment.

- The new treatment may not be more effective than the standard one. It may produce the same results. Occasionally it may have results that are not as good as the standard one.

- You may have some side effects or some risks from the new treatment that have not been anticipated.

- The additional tests and monitoring may not be covered by your insurance.

- Some treatments may not be covered by your insurance. You need to be sure to discuss costs because they vary from study to study.

What might disqualify me from participating in a clinical treatment trial?

Each study enrolls patients with certain types and stages of cancer and certain health conditions. There may not be a trial that is being done currently for your type and stage of cancer; you may not be eligible for the particular phase of the trial that is being conducted; you may have had previous treatment or a medical condition that precludes you from participating; the trial may not be done in your part of the country. However, you may be eligible for different phases of trials depending on your general condition and the type and stage of your cancer.

Will I be able to be on a clinical trial if I am on Medicare?

If you are on Medicare, it will probably pay for a cancer treatment clinical trial that is sponsored by the National Cancer Institute or another part of the Federal Government. All the routine costs that are part of the clinical trial should be covered, including visits to the doctor's office, tests you will need for your medical care, any stays in the hospital, surgery or tests and treatments for side effects. Not all other costs will be covered—only those that are reasonable and necessary, used to diagnose and treat complications arising from participation. It will not pay for your medical insurance and deductibles. Before you start or agree to be in any clinical trial, make sure that your Medicare plan will cover it, especially if you are in a Medicare + Choice plan. If you have any questions, call the Medicare toll-free line at 1-800-633-4277.

What are the different phases of clinical trials?

Clinical trials are carried out in three phases, each designed to find out certain information. Each new phase of a clinical trial depends on and builds on the information from an earlier phase.

- **Phase I** studies search for the best way to give a new treatment and how much of it can be given safely. The research treatment has been well tested in laboratory and animal studies but it is not known how patients will react to it. Harmful side effects are carefully watched. Since there may be significant risks, Phase I studies usually are offered only to patients whose cancer has spread and who would not be helped by standard treatments. The treatments may produce some effects and may help some people.

- **Phase II** studies determine the effect of a research treatment on various types of cancer.

- **Phase III** studies compare the new treatment with standard treatment to see which is more effective. Most often researchers use standard treatment as the basis for designing the new treatment.

How am I protected if I participate in a clinical trial?

Any well-run clinical trial is carefully reviewed for medical ethics, patient safety, and scientific merit by the research institution. In addition, most clinical research is federally regulated or federally funded (at least in part), with built-in safeguards to protect patients. (One can manufacture a drug and use it within the same state without federal regulation or manufacture and give the drug outside the U.S.) Your safeguards include regular review of the protocol (the study plan) and review of the progress of each study by researchers at other places. Federally supported or federally funded and federally regulated clinical trials (and in most major medical centers, all clinical trials) must first be approved by an Institutional Review Board located at the institution where the study is to take place. This board is designed to protect patients and is made up of scientists, doctors, clergy, and other people from the local community. It reviews each study to see that it is well designed with safeguards for patients and that the risks are reasonable in relation to the potential benefits. The federally supported or regulated studies also are reviewed by a government agency, such as the National Cancer Institute, which sponsors and monitors many trials around the country.

Is the quality of life ever measured in treatment clinical trials?

There are several trials that have added measurements of quality of life issues, such as depression, self-esteem, social support, and religious involvement to the trial. Nurses, either within the clinical trial itself or in separate studies, conduct most of the quality-of-life research. Questions that are being answered include: Must the patient make significant lifestyle changes because of the treatment? Is the patient anxious or depressed? Is the patient able to maintain relationships with family and friends?

What is informed consent?

Informed consent, which is required in federally conducted, funded, or regulated studies as well as by many state laws, is the formal process by which you learn about and understand the purpose and aspects of a clinical trial and then agree to participate. The nature of the trial is explained by the doctors and nurses who are involved in it. You need to make sure you understand what is involved in participating in your specific trial. You will be given an informed consent form that defines the potential benefits and risks. Read it and consider it carefully. Ask any questions you may have. Then, if you agree to take part, you can sign the form. Of course, you can also refuse.

Can I leave a trial at any time?

Signing a consent form does not bind you to the study. You can still choose to leave the study at any time. Your rights as an individual do not change because you are a patient in a clinical trial. You may choose to take part or not, and you can always change your mind later, even after you enter a trial. You may also refuse to take part in any aspect of the research. If you have any questions, be sure to discuss your concerns with your doctors. If you are not satisfied with the answers, you may consider leaving the study. If you decide to leave, it will not be held against you. You can freely discuss possible other care and treatments with your health care team.

How can I find out about the clinical treatment trials being done in my kind of cancer?

There are many ways to find out your treatment choices. Talk with your doctors. Get a second opinion from other cancer specialists. Go to or call a comprehensive cancer center if there is one in your area. Call the Cancer Information Service (1-800-4-CANCER) and ask the information specialists the questions you have about the treatment being offered. Request a PDQ search for clinical trials that pertain to your type and stage of cancer. Check the Internet. There are several sites, listed at the end of this chapter, on which you can do your own search.

What is a PDQ?

PDQ is a helpful treatment information database supported by the National Cancer Institute. PDQ offers state-of-the art treatment statements, compiled and updated monthly by panels of the country's leading cancer specialists, giving the range of effective treatment options that represent the best available therapy for a specific type or stage of cancer. PDQ also gives the latest information on over 1,000 active clinical treatment trials being offered around the country for each type and stage of cancer. It is a ready reference that is updated monthly by a review boards composed of cancer specialists.

What do I need to know in order to have a PDQ search of clinical trials for my kind of cancer?

If you call the Cancer Information Service and request a PDQ search, you will be asked a series of questions to get the information needed to complete the search for you:

- The first question will be whether or not you are currently receiving treatment. If you are already being treated, a search of potential clinical trials may not be appropriate.
- Whether you are interested in participating in a clinical trial.
- Whether you are able or willing to travel to a participating center and how far you are willing to travel for treatment.

- The primary site of your cancer, the stage, and if possible cell type and grade. In addition, breast cancer patients will be asked for hormonal and menopausal status.

- The site of metastases, if any.

- What previous treatments you have had, type of treatment, when and where, including names of drugs previously received and when.

- Major medical conditions that might preclude participation.

Can I be treated at the Clinical Center at the National Institutes of Health?

The National Institutes of Health, the Federal Government's agency for medical research, has a medical research center and hospital—the Warren Grant Magnuson Clinical Center—located in Bethesda, Maryland, just outside of Washington, D.C. The hospital portion of the Clinical Center, with room for 540 patients, is especially designed for medical research. All individuals treated at the hospital are participants on clinical trials. The number of beds available for a particular project and the length of the waiting list of qualified patients are important in determining whether and when you can be admitted. Research on a particular disease may allow only one or two patients to be studied at any given time.

How are patients selected for treatment at the Clinical Center?

Each project is designed to answer scientific questions and has specific medical eligibility requirements. You can be treated at the Clinical Center only if your case fits into a research project. To find out if there is a study available for a specific cancer, patients, and doctors can call the NCI's Clinical Studies Support Center at 1-888-624-1937 weekdays between 9:00 a.m. and 5:00 p.m. eastern time. You will talk with an oncology nurse or information specialist who can tell you what clinical trials may be appropriate. They can mail or fax you the summaries or other information about the trials, including the type of treatment being offered, the type of patient eligible for the trial and other useful information. You should then review the summaries with your doctor to decide which study you may wish to consider. Your doctor should then contact the Clinical Studies Support Center to talk with the NCI investigator in charge of the study.

Will I need to visit the Clinical Center before I am accepted into a trial?

If you meet the initial medical eligibility requirement, you may be asked to schedule a screening visit at the Clinical Center.

How much will it cost me to participate in a trial at the Clinical Center?

If you are asked to come for a screening visit, you will be responsible for the initial travel expenses. As part of the Federal Government, the Clinical Center provides treatment in clinical trials at no cost to the patient. If accepted, you may also receive some help to cover the cost of traveling to the Center for treatment and follow-up care.

BONE MARROW TRANSPLANTS AND PERIPHERAL STEM CELL SUPPORT

People in some 500 specialized transplant centers throughout the world are choosing to undergo bone marrow procedures, such as peripheral stem cell or bone marrow support, to allow the use of high-dose chemotherapy or radiation therapy treatments for their cancers. Sometimes the patient's own marrow or stem cells are used. Other times donor marrow is the best option. Using peripheral stem cells instead of bone marrow is making the process easier and sometimes less costly. However, there are many questions to ask and things to consider before you decide to have a transplant. Not only is it expensive and may not be covered by your health insurance, but it is a difficult treatment. Since most bone marrow transplants and stem cell support procedures are investigational treatments, it is important to have these procedures done in major medical centers, where you can participate in a clinical trial. Moreover, experience has shown that there is a greater chance for recovery if your doctor chooses a hospital that does at least ten bone marrow transplantations per year.

What You Need to Know About Bone Marrow Transplants and Peripheral Stem Cell Support

- Bone marrow is the soft, spongelike material that is found in the cavities of your bones. It contains stem cells that produce blood cells. The chief function of bone marrow is to produce the three types of cells found in the blood—red blood cells, white blood cells, and platelets. Chemotherapy and radiation therapy, when given at very high doses, destroy the bone marrow and the body's ability to produce new blood cells.

- Bone marrow transplants date back to the mid 1950s. They were developed as a potential therapy for fatal blood diseases such as leukemia and aplastic anemia. Healthy bone marrow from a donor—usually a family member (called an allogeneic transplant)—is transplanted into a patient whose diseased cells have been wiped out by radiation and chemotherapy.

- Autologous transplants, using the patient's own bone marrow, became possible in the 1970s, when the technique of freezing the marrow while the patient was given radiation and chemotherapy, thawing it and returning it to the patient was perfected.

- In the early 1990s, it became possible to replace blood cells by using a special type of cell that circulates in the blood vessels, called a peripheral stem cell. Peripheral stem cells, taken from the patient's own blood, began to be used to support patients undergoing high dose chemotherapy, making the process simpler and less expensive. Unlike bone marrow, which requires the patient to undergo general anesthesia to remove it, peripheral stem cells are easier to get. The process is similar to donating blood.

- Today, bone marrow and peripheral stem cell support are used to regenerate the bone marrow so that it can begin dividing and producing blood cells after high-dose treatments are given for such cancer as leukemia, lymphoma, childhood brain tumors, and nueroblastoma. It is being evaluated in clinical trials for various types of cancer including breast, ovary, multiple myeloma and Wilms' tumor.

- Since bone marrow and stem cell support are investigational treatments in some diseases, it is important to have these procedures done in major medical centers, where you can participate in a clinical trial. There are many hospitals that are now performing bone marrow transplants and peripheral stem cell support. It is essential that you ask how many of the procedures have been done in the institution where you are planning to have your transplant and how many have been done for your kind of cancer. The American Society of Clinical Oncologists has established minimum standards for bone marrow transplant programs that include a requirement that the facility conduct at least ten transplants a year.

- A specially trained support team, including nurses, pharmacists, social workers and other support staff, is also needed for bone marrow transplants. This team must be able to recognize and resolve complications that might arise.

Questions to Ask your Doctor About
Bone Marrow and Stem Cell Support

- **Am I a candidate for peripheral stem cell support or for bone marrow transplantation?**

- **What kind of bone marrow transplant will you do? Will you be using donated marrow?**

- **Is this the best treatment for my condition? Why?**

- Is this treatment part of a clinical trial? If not, why not?

- How many of these procedures have been done in this center? How many for my kind of cancer?

- Can you put me in touch with other people who have had this procedure?

- What are the risks and possible side effects? Can I die from the procedure?

- With my condition, what are my chances of being cured?

- If you will be using donated marrow, what are the chances that the donated material will not grow in me?

- If this procedure is done, will I need other treatment?

- What is the cost of the treatment and how does it compare with the cost of other possible therapy?

- Will my insurance pay for this treatment? Can you help me with dealing with my insurance company? Is there any other financial help available? Will I need to make a payment before this treatment can be started?

- How long will I have to stay in the hospital? Can any of it be done on an outpatient basis?

- Will I have to be treated far from home?

- What kind of support team is available? Do you have a support group for patients?

- Can friends and family visit me in the hospital? If so, are there special places for my family to stay while I'm in the hospital?

- How long will I be treated as an outpatient?

- How long will I be out of work?

- What changes in my normal activities will be required?

- How soon after the transplant will I be able to resume normal activity?

- What kind of complications may occur?

- After the transplant, how often will I need medical checkups?

- Has the hospital done at least ten bone marrow transplants this year?

Where are stem cells found?

Most stem cells, used for transplant in cancer, are found in the bone marrow. But some are found in the bloodstream. In addition, there are stem cells in umbilical cord blood. Stem cells can divide to form more stem cells or they can grow into white blood cells, red blood cells, or platelets.

Why is peripheral stem cell or bone marrow support being used in cancer treatment?

Although neither of these procedures is considered treatment itself, both are being done to allow you to receive very high doses of radiation or chemotherapy. The treatment doses that are given are so high that they severely damage the bone marrow or might even destroy it. The damaged marrow needs to be replaced with healthy marrow to allow you to produce new cells so you have the ability to fight off infections, clot blood, and transport oxygen.

What are the different kinds of transplants that can be done?

There are three main types:

- Autologus, in which patients receive their own stem cells.

- Syngeneic transplants, in which patients get stem cells from an identical twin.

- Allogeneic transplants, in which patients receive stem cells from somebody else—either from a family member or an unrelated person.

What kind of hospital should I go to if I am going to have a bone marrow transplant or peripheral stem cell support?

You must be sure that you are being treated at a major medical center that specializes in the kind of bone marrow transplant you will be having for your specific kind of cancer or that has done stem cell support for your kind of cancer. The doctor should be experienced in this specialized treatment, supported by a trained team. You will need to be at a center that has access to the blood products that may be needed if you have complications. Moreover, since for most cancers these are investigational treatments, it is important that you be at an institution that is carrying out clinical trials. The number of treatment centers that perform these procedures has grown considerably in recent years, but it is important to ask enough questions to make sure you are making the right choice. (The rule of thumb is the hospital should be doing a minimum of ten such procedures a year.)

Is the end result the same for autologous bone marrow transplant and peripheral stem cell support?

The end result of both stem cell and autologous bone marrow transplants is the same—your bone marrow function recovers. However, the early results from several major centers suggest that recovery after stem cells is faster than after bone marrow infusion. This more rapid recovery reduces side effects, such as serious infections, and the need for blood and platelet transfusions.

In addition, stem cell support does not usually mean a long hospital stay. Rather, you can be cared for at home during most of the process. The theory is the same but the stem cell procedure is less complex, has fewer side effects and is less costly. The rapid recovery after stem cell "rescue" makes it possible for some patients to be treated with multiple courses of high-dose chemotherapy.

How are the stem cells produced?

Usually you are injected with a substance, called a growth factor, to stimulate the bone marrow to produce greater numbers of "stem" cells than the body usually produces. As these stem cells are released by the bone marrow into the blood stream, they can be collected by a process called *apheresis*.

How is apheresis done?

It is usually done in a blood bank of a hospital. To collect the stem cells, your blood is withdrawn. You will be connected to a cell separator for about two to four hours for each of four or five collections. Sometimes these collections will be separated by several days, to allow your body to produce more cells in between the withdrawals.

What kind of growth factors are given?

Growth factors, also called cytokines, are routinely used to stimulate the bone marrow to begin dividing. Two types—granulocyte macrophage colony-stimulating factor (GM-CSF) or granulocyte colony-stimulating factor (G-CSF) are generally used. In stem cell support, growth factors may be given before and during the gathering of the stem cells.

Will I have any side effects during the process of collecting these stem cells?

You may experience some tingling, chilling sensations or lightheadedness during the procedure, similar to those felt when a person is giving blood.

What happens to the blood that is taken out?

The blood is separated and the red blood cells, platelets, and plasma are returned to your body. Once collected and separated, the stem cells are purified and frozen for storage, while you get your high-dose chemotherapy or whole body radiation treatments. This also may be done in an outpatient setting. If you have severe complications, you may be admitted to a hospital until they are under control. When the treatments are completed, the stem cells are reinjected into your system.

How are the peripheral stem cells then transplanted back into my body?

The cells are thawed and reinjected into your system through your veins. This procedure can take up to two hours and may be done in a hospital or in an outpatient facility. Sometimes patients complain that their rooms smell like garlic or that they experience a garlic taste in their mouths. This is due to the solution used to freeze the stem cells.

What kinds of complications might I have while the cells are being reinjected?

You may have shortness of breath, or problems with your liver or your heart. Once these complications are taken care of, your care will be similar to that of a bone marrow transplant patient. Some patients may not need to stay in the hospital because they may recover more quickly.

What are the long-term effects of peripheral stem cell transplants?

Long-term effects are not yet known since the procedure is relatively new. Both the advantages and disadvantages of this transplant method and the long-term side effects are presently being studied in major centers around the country. In addition, improved techniques of collecting and storing the stem cells and for adding growth factors to restore disease-free marrow function will be tested in the future. Further research will determine the optimal use of this treatment.

What is a mini–bone marrow transplant?

A mini-transplant, also referred to as a nonmyeloablative transplant, gives much lower doses of chemotherapy or of radiation. Therefore, the patient's marrow is not completely destroyed. This means that the recovery time is less. However, there are still potential side effects, including infection, graft versus host disease, or rejection. Bone marrow cells from both the patient and the donor may exist in the patient's body for some time before the transplanted marrow replaces the patient's own. You might be given an injection of the donor's white blood cells to boost the grafting.

What steps are involved in bone marrow transplantation?

It depends upon the institution and what kind of transplant. However, there are usually five steps you need to go through: evaluation, pretreatment and supportive care, the transplant itself, engraftment, and convalescence, which take place both in and out of the hospital.

How can I use my own bone marrow for support?

If you are having an autologous bone marrow transplant, you serve as your own donor. Usually, your bone marrow is removed, or *harvested*, when you are in remission or when no cancer cells can be found when looking at your cells under a microscope. The purpose of removing your bone marrow is to collect enough stem cells—cells from which blood cells develop—for the transplant. The stem cells will produce the new red blood cells, white blood cells, and platelets that you need.

How will I be evaluated?

The doctor carefully examines you and your history to make sure that the transplant is the best treatment. The doctor will discuss the complications and risks with you. You and your family, along with the doctor, will look at all the factors, especially your condition, outlook and what other treatments might be available, before making the decision to go ahead with the transplant.

What will happen to me during the pretreatment phase?

You will have several days of tests and other procedures. You will probably have a catheter inserted into one of the large veins in your chest. It will be used to withdraw blood samples as well as to give you blood, drugs, and nutrition. In addition, the catheter will be used in transplanting the new marrow. The catheter will probably stay in your vein for several months.

Will I also be given chemotherapy during this pretreatment phase?

Yes. Before you can have a transplant, the cancer cells must be killed. You will receive intensive chemotherapy. Some patients will also get radiation treatment. If you have leukemia, you may receive whole body radiation. These high-dose treatments will destroy your healthy marrow as well as the cancer cells. You will be given medicines to help manage and lessen the side effects of the high-dose chemotherapy and the radiation therapy. The pretreatment phases usually last from two to ten days, depending upon the procedures being used.

What side effects should I expect during this time?

You might experience nausea, vomiting, mouth sores, diarrhea, lowered blood counts, damage to your vital organs, loss of appetite, and loss of your hair. Since your bone marrow is being destroyed, your body will be unable to defend itself against infection.

DIFFERENCES BETWEEN PERIPHERAL STEM CELL AND AUTOLOGOUS BONE MARROW SUPPORT

ITEM	PERIPHERAL STEM CELL	AUTOLOGOUS BONE MARROW
How material is obtained for transplant	Four or five days before procedure, medication given to increase number of stem cells. Flexible tube put in large vein in neck, chest, or arm. Blood goes through machine that removes stem cells. Blood returned to patient. Stem cells frozen until transplanted back into patient.	General or local anesthesia; several incisions in skin over hip or breastbone. Needle inserted through opening. Marrow taken out of bone. Blood and fragments removed from bone marrow; marrow combined with preservative and placed in liquid nitrogen freezer to keep stem cells alive till needed.
Length of time for getting transplant material	About four to five hours, to take out blood and put it back.	About one hour to remove bone marrow.
Risks to donor	Medication given to stimulate stem cells may cause bone and muscle aches, headaches, and/or difficulty sleeping. Generally cease within two to three days of last dose. Procedure usually painless, but can cause lightheadedness, chills, numbness around lips, and cramping in hands.	Risk of anesthesia. Soreness in area where bone marrow was taken out. Recovery time varies from a few days to three to four weeks. Within a few weeks bone marrow replaced.
How transfused to patient	Patient receives after being treated with high-dose chemotherapy and/or radiation. Flexible tube placed in large neck in vein or chest area used.	Patient receives after being treated with high-dose chemotherapy and/or radiation. Flexible tube placed in large vein in neck or chest area.

**What kind of supportive care will I get during the
pretreatment phase?**
Usually you must stay in a hospital room where it is easier to keep the environment as free from infectious agents as possible. You will be given antibiotics to help prevent infections. In addition, you will need periodic blood transfusions because the chemotherapy and radiation will damage parts of the bone marrow that produce red blood cells and platelets. If you are unable to eat, you will be given nutrition through the catheter.

Will I feel very tired?
Yes, you probably will. Bone marrow transplants take a great deal of energy, not only for you but also for your family. You may get tired from the treatment itself, which is long and severe. You may also be tired and discouraged from not knowing what the final results will be. In addition, your family may need to travel a long distance to the treatment center or need to live away from home for an extended period of time. This adds a great deal of pressure and stress on both you and your family.

How is the actual transplant of the bone marrow done?
Soon after the chemotherapy and radiation treatments are finished, you will receive the bone marrow through the catheter. You might hear the health professionals calling this the transplant or the rescue process. The new marrow will travel through your blood to your bone marrow where it will begin to make new red and white blood cells and platelets. This is called engraftment. It will take from 14 to 30 days for this to happen. Your doctor will take blood tests or remove a small amount of marrow to make sure it is growing and that the cancer has not returned.

**How is the process of donating bone marrow
different if I am the donor myself?**
If you are having an autologous transplant and thus are the donor yourself, your bone marrow may be treated to remove malignant cells. Your bone marrow cells may be combined with a preservative to keep the cells alive when they are frozen and stored in a liquid nitrogen freezer until the day they will be transplanted. The marrow may also be purged with anticancer drugs, or other methods may be used to remove any cancer cells before it is frozen.

**If I am having an allogeneic transplant,
how will the donor be matched with me?**
The matching of bone marrow is a very complicated process. It is based on markers found on the white blood cells. Scientists look at six markers, called human leukocyte antigens or HLA, to judge whether there can be a good

match between you and the donor. These antigens are proteins that play a critical role in protecting the body from disease. Each person's antigens are a combination inherited from the mother and father. Related donors, such as brothers and sisters have a 35 to 40 percent of being a match. The chances of a match among unrelated donors are much lower—estimates range from one in a thousand to one in a million, depending on the frequency in the general population of your tissue type. Special blood tests show whether you and the other person share any of these antigens. Most institutions require a match on at least three antigens. The more matching antigens you have, the fewer the complications will be.

Who can help me find a bone marrow donor?
There are several resources to help find donors. However, although the number of donors increases constantly, there is still a possibility that you may not find a donor with enough matching antigens. The National Marrow Donor Program was created to help you find a suitable donor. It receives requests for bone marrow donors from transplant centers throughout the United States, searches its computer file for a match, coordinates additional testing of donors, helps with transplantation arrangements and collects and analyzes data. Local American Red Cross chapters may also be helpful in locating bone marrow donors. See Chapter 28, Where to Get Help, for further information.

Can I get information on bone marrow transplants on the Web?
One of the newer sites is BMT Net (www.bmtnet.org), a joint project of several BMT organizations—the American Society for Blood and Marrow Transplantation, Canadian Blood and Marrow Transplant Group, European Group for Blood and Marrow Transplantation, Foundation for accreditation of Cellular Therapy, International Bone Marrow Transplant Registry and Autologous Blood and Marrow Transplant Registry, International Society for Cellular Therapy and National Marrow Donor Program. Described as the "doorway" to bone marrow transplants on the Web, you can find information and will be able to move back and forth among the Web sites of these organizations. The site also links to many other Web sites. There are many other sites that you might wish to access. See "Resources" at the end of this chapter as well as Chapter 3, Searching for Answers on the Web, and Chapter 28, Where to Get Help.

What does the donor have to do during the transplant?
Donors for allogeneic or syngeneic transplants usually go into the hospital the day before or the day of the transplant. Depending on the hospital,

donors will get either local anesthesia to deaden the area of the body where the marrow will be removed or general anesthesia to put them to sleep. The process to extract the marrow takes about 45 minutes and must be done in an operating room under sterile conditions. The marrow is usually taken from the hipbones. The doctor makes six to ten punctures with a large needle and, using a series of smaller needles, draws about one to two pints of fluid, containing marrow, out of the donor's bones. The marrow is then strained to remove blood and bone fragments and put into the patient (the recipient) within two to four hours. Because there may be some blood loss, donors usually store two units of their own blood beforehand, to be used as needed during or after the procedure.

Does the donor have any side effects from giving the marrow?
Usually the donor has no problems. There may be some soreness around the puncture sites for a few days. Within a few weeks, the donated marrow will have been replaced by the donor's system. Most people are back to their regular routines within a day or two, although some may take a little longer. In some rare instances, there may be infection around the incision site.

How long do I need to stay in the hospital after the transplant has taken place?
Most people stay in the hospital, in a protective isolation room, for two weeks to two months after the transplant has taken place. It will depend on what type of transplant was done and how long it takes it to engraft. After you are discharged, you will be seen at the outpatient clinic several times a week for several weeks.

Why do I need to stay in the hospital so long?
You will need to be monitored to make sure that the new bone marrow is growing. You will also be watched for infections. If you had an allogeneic transplant, you will be watched carefully for acute graft-versus-host disease so that you can be treated if any problems develop. You will also be given high calorie, highly nutritious feedings through an intravenous line. In addition, you will be taught to take care of your catheter, which will be left in place for a while after the transplant, and you will be shown other techniques you will need to know to care for yourself after you go back home.

What side effects need to be considered?
There are many side effects. The extent of them will vary from one person to another and will depend upon what kind of bone marrow transplantation you have. Some, such as hair loss, are temporary. Others, such as infections and graft-versus-host disease (GVHD—a side effect of an allogeneic transplant), can be serious, and sometimes fatal. You may have bleeding in the

nose, mouth, under the skin or in the gastrointestinal tract. You may also have some liver damage. The period of highest risk is between 14 and 30 days after your transplant has taken place, as your body begins to manufacture new red and white blood cells and platelets.

What kind of infections am I at risk for?
You may get viral, bacterial, or fungal infections. For instance, herpes simplex, herpes zoster, and cytomegalovirus are frequent causes of infections. Pneumonia is another common complication. You may have inflammation in your mouth and intestinal tract, called mucositis. You can be treated with antibiotics or antiviral and antifungal therapies. You may also be given antibiotics to prevent infection.

Graft-versus-Host Disease

What is graft-versus-host disease?
When you have a bone marrow transplant, your immune system is replaced. If you are getting donor marrow, the new marrow, particularly its T cells, identifies you as foreign. It may launch an attack against you, just as whatever remains of your original immune system may reject the marrow graft. This is called graft-versus-host disease or GVHD.

Who gets GVHD?
It happens to people who have allogeneic transplants. If you are older, you are more likely to develop GVHD than if you are younger. If you have more matching antigens with your donor, you are less likely to develop GVHD. In addition, if your donor is of the same sex as you are, you are less likely to develop GVHD than if your donor is of the opposite sex. Nearly half of the people develop symptoms of GVHD soon after the transplant, some as soon as nine days after the procedure. When it happens soon after, it is called acute GVHD. When it develops later, it is called chronic GVHD.

What are the symptoms of GVHD?
If you have acute GVHD, you may have skin rashes, jaundice, liver disease, or diarrhea. These symptoms may be mild or they may be severe. If you have chronic GVHD, you may have temporary darkening of the skin and hardening and thickening of the patches of skin and the layers of tissues under it. You may also have bacterial infections and weight loss. GVHD affects the liver, the skin, and the gastrointestinal tract—you can have it in all three sites. Corticosteriods and other drugs are used for treatment.

Can anything be done to prevent GVHD?
Yes. Since the T lymphocytes are the major cause of the immune attack, drugs that help suppress them are given to patients routinely after transplantation. Also under study is the use of a procedure called T-cell depletion. Monoclonal antibodies or other processes are used to destroy T lymphocytes in donated marrow before it is given to the patient.

Are there any benefits to developing GVHD?
Many studies have shown that mild GVHD is actually beneficial over the long term because it kills tumor cells. People with leukemia and lymphoma who develop mild GVHD are less likely to have a relapse than are those who never have the reaction.

How can the doctor tell if the bone marrow transplant is failing?
There are several signs. If your body is rejecting the graft, the donor's cells will not grow and your own cells may not begin growing again. If you have leukemia, leukemia cells may show up again in your bone marrow.

**How long will it take for me to get back to
feeling like my normal self?**
You will probably need a full year to recover fully from your transplant. You need to understand, however, that you may have to change your normal habits to help you cope with the long-term effects of your treatment. You may feel tired, have dry eyes, skin sensitivity, and reproductive disorders. Because of changes in your liver, you may need modify your diet. You may also need to remain on medication for a long time.

**What are the major long-term side effects of
bone marrow transplants?**
There are several major long-term side effects. They include infertility, cataracts (especially for persons who have had allogeneic transplants) and second cancers. Persons who have had transplants complain most often about muscle spasms, leg cramps, numbness of extremities, eye problems, and infertility. Slow return of energy and memory loss are also frequent complaints. However, most people who have had transplants feel their overall health is good and that the benefits of the transplant outweigh the side effects.

Will the transplant affect my sexual ability?
It depends on your age, and the dose and length of treatment you have as part of the transplant procedure. If you receive whole-body radiation as part of your transplant procedure, you (both men and women) will most likely become sterile, that is, unable to produce a child. However, you will probably

still have the desire and will be able to be active sexually. Men who undergo chemotherapy for bone marrow transplants commonly become infertile. You may wish to discuss sperm banking before you begin the transplant procedure. Many women who receive chemotherapy alone as part of the transplant procedure will have irregular periods, which usually will return to normal within three to 28 months after the transplant. If you are a woman, are over 26 years old, and have both chemotherapy and whole-body radiation, you will probably develop early menopause because your ovaries will stop producing certain hormones.

How often do transplant patients get cataracts?
Cataracts are a common long-term side effect among allogeneic bone marrow transplant patients who have single-dose total body radiation, with about 75 percent of patients getting cataracts some three to six years later. If you had total body radiation in several small doses, your risk is reduced to 25 percent.

Do many patients who have transplants get secondary cancers?
It is not yet clear, because bone marrow transplants have been done for a relatively short period of time. However, there is concern that the high-dose chemotherapy, radiation therapy, and other factors related to the procedure could cause other cancers. The risk varies and depends on your age, general health, menopausal status, drug dose, and previous treatment.

Will my health insurance pay for the bone marrow or stem cell transplant?
It depends on your health plan. Even though the cost of these procedures has been reduced, mostly due to less time spent in the hospital, these are extremely expensive treatments. Some health plans cover some of the costs both in the hospital and if special care is required at home. You need to discuss your coverage with your health plan and the doctor before you decide to proceed with the treatment. A hospital social worker usually can help you explore these issues.

Is it normal to worry about relapse?
Yes, it is normal. Unfortunately, some people do have relapses, most from their original tumors although some persons may also develop new primaries from the chemotherapy and radiation. It is possible for some patients to get a second transplant, although it may involve a different regimen, without whole body irradiation. New immunologic agents, such as interleukin-2, interferon, and ricin are being evaluated for use in decreasing the risk of relapse.

New Prevention Techniques

The new term in the area of prevention is *chemoprevention*. It uses drugs and other substances to prevent cancer. There are several kinds of research studies being done in this new field. Some are directed at people who have been successfully treated for one cancer and are at high risk for getting a second cancer. Others are aimed at people who have a medical condition that may lead to cancer or are at risk for getting cancer. Still others enroll healthy, disease-free people who are studied to understand how to improve the comfort and quality of life of people who have cancer.

What are cancer prevention clinical trials based on?

They are based on the belief that various chemoprevention agents may stop or reverse cancer development or prevent it from ever starting. These agents need to be studied scientifically over time to find out if they can indeed prevent cancer.

Does everyone on the trial get the agent being tested?

People who take part in the trial are separated into different groups. In some studies, the chemoprevention agent will be tested against no agent at all. That means that one group will get the agent and others will receive an identical looking pill, called a placebo, that contains no drug at all. You will be put into one group or the other purely by chance and you will not usually be told what group you are in. Other times, the agent will be tested against another agent. The people in each group take a different agent or a different dose of the same agent.

What kinds of agents are being tested in chemoprevention trials?

They are drugs that have shown through research some success in preventing a type of cancer when given in a specified dose over an extended period of time. The agent may be a medicine, vitamin, mineral, nutritional supplement, such as Vitamins A or E, food supplement, or a combination of these. The prevention trials go through the same process of approval as do cancer treatment clinical trials.

Are there side effects or risks in cancer prevention trials?

There may be. Some agents used may cause side effects depending on what they are and how you respond to them. Every possible effort is made to identify the risks associated with the agents being used. Generally, they are not expected to cause serious side effects.

Are there any costs involved?

Each trial is different. Some are entirely cost-free to those who participate. In others, you may have to pay for some or all of the costs of the tests and examinations that are required. The trials, however, are designed so that most of the tests are considered to be part of routine medical care, so that if possible, they are costs that your insurance can pay for. These tests may include mammograms, Pap tests, or cholesterol tests—examinations that healthy people are encouraged to do on a regular basis. You need to discuss the costs with the doctor or nurse and check with your health insurance company before you decide whether or not you wish to participate.

Questions to Ask Before Joining
A Chemoprevention Trial

- **What is the purpose of the trial?**
- **What part of the trial is experimental?**
- **What kinds of tests are required?**
- **Whom do I contact with questions about the research?**
- **What are the potential risks and potential benefits?**
- **What are my responsibilities while on the trial?**
- **How long will the trial last?**
- **What costs may I expect?**
- **Will my records be confidential?**
- **How can the trial affect my daily life?**
- **What side effects could I expect from the agent being used?**
- **Do I have any further responsibilities after I have completed the study?**

What are some of the chemoprevention trials that are underway?

There are several, including:

- The Study of Tamoxifen and Raloxifene (STAR) trial comparing the osteoporosis drug raloxifene with tamoxifen in women at high risk for breast cancer. The original trial, the Breast Cancer Prevention trial showed that high-risk women given tamoxifen had 49 percent fewer diagnosed cases of breast cancer. However, there were serious side effects, such as endometrial cancer and blood clots, leading to the new trial.

- The Prostrate Cancer Prevention Trial, to evaluate whether taking the drug Proscar (finastride) will prevent prostate cancer from developing in men. This study has enrolled 18,000 men ages 55 and older, half of whom are receiving finastride each day and half of whom are receiving a placebo. The trial will last seven years.

- The Prostate, Lung, Colorectal and Ovarian Cancer Screening Trial, to determine whether the widespread use of certain screening tests for these cancers will save lives. This test is studying digital rectal exam and PSA (prostate), chest x-ray (lung), flexible sigmoidoscope (colorectal) and physical exam of the ovaries, CA–125 and transvaginal ultrasound (ovary). More than 154,000 men and women between the ages of 60 and 74 have been enrolled at 10 medical centers across the country. Results are expected in 2015.

- The SELECT trial, which is studying whether selenium and Vitamin E can reduce the risk of developing prostate cancer.

- Aspirin, piroxicam, celecoxib, and sulindac and calcium compounds are being studied alone or in combination in people with a family history of colon polyps or cancer.

- Budesonide, which has been used to treat asthma, is being studied to prevent the progression of precanceerous changes in lung tissue. It is being given as a spray.

- Other agents being investigated include selenium, Vitamin E, 2–difluoromethylornithene (DFMA) folic acid, oltipraz and genistein. See Chapter 14, Prostate Cancer and Other Male Cancers, for information on Vitamin D and prostate cancer.

Web Pages to Check Out

www.cancer.gov: For general up-to-date information, and for clinical trails.

www.cancer.org: For general up-to-date information and community resources.

www.cordblooddonor.org: Cord Blood Donor Foundation.

www.crir.org: Caitlin Ramond International Registry (University of Massachusetts Medical Center). Describes international registry and its services plus links to other sites.

www.marrow.org: Human Leukocyte Antigen Registry Foundation. Largest bone marrow donor registry in National Marrow Donor Program.

www.office.de.netcord.org/index.html: NETCORD Worldwide access to international cord blood registries.

www.redcross.org/services/biomed/blood/cord: International Bone Marrow Transplant Registry.

www.bmtnet.org: BMT Net. Joint project of several bone marrow transplant (BMT) organizations. Serves as portal to BMT resources on the Web.

www.marrow.org or 1–800–MARROW–2: National Marrow Donor Program. Has directory of participating transplant centers. Each entry includes description of center, summary of center's area of expertise, and contact information.

www.cancer.gov/cancerinfo/pdq/prevention: Information on clinical trails for cancer prevention.

www.clinicaltrailshelp.org: Coalition of National Cancer Cooperative groups. Searchable list of clinical trials. Links to National Cancer Institutes' PDQ.

www.clinicaltrials.cancer.org: Matching and referral service of American Cancer Society and EmergingMod.

www.cancer.gov/cancerinfo/pdq: National Cancer Institute site for clinical trials information.

www.acr.org or 1–800–ACR–LINE: American College of Radiology. CT/PET scan, diagnostic radiology.

www.radiologyinfo.org: Radiological Society of North American and American College of Radiology. Radiology Info Web site.

Also see Chapter 2, Searching for Answers on the Web, for more information.

Twelve

UNDERSTANDING COMPLEMENTARY AND ALTERNATIVE TREATMENTS

Many people (in fact, more than 70 percent) use some sort of complementary or alternative treatment to help them get through the cancer experience. Much of what is called complementary medicine has become integrated into conventional treatment (such as support groups and massage) and these activities can empower patients and improve their lives. The best way to fight cancer is to get the best conventional treatment and, if you're interested, to search out the complementary treatments that make sense to you. Many of these can safely be used along with conventional treatment to help relieve symptoms or side effects, to ease pain, and to help you relax. (Information about the specific complementary treatments can be found in Chapter 27, Living With Cancer). Most physicians are now open to helping their patients sort out the pros and cons of incorporating nondrug techniques into treatment. Our advice is that you discuss your ideas with your doctor. Just be sure you don't abandon a treatment where there is a known and proven response for a fly-by-night treatment that has no proven track record.

EVERYONE IS susceptible to the promises of a "sure cure" that is without risks or pain, using natural products with no side effects. And cancer patients and their families are no exception. The cures commonly offered by the proponents of many alternative methods include diets, devices, and drugs. This subject is a controversial one, with information that can be misleading and claims that can be difficult to interpret. Some people turn to alternative methods because they think the treatments will be easier for them to withstand. Others have a deep-seated mistrust of doctors or are afraid of the usual treatments for the disease. Sometimes friends or family members encourage the use of miracle cures they've heard or read about. In making your choices, you should be aware that there are many products and treatments that often promise a great deal but which produce little if any benefit. On the other hand, many lifestyle approaches, referred to as **complementary treatments,** can be used along with conventional treatment.

The Difference Between Conventional, Investigational, Complementary, and Alternative Treatments

Proven treatments or conventional approaches to cancer treatment have been studied for safety and effectiveness through a rigorous scientific process, including clinical trials with large numbers of patients. They represent the best hope for a cure. Surgery, radiation therapy, and chemotherapy are curative for many cancers.

Investigational treatments, sometimes called experimental treatments, are those treatments being studied in clinical trials to determine whether the treatment is effective and is safe for patients.

Complementary treatments, sometimes called integrative treatments, include a whole category of methods that complement or are used in addition to conventional treatments. They include spiritual, psychological, nutritional, and physical approaches such as meditation, acupuncture, biofeedback, hypnosis, massage, yoga, tai chi, and relaxation. Many medical centers are combining the use of complementary and proven treatments. You may hear the term integrative therapy to describe this combination. For more information on complementary treatments, see Chapter 27, Living With Cancer.

Alternative treatments, sometimes referred to as unproven or untested, are treatments that are used *instead of* conventional treatment. They have not been scientifically tested, or if tested, found to be ineffective. In addition, many of them are offered by unscrupulous marketing, are expensive, and most are not covered by health insurance. They can interact poorly with your conventional treatment or even be harmful.

How do investigational treatments differ from alternative methods?

Investigational treatments, sometimes called experimental treatments, are conducted using specific scientific methods and standards to evaluate new therapies or procedures. Although the standards being used for investigational treatment are complex and strict, they are necessary to ensure any new treatment offered to patients is effective and safe. These procedures are described in Chapter 11, New and Investigational Treatments.

What does the National Center for Complementary and Alternative Medicine do?

The National Center for Complementary and Alternative Medicine, a part of the National Institutes of Health, was established to investigate complementary and alternative treatments using the scientific methods used in conventional medicine. It supports a number of programs, including The Best Case series, which provides an opportunity for an individual to present case reports that give evidence of a successful alternative medical approach.

What You Need to Know About Complementary and Alternative Treatments

- Although the terms *complementary* and *alternative* are sometimes used interchangeably, they are different. Complementary therapies are those that are used along with conventional treatment. Alternative treatments are used instead of conventional treatments.

- There are many complementary methods that can be used along with conventional treatment to help you get through your treatments. You may want to try meditation, deep relaxation, massage, hypnosis, imagery, a wholesome balanced vegetarian diet, psychological or spiritual support, tai chi, yoga, or traditional Chinese medicine. For these, there are ethical and appropriately qualified practitioners available locally at moderate cost. Chapter 27, Living With Cancer, has more information about these methods.

- In most cases there is little scientific evidence presented by those promoting alternative methods. People may be encouraged to have the treatment even though there is no true evidence that it really works. There are some promoters who engage in unethical sales techniques, make misleading promises, charge high fees, and neglect prudent conventional medical supervision and care. Many times the writeups for the alternative treatments use scientific words or phrases in a misleading manner. Many alternative treatments can be found on the Web. In determining whether information is reliable or unreliable, you should follow the guidelines listed in Chapter 2, Searching for Answers on the Web.

- "Natural" does not mean safe. Many natural treatments have side effects and can interfere with your conventional treatments. Herbal extracts and supplements should be used with care. Check with your doctor before you take them.

- We have found that some treatments that have been tested and found useless, such as Laetrile, have been renamed and repackaged and continue to be sold to unsuspecting patients.

- Many treatments are being promoted by doctors with unrecognizable degrees such as DA BB-A (Diplomate of American Board of Bioanalysts), and MsD. (Doctor of Metaphysics). Be sure to check the credentials of doctors giving treatments.

- The greatest danger for cancer patients occurs when there is a possibility for a cure with conventional therapy, but it is abandoned in favor of alternative medicine. If you do decide not to follow the conventional route, be sure that you have a full understanding of the risks and that you keep a complete record of your treatment and the results. Be an informed consumer.

- Check out the costs of the treatment. Check out whether your insurance will cover any of these costs.

- If alternative therapy is something you're thinking about, it is important to discuss it with your doctor and your healthcare team. Educate yourself about the alternative method and ask your doctor what he knows about it, what experience he or his colleagues have had with it, and what he suggests you do. It is important for you to understand that many alternative treatments can interfere with your regular treatment and may have potential side effects. There may be a risk, for instance, in mixing some chemotherapy drugs with herbal medicines, large doses of vitamins, or other unorthodox substances. Dietary supplements, such as herbs, can affect conventional medicine and should not be taken without the doctor's consent.

ALTERNATIVE TREATMENTS

Cancer patients are frequently tempted to try untested methods of treatment by the promise of a simple, uncomplicated cure—treatments that seem less threatening than those offered by the medical establishment. If you are considering some of these treatments, it is important to be an informed consumer in assessing "cures." Ask the hard questions about the alternative methods being offered and do your own research into what is being promised. Use your own common sense and sound judgment—if it sounds too good to be true, it probably is. One of the reasons why alternative methods of treatment are considered risky is because, unfortunately, there have been very few independent interpretable scientific studies on them. The National Center for Complementary and Alternative Medicine at the National Institutes of Health was created to remedy this situation. Growing interest in all areas of alternative medicine has made even the most conventional physicians aware of other approaches. In this chapter we have tried to shed light on some of the more commonly known alternative treatments to help you assess them for yourself. We encourage you to discuss all treatments—be they conventional, complementary, or alternative—with those who are handling your health care.

Questions You Should Ask Before You Use Alternative Methods

- **Why do I want to use this kind of treatment?**
- **What do I think it will accomplish?**
- **Is there a clinical trial where this treatment is being studied?**
- **What evidence is there that the alternative method will work? How has it been evaluated?**
- **What claims are made for the treatment?**
- **What are the credentials of those giving the treatment?**
- **Has it been written up in a scientific journal? Why not?**
- **Do the practitioners of the method claim that the medical community is trying to keep their cure from the public?**
- **Does the treatment have a "secret formula" that only a small group of practitioners can use? Has the treatment been evaluated by an independent group of researchers?**
- **How long has the establishment been in operation? Is it certified by any authoritative body?**
- **What are the qualifications of the people who will be treating me? Have they graduated from accredited schools?**
- **Does it sound too good to be true?**
- **Have I discussed the treatment with my doctor?**
- **Will the doctor continue to care for me if I am using this treatment?**
- **Is there some way my doctor and I can come to a compromise?**
- **Can I continue my regular treatments and try the alternative method at the same time?**
- **Is there some kind of conventional investigational treatment that would give the same or better results?**
- **What costs will be associated with the unproven method?**
- **How do these costs compare to conventional treatment?**

Is the subject of unconventional methods new?

Untested cancer treatments are as old as the disease itself. In 1784, the House of Burgesses of the General Assembly of Virginia, of which George Washington was a member, passed a resolution appointing a committee to examine Mary Johnson's "receipt of curing cancer," consisting of garden sorrel, celandine, persimmon bark, and spring water, and to report on its effect. In 1754, upon hearing the testimony of many witnesses who said the remedy had cured them of cancer, the committee put the report into the minutes of the House of Burgesses and voted Mrs. Johnson a reward of 100 pounds.

Why are doctors so opposed to alternative treatments?

Most doctors think that unconventional methods have more risk associated to them than conventional treatments. The most substantial concern is the delay in getting proper treatment that has proven its effectiveness. (Many standard treatments are highly successful, especially in curing cancers that are found early.) If you use an unproven treatment first and it does not work, the next step would be to get a standard treatment. Unfortunately your cancer will probably be at a more advanced stage than when it was first discovered. The delay could result in the loss of valuable time in receiving a conventional treatment that could have cured your cancer or at least controlled it. You are also spending money for treatment, usually not covered by your insurance, that is not effective.

Is it difficult to get information about treatment results of untested methods into scientific journals?

Papers that are published in reputable medical and nursing journals require that scientifically sound methods be used and that objective evidence be presented so that the overall effectiveness of the treatment can be evaluated. The papers are read by professionals in the field, through a process called peer-review. Whether they are reporting on alternative methods or other treatments, the studies do not get published without hard evidence. There is no lack of places to present scientific data, with over 500 high-quality medical and nursing journals and nearly 3,000 health-science journals in which new medical developments are regularly published. In addition, there are thousands of regularly scheduled meetings of doctors and scientists at which to present well-documented scientific evidence.

Can those who provide untested treatments get any help from the government in conducting trials of their treatments?

The National Center for Complementary and Alternative Medicine, established in 1992 at the National Institutes of Health, is funding research in five different categories—mind, body, and spirit methods; manual and physical touch meth-

STANDARDS FOR ALTERNATIVE METHODS COMPARED TO INVESTIGATIONAL TREATMENTS

ALTERNATIVE	INVESTIGATIONAL
People giving treatment usually claim it has high degree of activity against cancers that are considered incurable with no basis for the claim.	Must have scientific evidence that treatment being used has some effectiveness against cancer.
Usually no study has been outlined with objectives.	Objectives of study must be clearly stated.
Usually no written protocol or standardized methods of giving drugs or medication. Even the same patient may get different doses given in different manners.	Methods used to achieve objectives must be stated in protocols and in reports of results.
No comparison groups.	Study includes comparison groups to determine whether treatment is better than standard treatment.
No review by human subjects committee. Institution normally not certified by usual authorizing agencies.	Must be reviewed by human subjects committee in qualified medical institution.
Most untested methods are used without any explanation and without your signing a consent form.	Informed consent, including written explanation of the purpose and aspects, the potential benefits and risks of the trials is required.
Many times no biopsy evidence to prove that person had cancer.	Must be clear evidence that patients have cancer.
No control groups used.	Patients randomly assigned to treatment and control groups to eliminate bias.
Unproven treatment being studied often used after or along with standard treatment. No way to tell which treatment caused improvement.	Response to treatment must be objectively assessed using sound, well-defined methods.

(continued)

STANDARDS FOR ALTERNATIVE METHODS COMPARED TO INVESTIGATIONAL TREATMENTS (continued)

ALTERNATIVE	INVESTIGATIONAL
Claims of treatment effectiveness based on stories of people who appear to be cured or on testimonials from people who believed they were cured.	Results enough to determine effects of must be analyzed thoroughly treatment.
Records often scanty, inadequate, or nonexistent. No means of replicating results or even of knowing what results have been.	Other researchers using same method must be able to achieve same results.
Results not reported in scientific journals and not reviewed by experts in field. Findings are reported directly to press.	Results must be published in reputable scientific journals.

ods; herb, vitamin, and mineral methods; diet and nutrition methods; and pharmacological and biological treatments. A major reason for the establishment of the office was to give those who are practicing alternative medicine an opportunity to demonstrate the scientific validity of their treatments.

What are antineoplastons?

Dr. S.R. Burzynski of the Burzynski Research Institute in Houston, Texas, has identified a group of peptides produced by the body, which he calls antineoplastons. He and his colleagues believe these peptides are produced in individuals as part of a "biochemical defense system" that inhibits cancer cell growth. According to Dr. Burzynski, "The failure and deficiency of antineoplastons will result in perpetuation of neoplastic growth and development of cancer." He asserts that giving antineoplastons to people with cancer will restore this "cancer defense system."

Has the National Cancer Institute reviewed
Dr. Burzynski's antineoplastons treatment?

The National Cancer Institute reviewed seven cases of primary brain tumor that were treated by Dr. Burzynski with antineoplastons. Some patients initially progressed on a study using oral antineoplastons with low-dose

SOME QUESTIONABLE ALTERNATIVE CANCER TREATMENTS

Alivazatos Greek cancer cure (see Greek Cancer Cure in this chapter)

Antineoplastons (Burzynski—see questions in this chapter)

Apitherapy (bee venom and other honeybee products)

Beard method (pancreatic enzymes)

Bonifacia anticancer (goat serum)

Bovine cartilage (see question in this chapter)

Burton method: Immunoaugmentive therapy (see questions in this chapter)

Burzynski method: Antineoplaston Therapy (see questions in this chapter)

Cancell (see question in this chapter)

Carcino and neocarcin (antibodies made from mouse, rabbit, goat extracts)

Carzodelin (nutritional therapy)

Cell specific therapy (magnetic donut-shaped device)

Cell therapy (injections of living tissue from animal organs, embryos, or fetuses—see question in this chapter)

Coley toxins (see question in this chapter)

DHEA (steroid hormone produced by adrenal gland; especially dangerous if used in people with hormone responsive cancers)

DiBella therapy (mixture of drugs, vitamins and other substances; clinical trials in Italy showed it ineffective in treating cancer.)

Dimethyl sulfoxide, also known as DMSO (industrial solvent medically approved for treatment of intersitial cystitis and to reduce swelling in horses and dogs).

Dotto electronic reactor (magnetic device)

Enzyme therapy (see question in this chapter)

Gerson method (fruit/vegetable diet, enemas)

Gonzalez protocol trial (gland extracts, coffee enemas, vitamin megadoses—see questions in this chapter)

Grape diet

Greek cancer cure (Alivizatos therapy includes blood test to diagnose location and extent of cancer, serum made of brown sugar, niacin, Vitamin C, and alanine, injected daily, special diet low in salts and acids; marketed under names Metbal and Cellbal)

(continued)

SOME QUESTIONABLE ALTERNATIVE
CANCER TREATMENTS *(continued)*

Hoxsey method (herbal mixture taken internally or applied externally)

Hydrazine sulfate (compound used to reverse weight loss in patients with advanced cancers)

Hyper-oxygen therapy (ozone blood infusion and absorption of oxygen water)

Immunoaugmentative therapy (IAT or Burton Therapy—see questions in this chapter)

Inositol hexaphosphate or IP6 (chemical found in brown rice, corn, sesame seeds, wheat bran; aids in metabolism of insulin and calcium.)

Iscador (mistletoe preparation with mistletoe collected at times and places determined by astrology)

Issel's combination therapy (fever therapy)

Krebiozen (also known as creatine and carcalon, manufactured in powder and liquid forms)

Laetrile (see question in this chapter)

Livingston-Wheeler (see questions in this chapter)

Macrobiotic diet (see questions in this chapter)

Metabolic therapy (Gonzalez [Kelley])

Mucorhicin (made from mold extracts—mucor and rhizopus)

Noni (fruit extract used by Asians and Pacific Islanders)

PC SPES (eight herbs containing plant chemicals and trace minerals used to treat prostate cancer. See questions in chapter.)

Recnac (intravenous ascorbate used as chemotherapeutic agent)

Revici method (lipid therapy formulations, urine interpretation)

Shark cartilage (see question in this chapter)

SV, Sun Soup, also called selected vegetable soup. Freeze-dried brown powder containing specific selection of vegetables and herbs promoted as cancer cure.

714X (chemical solution—one component is camphor—produced in Quebec) methotrexate. There was a marked decrease in tumor size and possible complete response lasting about four months in a 46-year-old female with glioblastoma multiforme, a type of brain cancer. Other patients showed decreases in tumor size. However, several of these patients received antineoplaston treatment shortly after taking radiation therapy, and some researchers questioned the effects of the radiation in evaluating the cases. To determine whether the antitumor activity was due to treatment with antineoplastons, NCI sponsored several clinical trials using antineoplastons, but only nine patients enrolled. Therefore no definitive conclusions could be drawn. The Burzynski Research Institute is conducting trials on several types of cancer (see www.clinicaltrials.gov).

What is Cancell?

Cancell is a liquid made up of common chemicals, including nitric acid, sodium sulfite, potassium hyroxide, sulfuric acid, inositol, and catechol. It is known as Entelev, Cantron, Sheridan's Formula, Jim's Juice, Croncinic Acid, and Radic. It is purported to change cancer cells to "foreign" cells that the body destroys. It may be taken orally or rectally, or is suggested for external use by being applied to the wrist or the ball of the foot with a cotton pad. There is no evidence that this substance is effective in treating cancer.

What is cell therapy?

Cell therapy involves the injection of living tissue from animal organs, animal embryos, or fetuses to supposedly repair cellular damage. Practitioners claim that healthy cells injected into the body find their way to unhealthy organs of the same kind and stimulate the body's own healing process. The treatment was invented in 1931 by Paul Niehans, MD, a Swiss physician. Though there has been rigorous scientific testing, claims have never been proven. Even proponents of cell therapy admit they don't understand how cell therapy works. Cell therapy, in fact, may be dangerous. Deaths have been reported as well as viral and bacterial infections caused by the animal cells. Complications such as encephalitis, immune vasculitis, and nerve inflammation have also been noted. The treatment is not legally available in the United States but is offered in clinics in Europe, Mexico, and the Bahamas.

What is Coley toxin?

William B. Coley, MD, developed Coley toxins in the 1890s. He is credited with pioneering in the field of immunotherapy, which is used today as an effective cancer treatment. Coley toxin is an injection of inactive bacterial cultures designed to stimulate the immune system. Several small research studies found that patients who received Coley toxins or MBV (mixed bacterial vaccines) in combination with conventional treatment, tended to live longer than patients who received conventional treatment alone. Newer methods of immunotherapy are being studied in treating cancer. The inactive bacteria in Coley toxins can produce fever and nausea and can cause serious infections among patients with weakened immune systems.

What is the Gonzales protocol trial?

This is a five-year clinical study funded by the National Institutes of Health's National Center for Complementary and Alternative Medicine. It is examining the standard treatment for advanced pancreatic cancer that cannot be removed surgically as compared to a regimen of pancreatic enzymes and dietary supplements known as the Gonzalez protocol.

Why was this enzyme treatment chosen?

It is known that chemotherapy can stop tumor cells from dividing so that they cease growing or die. Gonzalez felt that pancreatic enzymes could act like chemotherapy and kill cancer cells. Gonzalez based some of his protocol on theories derived from early-20th-century studies from the University of Edinburgh that showed that pancreatic enzymes had cancer-killing properties. Gonzalez's regimen is derived primarily from his experience working with William Kelley, DDS, who is said to have developed this treatment approach and reported it in a book called *One Answer to Cancer*.

What is the Greek cancer cure?

Dr. Hariton-Tzannis Alivizatos, a microbiologist in Athens, Greece, claimed to have developed a blood test that could diagnose, locate, and determine the extent of a person's cancer. He also asserted that a series of serum injections were successful in fighting the cancer found. His findings were never published in a scientific journal, his serum was never tested by other scientists, and he never allowed an independent review of his findings. The Greek government suspended his license several times because it could not establish that his serum was effective. Dr. Alivizatos died in 1991. Today, a few clinics in this country offer what they claim is the same treatment. The serum formula is marketed under the names Metbal and Cellbal. The stated ingredients are brown sugar, niacin, Vitamin C, and alanine. Like its predecessor, there is no indication that this treatment is effective in treating cancer.

What is immunoaugmentative therapy?

Immunoaugmentative therapy (IAT) is designed to stimulate a person's immune system and restore normal immune function. It involves daily injections of processed human blood products, a treatment that was developed by Lawrence Burton, PhD, given at the Immunology Researching Centre in the

Bahamas. Dr. Burton purported that this treatment was effective against cancer, multiple sclerosis and AIDS.

Has the therapy even been tested by the NCI for effectiveness?

Several attempts were made to plan a clinical trial in collaboration with Dr. Burton, but they were unsuccessful. However, other issues have resulted in the FDA banning the import of IAT. In 1985, at the request of the families of two patients who had returned to the United States from Dr. Burton's clinic, a Washington State blood bank examined 18 sealed IAT specimens. All tested positive for hepatitis B; some of the samples also were positive for HIV. The Centers for Disease Control and Prevention (CDC), the National Cancer Institute (NCI), and independent laboratories reviewed the results and confirmed the analysis. In July 1985, the Bahamian Ministry of Health requested that representatives from the CDC and the Pan American Health Organization (PAHO) visit the Immunology Researching Centre to investigate the IAT manufacturing process. The groups concluded that the manufacture of the substance represented a serious health hazard, and the Bahamian Government closed the clinic. It reopened in March 1986 after Dr. Burton had agreed to follow certain quality control procedures, including screening blood sources for HIV and hepatitis B, and conducting standard blood donor screening and collection practices. In July 1986, the FDA issued an import ban prohibiting anyone from bringing IAT into the United States. This ban is still in effect. Dr. Burton died in 1993. The Immunology Researching Centre remains open under the direction of Dr. R.J. Clement.

What is laetrile?

Laetrile is a compound made from the kernels of apricots, peaches, and almonds, which produces a chemical called amygdalin. Promoters of laetrile, which is also called Vitamin B17 or amygdalin, claim that it is a viable treatment for cancer and that it is useful in cancer prevention. However, no scientific evidence supports these claims. The National Cancer Institute tested laetrile in laboratory animals several times but found no convincing evidence that it is effective against animal cancers. However, because of widespread public use and interest in the subject, a clinical study of laetrile was conducted with cancer patients at medical centers around the country. Researchers who participated in the trial concluded that laetrile was ineffective as a treatment for cancer.

What is Livingston-Wheeler Therapy?

Dr. Virginia Livingston-Wheeler, who died in 1990, operated the Livingston-Wheeler Clinic in San Diego, California. She believed that cancer is caused by a bacterium she called *progenitor cyptocides* and published reports on her bacterium beginning in the 1950s. Dr. Livingston-Wheeler's treatment involves a vaccine derived from bacteria usually cultured from the patient's urine, along with a strict vegetarian diet, antibiotics, digestive enzymes, nutritional supplements, bile salts, enemas, laxatives, and blood transfusions. However, other researchers have not been able to confirm the existence of the unique organism that Dr. Livingston-Wheeler described. When she submitted cultures to the American Type Culture Collection, a private organization that collects, grows, preserves, and distributes authentic cultures of microorganisms, they identified the samples as *staphylococcus epidermidis*. The California Department of Health Services Cancer Advisory Council conducted a review of the available information and concluded that there is no scientific basis for believing that the Livingston-Wheeler vaccines are safe and effective in treating cancer. As a result, in 1990, the State of California ordered the clinic to stop treating cancer patients with these vaccines, which were not approved by the FDA. (Dr. Livingston-Wheeler had never sought FDA approval for her vaccine). However, the clinic remains in operation, no longer using vaccines but treating cancer patients with arthritis, lupus, allergies, and AIDS.

What is the macrobiotic diet?

Macrobiotic diets were not invented primarily as cancer treatments; they stem from the teachings of a Japanese philosopher who believed simplicity in diet was the key to good health. Those who recommend the diet for cancer patients believe that cancer is a toxic blood condition that has developed because of poor eating habits. There are many variations of the macrobiotic diet, but the standard macrobiotic diet consists of 50 to 60 percent organically grown whole grains, 20 to 25 percent locally and organically grown fruits and vegetables, five to ten percent soups made with vegetables, seaweed, grains, beans, and miso (a soy product).

Can the macrobiotic diet be harmful to cancer patients?

Strict macrobiotic diets that exclude animal products may lack in many vitamins and minerals. Since milk products are excluded, getting enough calcium can be a problem. An inadequate intake of protein, Vitamin D, zinc, calcium, iron, and Vitamin B12 can cause further problems for patients with cancer—many of whom already have difficulty in maintaining their weight, in eating enough calories and consuming the necessary protein. Persons on the macrobiotic diet need to eat large amounts of food, mostly bulky foods, just to obtain the number of calories required by the diet. Research using microbiotic studies in cancer patients is limited and controversial.

What are PC SPES and SPES?

These are dietary supplements and herbal products. PC SPES is a capsule that is marketed for "prostate health" and has been used by prostate cancer patients hoping to control their disease. The U.S. Food and Drug Administration (FDA) has warned consumers to stop taking the PC SPES and SPES because they contain undeclared prescription drug ingredients that could cause serious health effects if not taken under medical supervision. The California-based manufacturer of the product, BiotanicLab, voluntarily recalled PC SPES and SPES nationwide, and on June 1, 2002, BotanicLab officially closed.

Are there any trials being conducted with PC SPES and SPES?
NCCAM had funded four research studies of PC SPES to learn about its safety, efficacy, and mechanisms of action; one of them involved research with patients. After meeting with the scientists performing the major PC SPES studies, prostate cancer specialists, experts in herbal medicine, and representatives of government and industry, NCCAM has allowed the three laboratory studies of existing PC SPES supplied to resume. These studies will seek to learn the cellular and molecular mechanisms of action of the herbs as opposed to the drug ingredients that contaminated the product.

When will the PC SPES patient study resume?
Because of the promising data from the early studies of PC SPES and the importance of addressing advanced and harmone-refractory prostate cancer, NCCAM is interested in resuming studies of PC SPES with patients and in funding new laboratory studies of PC SPES. However, these trials will resume only when a fully characterized and standardized contaminant-free product using the original product formulation becomes available.

What is shark cartilage treatment?
The theory is that there is a protein in shark cartilage that can inhibit the development of the network of blood vessels that tumors need for nourishment. Scientists say that an insignificant number of sharks—one out of a million or less—get cancer. Sharks seem to resist tumors naturally. Rather than bones, the skeletons of sharks are made of pure cartilage, a hard gristly material formed from proteins and complex carbohydrates and toughened by rodlike fibers. Clinical trials are underway to determine whether shark cartilage has a role in cancer treatment. NCI and the National Center for Alternative and Complementary Medicine are sponsoring a multicenter phase III controlled trial of a liquid shark cartilage extract for the treatment of lung cancer along with conventional therapy. Shark cartilage is available in capsule, powder, or liquid form.

Are shark and bovine cartilage treatments similar?

Bovine cartilage is extracted from various parts of a cow. The theory is similar to that for shark cartilage. Like shark cartilage, studies are underway to evaluate the effectiveness of bovine cartilage in some solid tumors.

What is the substance in shark cartilage and bovine cartilage that is being studied?

The process, known as antiangiogenesis therapy, may hold some promise for people with certain types of cancer. A number of antiangiogenesis drugs have been developed and are currently under investigation. Some researchers are trying to purify antiangiogenic compounds from cartilage. The most promising are those that have been purified from sources other than cartilage or have been developed synthetically in laboratories. Possible complications from use of cartilage include the slowing down of the recovery from surgery. Researchers warn that people with a low white blood cell count should not take cartilage enemas because there is a risk of life-threatening infection.

Is tea being used for cancer prevention and treatment?

In China and India, tea drinking has long been regarded as an aid to good health. Researchers have found some promising early research in the laboratory that may reduce the primary risk of cancer. Catechins, antioxidants found in tea, have obstructed the growth of cancer cells in animals. They have also reduced the number and size of tumors. Some studies that compare tea drinkers to non-tea drinkers support the claim that drinking tea prevents cancer while other studies do not. Research on cancer patients is sparse. The recent National Cancer Institute study on prostate cancer patients showed no benefit from tea. Studies are continuing.

What is the wheatgrass diet?

Wheatgrass in its natural state, along with its roots and rhizomes, is said to have a therapeutic value. The diet was developed by Ann Wigmore, who emigrated to the United States from Lithuania. Her belief in the therapeutic value of wheatgrass came from her interpretation of the bible and observations that dogs and cats eat grass when they feel ill. The wheatgrass diet excludes all meat, dairy products, and cooked foods. Live foods—such as uncooked sprouts, raw vegetables, fruits, nuts, and seeds—are used exclusively. Though wheatgrass is considered safe, there is no scientific evidence to verify that wheatgrass or the wheatgrass diet can cure of prevent disease. Wheatgrass is available in tablets, capsules, liquid extracts, tinctures, and juices.

Web Pages to Check Out

www.cancer.gov: For general up-to-date information, and for clinical trials.

www.cancer.org: For general up-to-date information and community resources.

www.nccam.nih.gov: National Center for Complementary and Alternative Medicine.

www.quackwatch.com: Information about alternative treatments.

www3.cancer.gov/occam/bcs: information on best case reports.

www.inlm.nih/gov/nccam/camonpubmed.htm: National Library of Medicine research articles.

www.heall.com: Health Education Alliance for Life and Longevity. Resource center for body, mind and spirit treatments.

www.cancersource.com: Current information on complementary therapies including interactions with drugs.

www.mskcc.org: Information resource about herbs, botanicals, and other products.

www.hopkins-cam.org: Research studies being done at Johns Hopkins Center for Complementary and Alternative Medicine.

www.rosenthal.hs.columbia.edu: Information on research projects being conducted the Rosenthal Center for complementary and alternative medicine at Columbia. Includes directory of databases, such as CAM on PubMed (contains over 220,000 citations of journal articles related to CAM research) and other CAM databases throughout the world.

Also see Chapter 2, Searching for Answers on the Web, for more information.

Thirteen

BREAST CANCER

Finding a lump in your breast or being told you have a suspicious mammogram is a jolting, shocking, emotional experience. Today, with the new knowledge of how breast cancer behaves, there are many new options and alternatives available. What you need to do before making any decisions is to give yourself a "crash course" in what choices are available. Don't rush into making quick decisions. Most breast cancers take eight to ten years before they are large enough to be seen on a mammogram or felt in a breast exam.

DON'T PANIC. A confirmed diagnosis of breast cancer doesn't mean you will lose your breast. It is seldom a medical emergency that requires you to have treatment right this minute. Take the time to learn about the choices so you can pick what is right for you. What you need to do first of all is find out all the facts about your diagnosis and suggested treatment. What you choose is a personal decision, made in partnership with your medical team. But you need to be well-informed about your particular case and the pros and cons of the various treatments available to you before you do anything.

What You Need to Know About Breast Cancer

- **Most breast lumps turn out NOT to be cancerous. Eight out of ten lumps are found to be benign.**

- The majority of women with breast cancer now live long and productive lives. 63 percent of breast cancers are discovered at an early stage when the "cure" rate is over 90 percent.

- Having breast cancer does not mean you will lose your breast. More than half the women with breast cancer have lumpectomies. Those women who need a mastectomy can have their breast restored through reconstructive surgery.

- About 80 percent of breast cancers are diagnosed in women over age 50. Men do get breast cancer, but they are a small minority of cases.

- Any breast lump needs to be evaluated by a physician. New, less invasive, biopsy procedures (such as stereotactic core needle biopsy) permit removal and evaluation of the lump without any special preparation or recovery period.

- Sentinel node mapping, in which the surgeon finds and removes only the first lymph node—the one most likely to contain cancer cells—to determine whether or not the lymph nodes are affected. This lessens the possibility of serious side effects, such as lymphedema.

- Even if your general surgeon performed your breast biopsy, we recommend that, if possible, you arrange to have your treatment with someone whose main practice is breast cancer—an expert breast surgeon, a radiation oncologist, or medical oncologist.

- The two treatment options for early stage breast cancer are *lumpectomy* (can also be referred to as partial mastectomy or breast-conserving surgery) followed by radiation therapy or *modified radical mastectomy* (may also be referred to as total mastectomy). Research, now with 20 years of follow-up, shows that cure rates for both types of treatment are the same.

- Further treatment, such as radiation, chemotherapy, or hormonal therapy, is important in breast cancer. Designed to kill any cancer cells that may have spread, it increases your chances for long-term survival.

- There are treatments for all kinds of breast cancer.

- There are many new tests and treatments being studied for breast cancer, such as:

  Identifying genes that are linked to nonhereditary breast cancer.

A saliva test that measures levels of HER2, a protein that is sometimes higher in some cases of breast cancer

Using gene-expression signatures to determine prognosis

Ductal lavage, a method of getting cells from the milk duct to evaluate a person's risk for cancer

Ablation, which uses cold or heat inserted through tiny cuts to destroy the tumor

Aromatase inhibitors that hinder the development of estrogen

The use of hyperthermia (heat) to increase the uptake of chemotherapy to the breast

Giving higher doses of chemotherapy on a condensed schedule

The use of internal radiation targeted at the tumor.

UNDERSTANDING BREAST CANCER AND MAMMOGRAPHIES

Why is the breast susceptible to cancer?

Your breast is a very complicated organ. It is made up of glands (or lobules) that make milk, channels (ducts) that connect glands to the nipple, fibrous connective tissue, and fat. The breast is made up of 15 to 20 sections called lobes, each with many smaller lobules. Your muscles lie underneath the breast and cover your ribs. Each month, before and during menstruation, changes, such as swelling, tenderness, pain, and even lumps, may occur in your breasts.

Do most women have "lumpy" breasts?

Women's breasts come in all sizes and shapes. Most women's breasts are lumpy and uneven, especially in women under 35 years old. Sometimes, especially right before a menstrual period, they feel swollen and tender. Women's breasts also change because of age, pregnancy, menopause, birth control pills, or other hormones. By doing a breast self-exam every month, you will learn what is normal for your breasts and will be more likely to notice when something feels different.

If I have lumpy breasts, am I at a higher risk to get breast cancer?

At one time, doctors used to refer to women with lumpy breasts as having fibrocystic disease or benign breast disease or fibrocystic changes. They believed that these women were at a higher risk for developing breast cancer.

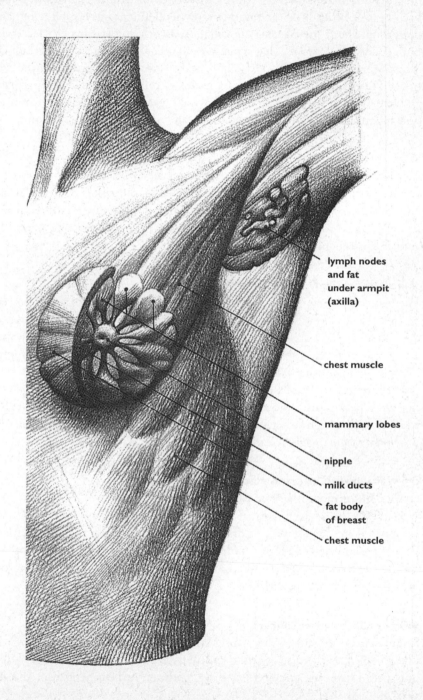

lymph nodes
and fat
under armpit
(axilla)

chest muscle

mammary lobes

nipple

milk ducts

fat body
of breast

chest muscle

Breast

Doctors now find that 70 percent of the women with such changes who have been biopsied have little increased risk of developing cancer. Of the remaining group, about five percent are diagnosed with atypical hyperplasia, with both excessive cell growth (hyperplasia) and cells that are not normal (atypia). These women have a moderately increased risk of getting breast cancer. The other 25 percent show signs only of excessive cell growth, called hyperplasia and have a slightly increased risk of having breast cancer. Women with intraductal papilloma and sclerosing adenosis are included in this last group.

What is my personal risk of getting breast cancer?

One woman in eight will develop breast cancer in her lifetime—this is the average lifetime risk assuming you live to age 85. Your risk is different at different times in your life. If you are between the ages of 30 and 40, your risk is one in 252. From age 30 to 40, its one in 68. If you are 50 to 60 years old, your risk is roughly one in 35.

Who is most likely to get breast cancer?

Women over the age of 50 are most likely to get breast cancer—80 percent of breast cancer is seen in women over 50. Women whose mother, sister, or daughter, has had breast cancer and women who have already had breast cancer in one breast are also at increased risk. White women, women with higher incomes, women who had their first period at an early age, and women who have children later in life, or who remain childless are more likely to get the disease. There is also evidence suggesting that women who are overweight, who eat a diet high in fat, who drink alcohol, or have taken estrogen plus progestin may have an increased risk of breast cancer.

Do women with inverted nipples have a greater chance of developing breast cancer?

No, not if this is your normal condition. Inverted nipples are subject to infection if not kept clean and dry, but there does not seem to be a relationship between inverted nipples and breast cancer. However, if your nipple is normally erect and retracts—or if you see dimpling or puckering in your breast—you should see the doctor to have it checked.

What causes breast cancer?

Scientists do not know what causes breast cancer and cannot explain why one person gets the disease while another does not. Breast cancer also does not spread from one person to another, and cannot be caught from another person.

WHO IS AT RISK FOR BREAST CANCER?

- Females.

- Over age 50, risk increases with age.

- Family history of breast cancer (mother, sister or daughter), especially if your relative's cancer developed before menopause or affected both breasts.

- Personal history of breast cancer.

- Period started at early age.

- Menopause started later than normal.

- Never had children or late age at first live birth.

- Changes in certain genes (BRCA1, BRCA2, and others).

- History of cancer of the endometrium, ovary or colon.

- Higher education and socioeconomic status.

- Post-menopausal obesity.

- Hormone replacement therapy—estrogen plus progestin.

- Use of DES during pregnancy.

- Alcohol consumption.

Can blows or injuries to the breast cause breast cancer?
No. Bumping, bruising, or touching the breast do not cause breast cancer. Such injuries often draw attention to a lump in the breast, which may then be diagnosed as cancer even though the lump is not a result of the injury.

Is breast cancer inherited?
A small proportion may be. If two or more relatives have breast cancer, if it occurs before age 50, especially with cancer of the ovary, or if it was in both breasts, you are more likely to develop the disease than women with no family history of the disease. If you are at higher risk, you should be checked regularly by a doctor who specializes in breast diseases.

What are BRCA1 and BRCA2?
These are the names of two genes located on chromosome 17 that are altered in certain families. (The names stand for BReast CAncer 1 and 2) When these genes are defective, they are passed onto relatives sometimes causing female breast and ovarian cancer, often at a young age. The likelihood of breast and ovarian cancers are highest in families with a history of multiple

cases of breast cancer, cases of both breast and ovarian cancer, one or more family members with two primary cancers at different sites or those with Ashkenazi (Eastern European) Jewish background.

How would having the BRCA1 or BRCA2 gene affect my changes of getting cancer?

You are three to17 times more likely to get breast cancer than someone in the general population if you have inherited an altered gene. You also risk getting the cancer at a younger age.

Where can I get genetic testing to tell me if I have the BRCA1 or BRCA2 gene?

You need to speak with a professional trained in genetics before you decide whether or not to be tested. Genetic testing requires blood samples from not just one, but several, family members. Most of the major cancer centers offer genetic testing and counseling services, which include doctors, nurses, psychologists, or social workers trained in genetics. To get more information on genetic testing or to get help in finding a health professional trained in genetics, contact the National Cancer Institute's Cancer Information Service at 1-800-4-CANCER.

What would a positive BRCA1 or BRCA2 test tell me?

It would tell you that you are at an increased risk for breast cancer. It will not tell you whether or not the cancer will actually develop or when it might develop. Not all women who have the inherited mutation will get cancer. On the other hand, a negative test will tell you that you probably have not inherited the mutation and that your chance of getting cancer is the same as the rest of the general population.

What can I do if my test is positive?

There are some things you might do, but at this time no one really understands how effective they might be. You can be closely watched and monitored, using mammography and clinical breast exam, so that the cancer can be found at an early stage. Some people have surgery to remove the healthy breasts in order to prevent cancer from developing. But because not all the tissue can be removed, you may still develop breast cancer. You can practice preventive habits, such as exercising regularly and not drinking alcohol (although there are no research studies yet completed of people with the BRCA1 and BRCA2 gene to show whether or not these are effective). Studies are ongoing to see if tamoxifen or raloxifene could be used as a chemoprevention agent.

What do the latest tamoxifen studies show?

One major trial that compared high risk women who took tamoxifen every day for five years with those who took a placebo pill found the risk of getting invasive breast cancer was reduced by 49 percent. These reductions in risk were seen among women with a family history of breast cancer and those without a family history. However, along with these benefits came some problems. The women over age 50 also had more endometrial cancers, strokes, and blood clots in their veins and lungs. There are some preliminary data from another trial that suggest that women with the BRCA2 gene are bene-fiting from tamoxifen to the same extent as those without this gene. Women with BRCA1 gene do not seem to be developing the ER-negative breast cancer for which they are at higher risk. However, these are early results, based on a small number of patients.

Can I have the altered gene repaired?

That may be possible some day in the future, but at the present time, there is no way to have the BRCA1 or BRCA2 gene repaired.

What is ductal lavage?

Most breast cancer starts in the cells that line the inside of the milk ducts. Researchers hope that by identifying changes in these cells during the begin-ning stages of breast cancer, they may be able to detect the disease earlier and develop new approaches to cancer prevention. Ductal lavage is a technique used to collect cells from the lining of the milk duct. A tiny catheter is put through the nipple into a milk duct. Cells are washed out and collected. A pathologist then examines the samples under a microscope for atypical cells or biomarkers to help determine the risk of breast cancer. Ductal lavage is presently in clinical trials. It is anticipated that the results of such tests would be used in conjunction with other risk factors, such as age and family history to make decisions about breast cancer prevention and screening.

What is the Li-Fraumeni syndrome?

This is a rare, inherited cancer syndrome found by scientists in 1990. It is due to an alteration of a gene called p53, that ordinarily controls normal cell growth. If this gene is damaged, cancer may occur. If you have this syndrome in your family, you inherit a predisposition for certain cancers, including breast cancer.

What is preventive mastectomy?

Preventive mastectomy—sometimes referred to by the doctor as a prophylactic mastectomy—is the removal of one or both breasts to reduce the risk of can-cer. Some women who have a very high risk for cancer choose this alternative.

This is a decision sometimes made by women who have had several biopsies or have a mother and sisters who have had breast cancer before menopause. Women, who have had cancer in one breast and have many lumps in the other breast or who have had several suspicious biopsies on one breast, sometimes opt to have this operation.

Are there reasons against having a preventive mastectomy?

There is some controversy about the advisability of this procedure, even for high risk women. You should be aware that in most women who have had this operation, no cancer has been found in the breasts that have been removed. In addition, some breast tissue is left behind when a mastectomy is done, so there is no guarantee that you will be free of cancer. Determining who is at high risk for the disease is also a very difficult issue, even when a woman has a BRCA1 or BRCA2 mutation. Most doctors will recommend that you perform monthly breast examinations and have checkups every three months instead of having this operation. If you are considering a preventive mastectomy, you should discuss the procedure, reconstructive surgery, possible complications, and follow-up care with your doctor and a plastic surgeon. You may want to get a second opinion and request a consultation with a genetic counseling service affiliated with a university medical school. Furthermore, you may wish to talk with someone who has had a preventive mastectomy. You need to study the pros and cons carefully before you decide.

Can breast feeding cause or prevent breast cancer?

For many years, it was thought that nursing helped to immunize women against breast cancer. Later studies seemed to indicate that women who nursed were more prone to cancer. The question continues to be asked, mainly because the individual studies have been too small to provide answers. The data have been pooled and reanalyzed and again it looks like the risk of breast cancer drops for every year a woman breastfeeds.

Do birth control pills cause breast cancer?

Several studies have been conducted on this subject, with conflicting results. Some studies show an increased risk of developing breast cancer among women under age 45 who used the birth control pills for long periods of time at a relatively young age, generally before age 25, or before their first full-term pregnancy. Others showed that women who have not had children, women who used certain high progesterone combinations of birth control pills, and women with a family history of breast cancer were at increased risk. It is not known whether the differences found in the studies are due to chance, to differences in the types of birth control pills, or to some undetected factor. However, at this time it is not possible to determine whether birth control pills cause an increase in breast cancer, or whether the risk is limited to certain subgroups of women or to certain types of birth control pills. If you fall into any of these groups, you should discuss the use of birth control pills with your doctor.

Are women who have had induced abortions or miscarriages at greater risk for developing breast cancer?

There is no evidence of a direct relationship between breast cancer and either induced or spontaneous abortion.

Does estrogen replacement therapy cause breast cancer?

The association between hormonal replacement therapy, either estrogen or a combination of estrogen and progestin, also is not clear. There is a controversy in the medical profession about whether the benefits of estrogen replacement, such as reduction in cardiovascular disease and osteoporosis, outweigh the risks (see Chapter 5, Cancer Controversies). But several studies are showing there are risks. Data released by the National Cancer Institute from the Women's Health Initiative in 2002 concluded that combined estrogen and progestin therapy increases the risk of invasive breast cancer. The part of the trial that looks at estrogen alone shows different results—five years of follow-up has found no indication of increased breast cancer in those women. However, a recent reanalysis of over 90 percent of breast cancer studies throughout the world showed an increased risk in breast cancer for women who used postmenopausal hormones for five years or longer—and most of these women were on estrogen alone. Women who have had breast cancer are usually advised not to take replacement therapy. You should discuss the question of hormone replacement therapy, along with how long you should use it, with your doctor.

Does diet play a role in breast cancer?

Research findings, especially of large population groups, indicate that diet may be a possible factor in breast cancer, but as of now, these epidemiologic studies have not yet been supported by stronger case control studies. However, in areas of the world where breast cancer is common, diets are high in fat and animal protein. Americans, for instance, consume three times as much fat and more animal protein than the Japanese, and have proportionately more breast cancer. When Japanese women move to the United States, their rate of breast cancer begins to rise and continues in each generation until the rate approaches that of American women. In addition, postmenopausal women who are overweight have an increased risk of developing breast cancer. The National Cancer Institute and the American Cancer Society both recommend cutting total fat intake to less than 30 percent of calories.

Research is underway to study whether reducing the amount of fat eaten by women at high risk for breast cancer will affect the number of breast cancer cases.

Does drinking alcohol cause breast cancer?

Several studies now suggest that women who drink alcohol even in moderate amounts (3–9 drinks per week) may have a slightly higher risk for breast cancer. The risk seems to go up with the amount of alcohol consumed, but the increase is mainly in women who had no other risk factors for the disease. Studies in France and Italy, where wine is consumed with meals by almost everybody, support this finding. Other studies found that the increased risk was only in women who begin drinking before the age of 30.

Do men ever get breast cancer?

Yes. However it is uncommon, with only 1,500 new cases diagnosed each year as compared to 204,000 new cases for women. The data on this rare cancer are limited, but it seems to have similar risk factors, as does female breast cancer. Most occur in middle age or older, with the most common kind being infiltrating ductal carcinoma. Male breast cancers are usually found in a more advanced stage than are female breast cancers. The majority of cases are estrogen receptor positive. Men also can develop Paget's disease and inflammatory carcinoma.

What are the symptoms of male breast cancer?

A painless lump, usually discovered by the man himself, is by far the most common first symptom. Nipple discharge, nipple retraction, and a lump under the arm are also symptoms commonly seen in male breast cancer. Diagnosis and staging are the same as for women.

Is breast cancer in men treated differently from that in women?

The treatments are similar to those used for women: surgery, radiation, and chemotherapy, depending on the stage of disease, because male breast cancer shares a similar natural history with female breast cancer. Modified radical mastectomy is the usual surgery, since saving the breast is not an issue in males. However, lumpectomy, with removal of some lymph nodes under the arm can be done if the patient is unable to undergo extensive surgery. Metastatic breast cancer involves hormonal treatment, with tamoxifen, or orchiectomy, adrenalectomy, or hypophysectomy.

SYMPTOMS OF BREAST CANCER

- A lump or thickening in the breast or under the arm.
- A change in the size or shape of the breast.
- Discharge from the nipple.
- A change in the color or feel of the skin of the breast or the skin around the nipple; this may be dimpling, puckering or scaliness of the skin.
- Other changes in skin color or texture, such as "orange peel" skin.
- Swelling, redness or feeling of heat in the breast.

What kind of doctor should I see if I have signs of breast cancer?
If you have a lump or notice any of the other symptoms, you should first see the doctor or nurse who normally takes care of you—your internist, family practitioner, gynecologist, or general or nurse practitioner. Your doctor will order whatever tests are necessary to determine whether or not your symptom is actually cancer or will refer you to a specialist for further testing.

Mammograms, breast exams, and breast self-examination

**What kinds of new advances have been made
with mammograms?**
There are many. Several techniques already in use, such as digital mammography, ultrasound, and MRI, are being tested in combination with other methods. A new use for digital mammography that converts breast x-rays into computer images makes it possible for radiologists to get a better look at suspicious areas and even to e-mail the x-rays to another radiologist for a second opinion. Other new approaches being tested include infrared imagining and time-lapse photography to detect the early vascular changes that can be a hallmark of cancer. A new, smart surgical probe, derived from space technology, is able to detect the differences between malignant and benign tissue without removing any tissue and can then display them on a computer screen. A system known as electrical impedance scanning (EIS) is based on low-level electrical signals transmitted through a probe that distinguishes the different electrical properties of normal and malignant breast tissues. A computer program, ImageChecker, used in conjunction with a regular mammogram, has helped to increase mammography accuracy rates.

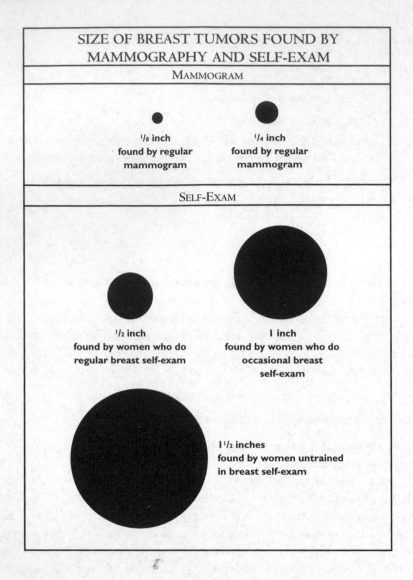

SIZE OF BREAST TUMORS FOUND BY MAMMOGRAPHY AND SELF-EXAM

MAMMOGRAM

$^1/_8$ inch
found by regular
mammogram

$^1/_4$ inch
found by regular
mammogram

SELF-EXAM

$^1/_2$ inch
found by women who do
regular breast self-exam

1 inch
found by women who do
occasional breast
self-exam

1$^1/_2$ inches
found by women untrained
in breast self-exam

How often should I be checking my breasts for cancer?

There is some controversy about the value of breast self-examination (BSE) with studies showing that BSE alone has so far not shown to reduce the number of deaths from breast cancer. There are some general guidelines. First, you should do breast self-examination every month, starting in your twenties. Second, you should have the basic screening exams—a breast exam by a doctor or a nurse, and a mammogram. Both are necessary. Third, if you have had breast cancer, or if your mother or sister has had breast cancer, you need to be under the care of a doctor who specializes in breast cancer, with your screening schedule tailored to your specific needs.

At what age should I start having a mammogram and a breast exam by a doctor or nurse?

Both the American Cancer Society and the National Cancer Institute recommend that, starting at age 40, you have a breast exam by a physician or nurse and a mammogram every one to two years. Women who are at a higher risk of breast cancer should talk to their doctors about whether they should begin screening earlier or have it done more often.

Where in the breast does most cancer develop?

Over half of all breast cancers develop in the upper outer portion of the breast, the part of the breast closest to the underarm. The second most common site is the area beneath the nipple. Breast cancer is more often found in the left than in the right breast.

Are there standards for mammography facilities?

As a result of the 1992 Mammography Quality Standards Act passed by Congress, all medical facilities that perform and interpret mammography tests must be certified by the Food and Drug Administration (FDA). Under these regulations mammography facilities must be certified by an accrediting body approved by the FDA and comply with the following:

- The personnel who perform mammography and physicians who interpret the mammograms must be certified or licensed and have adequate training and experience.

- All certified facilities must be inspected annually by federal inspectors or state inspectors working under contract to the FDA.

- Mammography units must be monitored closely to ensure proper radiation levels.

- Facilities must set up quality assurance programs to ensure that mammograms are as clear as possible and that positive results are followed up properly.

- Mammography and other patient records must be retained for five years.

How much radiation will I receive when I get my mammogram?

The Federal government has set standards that limit the amount of radiation used in mammograms—one-tenth of a rad per two views for one breast. The machines in most facilities deliver a lower dose than this. However, the amount needed depends on several factors. For instance, if your breasts are dense, they may require a higher dose to get a clear image. You need to be sure that you are in an institution that has good equipment, good technology, and expert technicians. These will assure quality mammograms with the lowest possible doses of radiation.

Does it hurt to have a mammogram done?

When you have a mammogram, your breast must be compressed between two flat plates in order to get a good picture. While most women feel uncomfortable while this is being done, it lasts only for a few seconds. It is a good idea to schedule your mammogram after your menstrual period, when your breasts are less likely to be as tender. Those few women for whom mammography is very painful should discuss the problem with the technologist and the radiologist before the mammogram is done.

What preparations are necessary before having my mammogram?

On the day of the examination, you may be asked not to use any deodorant, perfume, powders, ointment, or preparation of any sort in the underarm area or on your breasts. Also, it is more convenient to wear a blouse or sweater with a skirt or slacks, since you will be asked to undress to the waist for the examination.

What is digital mammography?

Digital mammography records x-ray images in computer code instead of placing them on film. Using computer software, the radiologist enhances subtle variations in the image, making tumors easier to spot. Digital mammograms also can be sent electronically (called telemammography), allowing consultation with experts. A study is presently being carried out involving 49,500 women in the United States and Canada comparing digital mammography with standard film mammography.

What is contour mammography?

Contour mammography is done with a special type of equipment that makes the exam more comfortable, photographs more breast tissue, and uses lower doses of radiation.

What does a mammogram show?

Mammograms are x-rays of the breast. You will usually have two taken of each of your breasts, one from above and one from a side angle. A mammogram can show a lump as early as two years before it can be felt. If it is cancer, it is usually at an early stage, has not spread, and is usually curable. It is important to have a doctor or a nurse examine your breasts each year, because some changes, including lumps that can be felt, **may not** show up on a mammogram.

Are mammograms difficult to interpret?
The radiologist looks for unusual shadows, clusters of white specks, distortions, special patterns of tissue density, any mass and its shape, and the differences between the images of the two breasts. The radiologist must have experience in interpreting these different areas, which can be difficult, depending on the size, shape, and density of your breasts. For instance, mammograms of younger women are more difficult to interpret because their tissue is more dense. As you grow older, your breasts become less dense. It is important that your mammogram be "read" by a radiologist who is an expert in this field.

Can two radiologists read the same mammogram differently?
There have been several recent studies looking at this issue that have found that trained radiologists can disagree on the diagnosis of more than 20 percent of the mammograms. That's why it is important to be certain that your mammogram has been read by someone who is an expert and why you may want to get a second opinion on a reading.

How many mammograms should a radiolgist read to be proficient?
There is a federal law that sets the guidelines and standards for mammography, including the number of mammograms to be read. By this law, physicians need to read 480 studies per year. However, experts say that doctors need to read at least 2,500 a year to keep their skills keen.

Will the radiologist compare my mammograms from year to year?
It is essential for the radiologist to be able to compare earlier mammograms with new ones, in order to evaluate the areas that look suspicious. If you change the place where you have your mammograms taken or you move, be sure to ask your radiologist for your films so they can be put on file. They are an important part of your health record and cannot be replaced.

Should I have a mammogram if I have had a breast implant?
If you have had a breast implant after you have had surgery for breast cancer, you should check with your doctor to find out whether you need to have a mammogram on that side. If you have had implants for other reasons, you should talk with the professionals at the facility to make sure that they are experienced in doing mammography in women with implants. There are special techniques that must be used, both in taking the x-rays and in reading them.

What special mammography techniques need to be used if I have had a silicone implant?

First of all, silicone implants are extremely dense on x-rays, so they can block the view of the tissues that are behind them. The breast needs to be positioned in certain ways in order to detect any abnormal areas. Secondly, the technician needs to take special care to avoid rupturing the implant when compressing the breasts. Lastly, reading these mammograms is more difficult. You must be sure that the radiologist has had experience in interpreting mammograms in implant patients. Unless it is done properly, the screening may be inadequate and cancers missed.

How much does a screening mammogram cost?

It depends on where you live and the facility you are using. Most mammograms used for screening cost between $100 and $150. Remember, that high cost does not always mean high quality. Many insurance companies cover all or part of the cost of screening mammograms. For women 65 and older, Medicare will cover one screening mammogram each year.

What to Do When You Have Symptoms of Breast Cancer?

What should I do if I find a lump in my breast?

First of all, examine your other breast to see if it feels the same. If it does, what you are feeling is probably a normal part of your breast. You should make sure, however, that you mention what you have found to your doctor. If the lump does not go away after your period, see your doctor. If you are past menopause and you find a new lump or a thickening in your breast, you should see your doctor. Most often, the problems are not breast cancer, but only a doctor can tell for sure.

Does breast pain mean I have breast cancer?

Almost all women experience breast pain at times. Often it occurs before the menstrual period. Some women report stinging, burning, or throbbing at the spot. This pain is called mastalgia or mastodynia. It may appear suddenly, last a few months and disappear. If the pain comes and goes with your menstrual cycle, it is probably not cancer. If pain starts suddenly, in one spot, especially after menopause, you should report it to your doctor.

Questions to Ask Your Doctor If You Have a Suspicious Lump in Your Breast

- **What does the lump feel like?**
- **What do you think it is?**

- **Will I need to get a mammogram? What will it show?**

- **Who gets the report of my mammogram? How long will it be before you let me know the results?**

- **What other tests should I have? How will these tests be done? Where will I go to get these tests? Will these tests have any side effects?**

- **How long will it take to get the results of each of these tests? What will they show?**

What is a cyst?

A cyst is a sac filled with fluid. It can be as tiny as a pinhead or as big as an egg. Sometimes a cyst appears and disappears practically overnight. Cysts are caused by a buildup of tissue related to the changes that normally take place in the breast during each menstrual cycle. They are usually found in both breasts. Cysts tend to get larger toward the end of the menstrual cycle and shrink or disappear after it. These changes may be exaggerated if the menstrual cycle becomes irregular, particularly if there is a long time between periods. You are more likely to develop cysts as you approach menopause. If you take estrogen after menopause you may also develop cysts. Cysts are rarely cancerous.

Can a doctor tell the difference between cancer and cysts by feeling them?

Sometimes. Cysts feel different from cancerous lumps. A large cyst near the surface of the breast feels smooth, slightly squishy and may be somewhat movable. Cancers are usually harder and more irregular in shape and tend to be more fixed. If the cyst is deep in the breast, it cannot be felt but may be found through a mammogram. One way to determine whether or not it is a cyst or cancer is to do needle aspiration.

Will ultrasound be used if I have a cyst?

Ultrasound is most useful in telling the difference between solid masses and cysts, especially in younger women whose breasts are very dense. It may also be used for pregnant women or a woman who has been recently nursing whose breasts are extremely dense. The doctor may order an ultrasound if your cyst does not disappear when the fluid is taken out (aspirated). Some cysts are very small or have thick walls or may have thick fluid that does not flow through the needle. Ultrasound does not, however, show microcalcifications or identify very small cancers, so it is not as good as mammography for general screening.

If the doctor finds a solid tumor on the ultrasound does it mean I have breast cancer?

No. Sometimes the doctor will find a benign tumor in the breast—that is one that does not have any cancer cells in it. These tumors, called fibroadenomas, are harmless growths. They are not usually found in women who have had menopause, unless they are taking estrogen. However, the only way to know whether the solid tumor has cancer cells in it is to have a biopsy.

Are there other kinds of breast lumps that are not cancer?

Yes, there are several other conditions that the doctor might mention, such as fat necrosis, sclerosing adenosis, intraductal papilloma, mastitis, and mammary duct ectasia. Some of these conditions, such as fat necrosis, sclerosing adenosis, and intraductal papilloma, will require a biopsy to make sure the lumps are not cancerous.

Are most breast lumps cancerous?

No, they are not. In fact, eight out of ten lumps are found to be benign. However, it also is important to know that lumps found in post-menopausal women are more likely to be cancerous than those found in women who are still menstruating. About 80 percent of breast cancers are diagnosed in women over the age of 50.

What if my mammogram does not show the lump I can feel in my breast?

If you have a lump that does not go away, it needs to be tested further and biopsied, even if it **does not** show on the mammogram. About 10 percent of mammograms do not show lumps even when they are there. These are called "false-negative" results.

Is discharge from the nipples of the breast a cause for alarm?

It is wise to tell your doctor about any discharge from the nipples. If the discharge is pink or bloody or comes on suddenly and is from only one breast, you need to have a doctor look at it immediately to determine its cause. Some young women may have a slight clear or yellowish nipple discharge at the time of menstruation. This is not unusual and should not cause alarm but should be mentioned to the doctor. Breast discharges may occur prior to menopause when other changes are taking place in the body and should be checked by the doctor to determine if you have a problem. Some of the fluid can be put on a slide and analyzed.

Are any new tests being used to detect and diagnose breast cancer?
There are some studies looking into the use of new technologies in this area but they are not a standard part of testing at the present time. Positron emission tomography (PET), magnetic resonance imaging (MRI) and laser scans, along with ultrasound and CT scans, all seem to have some potential when added to mammography for diagnosing breast cancer. PET, for instance, may be useful as a problem-solving tool to detect tumors in women whose screening mammograms do not reveal them. Early results from MRI studies are showing a benefit for MRI screening for high-risk women when used in conjunction with mammography. MRI may also play a role for women who have silicone implants. Laser beams along with a camera to record the image are also being used. Ultrasound can often show whether a lump is solid or filled with fluid. CT scans sometimes locate tumors that are hard to find. However, these tests are more expensive than mammography—PET, for instance, costs about $1,500 per test. They are not used routinely for diagnosis of breast cancer.

**Are thermography, transillumination, microwaves,
or lasers being used to diagnose breast cancer?**
Although research has been done with thermography, transillumination, microwaves, or lasers, none has been shown to be essential, either in screening or in diagnosing breast cancer.

What is meant by the term *calcifications*?
Calcifications are deposits of calcium that can be seen on a mammogram of the breast. There are two kinds—macrocalcifications, which are large deposits and are usually not related to cancer, and microcalcifications, which are specks of calcium that may be found in an area of rapidly dividing cells. When these specks form a certain pattern, it is called a cluster. A cluster signifies to a doctor that the tissues surrounding the calcium specks may be cancerous. If the pattern is not clear, the doctor may advise you to have another mammogram in three to six months. If the pattern of calcifications looks suspicious to the doctor, you will have a biopsy. About half of the cancers detected by mammography are seen as these clusters on the mammogram.

**What will the doctor do if there are any doubts
about my lump or suspicious cluster of cells?**
If the doctor has any doubts, further studies will be suggested. These may include more mammograms or one of several procedures to determine whether or not the lump is cancer. Remind yourself again that eight times out of ten the lump is not cancer.

A lump should not be ignored just because it cannot be seen on a mammogram. About 10 percent of mammograms do not show lumps even when they are there.

What is a diagnostic mammogram?

This mammogram is done when you have specific symptoms, such as a lump or a thickening, or when an irregularity is found on your screening mammogram. The technician will take different views, from different angles. The area in question may be magnified to allow the doctor to see the details more clearly so that an accurate diagnosis can be made.

Can the mammogram tell whether or not cancer is present?

Mammograms indicate to a trained doctor a suspicion that cancer may or may not be present. They can be used by surgeons to locate the site of the tumor and to check if there are additional tumors in the breast. However, they should not be used alone to definitely tell whether there is cancer in the breast. Only the pathologist, looking at cells under a microscope, can tell whether they are cancerous. In addition, even a negative mammogram **does not** guarantee that there is no cancer in the breast.

What kind of examination will the doctor do if I have symptoms?

The doctor will ask about your health and medical history and will do a physical examination. In addition, the doctor will carefully feel the lump and tissue around it (called *palpation*). If you have had a recent mammogram, it will be compared with ones done in the past. A new mammogram or additional views may be needed. Sometimes a doctor will order an ultrasound, also called a sonogram, which can show whether the lump is filled with fluid or is solid. Lumps that are filled with fluid are usually not cancer. Depending on the results of these tests, you may need to have a biopsy done.

What happens after either the doctor or I find a breast lump?

There are numbers of ways in which your case can proceed. This is an important decision point. You must prepare yourself to make a decision about how you want to proceed if, after the examination, the doctor suggests there is a possibility that the lump may be cancer. You need to decide, for example, whether you wish to have a second opinion on the kind of treatment you will have.

What kinds of treatments are used for breast cancer?

Generally, a number of different treatments can be used, alone or with one another: surgery, taking out the cancer in an operation—either removing

TESTS THAT MAY BE DONE TO DETERMINE IF YOU HAVE BREAST CANCER

- Complete history and physical exam.
- Careful inspection of breast and lymph node areas.
- Mammography.
- Ultrasound.
- Aspiration biopsy to remove fluid from cyst.
- Fine-needle aspiration for cytology.
- Needle biopsy.
- Stereotactic biopsy.
- Mammographic localization with biopsy.
- Excisional or incisional biopsy.
- Chest x-rays and blood tests.
- Estrogen and progesterone receptor tests.
- MRI or CT scan.

only the cancerous area or removing the entire breast; radiation therapy, using high-dose x-rays to kill cancer cells; chemotherapy, using drugs to kill cancer cells; and hormone therapy, using hormones to stop the cells from growing. Biological therapy uses your body's immune system to fight cancer. For those who are dealing with advanced breast cancer, bone marrow transplants and peripheral stem cell support are sometimes being used as treatments.

Are radiation seeds being used for breast cancer?

The FDA has recently approved the use of radiation seeds (referred to by the medical profession as brachytherapy or seed implants). It is being suggested for those with early-stage breast cancer. Usually it is given shortly after a lumpectomy or following completion of chemotherapy. Radiation seeds are injected into the breast in the area where the cancer was removed. Performed twice daily for five days, it replaces the six-week external radiation therapy that is popularly used as standard treatment.

Who are the best candidates for radiation seed treatment?

Women with early-stage breast cancer who meet these criteria are the best candidates:

WHAT HAPPENS NEXT IF YOU HAVE SIGNS OF BREAST CANCER

Problem is compared with a prior mammogram	Changes, if any, are noted. Additional tests may be done. It is important to make sure your mammograms are kept on file and sent to your new doctor when you change doctors.
Additional mammograms or tests done	The doctor may order another mammogram or different views. Ultrasound may be done to see if lump is solid or filled with fluid.
Stereotactic fine needle biopsy or needle core biopsy done	These types of biopsies are used to take fluid out of cyst or to take cells out of breast, after numbing breast. Usually used if the doctor suspects that a problem may be present. May be followed by excisional or incisional biopsy.
Excisional or incisional biopsy done	If the doctor is highly suspicious that a problem is present, an excisional or incisional biopsy may be done immediately rather than the stereotactic fine needle or core biopsy.
Second opinion consultation	Many women, unless their diagnosis was made in a center that has multidisciplinary opinions, decide they wish to get a second opinion at this time.

- The tumor is three centimeters in size or less.
- There are three or less positive lymph nodes.
- Margins around the tumor are negative or clear.
- It is within eight weeks of lumpectomy or within three weeks after finishing chemotherapy.

Questions to Ask About Your Type of Breast Cancer

- **What is the exact type of breast cancer I have?**
- **Is it a frequently seen or rare type?**
- **What stage is my cancer and what does that mean?**
- **Were estrogen and progesterone receptor tests done on my tumor? What were the results?**
- **Did you look at my pathology slides and what is your opinion? Has a pathologist who specializes in this type of cancer also reviewed the slides? If not, can that be arranged?**

MAJOR DECISIONS YOU'LL HAVE TO MAKE

- Should you have a lumpectomy (breast conserving surgery) or a mastectomy?

- Is it possible or advisable for you to have radiation or chemotherapy prior to surgery to reduce the lump?

- Are you a candidate for surgery near the nipple that barely leaves a scar?

- If you decide to have a mastectomy, do you wish to have reconstructive surgery immediately along with the mastectomy, wait until later after the mastectomy, or not have it at all?

- What kind of other treatment you will need following surgery?

- **Is there an indication that the cancer has spread outside the breast to the lymph nodes or other areas?**

- **How many lymph nodes were affected?**

- **Will I need to undergo other tests?**

- **What kind of treatment do you think I will need?**

- **Am I a good candidate for a lumpectomy?**

- **Am I a candidate for seed implant treatment?**

Is a second opinion important in breast cancer?

In our view, a second opinion is important in cancer because it is such a complex disease, and in breast cancer, there are many options and differences of opinion. Unless you are at a comprehensive breast center or a medical center where you are getting a multidisciplinary consultation, a second opinion would probably be useful for you to help you think through and sort out your choices.

What does a multidisciplinary consultation consist of?

You will be seen by a team of specialists, usually at the same time or at least during the same visit. The team will include a surgeon, radiation oncologist, and a medical oncologist. Sometimes a diagnostic radiologist, plastic surgeon, pathologist, oncology nurse, and a social worker also may be included. You should be told by the team what treatment would be best, in its opinion, for your kind of breast cancer. Some women use this team for a second opinion only, while others wish to use it for their entire treatment.

TYPES OF PROCEDURES TO DETERMINE IF A LUMP OR SUSPICIOUS CLUSTER IS CANCER

Fine needle aspiration (tissue aspiration)	Uses fine-gauge needle to take fluid out of cyst or to take cells out of lump. Usually done in doctor's office or outpatient area of hospital. No scar. May be followed by excisional or incisional biopsy.
Core needle biopsy (percutaneous)	Uses larger needle with special cutting edge to take a core of tissue out of breast. Uses local anesthesia. Not used for very small lumps. Usually done in doctor's office or outpatient area of hospital. Usually no scar.
Needle localization May also be called localization biopsy or mammographic localization with biopsy	Fine needle containing a wire put in breast so that tip rests in area of change seen on mammogram. Second mammogram confirms needle is in right place. Surgeon, in operating room takes out lump or cluster in area where wire is located. Fine needle portion done in radiology department, with surgery in operating room with local anesthesia. Scar depends upon amount of tissue taken out.
Stereotactic biopsy, or **Stereotactic localization biopsy,** or **Stereotactic needle-guided biopsy**	Patient may be sitting up or lying on table with hole in it to accommodate breast. Computer guides exact position for needle. Either fluid or cells are taken from lump. Local anesthesia may be needed. No scar.
Incisional	Since the advent of fine needle and core biopsy, rarely used for breast cancer. Takes out part of the lump to be examined by a pathologist. Uses local or general anesthesia. Usually done in outpatient department of hospital. Operation lasts less than one hour, followed by an hour or two in the recovery room. Small scar.
Excisional	Takes out the entire lump or the suspicious area. Used for lumps that are small. Uses local or general anesthesia. Usually done in the outpatient department of a hospital. Operation lasts less than one hour, followed by an hour or two in the recovery room. May change the shape of your breast, depending on size of lump, where located, and how much additional tissue is removed. Scar depends on type of surgery done.

Questions to Ask Your Doctor if You Are Going to Have a Biopsy

- **What type of biopsy will I have? Please explain exactly what you will be doing.**
- **How long will the biopsy take? Will I be awake? Will it hurt?**
- **Where will you do the biopsy? Will I be able to drive myself home after I have it done?**
- **How much tissue will be taken out?**
- **Will you do estrogen and progesterone receptor tests before the biopsy?**
- **Will the biopsy leave a scar? Will it change the shape of my breast?**
- **How soon will I know the results of the biopsy?**

How will the doctor determine whether or not the growth is breast cancer?
The only certain way to tell is for the doctor to do a biopsy—removing all or part of the lump and sending it to the laboratory to be analyzed. You may have one of several kinds of biopsies: needle, incisional, excisional, stereotactic, or needle localization.

What is fine needle aspiration?
The doctor uses a long, thin needle to draw out any fluid that may be present in the lump. Once the fluid is gone, the cyst collapses. If the lump is solid, the doctor may remove some cells with the needle and send them to the laboratory for further testing. Fine needle aspiration, also called aspiration or needle aspiration, is usually done in the office and is relatively painless.

What is a core needle biopsy?
A core needle biopsy is done much the same way as the needle aspiration but uses a bigger needle to remove a sample of tissue, called a core, from the lump. It differs from a needle biopsy in that it removes a piece of tissue rather than just cells.

What is needle localization?
This procedure is also called mammographic localization with biopsy. If the doctor sees a definite area of change on your mammogram that cannot be felt manually, a surgical biopsy may be necessary. The area that is to be removed must be pinpointed and marked by the radiologist before the surgeon can perform the biopsy.

How is needle localization done?

Using your mammogram as a guide, a needle is placed in the breast with its tip at the abnormal spot. The wire is placed through the needle. The needle is removed, leaving the wire in place. The top of the wire may be taped to your breast so that it won't move. At this point, you will be brought to wherever the surgery will be done.

The wire is about the size of a strand of hair, with a tiny hook at the tip holding it in place in the breast. During the biopsy, this wire guides the surgeon, who will cut along the wire and follow it inside your breast to the suspicious area that cannot be seen with the naked eye. The surgeon will remove the area along with the marker wire.

Is needle localization painful?

Not usually. Before placing the needle, the doctor numbs your skin with a painkiller. The skin of the breast is sensitive to pain but the tissue inside the breast is not. Many women say the insertion of the needle is painless. Others find it rather uncomfortable. You may feel some tugging if the needle needs to be moved into a different position.

What is a stereotactic biopsy?

The stereotactic biopsy, sometimes called a stereotactic needle-guided biopsy, is a newer procedure, used when something is seen on the mammogram that cannot be felt. It can be used to tell whether the cells are benign or malignant, without leaving a scar. The procedure is done in the radiology department. During the procedure, you may be sitting up, or you may be lying on an examining table that has an opening in the front end to accommodate the breast. You will be given local anesthesia to numb your breast. The radiologist will use imaging equipment to position the needle, and take both aspiration and core biopsy samples. If a surgical biopsy is needed, a small hook wire is inserted into the area where the samples are taken.

When is an excisional biopsy recommended?

There are several circumstances when a doctor may want to do an excisional biopsy, including: if the ultrasound shows the lump to be solid; if the results of the other procedures are not definitive enough to allow the doctor to make a diagnosis; or if the doctor, when looking at the mammogram, becomes highly suspicious that the problem is cancer.

Are there any new methods of detecting breast cancer without doing a biopsy?

There are some presently under study. Dynamic contrast-enhanced MRI, also called DCE-MRI, 3TP MRI, or three-time-point MRI, uses high resolution imaging, a contrast material (low molecular weight Gd-based extracellular contrast agent) and data from three strategically chosen time points (before contrast material given, two minutes, and six minutes after) to produce color maps of the tumor. 3TP MRI helps doctors pinpoint exactly where the cancer is. It also helps to differentiate between benign and malignant disease. It is anticipated that this new method will offer a standardized, reproducible technique for using MRI to diagnose breast and prostate cancer. This procedure is now in clinical trials.

Is contrast-enhanced MRI being used in any other way?

Contrast-enhanced MRI, in combination with molecular tumor markers, is also being studied in clinical trials to see whether it can predict tumor response and disease-free survival in women with breast cancer who are getting adjuvant chemotherapy.

What kind of doctor will perform a breast biopsy?

The biopsy is done by a surgeon. You need to be sure that the surgeon doing it is skilled in performing breast biopsies.

What should I expect as side effects from a biopsy?

It depends on what kind of biopsy is done. In general, however, you might have some mild pain that can be relieved by pain medicine, you may need to wear a soft bra for 24 hours for support, you might not be able to use your arm on the side of the biopsy for a few days, and the area where the biopsy was done will be tender for a while. You may also have some bruising and an indentation in your breast where the biopsy was done. However, within a month or two it should fill in, unless you have additional surgery at the same site.

Will I have to go to the hospital for the excisional biopsy?

It depends on your doctor and the kind of procedure being done. It is usually done on an outpatient basis, either in a surgical center or in a hospital. It is usually done with local anesthesia, and you will go home the same day.

Is the biopsy ever done as part of the operation for breast removal?

A few doctors and some women prefer to have the biopsy done as part of the mastectomy. If it is done in this manner, it is known as a one-step procedure. If the biopsy is done separately, it is known as a two-step procedure.

Is there an advantage to having a two-step procedure rather than a one-step procedure?

There are some differences between the two procedures. Approximately 80 percent of the women who have a suspicious lump biopsied will not have cancer. The two-step procedure allows you to have the biopsy, go home, and wait for the results. If it turns out to be cancer, you will have time for needed additional tests to be done. You will be able to have hormonal testing. If you wish, you will be able to get another opinion on what kind of treatment you should have. You will have time to make arrangements at work and at home for your recovery period and time to prepare yourself emotionally for your surgery. In addition, the doctor will be able to read both the frozen-section biopsy as well as the regular biopsy, which will assure you a more accurate reading.

Are there any women for whom the one-step procedure makes sense?

There was a time when all breast cancer surgery was done as a one-step procedure, allowing the doctor to do an immediate mastectomy if the frozen section showed cancer. Now, most breast cancer operations are done as two-step procedures. However, there are still a few women and doctors who favor the one-step procedure. If you have already decided on your choice of treatment if cancer is found, a one-step procedure may be the right choice for you. It means that you will have surgery only once. You will not have to wait between knowing you have cancer and having the final operation. On the other hand, you will not have the ability to get a second opinion or to have additional tests done.

What is the difference between a frozen section biopsy and a regular biopsy?

A frozen section refers to the procedure of preparing the tissue for the pathologist to read. There are two ways of preparing the tissue—via frozen section, which is a quick procedure taking 15 to 20 minutes, or via permanent section, which takes several days. The frozen section is a quick-reference method of determining whether or not cancer is present. The permanent section is a more accurate method. A full discussion of the two kinds of biopsies is in Chapter 6, How Cancers are Diagnosed.

If the doctor has found that I have breast cancer, what other tests need to be performed?

If the pathologist looking at your breast cells under the microscope determines they are cancerous, several other tests may be called for. There may be hormonal receptor tests, called estrogen and progesterone receptor tests, done in a special laboratory to show whether the cancer is sensitive to hormones. Since breast cancer can spread to the lungs, liver, or bones, the doctor usually orders x-rays of the lungs and blood tests and a bone scan. The additional testing is important to help the doctor recommend what kind of treatment should be done.

Why are estrogen and progesterone receptor tests important?
They can predict if the cancer is dependent on hormones for growth and whether or not you will respond to hormonal treatment. Estrogen or progesterone-positive cancers tend to grow relatively slowly and can be treated by modifying the hormonal environment in your body. If the tests are positive, the doctor may treat you with hormonal drugs, or, in rare cases, may remove one of your hormone-secreting organs (such as the ovaries, adrenal glands, or pituitary gland). Women who are estrogen-receptor-positive have a 50 to 60 percent chance of responding to hormonal therapy. If you are both estrogen and progesterone-receptor-positive, you have nearly an 80 percent chance of responding to this kind of treatment.

How is an estrogen receptor test done?
Preparations for the test must be done before the tumor is removed, because the cells must be tested immediately after being removed from the breast. The doctor sends a sample of the tumor (about 1 gram) to the laboratory to determine whether the cells are sensitive to estrogen. A score of two means the tumor is positive for estrogen. Five is the highest possible score. If chemotherapy is being planned to shrink the tumor before the operation, the test should be done before starting chemotherapy treatments, since chemotherapy may alter its accuracy.

What is a progesterone receptor test?
It is similar to the estrogen receptor test, but it measures the progesterone receptors. If progesterone is not detected, your report will show it as negative; if it is detected, it will show it as a positive.

**Do most women with breast cancer have
positive estrogen receptors?**
Yes. Studies show that about two-thirds of all breast cancers are estrogen-receptor-positive (ER+). In addition, about two-thirds of ER+ are also progesterone-receptor-positive (PR+). Generally women who are past menopause are more likely to be estrogen-receptor-positive, while premenopausal women are more likely to be estrogen-receptor negative (ER−).

Is there more than one type of breast cancer?
There are at least fifteen different varieties. However, more than 80 percent of breast cancers start in the lining of the ducts and are called ductal carcinoma. The next most common (about 12 percent) start in the lining of the lobules of the breast and are called lobular carcinoma. The remaining start in the surrounding tissue. Cancer *in situ* is early cancer that has not spread to neighboring tissues.

If I have lobular cancer *in situ*, am I at higher risk for getting cancer in the other breast?

If you have lobular cancer *in situ*, you are at higher risk for getting invasive cancer in both breasts.

What is meant by the term *infiltrating* or *invasive*?

Infiltrating—sometimes the word *invasive* is used—means that the cancer has grown outside of the duct or lobule where it started, into the surrounding tissue. You can have infiltrating (or invasive) ductal cancer or infiltrating (or invasive) lobular cancer.

What is inflammatory breast cancer?

This is an uncommon type of breast cancer that often spreads rapidly to other parts of the body. The breast is warm, red, and swollen. You may feel a lump in your breast, an enlargement or thickness, discharge from or a pulling back of your nipple or a pain in your breast or nipple. Ridges may appear on the skin, or it may have a pitted appearance known as *peau d'orange*. Generally, this type of breast cancer is treated with all three types of treatment—chemotherapy, surgery, and radiation therapy. Sometimes, the chemotherapy is given first, followed by mastectomy and radiation therapy. The order of the treatment varies.

What is Paget's disease?

Paget's disease is a form of breast cancer that involves the nipple. The tumor is in the ducts under the nipple. The tumor cells grow through the ducts onto the nipple's surface.

Are there any other types of breast cancer?

There are some other cell types of ductal cancer—comedo, medullary, mucinous (colloid), papillary, scirrhous, and tubular. In addition, phyllodes is a rare type of breast disease that is usually benign but in some cases has been found to be malignant.

What is meant by lymph node involvement?

The doctor checks to see whether or not the cancer that started in the breast has spread to the lymph nodes under the arm. The treatment used for breast cancer that has spread to the lymph nodes is different from treatment for localized breast cancer that has not yet begun to spread.

The Stages and Treatments for Breast Cancer

How will the doctor decide on what treatments will be used for my breast cancer?

There are many factors that your doctor will consider in helping you make a choice , such as the size and location of your tumor, cell type of your cancer, the stage of your disease, size of your breast, your age, and menopausal status, and your overall health. In addition, estrogen and progesterone receptor levels, tumor grade (nuclear and histologic), the doctor's experience, and your personal preference will have a role in making these decisions.

Why does the doctor want to find out the stage of my breast cancer?

The most important factor in making the decision about the right treatment for your cancer is to understand the stage of your disease. The stage is based on the size of the tumor and whether the cancer has spread to other organs.

What is meant by tumor grade?

Grading takes into account the structure of the cells and their growth patterns. Histologic grade refers to how much the tumor cells resemble normal cells (called differentiation). The lower the grade, the more the tumor cells resemble normal cells. Nuclear grade refers to the rate at which the cancer cells in the tumor are dividing to form more cells (called proliferation). Cancer cells that divide more often are faster growing and more aggressive than those that divide less often. The nuclear grade is determined by the percentage of cells that are dividing. Again, the lower the grade, the more normal. Differentiation is discussed in Chapter 4, What Is Cancer?

What does flow cytometry measure?

Flow cytometry, an instrument with a computer system, measures several features of cells. It can evaluate the amount of DNA, determining whether tumor cells have too many or too few pairs of chromosomes. If the cells have the expected amount, they are known as diploid tumors. If they have too much or too little DNA, they are known as aneuploid. In addition, flow cytometry can also measure the growth rate of the tumor—the percentage of cells that are dividing and producing new cancer cells, called the S-phase fraction. Diploid tumors and those with a low S-phase fraction are considered less aggressive. This information can be useful in deciding treatment, especially for women with breast cancer in whom no cancer was found in the lymph nodes.

Are there any other indicators that doctors use to tell whether a patient will do well with breast cancer treatment?

There are several other biomarkers. They include cathepsin-D, Ki-67, NM23, SPF (S-phase fraction), epidermal growth factor, heat shock protein, and the HER2-neu gene. These markers can tell doctors such things a how fast the cells are growing and how likely the cancer is to spread or recur. Some of these are already being used in routine testing, while others are being tested and refined.

What is breast cancer *in situ*?

The term *in situ* means early cancer that has not spread to neighboring tissue. With the increasing numbers of women being screened with mammography, cancers are being found at an early stage. There are two common types of breast cancer *in situ*: intraductal carcinoma *in situ* and lobular carcinoma *in situ*.

How is lobular carcinoma *in situ* treated?

Many doctors feel that rather than being a premalignant tumor, lobular carcinoma *in situ* is a marker for the invasive cancer at some later time—since about a quarter of the women who have it will develop invasive cancer of the breast within 25 years. There are differing opinions on how to treat this cancer. X-rays should be taken of both breasts to see whether there are any other abnormal areas in either breast. A second (or even third) opinion on the biopsy should be done to be certain that the diagnosis is indeed lobular cancer *in situ* and not an invasive cancer or a benign condition. The preferred option for lobular cancer *in situ* is no treatment, with careful followup by physical examination, pelvic exam and mammography (usually every six to 12 months). In some women with special circumstances, such as an extensive family history of breast cancer, a mastectomy of either one or both breasts may be advised. This is a decision that must be made with your physician and with all of the facts at hand. For those who choose careful follow-up as their treatment, there is evidence that tamoxifin, taken daily by mouth for five years can lower the risk of an invasive breast cancer developing.

How is ductal cancer *in situ* treated?

Treatment for ductal cancer *in situ* depends on how widespread the disease is. If it is found in only one-fourth of the breast (known as one quadrant) and is not found at the edges of the surgery, usually a lumpectomy plus radiation is done. If it cannot be completely removed by breast-conserving surgery, or if it is found in two or more quadrants of the breast, then a mastectomy may be the treatment. Studies have shown that women with ductal cancer *in situ*, who are treated with a lumpectomy plus radiation, appear to have the same long-term survival as those who undergo mastectomy. Women with ductal

STAGES OF BREAST CANCER

STAGE	DESCRIPTION
In situ	Very early cancer is found in only a few layers of cells. It has not spread to nearby tissues. Two types—ductal (DSIC), which may develop into an invasive type of breast cancer, or lobular (LCIS), which is not considered to be cancer but is an indicator of an increased risk for developing invasive breast cancer. LCIS can affect both breasts.
Stage I	Cancer is no bigger than about one inch across (two centimeters) and has not spread outside the breast.
Stage II A	Cancer is no bigger than about one inch across (two centimeters) but has spread to lymph nodes under arm (axillary lymph nodes); **or**
	Cancer is between one and two inches across (two to five centimeters) and has spread to lymph nodes under the arm; **or**
	Cancer is bigger than two inches across (five centimeters) but has not spread to lymph nodes under arm.
Stage IIB	Cancer is one to two inches across (two to five centimeters) and has spread to lymph nodes under the arm **or**
	Cancer is bigger than two inches across (five centimeters) but has not spread to lymph nodes under arm.
Stage IIIA	Cancer is smaller than two inches (five centimeters) and has spread to lymph nodes under the arm and the lymph nodes are attached to each other or to other structures; **or**
	Cancer is larger than two inches (five centimeters) and has spread to the lymph nodes under the arm and the lymph nodes may be attached to each other or other structures.
Stage IIIB	Cancer has spread to tissues near breast—skin or chest wall, including ribs and muscles in chest; **or**
	Cancer has spread to lymph nodes inside chest wall along breastbone.
Stage IV	Cancer has spread to other organs of body, most often the bones, lungs, liver or brain; **or**
	Cancer has spread to lymph nodes in neck, near collarbone

(continued)

STAGES OF BREAST CANCER (continued)

STAGE	DESCRIPTION
Inflammatory breast cancer	Rare breast cancer. Breast has red appearance and feels warm. Skin may show signs of ridges and wheals or may have pitted appearance called *peau d'orange* (like the skin of an orange.)
Recurrent	Means cancer has come back after it has been treated. May come back in breast, in muscles of chest (chest wall), or in another part of body.

cancer *in situ* do not need lymph node dissection. There is evidence that using taxomifen as an additional preventive treatment can lower the risk of invasive cancer from developing. Followup should include a medical history, physical and pelvic exam every six months for five years and yearly thereafter.

Is surgery always needed in treating breast cancer?
Most breast cancer is treated by surgery although other treatments may be given before or after the surgery. However, cell types, such as lobular cancer *in situ*, and Stage IIIB and Stage IV breast cancers are sometimes treated with chemotherapy or hormonal therapy alone.

Treatment Before Surgery

Is chemotherapy sometimes given before surgery so that a mastectomy can be avoided?
Chemotherapy before surgery (referred to as neoadjuvant treatment) is an option that can enable some women who would otherwise need a mastectomy to have a lumpectomy. Cancers that are too large for lumpectomy may shrink enough during this pretreatment chemotherapy to permit a lumpectomy that completely removes the main tumor and still preserves the size and shape of the breast. Before starting the chemotherapy treatments it is important to have blood and chemical tests, a chest x-ray, mammography of both breasts, breast ultrasound if needed, pathology review, estrogen/progesterone receptor tests, and a HER2/neu test. A bone scan is also recommended for those with Stage IIIA and for Stage II patients with symptoms of distant spread. These tests are considered optional for other women with Stage II cancers. A CT, MRI, or ultrasound of the abdomen is recommended for Stage IIIA patients but not for Stage II patients. After surgery, more chemotherapy may be prescribed.

HISTOLOGIC AND NUCLEAR GRADES OF BREAST CANCER

GRADE NUMBER	HISTOLOGIC	NUCLEAR
Grade I	Well-differentiated cellular features and growth patterns.	Cells have low proliferation capacity with well differentiated tumor nuclei.
Grade 2	Intermediate changes in cellular features and growth patterns.	Cells have intermediate proliferation capacity with intermediate changes in tumor nuclei.
Grade 3	Poorly differentiated cellular features and growth patterns.	Cells have high proliferation capacity with poorly differentiated tumor nuclei.
Grade 4	Undifferentiated.	No nuclear grade 4.

What is HER2/neu testing?

HER2/neu is the name of a gene that produces a type of receptor that helps cells grow. Breast cancer cells with too many of these gene receptors tend to be exceptionally fast-growing and tend to respond better to chemotherapy combinations that include doxorubicin. A drug called Herceptin (transtuzumab) acts against tumors with an abundance of HER2/neu receptors. Tests are performed on a portion of the breast biopsy specimen to determine if this receptor is present.

Understanding the Operations for Breast Cancer

One of the most difficult decisions you will make is determining the kind of operation you will have for your breast cancer. You will have several choices. Doctors may use different terms for the same operation, which makes it very confusing. We have described them, using the terms as they are most commonly referred to today. However, you need to be sure you ask your doctor to explain exactly what is going to be done, how much tissue will be removed, and what your breast will look like after the operation.

What choices do I have for surgery?

You may have one of several operations:

- **Lumpectomy** (sometimes called partial mastectomy, breast-sparing or -conserving surgery, or segmental mastectomy) removes the lump and leaves most of the breast intact. Sometimes chemotherapy is given before the surgery if the tumor is large and the person wants breast-conserving surgery.

- **Lymph node dissection** takes out the lymph nodes underneath your arm. Sentinel node biopsy involves the removal of only one or two lymph nodes.

- **Modified radical mastectomy**, also referred to as total mastectomy, removes the breast and lymph nodes.

- **Radical mastectomy**, sometimes called the Halsted radical mastectomy, is not performed today.

Questions to Ask Yourself Before Deciding on a Breast Operation

- **How important is it for me to save my breasts?**

- **Is the tumor of a size and in a position that makes it possible to save my breasts?**

- **Am I willing to have breast-conserving surgery followed by six weeks of radiation treatment?**

- **Do I want to get another opinion?**

- **If I have the breast removed, do I want to have immediate reconstruction?**

What is the difference in results between a mastectomy and a lumpectomy?

For years, mastectomy was the only surgery performed for breast cancer. During the past 20 years, research has shown that a lumpectomy is a safe and appropriate option for the vast majority of early-stage invasive breast cancers. The survival rate for women who choose lumpectomy with radiation is the same as the rate for those who have mastectomies. But, many women who are candidates for lumpectomy are not getting them, and a large number may be undergoing more extensive and disfiguring surgery than is necessary. Of women with Stage I disease, 90 percent are candidates but only about 70 percent of them get lumpectomies. Women with Stage II disease, 75 percent of whom are possible candidates, fewer than 40 percent are treated with this surgery.

Are there reasons why a mastectomy would be the first choice for some people?

There are many cases in which a mastectomy would be preferable. Mastectomy is usually the more appropriate treatment for women with Stage III and Stage IV breast cancer. If you are small-breasted and have a large tumor, a lumpectomy may be more disfiguring than mastectomy. Some women may choose to have a mastectomy, because getting to radiation

TREATMENTS FOR BREAST CANCER

STAGE	DESCRIPTION
In situ	*If you have ductal cancer (DCIS):* Breast-conserving surgery with or without radiation therapy or hormone therapy; **or** removal of breast with or without hormone therapy; **or** clinical trials. *If you have lobular carcinoma* in situ *(LCIS):* Biopsy to diagnose the LCIS, followed by observation which includes regular examinations and mammograms; **or** Tamoxifen to reduce risk of developing breast cancer; **or** surgery to remove both breasts. (Even though there is a higher risk of invasive cancer in both breasts with lobular cancer, most surgeons believe that this is a more aggressive treatment than is needed.)
Stage I, II and Stage IIIA	Breast-conserving surgery to remove only the cancer and some surrounding breast tissue, followed by radiation therapy. Some of the lymph nodes under the arm are removed; **or** Modified radical mastectomy (removal of the whole breast and lining over chest muscles and some lymph nodes under arm), with or without breast reconstruction; **or** clinical trial evaluating sentinel lymph node biopsy (removal of the first lymph node to which cancer is likely to spread) followed by surgery **or** other clinical trials.
Followup Treatment	Radiation to lymph nodes near breast and to chest wall after modified radical mastectomy; **or** systemic chemotherapy, with or without hormone therapy; **or** hormone therapy alone; **or** clinical trials.
Stage IIIB	Systemic chemotherapy; **or** Systemic chemotherapy followed by surgery (either breast-conserving or mastectomy) with lymph node removal followed by radiation. Additional chemotherapy, hormone therapy, or both may be given; **or** *Clinical trials:* new anticancer drugs, drug combinations, new ways of giving treatment.

(continued)

TREATMENTS FOR BREAST CANCER *(continued)*

STAGE	DESCRIPTION
Stage IV (metastatic cancer)	Hormonal therapy or chemotherapy with or without Herceptin (trastuzumab); **or**
	radiation and/or surgery for relief of symptoms or pain; **or**
	Clinical trials: New chemotherapy and hormonal drugs and new combinations of Herceptin with anticancer drugs; **or** high-dose chemotherapy with bone marrow transplants or peripheral stem cell transplants.
Inflammatory breast cancer	Systemic chemotherapy; **or** Systemic chemotherapy followed by surgery (either breast-conserving or mastectomy) with lymph node removal followed by radiation. Further treatment with chemotherapy or hormone therapy or both may be used; **or**
	Clinical trials: New anticancer drugs, drug combinations, new ways of giving treatment.
Recurrent	*If it has come back after treatment in breast or chest wall:*
	Surgery (modified radical mastectomy if had lumpectomy or local surgery if recurrence at chest wall or scar), radiation therapy or both; **or**
	systemic chemotherapy or hormone therapy; **or** Clinical trials

treatment facilities can be difficult for those who live in rural areas or they wish to avoid the inconvenience of repeated visits for radiation treatments. Many women also think they need to have this operation to "get it all out" of their bodies.

When is a lumpectomy NOT recommended?
Lumpectomy is not usually recommended for women who:

- Have two or more areas of cancer in the same breast that are too far apart to be removed in a single operation.
- Have a small breast and a large tumor, which means that removing the tumor would be extremely disfiguring.
- Have had radiation treatment in that area.
- Have had an excisional biopsy that did not completely remove the cancer.

Many women assume that if they have a mastectomy, it means that the doctor will get all of the cancer out of the body. However, scientists now believe that cancer cells may break away from the primary tumor and spread to other parts of the body even when the disease is at an early stage. Studies over the past 20 years show that survival rates are the same for either operation. If the doctor tells you that you can have an operation for breast cancer that can save your breast, you should understand that a mastectomy (taking out the breast) will not increase your chances of being cured or of living longer.

- Have a connective tissue disease that causes sensitivity to the side effects of radiation.
- Are pregnant and would require radiation during the pregnancy.

Will I be able to have an operation that saves my breast?

If the *microcalcifications* in your breast are not extensive, or if your tumor is less than four centimeters in diameter and can be totally taken out, you will probably be able to have a lumpectomy, if you wish. Most of the time, breast-conserving surgery is done for early (Stage I, Stage II and Stage IIIA) breast cancer. If you have more than one primary tumor in your breast, or if you have extensive microcalcifications on your mammogram, you probably will not be able to have this kind of operation. The doctor will also have to take into account several other factors, such as the size of your breast, the technique used to do the biopsy, the amount of breast tissue that will be taken out along with the tumor and whether or not you are willing to have radiation therapy after the surgery. If the tumor is too large for lumpectomy, chemotherapy may be given to shrink the tumor before the operation is performed.

What is involved in having a lumpectomy (breast-conserving surgery)?

The doctor will take out the entire tumor along with some of the normal tissue surrounding it, and, depending on the procedure, some of the lymph nodes under the arm. After two to four weeks of recovery, external radiation will be delivered to the entire breast. For some patients, a boost of radiation to the area where the tumor was found will also be needed.

Will my breast look different after I have breast-conserving surgery?

Yes, it will. How different it will look depends upon the size of your breasts and amount of tissue that has been taken out.

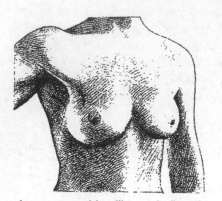

lumpectomy with axillary node dissection

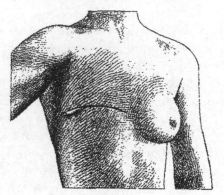

total mastectomy

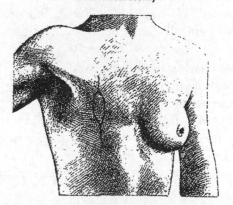

radical mastectomy with skin graft

Examples of breast operation scars

KINDS OF OPERATIONS

NAME	DESCRIPTION
Lumpectomy. Also called partial or breast-saving or -conserving surgery.	The lump in your breast is taken out, along with some of the normal breast tissue around it to get clear margins. Sentinel node biopsy or lymph node dissection, followed by radiation therapy to the part of the breast that remains. Survival rates are the same as with the modified radical mastectomy when cancer is treated in its early stages. *Advantages*: If you are large-breasted, most of your breast is preserved. You'll have a better appearance than with a modified radical mastectomy. There is little possibility of loss of muscle strength. *Disadvantages*: If you have small or medium-size breasts, you will have a noticeable change in your breast shape. You must undergo radiation treatments following the lumpectomy. If lymph nodes are not taken out, cancer may spread undetected.
Lymph node dissection. Also called axillary lymph node dissection.	Lymph nodes are taken out in the hollow of your armpit. Usually done at the same time as breast operation. *Advantages*: Doctor can check to see if there is cancer in nodes. *Disadvantages*: You have a slight risk of getting lymphedema. Sentinel node biopsy which removes only one or two lymph nodes may be used.
Modified radical mastectomy. May also be referred to as total mastectomy.	Entire breast, lining over chest muscles removed. Lymph nodes under arm taken out. Sentinel node biopsy which removes only one or two lymph nodes may be used. Survival rates are the same as with the lumpectomy plus radiation therapy when cancer is treated in its early stages. *Advantages*: Your chest muscles are not taken out. You can have breast reconstruction and you can plan it before your operation. *Disadvantages*: Your breast is removed.

What is a laser lumpectomy?

Laser lumpectomy, still considered experimental treatment, is being done in a number of hospitals. A special MRI technique, known as RODEO, is being used with a dye to make the tumor stand out. During the procedure the patient lies face down on a special x-ray table. The laser needle is inserted into the tumor. Laser light is used to vaporize the tumor.

Can I have breast-conserving surgery even if I'm older?

Your age should not be a factor in deciding whether to have a lumpectomy versus a mastectomy. Survival rate, and rates of being free from recurrence for women 65 years of age and older, have been similar to those for women 45 years of age.

Are there some cases where it makes sense to choose a modified radical mastectomy instead of a lumpectomy?

There are several reasons why you and your doctor might decide to have a modified radical mastectomy rather than breast-conserving surgery:

- If you have many microcalcifications in different parts of your breast, or if you have tumors in more than one area of your breast.

- If too great a proportion of your breast must be removed either because the tumor is large or your breast is very small.

- If you are in your first or second trimester of pregnancy, you would not be able to have breast conservation because you could not have the radiation therapy. (Women in their third trimester might be able to have the breast-conserving surgery, with the radiation treatments done after delivery.)

- If you have a schedule that would not allow you to have radiation therapy every day for five or six weeks; or if suitable medical facilities for radiation treatments are too far away or require extended travel time.

- If you have a prior history of high-dose radiation to the breast area.

- If the tumor is directly beneath the nipple and the surgery would require taking out all or part of the nipple areola complex.

Some women believe that in order to get rid of all the cancer the entire breast has to be removed. But remember, a mastectomy will not increase your chances of being cured if breast-conserving surgery is a viable option.

Questions to Ask Your Doctor If the Biopsy Shows There Is Cancer in Your Breast

- **How big is the tumor? Where is it in my breast?**

- **What kind of breast cancer do I have? Is it invasive?**

- **Have estrogen and progesterone receptor tests been done? What do they show?**

- **What other laboratory tests were done on the tumor tissue and what did they show?**

- **What other tests will need to be done before we decide on the treatment?**

- **What kind of operation do you recommend? Am I a candidate for a lumpectomy?**

- **Is there another type of surgery I should consider?**

- **What are the pros and cons for each one?**

- **Can the operation be timed to the later phase of my menstrual cycle?**

- **Will you take out some lymph nodes under my arm? How many? Why? What are the risks and side effects of doing this? Am I a candidate for sentinel node dissection?**

- **How many sentinel node dissections have you performed?**

- **Will you be using dye *and* radioactive tracer? Will it be injected under the skin or into the tumor region? How many nodes will you remove? Only the sentinel node or the cluster that turns blue or concentrates the most tracer?**

- **If I need radiation, how long will the treatment be and where will it be done?**

- **What will my breast look like after the operation? How much tissue will be taken out? Where will the scar be? How big will it be?**

- **Do you recommend that I have breast reconstruction? Now? Later?**

- **How will we decide on the operation? How long can I take to make this decision? How long will it take to schedule the surgery?**

- **Where can I go for another opinion?**

How long can I wait to have my operation for breast cancer?

Most doctors agree that you can delay two to four weeks without any problem. Studies have shown that a short delay between biopsy and treatment will not affect the spread of disease or reduce the chances for successful treatment. Many women want time to think and to get a second opinion on treatment, looking at all the alternatives. For these women, getting all of the necessary information about the extent of the cancer is well worth the time it takes. On the other hand, if you are the kind of person who wants to have it done and over with and feel comfortable with your choice, you should proceed with your treatment.

Is there any validity to the idea that timing my breast operation to my menstrual cycle makes a difference?

Although studies that have been done are not definitive, there is a new study underway (Menstrual Timing Protocol) that is trying to determine whether the stage of your menstrual cycle has any bearing on breast cancer prognosis. If you and your surgeon agree, you can schedule your surgery during the later phase of your menstrual cycle—after ovulation.

Are lasers ever used for a mastectomy?
Some doctors do use a laser instead of the traditional scalpel for a mastectomy, feeling that it reduces pain and the length of the hospital stay.

Will I have to have treatments after the operation?
There are many factors that your doctor will consider in making this decision. They are discussed later in the chapter under the heading Adjuvant Treatment.

Having the Operation

Will I need to bank my blood for my operation?
Most breast cancer operations (except for some of the flap operations done in reconstruction) do not need blood transfusions. However, it is a question you need to ask your doctor. If your doctor thinks you will need blood transfusions during your operation, it would be wise to make plans to bank your own blood.

Is lymph node surgery always performed as part of breast surgery?
Whether you have a lumpectomy or mastectomy, lymph node surgery is usually part of the procedure except for women who have ductal or lobular cancer *in situ*. It was once believed that removing as many lymph nodes as possible reduced the possibility of the cancer spreading. It is now known that lymph node surgery itself does not improve chances for a cure but that surgery can accurately determine if the cancer has spread to the lymph nodes. In a standard axillary lymph node dissection, ten to 20 lymph nodes in the armpit are removed for investigation. This requires a four-to-six-inch incision. During this "standard" axillary lymph node dissection, the surgeon removes an irregular pad of fatty tissue in the armpit that contains the lymph nodes. The lymph nodes themselves are embedded in this fat and cannot be clearly seen or felt individually. Until the pathologist analyzes the tissues, it is not usually known how many nodes were actually removed and how many were found to be cancerous.

Can lymph node surgery cause problems?
Lymph node surgery (axillary node dissection) can cause complications including numbness, a persistent burning sensation, infection, limited movement of the shoulder, and lymphedema (swelling in the arm caused by excess fluid buildup). Newer techniques have been developed, such as sentinel lymph node biopsy, to minimize the consequences of lymph node surgery.

What is a sentinel lymph node biopsy?
This is a relatively new procedure in which the surgeon finds and removes *only* the sentinel node—the first lymph node into which a tumor drains, and the one most likely to contain cancer cells. Studies continue to show that if no cancer cells are found in the sentinel node, there probably are no tumor cells in the remaining axillary nodes. Because sentinel lymph node biopsy involves removal of fewer lymph nodes than the standard lymph node dissection, the potential for side effects such as lymphedema is much lower. In addition, the sentinel node biopsy leaves only a half-inch scar. Sentinel node biopsy may be done on an outpatient basis or may require a one day stay in the hospital.

What is the procedure for doing sentinel lymph node biopsy?
A blue dye and a low-level radioactive tracer are injected near the breast tumor. After the dye and tracer have traveled from the tumor region to the lymph nodes (the wait may take from 45 minutes to eight hours), the biopsy is performed. A gamma ray counter locates the sentinel node or nodes. Once the area is pinpointed, the surgeon makes a small incision (usually one-half inch) and removes the suspected node. The node is then examined by the pathologist. If no cancer is found, further lymph node surgery is avoided. This surgery should be performed only by a team experienced in the procedure. **Be sure to ask beforehand how many sentinel node procedures your doctor has done.** (The answer should be at least 20.) Investigational trials are presently under way to determine if survival of patients with positive sentinel nodes who do not undergo node removal is different from survival for those who have a complete axillary node dissection.

What happens if cancer is found during sentinel lymph node surgery?
If the node is found to be cancerous during the surgery, the surgeon will usually remove additional lymph nodes. However, if the final pathology report is not available until after the surgery has been completed and cancer is found, followup surgery may be necessary to remove more nodes.

What should I expect my breast operation to be like?
It depends on what operation you are having, where you are having it and what your hospital's procedures are like. You may be asked to go to the hospital prior to your surgery in order to have the routine tests done, such as chest x-rays and blood work. On the day of the operation, you will probably be given some medicine to make you relax. Then you will be taken to the operating room, where electrocardiogram sensors will be attached to your arms and legs to check your heart rate during surgery. You will be put to sleep. After you are asleep, a tube will be placed in your throat to carry air to

your lungs. Your operation should take about two to four hours, depending on what is being done. You will be awakened in the recovery room.

Questions to Ask Your Doctor Before Your Breast Operation

- **What kind of operation will you do?**
- **How long will the operation take?**
- **How should I expect to feel after my operation?**
- **Will I need blood transfusions during the operation and should I bank my own blood before going to the hospital?**
- **What will the scar look like? Please show me where it will be.**
- **Will you be doing a sentinel lymph node biopsy? If not, how many lymph nodes will you be removing? How many of these sentinel node biopsies have you done? (Answer should be at least 20.)**
- **Can you insert the port for chemotherapy treatments at the time of the operation?**
- **Can the chemo port be placed so that it does not interfere with my bra strap?**
- **Will I be in pain? What will you do for my pain?**
- **How long will I be in the hospital?**
- **Will I need special care at home after surgery?**
- **When can I get back to my regular routine? Will I have to take any special precautions?**
- **What kind of exercises should I do?**
- **If I decide to have breast reconstruction, can it be done as part of this operation?**
- **If I decide not to have reconstruction, what other choices will I have?**
- **What kind of treatment will I need after surgery?**

How long will I be in the recovery room?

You will probably spend an hour or so in the recovery room. Don't be surprised if your mouth feels dry and you feel drowsy and a little nauseated—these are common side effects of the anesthesia. There will, in all likelihood, be tubes in the area of your operation to drain away fluid, an IV (intravenous) tube in your arm so you can get liquid nourishment, wires taped to your chest to measure your heartbeat, and bandages on the area of the operation.

Will I stay in the hospital?

It depends on the surgery and the hospital. Many are letting patients, including those who had mastectomies, go home the same day as the operation. If you stay in the hospital, what happens when you go back to your room depends on the type of surgery you have had and the practices in that hospital. Usually, the nurse will be in often to take your temperature, pulse, and blood pressure. The area where you have been operated on will also be checked. You will be asked to turn, cough and breathe deeply to keep your lungs clear and to move your legs and feet, to improve your blood circulation. By the next day, you will probably get up out of bed, with help, and walk around. You will soon start eating solid foods and be able to take a sponge bath. Usually you will go home with the drains that are taking fluid out of the underarm area still in place.

Will I feel any pain?

You will probably feel some pain in the area of the operation. You may also feel some numbness, tingling, or pain in your chest, shoulder area, upper arm, or armpit. If you are in pain, do not hesitate to ask for medication to relieve it. Many hospitals are using pain pumps that let patients control the amount of pain medication they need.

If I am not staying in the hospital, are there any precautions I need to take?

If you are not staying in the hospital, you need to make arrangements for someone to listen to the instructions that will be given to you about your care and to drive you home. Wear warm comfortable clothing, including a cotton undershirt and a soft bra. It would be useful to ask your doctor for a referral to the Visiting Nurses Association if you think you will need help.

How will I take care of the area where the operation was done?

You need to take special care of the armpit where lymph nodes were taken out. You will be taught how to clean the area and put on a new dressing, how to take care of the drains and how to measure and record the volume of drainage, if drains are not removed before you go home from the surgery. You will need to be gentle with the site of your operation. Gently pat it dry, rather than rubbing. It is important for you to protect the area of your operation from any friction or bumps until it is completely healed. Healing will take anywhere from five to seven weeks.

When will the stitches be taken out?

The stitches are usually taken out seven to ten days after the operation. After they are removed, use lanolin cream, aloe gel, or Vitamin E cream to keep the scar from drying and shrinking. Cornstarch can be used to lessen itching or friction from your clothes.

When can I take a bath or a shower?

You can usually take a sponge bath or a tub bath a few days after the operation as long as you make certain that the area of the drain and incision stay dry. You will not be able to shower until after the stitches and drains are taken out.

What problems might I have after the operation?

You may have swelling in your arm, infection around the area of your operation, weakness in your upper body, a tired feeling, or shoulder pain.

Why do I need to exercise after my operation?

You need to exercise for several reasons. Exercises can help you regain motion and strength in your shoulder and your arm. They can also help decrease the stiffness and the pain in your neck and your back. If you have had the lymph nodes taken out under your arm, there are certain kinds of exercises you will need to do to help prevent or reduce lymphedema—a swelling of your arm and hand due to buildup of fluid.

When can I begin to do exercises after my operation?

You can usually begin carefully planned exercises as early as 24 hours after surgery. You need to discuss with your nurse and your doctor what exercises you can do and when you can begin to do them. Here are a few simple ones that you may be able to do within a day after surgery. Be sure that you do these only to the point of pulling or pain. Do not push yourself.

- Breathing exercises. Practice deep breathing. Lying on your back, breathe in deeply, expanding your lower chest as much as possible. Then let the air out and relax. Concentrate on relaxing while letting the air out. Do this three or four times, breathing in deeply and relaxing.

- Hand stretches. Flex your fingers. Rotate your wrist in a circle. Touch your fingers to your shoulder and, holding them there, lift your bent arm straight out.

- Shoulder and head rotations. Raise your shoulders and rotate them to the front. Now rotate them to the back. Try going from back to front in a circular motion. Slowly rotate your head in a circular direction, then move it

from left to right, then move it from front to back. This helps to loosen
your neck, back, chest, and shoulder muscles.

- Use your elbow and hand as much as you can for normal activities.

When can I do more active exercising?

Usually you can begin doing more active exercises after the stitches and drains
have been taken out. Again, you need to talk with your nurse and doctor about
your exercises. A Reach to Recovery volunteer from the American Cancer
Society may also give you exercise information (call 1-800-ACS-2345 to
schedule a visit or phone call from one of their volunteers). Here are some
suggested exercises to try. Start gradually and work up to doing each exercise
five times a day, then increasing until you do a maximum of 20 times per day
per exercise. If you get tired, be sure to rest before continuing.

- Stand up straight, feet apart, with toes 6 to 12 inches from and facing the
  wall. Bend your elbows and place your palms against the wall at shoulder
  level. Work both hands up the wall parallel to each other until the incision
  pulls or pain occurs. Mark the spot so that you can check your progress.
  Work your hands down to shoulder level. Move your feel and body closer
  to the wall if it is more comfortable. Rest and repeat.

- Stand straight, feet apart. Place your hand on your hip of the side that was
  not operated on for balance. Bend the elbow of your arm on the operated
  side, placing the back of your hand on the small of your back. Gradually
  work your hand up your back until your fingers reach the opposite shoulder blade. Slowly lower your arm. Rest and repeat.

- Lying in bed, clasp your hands behind your head and push your elbows
  into the mattress.

Will I do different exercises depending on the operation?

If you have breast reconstruction immediately after your mastectomy, you
will need special exercises. Be sure to ask your doctor and nurse to give you
specific instructions tailored to your own situation.

Is there any special care I should take of my arm
where I had the lymph node dissection?

Yes. You should elevate that arm, resting it on a pillow or on the back of a
sofa (your elbow should be level with your heart) for 30 to 45 minutes every
two hours for the first two to three weeks and then two to three times a day for
an additional six weeks. For the first eight weeks, you should limit the use of
this arm to 30 minutes at any one task. When you are sleeping, your forearm

should be higher than your elbow and your elbow higher than or level with your heart. If you sleep on your side, be sure it is on the side opposite your operation.

How long will it take before I get the full motion and strength back to my arm and shoulder?

It could be two or three months, depending on the kind of treatment you have had. The stiffness and tightness felt in the tissues of the chest and armpit after surgery or radiation therapy will come and go for a while. It is important to concentrate on activities that involve your shoulder on the side of the surgery, doing the stretching exercises slowly and smoothly. Continue to work at exercising at least three times a day, gradually improving your motion, until the feeling of tightness is no longer a problem. Over time, the numbness under your arm will decrease, but total feeling may not return for a long time.

How will I know when I have my normal shoulder motion back?

You will know that you have normal shoulder motion when you can do the same things with your arm on the side of the operation as you can on the non-operated side.

Will all the pain, numbness, and tingling sensations ever disappear?

Yes, they most likely will. However, some women continue to have symptoms up to a year after the operation. Some say that when they touch under their armpit, they have pain radiating from under the arm to the waist. Some describe the sensations as heaviness or a feeling of "pins and needles" and skin sensitivity. Others say that the sensations change from time to time. Some women who have had a mastectomy feel pain in the breast that was removed. Doctors and nurses are not sure why this "phantom pain" occurs, but it does exist. It is not imaginary. As with other operations, the symptoms are affected by the weather. If you have unusual sensations, discuss them with your doctor.

Will I have trouble sleeping?

Some women do have trouble sleeping, for a time, on the side where the operation was done. Others say that they cannot wear their prosthesis (a form to replace the missing breast) to bed because the elastic in the bra is too tight. (You can get a "sleeping bra" which is much softer and more comfortable to wear.) Some women describe the feeling as like being in a case, saying it is difficult to sleep because it is hard to find a comfortable position. Others talk about the difficulty of lying flat on their backs because of the pulling sensation. Yet others experience very little difficulty with this problem.

Will I be able to shave under the arm where I have had the lymph node dissection?

You should probably refrain from shaving and from using deodorants for two to four weeks. You need to ask the doctor and nurse when you can start using strong deodorants, or depilatory creams, and when you can shave under the affected arm.

How long will it be before I can return to my regular activities?

You will probably find that two or three weeks after your operation you will be doing many of the things you have always done. After six weeks, you probably will be able to go back to all your normal activities. However, listen to your own body. When you get tired, be sure to rest. Be careful not to overdo. This is a time to be good to yourself.

Is swimming a good exercise for me?

Yes, swimming, aerobics, and dance exercises are all good for you, but should not be started until about six weeks after your operation. Many communities offer swimming, exercise, and dance classes specifically for breast cancer patients. You need to discuss with your doctor and nurse how soon after your surgery you will be able resume these activities. The use of the sentinel node biopsy has lessened the occurrence of lymphadema for breast cancer patients.

Will I be able to play tennis or golf?

Yes, but you should check with your doctor as to when you can take up these active sports again.

Will I have a swollen arm after my operation?

Removing the lymph nodes under the arm interrupts the flow of lymph fluid. In some women, the buildup of this fluid in the arm and hand causes them to swell. This swelling is referred to by the health professionals as lymphedema. The swelling might occur shortly after your operation or many years later. If it occurs shortly after your operation, it is more likely to come and go. If it happens many years later, it is more likely to be a permanent condition. If you have radiation to the area under your arm after your operation, had an infection, or are greatly overweight, you are more likely to get lymphedema. If you notice that your arm is beginning to swell, get in touch with your doctor or nurse as soon as possible.

What causes lymphedema?

Lymphedema can be caused by the removal of lymph nodes, by radiation to the lymph node areas after surgery, and by chemotherapy. The lymph channels are one of three channels in the body that move fluids. Two of the channels, veins and arteries, move blood. The lymph channels move clear fluids. Treatment, be it surgery, radiation, or chemotherapy in the lymph node area, interrupts or destroys the paths that are used to drain the fluid. What is not clear is why two women who have identical treatment have different side effects—with one getting lymphedema and the other one not getting it.

Does this swelling mean that cancer has come back?

Normally, this swelling does not mean that your cancer has come back. Rather, it is a side effect that some women experience after treatment for breast cancer.

Will exercise help my lymphedema?

It might. General physical activity is essential for improved circulation. It is good for you to move around and use your swollen limb. Swimming, walking, and biking are particularly good exercises. But exercise when it is cool since heat and humidity can aggravate lymphedema.

What can be done for the swelling?

Your doctor will probably check to see if you have an infection. If so, you will need to take medicine to control the infection. If not, there are several steps you can take.

- Consult with a physical therapist.
- Elevate your arm to help reduce the swelling.
- You may need to wear an elastic sleeve or use an elastic cuff to improve the circulation of the lymph fluid.
- You may need to use an air driven pump that pushes the fluid out of your arm, along with a compression garment that prevents the fluid from returning.

Although all of these may help control the swelling, they will not cure it. When you stop using them, the swelling usually will return.

Why can't the doctor put a needle in and drain the fluid out?

It is not possible to do this because the fluid is within the tissues. What you need to do is to move the fluid from the affected area, past the obstruction and back into the venous system to get rid of it.

Are there any new treatments for lymphedema?

A type of massage, called manual lymph drainage, which has been used in Europe for many years, is now also being used in the United States. A therapist, using her hands like a milking device, milks the fluid out of the affected limb. Sometimes the limb is then bandaged overnight until the next massage session. When the limb is close to normal, a made-to-measure elastic support garment is used. In the research stages are treatments such as microsurgery, to reconnect the damaged lymph channels; cold laser, to promote the production of new channels, freeing up the existing ones; and drug treatment.

What is the National Lymphedema Network?

The National Lymphedema Network provides information about lymphedema and locations of centers in the country for its treatment. See Chapter 28, Where to Get Help, for additional information.

Will I be more susceptible to infections after my operation?

It is more difficult for your body to fight infection after lymph nodes have been taken out. You will need to protect your arm and hand on the side of your operation from any kind of injury for the rest of your life. If you get an infection, you should call the doctor immediately. You should also be careful about any cuts, scratches, insect bites, or other injuries you get on your arm and hand on that side of your body.

What will I need to do take special care of my affected arm?

There are several lifelong precautions that will help pamper the arm if you had the lymph nodes taken out:

- Don't carry suitcases or a briefcase with that arm.
- Do not wear tight-fitting or elasticized cuffs, tight sleeves, or tight jewelry, such as rings, wristwatches, or bracelets, on that side.
- Whenever possible, avoid injections, vaccinations, and drawing of blood from the affected arm.
- Wear loose rubber gloves when washing dishes. Do not expose the hand or arm to excessive temperatures.
- Keep the affected side covered when you are out in the sun. Use sunscreen and avoid sunburn.
- Avoid insect bites and stings by using protective insect repellent.
- Pamper your arm by carrying your purse or packages on the other side. Don't push heavy furniture with the arm.

- Wash cuts promptly, treat them with antibacterial medication and cover them with sterile dressing. Change the dressing and check cuts often for redness, soreness, or other signs of infection.

- Avoid burns while cooking or smoking.

- Wear a thimble when sewing to avoid pinpricks.

- Wear gloves or mitts when gardening and working with sharp objects or hot objects. Use a mitt when taking hot dishes out of the oven.

- Use an electric razor to avoid cutting this area. Underarm shaving may be a problem for a while because of the lack of mobility or numbness, so take great care.

- Never pick or cut cuticles or hangnails. Use cream cuticle remover for nail care. Apply lanolin hand cream to hand and arm several times a day.

- Though you should be cautious, it is also important to use your arm normally. Don't favor it or keep it dependent.

- If you do notice pain, swelling, or redness on your scar or arm, with or without fever being present, call your doctor.

Why do I have pain in my neck and back?

When your breast is removed, your weight may shift and be out of balance, particularly if you have large breasts. This can cause you to have some pain in your neck and back.

Why do I feel numbness and tingling in my arm?

Sometimes during the operation, some nerves may be injured or cut. You may feel some numbness and tingling in your arms, shoulder, underarm, and chest, especially in the first few weeks after your surgery. Most likely, the numbness and tingling will go away over time, but the total feeling may not return for a long time and some numbness may be permanent.

Having Radiation Treatment After Breast-conserving Surgery

Is it possible to have breast-conserving surgery without having radiation therapy?

It is not recommended, since studies have shown that women who have only the breast-conserving surgery are more likely to have a local recurrence in the breast.

Questions to Ask About Radiation with Breast-Conserving Surgery

- **When will the treatments begin? How long will each treatment take? How soon will the treatment begin? When will the treatments end?**

- **Who will be responsible for my radiation treatment? Who will be giving them? Where will they be done?**

- **What kind of short-term and long-term side effects will I have? What are the risks to this treatment?**

- **How many treatments will I have?**

- **Will I have to spend any time in the hospital as part of these treatments? How long?**

- **Can I continue my normal lifestyle during treatments? Is there anything special I can do to take care of myself during these treatments? Should someone come with me to the treatments?**

- **Will my breast change in appearance after treatment? How?**

- **Will the costs of the treatment be covered by my health insurance?**

- **How often will I have to have checkups and tests after my treatment is finished?**

If I have breast-conserving surgery, what kind of radiation treatment is used?

High-energy x-rays are aimed at your breast and sometimes at nearby areas that still contain some lymph nodes, such as under the arm (if only a sample of lymph nodes was taken during surgery), above the collarbone, and along the breastbone. The goal is to destroy any cancer cells that may still remain in the breast and surrounding areas. The high-energy x-rays are delivered by a linear accelerator or cobalt machine. You may get treatment in four areas: different sides of your breast, around your collarbone, in the center of your chest, and under your arm.

Is internal radiation ever used in treating breast cancer?

Internal radiation, sometimes called brachytherapy, can be used. The FDA has approved a device, a hollow catheter to which an inflatable balloon is attached. It is implanted into the breast where the lumpectomy was done. The balloon is inflated. A radioactive source is put into the catether. The balloon centers the radiation source within a wound. After a series of treatments, usually over several days, the catheter is removed. This treatment is for early-stage breast cancer and its effectiveness and safety has not yet been proven.

What is high dose rate brachytherapy?

High dose rate brachytherapy may be used after a lumpectomy, instead of external radiation, to deliver a precise target dose of radiation to tissues in the breast. Rows of thin hollow tubes, called treatment catheters, are placed in the breast when the lumpectomy is done or after the incision has healed. The ends of the tubes, which will later hold the radioactive source, come out through the skin. When treatment is to begin, the ends of the tubes are attached to the treatment unit, called an afterloader. The breasts are usually treated twice a day for five days, after which the tubes are taken out.

How is external radiation treatment done?

After you have had your operation and you have recovered from it—usually two to four weeks after the operation—you will start on radiation treatment. You will lie on your back, usually with your hand under your head, under a machine that will beam the x-rays.

How often will I go for my radiation treatments?

You will usually go for five days each week, for about five weeks. Each treatment takes about 20 to 25 minutes. Only a few minutes of this time are for the treatment; most of the time is spent putting you in the proper position. Many people continue with work or go about their regular activities during the treatment period. There are more details about radiation treatment and its side effects in Chapter 9, Radiation Treatment.

How is the boost done?

One to two weeks after the radiation treatment has been completed, most women receive a concentrated booster dose of radiation to the area where the breast lump was located. The boost is usually done with external radiation. If you have the external radiation boost, it is usually given for five consecutive days using a linear accelerator machine.

Will my breast feel firmer after radiation treatment?

Your breast, after being treated with radiation, may be different. It may feel firmer. It may be larger because of the buildup of fluid. Or it may be smaller because of tissue changes. Some women say that the skin of their treated breast is more sensitive after treatment, while other women say it is less sensitive. You may find you have itchy, red, or dry skin. If your skin blisters, be sure to report it to the doctor and nurse. If you have the boost with external beam radiation, you may notice an increase in skin redness at the site of the treatment.

Are there any other side effects from the radiation treatments?
Other side effects depend upon where the radiation is given and how much is used. Many women find their breasts are sore or tender. They report feeling tired. There are more details about radiation therapy and its side effects in Chapter 9, Radiation Treatment.

Adjuvant (Additional) Treatment

What is meant by adjuvant treatment?
An adjuvant treatment is one that is being used in addition to a primary form of treatment.

Why is adjuvant treatment important in breast cancer?
Adjuvant treatment is an important part of the treatment for breast cancer based on studies that have changed the thinking on how breast cancer spreads. Scientists once thought that breast cancer first spread to nearby tissue and underarm lymph nodes before extending to other parts of the body. Therefore, doctors believed that the spread of breast cancer could be controlled with extensive surgery to remove the breast, chest muscles, and underarm lymph nodes. However, researchers now believe that cancer cells may break away from the primary tumor in the breast and begin to metastasize even when the disease is in an early stage. Adjuvant treatment is designed to kill any cancer cells that have spread. Studies have shown that adjuvant treatment, given in addition to the primary treatment in breast cancer, increases chances for long-term survival.

What kind of adjuvant treatment is used for breast cancer?
Usually chemotherapy or hormones are used because they can affect cancer cells throughout the body (called systemic treatment). In some cases, such as before or after a mastectomy, radiation therapy might be used as an adjuvant treatment to kill breast cancer cells that have spread to nearby parts of the body, such as the chest wall.

What factors determine the kind of adjuvant treatment I am given?
The kind of adjuvant treatment you will be given depends on the stage of your disease, your general health, and other prognostic factors. These factors include whether or not you have lymph node involvement, the size and grade of your tumor, whether you have undergone menopause, and whether your tumor is positive or negative for estrogen or progesterone receptors. In addition, the doctor may look at the rate at which the cells in your tumor are dividing, sometimes referred to as nuclear grading. In some medical centers, testing for oncogenes will also be done.

**Do these factors affect my chance of recovery
from my breast cancer?**

These factors are used by the doctor to plan your treatment. Some of them also
tell your doctor how well you might do on different kinds of treatment. For
instance, if your breast cancer has not spread to the lymph nodes under the arm
(called node-negative), you are less likely to have a recurrence of breast cancer
than those women who do have cancer in their lymph nodes. If you have a smaller
tumor, you have a better chance of recovery than those who have a large tumor. If
your breast cancer is hormone-receptor-positive your tumor tends to grow less
aggressively and you are more likely to respond to hormone therapy. A low histologic or nuclear grade (Grade 1) is more favorable than a higher one (Grade 3).

**When will my adjuvant treatment begin and
how long will it last?**

Your adjuvant treatment usually begins between four and six weeks after surgery. If you are having chemotherapy treatment, it usually lasts for four to six
months, with a cycle of treatment followed by a recovery period, then
another cycle of treatment and so on. You will get the drugs either by mouth
or by injection into your blood vessel, usually in a doctor's office or in the
outpatient area of a hospital. If you are having hormonal treatment, you will
take a drug, usually tamoxifen, in pill form each day for up to five years. The
ideal drug and length of treatment is still under study.

*Questions to Ask Your Medical Oncologist Before Starting
Chemotherapy or Hormone Treatment*

- **Why do I need this treatment?**
- **Are there any other treatments for my stage of disease?**
- **Why have you chosen the one you are recommending?**
- **What are the benefits and risks of each of the treatments?**
- **Will you be inserting a port for my chemotherapy treatments? What
  are the pros and cons in my case of having this done? Can it be done
  at the time I have my surgery?**
- **Do I need hormone treatment?**
- **What regimen of drugs will I be taking?**
- **Are there any other regimens you considered?**
- **What side effects will I have?**
- **How long would I have to stay on them?**
- **How will it affect my normal lifestyle?**
- **Are there any clinical trials I should consider for my stage of disease?**

**What kind of adjuvant treatment will I have if
I am node-positive?**

 If you are node-positive, ER-positive, or PR-positive and are premenopausal, you may have chemotherapy plus hormonal treatment or
chemotherapy plus ovarian ablation; or chemotherapy plus hormonal
treatment plus ovarian ablation or GnRH analogue.

▪ If you are node-positive, premenopausál, ER-negative, or PR-negative, you
will probably have chemotherapy.

▪ If you are node-positive, ER-positive, or PR-positive and are postmenopausal, you will probably get hormonal treatment with or without
chemotherapy.

▪ If you are node-positive, ER-negative, or PR-negative, you will probably
get chemotherapy.

▪ If you are node-positive and over 70 years old, you will probably get
hormonal treatment, with chemotherapy considered if receptors are
negative.

Will I have adjuvant treatment if I am node-negative?
This is a very complex issue, and it has been studied by an international
panel. The panel has proposed categorizing women with node-negative breast
cancer in three groups: low risk (tumor less than one centimeter, tumor grade
1, positive ER/PR,); intermediate risk (tumor one to two centimeters, grade
1–2, ER or PR positive, and high risk (tumor more than two centimeters,
tumor grade 2–3, ER or PR negative).

**What are the guidelines for making treatment choices for
node-negative women in these three groups?**

▪ If you in the low risk group, you may receive no further treatment or will
receive just hormonal therapy.

▪ If you are in the intermediate group, you may receive hormonal treatment
with or without chemotherapy.

▪ If you are in the high risk group, you may receive chemotherapy with
or without hormonal treatment or chemotherapy with or without
ablation.

What is ovarian ablation?
Ovarian ablation means making the ovaries stop working, either by having
them out or by taking drugs that will cause them to cease functioning.

What are the side effects of having my ovaries taken out as a hormonal treatment for breast cancer?

If you have your ovaries removed as a hormonal treatment for breast cancer, you will no longer be able to have children. This is referred to as surgical menopause and, if you are premenopausal, the side effects will probably be more sudden and intense than those of people who have natural menopause. You may have hot flashes, dryness, or irritation of your vagina among other possible symptoms.

What is hormonal treatment?

Hormonal treatment is used to keep the cancer cells from getting the hormones they need to grow. You may need to take drugs to change the way hormones work. Another type of hormonal treatment is the removal of organs that make hormones, such as ovaries.

What hormone drug is usually used?

Tamoxifen is the drug most commonly used for hormone treatment, although the use of other drugs is under study. Taken in pill form, tamoxifen (its trade name is Nolvadex) blocks your body's use of estrogen, but does not stop your own estrogen production. It has been used for almost 20 years to treat patients with advanced breast cancer. More recently, it has been used as an adjuvant therapy following primary treatment for early stage breast cancer to reduce the risk of recurrence of the original cancer and also the risk of developing new cancers in the other breast.

Has tamoxifen been studied in clinical trials?

The National Cancer Institute funded a large research study, the Breast Cancer Prevention Trial (BCPT), to determine the usefulness of tamoxifen in preventing breast cancer in women who have an increased risk of developing the disease. This study found a 49 percent reduction in invasive breast cancer among women who took tamoxifen. Women who took tamoxifen also had 50 percent fewer diagnoses of noninvasive breast tumors such as ductal or lobular carcinoma *in situ*.

Are other hormonal drugs being studied?

The National Cancer Institute is presently conducting a clinical trial called STAR, comparing tamoxifen and raloxifene (an osteoporosis drug) to see whether raloxifene is more or less effective than tamoxifen in reducing the chance of developing breast cancer in women who are at an increased risk. The study is looking at whether raloxifene reduces breast cancer risk similar to tamoxifen and whether raloxifene has benefits over tamoxifen, such as fewer side effects. In addition, several drugs that are aromatase inhibitors (such as arnastrozole) are being tested. At present, tamoxifen is still the drug of choice for prevention of breast cancer recurrence.

When are the aromatase inhibitors used?
These drugs, which hinder the development of estrogen, are often used in women who need hormonal therapy if tamoxifen cannot be used. However, aromatase inhibitors are only useful for women who are postmenopausal.

What do aromatase inhibitors do?
Aromatase inhibitors block an enzyme found in many breast cancers. Called aromatase, it is the final enzyme involved in the conversion of adrenal androgens to estrogens, Anastrazole (Armidex), letrozole, and exemestane are the hormones most often used. The hormone targets only the aromatase and is being studied for use in women with ER-positive breast cancer. Aminoglutethimide therapy, which was once the major aromatase inhibitor used, is used today only for women without ovarian function.

Are there other beneficial effects of tamoxifen?
Yes. While tamoxifen acts against the effects of estrogen in breast tissue, it acts like estrogen in other body systems. If you take tamoxifen, you may share many of the beneficial effects of menopausal estrogen replacement therapy, such as a lowering of blood cholesterol and a slowing of bone loss.

What are the side effects of tamoxifen?
The side effects are not usually severe and not all women experience them. They are similar to some of the symptoms of menopause. You may have hot flashes and discharge from or irritation of your vagina. Some women have headaches, fatigue, nausea, vomiting, or skin rash. Your periods may become irregular, but they usually will not stop completely. You will not go into menopause or become infertile. If you are premenopausal, you may become more fertile, so you should use some type of birth control while taking tamoxifen. (You should not take oral contraceptives because they may change the effects of tamoxifen.) If you do become pregnant, you should not take tamoxifen during pregnancy or while breast feeding.

If I take tamoxifen, will I begin my menopause?
No. Tamoxifen does not cause a women to begin menopause, although it can cause some symptoms that occur during menopause. Your ovaries should continue to act normally and produce female hormones in the same or slightly increased amount.

**Are there any side effects of taking
tamoxifen over a long period of time?**

Tamoxifen is being recommended for a five year period. When tamoxifen first became available, a few women who had taken very high doses of tamoxifen reported vision and other eye problems. A few developed blood clots, particularly if they were also having chemotherapy while taking the tamoxifen. In one trial, depression was reported by about one percent of postmenopausal women using tamoxifen as adjuvant therapy. It has been found that postmenopausal women taking tamoxifen have a slightly increased risk of developing endometrial cancer or uterine sarcoma (an increase similar to that associated with women taking single-agent estrogen replacement therapy). Therefore, it is recommended that women taking tamoxifen should have an annual pelvic exam and should promptly report any abnormal uterine bleeding. If you have had a hysterectomy and are taking tamoxifen, you are not at increased risk for endometrial cancer or uterine sarcoma.

**What chemotherapy drugs are used as
adjuvant breast cancer treatment?**

Adjuvant chemotherapy involves a combination of anticancer drugs, which usually include some of the following: cyclophosphamide, methotrexate, fluoruracil, Adriamycin, paclitaxel with the hormonal drug tamoxifen added.

What is dose-dense chemotherapy?

The words "dose-dense" are used to describe chemotherapy that is given on a condensed schedule. New drugs, now available to control some of the more serious complications, allow doctors to give chemotherapy at reduced intervals. A clinical trial has shown that by using the granulocyte-colony stimulating factor, filgrastim, to stimulate the formation of white blood cells, breast cancer patients can be given the chemotherapy drugs every two weeks rather than every three weeks. The trial tested the dose-dense and the conventional chemotherapy on nearly 2,000 women with node-positive primary breast cancer. After four years, it was found that there was a 26 percent overall reduction in the risk of cancer recurrence in the women who had the dose-density chemotherapy.

Is Herceptin being used to treat breast cancer?

Herceptin (trastuzumab) is a drug that attacks the HER2 neu protein, which is found at high levels in about 30 percent of tumors of women with breast cancer. The drug is not toxic. It does not produce hair loss, vomiting, and the other severe side effects seen with other chemotherapy drugs. This drug is being tested and the results are very promising. Trials show that women with advanced cancer live 25 percent longer when the drug is added to standard chemotherapy. Further testing is being done to determine if Herceptin alone produces the same results.

Will I have menopause due to my chemotherapy treatments?

Some of the drugs used as treatment for breast cancer can damage your ovaries. If your ovaries stop producing hormones, you may have symptoms of menopause, such as hot flashes and dryness of your vagina. Your periods may become irregular or may stop completely. You may become infertile and unable to become pregnant. If you are over the age of 35, some of these side effects, such as infertility, may be permanent. There is more information on side effects in Chapter 10, Chemotherapy.

Are there any other side effects if my ovaries stop producing hormones?

Having your ovaries suddenly stop producing hormones means the symptoms of menopause will be exaggerated. You may feel less sexual desire, have soreness and dryness in your vulva or vagina, burning in the vagina during intercourse, or light spotting after intercourse. You may have persistent hot flashes and sweats. You should use a water-soluble lubricant during vaginal intercourse. You might try avoiding highly seasoned foods, caffeine, and alcohol to minimize your hot flashes. In addition, you may want to consult a specialist to help treat your symptoms, such as a gynecologic-endocrinologist, who has knowledge of menopause and nonestrogen replacement therapies.

Will I lose my hair as a result of the chemotherapy treatments?

It depends on the specific chemotherapy drugs you are taking. Your doctor and nurse will give you information on side effects of your specific drug protocol.

What is a chemotherapy port and how does it work?

There are various ways of giving chemotherapy, depending on the number of treatments, the dosage, personal preferences, and the treatment schedule. Some doctors and many patients, who are facing a long treatment plan, prefer to have a port implanted near the collarbone. The device gives direct access into a vein and provides a permanent port for the IV needle, making finding new veins in which to insert the IV needle unnecessary. Implanting the port requires a small incision and caring for it is simple. Because of risk of infection, having the port implanted is an excellent way to protect your veins especially since you aren't drawing blood from the arm where you had lymph nodes removed. **Tip:** Mark your bra line so that when the doctor inserts the catheter it will not be irritated by your bra strap.

Will I gain weight as a result of my chemotherapy?

Some women do gain weight, but research indicates that weight gain is often due to eating more calories rather than to the treatment itself. The women who gained weight reported feeling more unhappy, more worried, and more distressed about their appearance than those women with breast cancer who did not gain weight while on treatment. However, weight gain can be due to treatment if it includes prednisone or oral cyclophosphamide. If you are having problems with gaining weight, you may need to get help from a dietitian and begin a physical exercise program.

What kind of new treatments are being studied for breast cancer?

There are studies on many new kinds of treatments for all stages of breast cancer. They include new treatment methods, new doses, and treatment schedules and new ways of combining treatment. In addition, work is underway with various anticancer drugs and drug combinations as well as several types of hormone treatments and new ways of combining chemotherapy with hormone treatment and radiation therapy. Biological therapy—treatment with substances that boost the immune system's response to cancer—is also being studied in clinical trials. New approaches such as bone marrow transplants, peripheral stem cell support and colony-stimulating factors are also being researched.

Are bone marrow transplants or peripheral stem cell support being used for breast cancer patients?

The use of high-dose chemotherapy followed by bone marrow transplantation or peripheral blood stem cell transplantation has not been shown to work better than standard chemotherapy in the treatment of breast cancer. Doctors have decided that, for now, high-dose chemotherapy should only be tested in clinical trials. Before taking part in such a trial, women should talk with their doctors about the serious side effects caused by high-dose chemotherapy. You will find more information on this procedure in Chapter 11, New Advances and Investigational Treatments.

Is it possible to treat Stage II, or Stage III breast cancer with only tamoxifen instead of having an operation plus adjuvant treatment?

If you only take tamoxifen, you have a very high risk of having a local recurrence. This choice is only for women who cannot have a mastectomy or breast-conserving surgery plus radiation therapy because of their age or other complications that make an operation impossible.

Buying a Prosthesis

If I have had a mastectomy, are there medical reasons why I should wear a prosthesis?

There are reasons why you should wear a prosthesis—a form to replace the missing breast. The weight of the remaining breast, particularly if you have a medium-to-large breast, can cause shoulder, neck, and back pain. You may find that your posture will change, with the affected shoulder rising, if you do not have a prosthesis. The larger the remaining breast, the more vital the need, not only for appearance but also for the weight. In many cases, a well-fitted prosthetic device means the difference between a prompt, cheerful, total recovery and long-term personal distress.

What does a prosthesis look like?

Usually the prosthesis is flesh-colored. It is sized to match the remaining breast both in shape and weight. Normally it is shaped like a teardrop. The flat side goes against the wall of the chest and the tail end goes toward the armpit. Some companies make reversible ones that can be used on either side.

Does a prosthesis feel cold against the chest?

It depends on the type of prosthesis, what it is made of, and how it is supposed to be worn. Many of them feel a little cold when they are first put on. After they have been worn for a few minutes, they warm to body temperature and feel like a normal breast to the touch.

When should I plan on being fitted for a breast prosthesis?

Most doctors will tell you to wait until the scar is fully healed before you get fitted for a breast prosthesis. Most patients can begin using a full prosthesis a month or six weeks after surgery. However, soft forms, such as simple clean padding in your brassiere, can be worn from the very beginning. A Reach to Recovery volunteer may provide you with a temporary Dacron-filled prosthesis to wear while the wound is healing and the area is tender and swollen. (See information on Reach to Recovery in this chapter under "Getting Support.") Some patients tell us they use items such as cotton balls, lamb's wool, handkerchiefs, sanitary napkins, or padded bras during the period between their operation and being fitted for a prosthesis. You should check with your doctor before you start wearing a permanent prosthesis.

How can I be sure I find the right prosthesis?
First of all, you should not shop for the prosthesis by yourself. It is much better if an involved person, such as your sister, mother, husband, or a good friend, goes along with you. Second, you should make sure you try on several different kinds and models so that you can be sure the one you finally buy is what you really want. There are several dozen different breast forms on the market. You should try on several to compare the way they feel and look.

What should I be looking for in a prosthesis?
The breast form should feel comfortable, have a natural contour and consistency, and should remain in place when you stretch, bend, or reach. A properly weighted form provides the balance your body needs for correct posture and anchors your bra, preventing it from riding up. There are even forms that are designed with adhesive skin supports, and include an optional nipple, that you can wear without a bra, if you choose to. It is important to pay close attention to how the prosthesis feels and how it fits—the form should match your other breast when seen from the side, the bottom and the front. Your clothes should fit the way they did before you had your operation. The form may feel too heavy at first, but will feel natural in time. Take your time in choosing a form. Remember you will be wearing it every day for a long time to come. Make sure you shop around and try on different types and different brands.

What are the different kinds of prostheses available?
There are several different kinds of breast forms made by several companies. Generally they fall into these classifications:

- **Silicone:** Form made of silicone skin or polyurethane and filled with silicone gel or glycerin or fluid. Very soft and flexible with the look, feel, and weight of the natural breast. Some have different forms for left and right breasts, with side wings. Available with or without nipples. Depending on manufacturer, made to be worn on the skin, with or without regular bra or bra with pocket. Adjusts to body temperature; may need to be warmed before using. Some can leak if fingernail or pin pricks it. May be worn for swimming. Also available in customized model using preoperative impression. Silicone filled prostheses range in cost from $75 to $300; silicone gel from $150 to $450, with customized forms costing up to $1400.

- **Organic:** Made of cotton or other organic material. Filling is organic fiber, with glass beads or other weights cushioned into the form. Made in left and right breast forms. Warms quickly and remains at room temperature. Some can be worn directly on skin. Odorless. May be worn for swimming. Cost ranges from $60 to $200.

- **Foam:** Made of lightweight molded foam or foam chips; weights can be added. Spongy feeling. May get stiff and yellow with wear. Good for leisure wear or swimming (need waterproof cover). Especially useful with lounging bra for postoperative period, although some women like them for general wear. Cost ranges from $30 to $175.

- **Temporary:** Lightweight and long-wearing. Soft pads with tricot filling. Can also be cotton with cotton filling. Good for sleepwear and postoperative wear. Cost ranges from $5 to $50.

Where do I go to buy a prosthesis?

There are several places: corset shops, surgical supply houses, foundation departments of some large department stores, and some special outlets. Some American Cancer Society offices offer a variety of forms that a woman can examine (they are not for sale) in a noncommercial setting. The Reach to Recovery volunteer or the American Cancer Society office can give you material describing the various forms, their manufacturers and a list of suggested outlets available. Most of the outlets have fitters who can help you. The large mail-order houses also have prostheses available.

What should I wear when I shop for the prosthesis?

You should bring along some figure-revealing clothes to see how natural the form will look—a sweater or one of your more revealing dresses. If you want to use your own bras, make sure you bring them along so they can be altered if needed.

Can I make my own prosthesis?

Some people do make their own prostheses. Some small-breasted women or women who have had both breasts removed find that they can use homemade forms. However, in many cases, the homemade forms are too lightweight and tend to ride up. Again, you must be careful because you can end up with posture changes and discomfort in your shoulders or back if you wear a prosthesis that isn't the proper weight for you.

What is a special mastectomy bra?

It is a bra with a built-in pocket to hold the form in place. It also has extra material under the arm and above the breast. The form is placed in the pocket of the bra, which holds it in place. You can bend, stretch, or stoop without jarring it out of place. Some patients have complained that special mastectomy bras do not fit properly. Many patients have altered their own bras with pockets, and still others have had seamstresses make pockets for their regular bras. In some stores, fitters will sew pockets into your bras to hold the prosthesis. Some companies make mastectomy bras that are individually fitted.

What kinds of covers are available for the form?

Some of the forms, both lightweight and heavy ones, have nylon or cloth covers. The covers are made of washable, fast-drying materials. The cover allows the forms to be pinned directly into regular brassieres. Some women prefer to leave the covers on the forms at all times. They like the way they feel. The tricot covers, especially, are easy to wash out and dry.

Can I get a breast form with a nipple?

Some forms are made with nipples. Nipples also are sold separately and can be easily attached either to the prosthesis, or directly to the skin. Some women who have had breast reconstruction without having the nipple reconstructed use these separate nipples.

Can I get a form in a dark skin color?

Some forms are made in both light and dark skin colors.

Can I wear my prosthesis all the time?

Many women do wear their prostheses around the clock. Some women start by wearing it a few hours a day and gradually increasing the number of hours of wear. Wearing the form to bed at night may help prevent a stiff neck and shoulder problems. Waterbeds also have been recommended by some, since they provide support and conform to the body.

Are there any cosmetics to cover the scars I have after surgery?

There is a special brand of cosmetics, Covermark, which is designed to hide any skin flaw or blemish, no matter how severe the problems may be. The cosmetics are long-lasting, waterproof, sweatproof, contain SPF higher than 15, and are particularly useful for swimming. Made originally by Lydia O'Leary to cover her port-wine stain blemish, the brand is available in many drug and department stores and on the Web (www.covermark.com).

Is there anything I can do about the tightness of the elastic in my bra?

Notion stores and girdle and corset shops sell bra extenders that can be used to make a bra more comfortable. They also sell shoulder-strap pads that some women use to relieve discomfort on the shoulder-strap area.

Will my insurance cover a prosthesis?

It depends on your insurance plan. Some health insurances (and Medicare) cover part or all of the cost of the first prosthesis. Some will pay for a prosthesis every one or two years with a doctor's prescription. You will need the doctor to write the prescription for both the form and for mastectomy bras. When you are buying them, ask that the term "surgical" be written on the bill. You should also write "surgical" on your check. Breast forms, mastectomy bras, and even bra alterations may be tax deductible when medically prescribed. Be sure to read your insurance policy, because some say you must buy the form within a specific period of time and buy a certain type. If you are planning to have reconstruction, ask your insurance company whether they will also pay for a prosthesis and mastectomy bras. Some women have found that submitting a claim for a prosthesis and mastectomy bras makes them ineligible for payment for subsequent reconstruction. You also need to keep all your receipts, since most prostheses are covered by warranty.

Can I do anything about the perspiration under my prosthesis during the summertime?

You can buy a thin sheepskin pad, which you wear with the wool facing your body, behind the form, to absorb perspiration. Some women find using facial tissue under the form during the summer will also do the trick.

Is anyone making special bathing suits for women with mastectomies?

Many of the major bathing suit companies make special bathing suits for mastectomy patients. You can usually get them through the same source where you got your prosthesis, or in large department stores.

Breast Reconstruction

If I plan to have breast reconstruction when should I see the plastic surgeon?

If you plan to have breast reconstruction it is a good idea to contact the plastic surgeon before you have your mastectomy operation. You can choose to have the reconstruction done at the same time as the mastectomy or at some future time. If it is done after the mastectomy, you will have to wait three to six months.

Who is a candidate for breast reconstruction?

Breast reconstruction is designed for women who have had a mastectomy, regardless of age, the type of surgery performed, or the number of years since the surgery. Lumpectomy patients usually do not need breast reconstruction.

Questions to Ask Your Plastic Surgeon Before You Have
Reconstructive Surgery on Your Breast

- What are the different choices of reconstructive surgery? What type do you think is best for me? Why?

- Should I have the reconstruction at the time of my mastectomy or should I wait until later? How much later can I have it done? If I need to have chemotherapy, should I wait to have the reconstruction until I have finished chemo treatments?

- What are the advantages and disadvantages of having reconstruction at the time of my mastectomy? Of waiting to have it until later?

- What are the side effects and risks that I should consider?

- Will you be using tissue expanders? A saline-filled implant? What has your experience been with silicone gel implants? Can you use tissue from my body instead? What are my options?

- Will you explain how the surgery will be done? What kind of anesthesia will you use?

- What will I look like after the surgery? What kind of scars will I have and where will they be?

- What will my new breast look like? Will it match my other breast? Will it change over time? Will I have to have anything done to my other breast?

- Can I have my nipple reconstructed? How will it be done?

- What is your experience with this operation? How many reconstruction surgeries have you done?

- May I see before-and-after pictures of your patients?

- May I talk with someone who has had the operation?

- How many operations will I have to have? Will I need to be in the hospital each time? For how long? How long will I need for recovery?

- Will I be in much pain? For how long?

- What possible complications should I know about?

- Will I need blood transfusions? Can I donate my own blood?

- What can be done if the surgery is not successful?

- Will I need to wear a special bra after my operation? Where will I be able to buy it?

- How much will it cost? Will my insurance cover any part of it?

**Can I have breast reconstruction at the same
time I have my mastectomy?**
That is certainly a possibility, depending upon what stage and type of breast
cancer you have and your general health. Generally, if you have breast cancer
in situ or Stage I and II infiltrating cancer, reconstruction may be done. You
should ask your surgeon for a consultation with a plastic surgeon before the
mastectomy. The plastic surgeon will determine whether you are a candidate
for immediate reconstruction or whether you would be better off waiting. If
you don't have immediate reconstruction, you will probably have to wait
three to six months until your scar has healed. If you are having chemotherapy or radiation treatments, most doctors prefer to wait one to three months
after completing them. If you smoke, the doctor will ask you to stop smoking in order to ensure an adequate blood supply.

Why will the doctor ask me to stop smoking?
Cigarette smoking can narrow your blood vessels, reduce blood flow to the
tissues, and impair healing. Because it can seriously affect the results of the
reconstruction, the plastic surgeon usually will insist that you not smoke for
at least three weeks before your surgery and for several months after it.

**Are there advantages to my having the reconstruction
at the same time as my mastectomy?**
Having the reconstruction at the same time may make you feel better psychologically, make you feel attractive and may help with your sexual life. It
means, however, that your doctors must cooperate with each other, including
scheduling the operating room for two operations instead of one. You will be
in surgery and under anesthesia for a longer time and you may have additional complications from having two surgeries. It is important to be sure
that the plastic surgeon has had experience in performing immediate reconstruction. There is no evidence of harmful effects—that is, having the two
operations at the same time does not interfere with or delay adjuvant treatment and does not interfere with the management of recurrent disease. However, you may find that your doctor still prefers to do the reconstruction as a
separate operation.

Will my breast look like it did before the mastectomy?
You should not expect that it will. The new breast will probably look more
flattened than tapered. It may be firmer than your natural breast and it may
not match it exactly. There is a limit to the size of the constructed breast,
based on what the skin can support. Sometimes, women choose to have the
remaining breast reduced, or in some cases augmented, to more closely match

the new reconstructed breast. However, under clothing, you will probably not notice the difference between the two. Most women are pleased with the results of the reconstruction. Although the new breast will not be a perfect replica of the old one, most women who have the reconstructive surgery can wear a normal bra or a bikini. You need to talk to the plastic surgeon about your expectations. Ask to see before-and-after pictures of women who have had this surgery. If your expectations are not realistic, you may be better off not having the reconstruction.

What are the chances that I will have a good result?

It is difficult to know, but there are some factors that will give you and your doctors some clues. They include your overall health, your chest structure and body shape, how your body heals, the effects of other breast surgery you have had, the skill of your plastic surgeon, and the type of reconstruction operation you will be having.

Will I have scars as a result of the reconstruction?

You will have some scars, but the doctor will try to hide them as much as possible. The scars will depend upon the kind and extent of the surgery. When you talk with your plastic surgeon, ask where the scars will be, how long they will be, and what they might look like. Like most scars, they will fade in time, but probably they will never disappear completely. In people with darker skin, the scars usually look more prominent.

What is involved in breast reconstruction?

Breast reconstruction usually means one or more operations, even when you have it done at the same time as the mastectomy. You may have an implant (tissue expansion or simple breast reconstruction) or your own tissue. If you are going to use your own tissue, there are three operations that can be done— latissimus dorsi reconstruction, transverse rectus abdominus muscle flap, and free flap reconstruction. Having a nipple reconstructed or decreasing the size of the other breast means additional surgery.

What is expansion reconstructive surgery?

This is the most common reconstructive surgical approach. It can be done using one of several types of expanders. The expander, with a valve attached to it, is implanted behind the chest wall muscles, using the lines of the mastectomy incision. After a few weeks, when the wound has healed, you will return to the doctor's office every week or two, where sterile saline (saltwater) is injected into the valve until the expander is slightly larger than the desired final size. The filled expander is left in place for several months to stretch the breast tissue. The surgeon operates again, taking out the expander and inserting a permanent breast implant. This process results in a more natural, supple contour to the reconstructed breast. The entire process takes from four to six months to complete.

What does a simple breast reconstruction entail?

After you have had a mastectomy, the surgeon makes a small incision along the lower part of the breast area near the mastectomy scar (or the mastectomy incision may be used) and puts the implant into a pocket created under the chest muscle. Different types of implants can be used—saline, silicone gel, or double lumen implants. A drain may be put in to take away the fluid that may accumulate during the first few days, and the incision is closed. The operation takes about one to two hours and is usually done under general anesthesia. (According to the FDA, you can have silicone gel only if you are participating in a clinical trial. As for saline-filled implants, only two have been approved by the FDA—Mentor and INAMED.)

What is latissimus dorsal reconstruction?

This operation is used when chest muscles have been removed and there is too little skin to hold and cover an implant. The surgeon transfers skin, muscle, and other tissue from the back to the mastectomy site. To create a new muscle on the front of the chest, a broad flat muscle on the back, below the shoulder blade—called the latissimus dorsal—is used. An implant is then placed under the new chest muscle. Drains may be put in and kept in place for several days after the surgery, to remove fluid. This operation takes three to four hours. You will probably stay in the hospital for several days. You will have a scar on your back as well as on your chest.

What is transverse rectus abdominus muscle flap
(also called the TRAM flap)?

This operation is sometimes called the "tummy tuck." The surgeon transfers one of the two abdominal muscles (the rectus abdominus) to the breast along with skin and fat from the abdomen. This flap of muscle, skin, and fat is shaped into the contour of a breast. If there is enough abdominal tissue available, no implant is needed. Transferring tissue in this way also results in tightening of the stomach, thus the use of the term tummy tuck. This operation usually offers you a better cosmetic result. However, it is considerably more complicated and you will be in the operating room a longer time. You will have a horizontal scar across the lower abdomen plus the scar on your chest.

What is free flap reconstruction?

This is the most difficult type of reconstruction. You need two teams of surgeons, using microsurgical techniques. The first team removes the flap and

TYPES OF OPERATIONS FOR BREAST RECONSTRUCTION

DESCRIPTION	COMMENTS
Expansion Reconstruction Surgery. Can be of several types. Empty silicone sack, or double envelope with silicone layer and empty sack implanted under skin and muscle, gradually filled with saline (saltwater) solution through a valve over a period of weeks, stretching skin. Local or general anesthesia. Inpatient or outpatient. Surgery takes one to two hours.	Most common type of reconstruction. Provides greatest flexibility in breast size. Requires additional office visits (15 to 30 minutes) to add saltwater solution to stretch skin. May be uncomfortable for some women. Can have problems with valve. Another operation often needed to convert expander to permanent implant.
Simple Breast Reconstruction, also called **Implant** or **Fixed-Volume Implant.** Sack filled with silicone gel or saline fluid, implanted under skin and chest muscle. General or local anesthesia used. Can be outpatient or inpatient. Surgery takes one to two hours. Short recovery time. Low rate of complications.	Can use saline, silicone gel, or double lumen implants. Those filled with silicone gel can be used only if a woman is enrolled in a clinical trial. Saline filled have silicone layer or envelope that contains filling; two manufacturers of saline-filled implants have been approved by the FDA.
Dorsal Reconstruction, Latissimus Flap, also called **Back Flap.** Muscle, called latissimus dorsal, and an eye-shaped wedge of skin moved from back to chest wall and sewn in place, leaving tissue attached to original blood supply. Inpatient with general anesthesia. Surgery takes two to four hours.	May need blood transfusion. Major surgery that can be painful. Requires hospital stay. Scar left on back or side. May have drain in for several weeks. May have fluid buildup in back area. May have slight bulge under arm that will shrink in time.
Free Flap or **Microsurgery.** Muscle and fat from other parts of body, such as buttock or thigh, are cut free from blood supply, moved to breast and reattached to breast blood supply by microsurgery. Inpatient with general anesthesia. Surgery takes three to eight hours.	May need blood transfusion. Most complex of all operations for reconstruction. Needs surgeon with great expertise in procedure. Hospital stay. Scar in donor area. May have serious complications. Longer recovery period.

TYPES OF OPERATIONS FOR BREAST RECONSTRUCTION

DESCRIPTION	COMMENTS
Nipple Reconstruction. Can be made from existing skin, pinched and tacked to make nipple or created from tissue from other nipple or groin and attached to breast mound.	Areola reconstruction may also be done. May need tattoo to match color of other breast. If donor site used, area will feel tender for about two weeks.
TRAM flap (Transverse rectus abdominis muscle) also called **tummy tuck.** Fat, skin, and muscle taken from stomach area and moved up to form breast. Tissue usually remains connected to abdominal blood supply, although in some cases microsurgery used. Inpatient, with general anesthesia. Surgery takes three to five hours.	May need blood transfusion. Major surgery that can be painful. Long scar— from hipbone to hipbone. Possible distortion of belly button. Hospital stay. Recovery period may take several weeks, including inability of patient to stand straight for days or even weeks. Healing problems may occur, including thick tissue on flap.

the second prepares the blood vessels. A portion of the skin and fat is taken from your buttocks or lower abdomen and grafted onto the mastectomy site. The success of this surgery depends on the tissues getting enough nourishment from the blood vessels after the operation and the experience of the surgeon doing this procedure.

How is the nipple reconstructed?
The nipple is usually rebuilt by shifting a layer of skin and fat on the reconstructed breast to the place where the nipple and areola (the circle of darker skin that surrounds the nipple) will be formed. It can also be reconstructed by using tissue from the nipple of your opposite breast or tissue from other areas, such as your upper inner thigh or from the skin folds of the vulva, just outside the vagina. (NOTE: Since reconstructed nipples have very little sensation or sensitivity, it may not be a good idea to use part of your existing, natural nipple to create a new nipple since both nipples may then feel numb.) Most doctors recommend that you wait at least two months after surgery to have the nipple reconstructed. The surgery can also be done after a number

of years. There also are prosthetic nipples that can be attached directly to the skin, available in stores that sell prostheses.

Is tattooing a procedure in nipple reconstruction?

Tattooing may be used to match the color of the area of the areola. If it is done, a local anesthetic is often used. The pigment is placed directly onto the skin, using a tattooing device that has been dipped into the pigment. Since there is little feeling or sensation in the reconstructed breast, this procedure is not painful. The new tattoo usually look darker than the selected color when first applied but fades in time.

Can I have an operation on my opposite breast if it is larger than my reconstructed breast?

The surgeon can reduce the size of your remaining breast so that it will better match the new breast. This operation may be done at the time of reconstruction or as a second operation. The operation to reduce the size of the remaining breast is called reduction mammoplasty.

What is the difference between different kinds of breast implants?

There are two general types of implants—the saline (saltwater) implant and the silicone gel implant. The saline implant is a silicone rubber envelope filled with sterile saltwater during surgery. The silicone implant is a silicone rubber envelope filled with soft silicone gel that feels like thick jelly. The envelope may have either a textured or a smooth surface.

What is a double lumen implant?

The double lumen implant has two silicone rubber envelopes, one inside the other. One is filled with silicone gel and the other is filled during surgery with a small amount of saline water that allows the surgeon to adjust the size.

What is capsular contracture?

Capsular contracture is the term used by health professionals to describe the hard scar the body forms around an implant, resulting in a hard breast. Some of the newer implants have textured surfaces that help reduce the chances of the scar forming. These textured surfaces also seem to produce a softer breast.

What are the health risks of breast implants?

All of the implants have some health risks associated with them. They continue to be monitored and restricted by the Food and Drug Administration (FDA). There are several possible side effects. You may find some hardening of the scar tissue that normally forms around the implant. This can sometimes cause you to have pain, hardening of the breast, or changes in the appearance of your breast. Calcium deposits can also form in surrounding tissue, which also can cause you pain and hardening of the breast. The saline implant is more likely to rupture, so you need to be careful not to hit it, for instance, if you play sports. The silicone implant can leak, "sweat," or rupture, allowing the gel filling to be released into surrounding tissue. You should have your breast implant checked regularly.

What are the risks if the silicone gel is released in my body?

It is possible that if silicone gel escapes from the implant it may reach distant parts of the body. Although there is no data that link the implants to serious diseases, it has been suggested that even very small amounts of gel might affect autoimmune (connective tissue) diseases, such as fibromyalgia, lupus, scleroderma, and rheumatoid arthritis in some women. Although some doctors have reported that a few patients have developed arthritis-like diseases after receiving breast implants, it is not clear whether women with implants are more likely to develop these conditions than those without implants. There are also questions as to whether the silicone can increase the risk of cancer or pose a risk to unborn babies.

What are the symptoms of these autoimmune diseases reported by implant patients?

The symptoms include pain or swelling of joints, tightness, redness or swelling of the skin, swollen glands or lymph nodes, unusual or unexplained fatigue, swelling of the hands and feet, and excessive hair loss. There may be a combination of these symptoms. But you need to remember that these immune-related disorders are relatively rare.

Will I be able to have a silicone gel-filled implant for my reconstruction?

You probably will. The Federal Drug Administration (FDA) has issued guidelines that limit the use of these implants to reconstruction and has imposed a moratorium on the use of silicone gel-filled implants for breast enlargement. You can have a silicone gel-filled implant only if you are enrolled in a clinical scientific study through the surgeon who is doing your reconstruction. Enrollment is simple. Your doctor agrees to collect certain information and conduct periodic blood tests. Under the guidelines, if you have had breast cancer, you may still, if you wish, choose to have immediate or delayed reconstruction, using silicone gel-filled implants.

Is a saline-filled implant safer than a silicone-gel-filled implant?

This issue is not completely settled at this time. The Food and Drug Administration has asked the manufacturers of the saline-filled implants to submit safety and effectiveness information on them, especially since saline-filled implants use a silicone rubber envelope, whose long-term safety is unproven. Two manufacturers of saline-filled breast implants—Mentor and INAMED—have been approved by the FDA. Leakage or rupture of a saline implant would result in release of saltwater. Since saltwater is not foreign to your body, it is assumed that it would not present the risks that are associated with the gel.

Where would the saltwater in the saline implant go?
The salt water would be absorbed in your body within a few hours. The implant would be deflated quickly and would need to be removed surgically.

What are the results of the studies on the silicone implants at this time?
The National Cancer Institute conducted one study of 13,500 women who had silicone implant surgery for cosmetic reasons (not for reconstruction after breast surgery) and, for comparison, 4,000 women similar in age who had some other type of plastic surgery. This study, which followed the women for 13 years through medical records, found that the women with silicone breast implants were not at increased risk for most cancers, although they did find small increases in the risks for cancers of the lung, larynx, and brain. A follow-up study on 907 of these women found that one third of them reported that they had at least one surgery in which their implant was removed or replaced. The most common reason for surgery was for local problems with the implant (103 out of 303); the second most common reason was because of concern over the saftey of silicone (92 out of 303).

Are there results from the studies of the saline-filled implants?
About 9,000 women who had implant surgery for cosmetic reasons, for breast cancer reconstruction, or for other problems have been enrolled in five studies on implants that are made of a silicone shield filled with sterile salt water. Two of the studies that looked at women who received the implants after surgery for breast cancer or other problems had relatively similar results. In the first one, 237 women who received implants after breast or other surgery, were enrolled, and after three years, 39 percent had had additional surgery for complications—33 percent for asymmetry, 25 percent for capsule contracture, 23 percent for implant removal, 23 percent for wrinkling, and 6 percent for leakage or deflation. Some women experienced more than one of these complications. The second study, which enrolled 416 patients, found that after three years, 40 percent had had reoperations—35 percent for loss of nipple sensation, 30 percent for capsule contracture, 28 percent for asymmetry, 27 percent for implant removal, and 8 percent for leakage or deflation. The FDA has decided to allow the two companies to continue marketing their saline-filled implants, as long as information is given to the patients

about the possibility that a substantial number will require additional surgery at some point to remove or replace their implants because of complications.

What should I know before I decide to have either a saline or silicone implant?

There are several things you should ask about and keep in your records:

- A brochure that helps you make the decision as to whether or not to have the implant.

- Information about the manufacturer or the implant that is going to be used.

- A copy of the sticker that identifies the brand of implant you are going to get, its size, and the manufacturer's number.

- Information, in writing, from your insurance company about coverage for the implant. Will your policy cover the cost of the surgery, anesthesia, and other hospital costs? Will it cover the cost of having it taken out or replaced if needed? Will it cover the cost of detecting or treating a complication resulting from the implant or the surgery? Make sure you understand whether or not your insurance might be increased if you have the surgery or how future coverage may be affected.

How can I enroll in a study?

You first need to contact the doctor you choose to do the implant surgery. The doctor then makes the necessary arrangements with the implant manufacturer. The doctor will need to certify that you qualify medically for the implant. You will need to sign a special informed consent form, certifying that you have been told about the risks. You will be enrolled in a registry so that you can be notified in the future, if needed, about new information on implants. (You can get additional information by contacting the FDA Breast Implant Information Service at 1–800–532–4440, or visit the FDA's Web site: www.fda.gov.)

Is a soybean oil implant available?

Soybean oil implants have been manufactured, using soy triglyceride oils to fill the implant. They have been available in Europe for a few years. The soybean oil was thought to be less dense than silicone gel or saline solution, would be easier to see in mammograms, and could be safe if the implants failed and leaked. The manufacturer began a clinical trial in the United States but closed it before it was completed and has never submitted data to the FDA for approval of the device.

What other complications may result from breast reconstruction?
You must remember that there is always the possibility of complications from any surgery, even with the best surgeon. You might have an infection at the breast site, or large areas of the skin might die. Part or all of a transferred muscle may fail to survive. If you have had an implant and these complications happen, the implant may need to be removed temporarily and then replaced. You should not expect that the reconstruction will restore the sensation lost through your mastectomy. Make sure you discuss the possible complications with your plastic surgeon before the operation, realizing that as with any type of plastic surgery, it is difficult to predict the overall results.

Are most women satisfied with their breast reconstruction?
There have been several studies of women who have had breast reconstruction. Most women are satisfied that they had it done because of body image, the feeling of normalcy, and the ability to move on with life. However, even though they are content that they had the operation, many of them are not completely satisfied with the way their breasts looked after surgery, complaining that they did not look natural or that they were not symmetrical. Some women also felt that they had not asked enough questions before having the surgery or had not even known the right questions to ask. Areas of concern included the amount of time the drains were left in, the amount of pain with tissue expansion, lack of sensation in the reconstructed breast, the pulling sensation in the stomach area after a TRAM flap operation, types of bras they would be using, and the fact that the nipple was removed. Some women have had hardening of the reconstructed breast, and some have had additional surgeries for reasons such as to construct a nipple or to reduce the size of the other breast.

Will I have to do anything to care for my breast after reconstruction?
If you have had an implant, you will be taught how to massage it after the operation and how to exercise the muscles surrounding your implant. It will take a few months for the skin and muscle to stretch and for the reconstructed breast to take on a natural appearance. It is important that you continue to have your implant monitored for any leaking.

How long is the recovery period after reconstruction?
You will generally have a large bulky dressing and a drain, and will probably need pain medicine for the first couple of days. You may have more pain and discomfort from this operation than from your mastectomy, especially if the

surgery involves the transplanting of muscle and tissue from other parts of the body. Most women are able to resume normal activities in two to three weeks, although it is usually several more weeks before they can do strenuous exercise.

Should I be doing breast self-examination if I have a breast implant?

Yes, you should be doing monthly breast self-examination so you will be familiar with how your breasts normally feel and so you would be able to detect any complications that are due to your implant. It is particularly important for you to pay attention to changes in the firmness, size, or shape of your breast. You should also be attentive to pain, tenderness, or color changes in the breast area or any discharge or unusual sensation around the nipple. You should report these changes promptly to your doctor. In addition, you need to pay attention to the other breast.

Will I need to have mammograms on my reconstructed breast?

You should continue to have your mammograms at your regularly scheduled times. When you go for your mammogram, make sure you ask for a diagnostic mammogram (rather than a screening mammogram) and that you are in a facility that has personnel trained in doing mammograms for people with implants. Tell the technician where your implant is so that special care can be taken when the breast is flattened.

If I have surgery to reduce my other breast, will I need a special mammogram?

If you have had breast reduction surgery, you need to tell the technician and the radiologist before the mammogram is done. Usually the scar tissue that is seen in the reduced breast does not present a problem in reading the mammogram. If an implant was placed in the other breast at the time of the reduction surgery, you need to have special views taken.

How long does an implant last?

This can vary from woman to woman. Most implants last for many years. However, studies have shown that leakage or ruptures do occur after a period of time—sometimes after six to ten years. There is no guarantee on the exact length of time an implant lasts. Sometimes it is necessary to replace an implant to adjust the shape, size, or position if you lose weight or gain weight. One thing you should be aware of however is that it is very difficult to damage an implant under ordinary circumstances. It would take a very severe chest injury to impact the implant.

Can I have breast reconstruction if I had my mastectomy ten years ago?

There are women who have had successful reconstruction 20 years after their mastectomies. The fact that you had a mastectomy many years ago does not disqualify you as a candidate for the operation, nor does your age.

Can I have breast reconstruction after I have had radiation treatments?

It depends on many factors. However, radiation-damaged skin, grafted, thin, or tight skin, or the absence of chest muscles are not the obstacles to breast reconstruction that they once were.

Can I have breast reconstruction if I have had breast implants removed?

Yes. Breast reconstruction can be done after having the implants removed.

If I have a problem with my breast implant what should I do?

If you believe that you have a problem related to your breast implants, you should report it to your physician and ask the doctor to report it to Med-Watch, a voluntary reporting system. As a consumer, you can send your report to the FDA Medical Products Reporting Program, Food and Drug Administration, 5600 Fishers Lane, Rockville, MD 20852-9787, or fax it to 1–800–322–1088.

How much does breast reconstruction cost?

The operations are expensive and depend upon the extent of the surgery as well as other factors. The surgeon's fee can run from $2,500 to over $10,000, with hospital costs ranging from $3,000 upward. It can double if flap surgery is done at a later time because of the costs of the additional hospital stay. If you are eligible, Medicare and Medicaid will cover costs of reconstruction as well as breast prosthesis. Since 1999, insurance companies are required to pay for reconstruction and breast augmentation following breast surgery. Be sure you know the cost and what your policy will cover before deciding on the operation.

Getting Support

What is Reach to Recovery?

This is a volunteer program sponsored by the American Cancer Society. Its members are breast cancer survivors who, having experienced the pain, anxiety, and convalescence, are able to help others who are going through the same experiences. Trained volunteers offer emotional support and furnish information, including a kit with a realistically written manual of information and exercise materials. For women who have had a mastectomy, a temporary breast form and bra may be supplied. Call the American Cancer Society at 1–800–ACS–2345.

What is Look Good . . . Feel Better?

Look Good . . . Feel Better is a nationwide program that has been developed by the Cosmetic, Toiletry, and Fragrance Association in cooperation with the American Cancer Society (ACS) and the National Cosmetology Association. It helps women deal with the changes in their appearances that may result from chemotherapy or radiation treatments or from the illness itself, such as loss of hair, eyebrows and lashes, changes in skin tone, and texture or brittleness of nails. Cosmetologists give practical, one-on-one advice on appearance changes, including specific recommendations for skin care, hair styles, wigs and accessories, eyebrow and eye makeup and nail care, taking into consideration the changes you may have in your skin and nails. You can learn how to use scarves and turbans and about the different styles of wigs that are available. The American Cancer Society, along with cancer centers and hospitals around the country, run the program locally with members of the National Cosmetology Association offering their services on a voluntary basis to help women with cancer learn the beauty techniques. You can call 1–800–395–LOOK to find programs located near you.

Would it be useful for me to go to a support group?

Joining a support group can help you discuss your feelings with others who have shared your experience. A study, conducted in California with women with metastatic breast cancer, concluded that group therapy might help patients adapt to their disease and possibly prolong survival. Today, there are many different kinds of groups, from those that you go to in person locally, to support groups on the Internet, and telephone support groups. Your nurse, social worker, your local American Cancer Society, or the Cancer Information Service (1–800–4–CANCER) can assist you with finding a group. The Web site for Cancer Care has a nationwide listing of support groups (www.cancercare.org).

Why am I afraid to let my partner get near me since my operation?

This happens to some after breast surgery. You may worry about the scar hurting or you may be afraid of letting your partner see your new body. Sexual relations can be resumed as soon as you feel ready. The body's ability to heal is quite rapid. Intimacy can help to make you feel better psychologically.

A small, soft pillow to protect the scar may be helpful at first. You may need to experiment to find comfortable positions that do not put pressure on the area where you had surgery. Be honest with your partner. Explain your fears and enlist your partner's help. Your partner may also be nervous and scared.

Why it is that since my mastectomy I seem to be having difficulties with my partner—having sex less often and not enjoying it as much?

Several studies have shown that some, but certainly not all, women who have had breast surgery, may be faced with a problem involving their sexuality. There seems to be several parts to it, depending upon what kind of surgery you have had:

- You may be afraid of showing your scars to your partner.

- You may be afraid of having your partner see you with only one breast, or with a breast that is not as perfect as before.

- You may feel you will never be the same person sexually as you were before.

- Your partner may be afraid of causing you pain.

- Your partner may be unable to deal with the change in your body.

- Your emotional problems may be more involved than having the breast operation.

For some, the loss is so great they cannot overcome it alone. If you are having a problem of this kind, it is important for you to get some professional help. Also see the section on Sexuality in Chapter 27, Living with Cancer.

Are there any other activities that will make me feel better about myself?

Physical exercise, such as tennis, swimming, dance classes, or exercise classes, can help to improve your feelings about yourself. Your sense of grace and balance can be enhanced through dance-exercise classes. Yoga has been recommended as a way of achieving a sense of wholeness about the body. Many persons have taken up such challenging new activities as skiing. Others have returned to college and found a whole new sense of self-worth. Creative activities, such as music, painting, sewing, needlepoint, and writing are excellent fields to explore to help strengthen your self-image. In addition, you may want to explore the possibility of breast reconstruction if you have not already done so.

Is there anything a family member or friend can do to help someone who has gone through a breast cancer experience?
People who have gone through the experience tell us that several things have been helpful to them. Of course different things are beneficial to different people:

- Many women find that talking about their experience and their feelings is very helpful.

- A partner who tells you that you are still loved and needed will help you get through the difficult days and make you feel worthwhile.

- Friends and family members who are willing to talk and who are not afraid to bring up the subject make it easier for conversation to begin.

- Nurses who encourage the patient to look at the site of the operation, who listen, and make you feel at ease.

- People who are willing to go with you to buy your prosthesis or wig make a difficult decision easier.

Is it normal for me to feel depressed after a few weeks, when earlier I felt like I was facing the facts well?
People react to breast surgery in very different ways. Much of the reaction, it has been found, depends upon the expectations you have and how you approached the operation. It is not unusual to have emotional distress. It may be a feeling of panic. Some cry. Others say they don't feel like eating. Some cannot sleep or concentrate. Still others cannot talk about their cancer to anyone. Many women have a "why did this have to happen to me" feeling. These are normal kinds of feelings for breast cancer patients. Some people reach this stage directly after the operations, others not until a month or several months have gone by. Just understand that these are normal reactions to having a cancer diagnosis and to the feeling of helplessness about it. Above all, don't feel that you are strange because you have these feelings. It is normal to have them. Find someone to talk to—either a family member, a good friend, the Cancer Information Service, the American Cancer Society, a social worker, a nurse, doctor, or clergyman.

Do younger women have more difficulty coping with breast cancer?
It seems that they do and understandably so. Younger women seem to be more likely to be depressed, angry, and resentful, have more sexual problems, and more fears about recurrence than do older women with breast cancer. Even though there are many fewer young women who get breast cancer—the disease is usually more aggressive in this age group.

Are there any special groups for younger women?
The Young Survival Coalition was started in 1998 by three young women living in New York who had been diagnosed with breast cancer before they were age 35. They now have a registry of medical and family histories of over 1500 members that is being used as a basis for studies to determine what common factors there may be among them. The Coalition now has branches throughout the country (www.youngsurvival.org). Sharsheret (www.sharsheret.org) supports young Jewish women diagnosed with breast cancer by matching them with others who are having similar treatments. They correspond by phone or e-mail. The American Cancer Society and the Susan G. Komen Breast Cancer Foundation have each launched special programs also targeted at this group.

What can I do to help my children cope with my situation?
Children react in different ways and are influenced by their age and stage of development. Some are angry because you are ill. Others are frightened or worried. Some wonder whether or not they have caused your illness. It is better to tell them what is going on, because even young children know when something is happening. It's a good idea to tell your children the truth as simply and positively as possible. Ask for their questions and answer them honestly, but be careful not to burden them with any more information than is necessary. There is more information on helping your family cope with your illness in Chapter 27, Living with Cancer.

Pregnancy After Breast Cancer

Can a woman who has had breast cancer safely have a baby?
This is becoming a more common question, since about a quarter of all breast cancer patients will develop their disease during their childbearing years. There have been several studies assessing the possible effects of pregnancy on breast cancer patients. A summary of those studies shows that pregnancy after breast cancer treatment has no effect on recurrence or on survival rates. This appears to be true regardless of the number of pregnancies, the time between treatment and the pregnancy, lymph node status, or the stage of the initial breast cancer.

Should I get pregnant while I am getting my treatment?
You should not get pregnant while you are still undergoing treatment. Therefore, it is important to practice family planning while you are being treated.

How long should I wait after my treatment before I become pregnant?

Many doctors suggest that you wait a minimum of one year. The most important consideration is your overall risk for recurrent cancer based on your initial stage of disease. If, for instance, you have node-negative disease, there is no scientific evidence that you need to wait more than a year before attempting to get pregnant. You need to consider the time you need to get back to your normal activities before you decide to get pregnant. You and your partner should discuss the risks involved with your doctor. A consultation with a genetic counselor may also be useful. Of course, the decision of whether or not or when to attempt to become pregnant is one that only you can make.

Where can I find support during my pregnancy?

This is a difficult issue. Family members may not be supportive of your decision to become pregnant. You may have additional concerns, especially about your breasts, since they become fuller than normal during pregnancy. It is useful to find professionals who can be supportive during this time. You may need to go back to the health professional team that took care of you during your cancer treatment. You might also ask for help from an oncology nurse or social worker at a cancer center, or a genetic counselor. If they cannot help you, they can suggest others who can.

Will I be able to breast feed my baby and will it be safe for the baby?

Most women do not produce milk from a breast that has been radiated. Many find that they can breast feed from the other breast and that enough milk is made in that breast alone. If you plan to breast feed, you need to know that breastfeeding has not been shown to increase the risk of breast cancer in the infant.

Breast Cancer During Pregnancy

How is breast cancer detected during pregnancy?

It is usually a painless lump that has been felt by the doctor or the woman herself. Mammograms in pregnant women are difficult to read because of the increased water density of the breast.

What is the outlook for women who discover breast cancer during pregnancy?

About seven percent of women who develop breast cancer happen to be pregnant at the time of the diagnosis. The outlook for a pregnant woman is just as favorable as that for a nonpregnant woman of the same age with a similar stage of disease—provided that the cancer is diagnosed and treated promptly.

What kind of doctor should be taking care of me if I am diagnosed with breast cancer during my pregnancy?
It is important that you have a multidisciplinary group of doctors taking care of you, including your obstetrician, an experienced breast surgeon, and a medical oncologist. In addition, it may be necessary for a radiation oncologist to be involved.

How is a biopsy done if the doctor finds a suspicious lump in my breast while I am pregnant?
As with nonpregnant women, a prompt biopsy is essential to establish a diagnosis of breast cancer. Breast biopsy under local anesthesia is safe any time during pregnancy.

Should I have a bone scan?
This is a difficult decision to make. Under most circumstances, a bone scan will not be done because of the danger to the fetus from radiation exposure. However, if there is evidence that suggests you may have bone metastases, there are some ways of doing a bone scan with decreased radiation exposure to the fetus.

Will estrogen and progesterone receptor tests be done?
Very few studies have been done on this question. So it is not clear whether estrogen and progesterone receptor tests taken during pregnancy are as valid a predictor as they are in nonpregnant breast cancer patients.

Should I terminate my pregnancy if breast cancer is detected?
The types of biologic changes that occur during pregnancy—high output of hormones like estrogen and prolactin—are known to favor breast tumor growth. However, there have been several small studies that show that having an abortion does not change the course of your breast cancer nor does it improve your survival rates. Breast cancer has never been known to spread across the placenta to the fetus.

Will I be able to have a healthy baby?
Breast cancer does not seem to affect the developing fetus.

Can I have an operation for breast cancer while I am pregnant?

Most doctors will recommend mastectomy during the first six or seven months of your pregnancy. Later in your pregnancy, lesser surgery may be recommended, with your radiation treatment delayed until after your delivery. Radiation poses hazards to the baby and its use is discouraged during pregnancy.

Will I have general anesthesia for my operation?

You probably will, particularly if you are having a mastectomy. Studies have found that it is safe for you to have general anesthesia after your first trimester, so long as the usual precautions are taken to compensate for the normal changes that occur to your body functions during pregnancy.

Will I be able to have chemotherapy treatment while I am pregnant?

Chemotherapy is hazardous to the development of the baby during the first three months. Therefore, chemotherapy should be avoided at that time, if possible. If this is not feasible, then your doctor needs to decide whether treatment can be safely postponed until the second trimester or later. Studies show that single and combination chemotherapy can be given during the second and third trimester with a very low risk of fetal damage, although other side effects such as premature labor may be a risk. However, many doctors feel that chemotherapy should be delayed until after delivery. Your doctor may also recommend an early induced delivery or a cesarean delivery. You and your doctor need to discuss the advantages and disadvantages of each choice.

What if advanced local disease or metastatic breast cancer is discovered early in my pregnancy?

Advanced local disease or metastatic breast cancer in nonpregnant women is usually treated with both chemotherapy and radiation therapy. As a pregnant woman, you will need to think about whether or not you wish to end the pregnancy in order to begin the treatment. Although there is no evidence that termination of the pregnancy improves the outcome for breast cancer patients, it does permit standard aggressive treatment to be given for advanced disease.

Can I breast feed if I am taking chemotherapy?

Probably not. This is another question you need to discuss with your doctors. Systemic chemotherapy drugs may reach significant levels in your milk, especially if you are being treated with cyclophosphamide or methotrexate or some hormonal drugs. In addition, if you are scheduled to have breast surgery after you deliver, it is safer if you have not been breast feeding. **Important:** Pregnant and breastfeeding women should not take tamoxifen.

Is there any special care that a pregnant woman needs during treatment?

There are several issues that are especially important for pregnant women with cancer:

- You may need to increase the amount of food you eat so that you can maintain the appropriate weight gain during your pregnancy.

- If nausea and vomiting are potential side effects, you may need to take antinausea medicine. Your doctor will need to determine which medicines are appropriate to control it.

- You need to make sure you are getting good dental care and oral hygiene to prevent oral infections.

- You will need to pay greater attention to constipation, since this is a problem associated with both pregnancy and some chemotherapeutic drugs.

- If infection or hemorrhage are potential side effects, you will need to be especially watchful.

Will my delivery be specially timed if I am taking chemotherapy?

The doctor will time your delivery so that your blood counts are not dangerously low, thus putting you at risk. Following delivery, the doctor will reassess your treatment, particularly if it was planned to avoid risks to the fetus.

Are there any support groups for women with breast cancer who are pregnant?

There is one group, called Pregnant with Cancer (www.pregnantwithcancer.org) that was started by three young women in Buffalo who were diagnosed with cancer while they were pregnant. The group, which is endorsed by the American Cancer Society, matches pregnant women with cancer to each other.

Follow-up After Breast Cancer

How often will I need to return for checkups following breast cancer?

Your doctor will tailor a follow-up schedule for you. Generally, the doctor will ask you to come back every three to six months for the first year and then every six to twelve months. After five years, you will probably have yearly visits. There is some discussion among doctors about whether it is necessary for patients with no symptoms to have bone scans and a chest x-ray yearly. However, it is important that you have a physical examination and mammogram every year.

Why are these checkups important?

You need to make sure you have the checkups to see whether or not your cancer has reappeared (or recurred, as the medical community says). Even when a tumor in the breast appears to have been completely removed or destroyed, the disease sometimes returns because undetected cancer cells have remained in the area after treatment or because the disease had already spread before treatment. Most of the recurrences, about 60 percent, happen within the first three years after your first treatment. Another 20 percent happen within the next two years with 20 percent happening in the later years. It is important that you continue to be checked by the doctor on a regular schedule.

Questions to Ask Your Doctor About Follow-up Exams

- **How often will I need to be checked and to whom will I go for checkups? What kind of tests will be done then?**

- **Who will be in charge of my follow-up care? Will I have to go to more than one doctor?**

- **What kinds of tests will I need during my follow-up exam? Can they be done at the same time as my visit with you?**

- **Will I need a mammogram?**

- **Should I be doing breast self exam? Can you show me what to look for?**

- **What symptoms should I be checking for between examinations with you?**

- **Are there any specific symptoms or problems I should report to you?**

What kind of doctor will be doing the follow-up exams?

There are differing opinions on this issue. Studies are showing that a primary doctor can provide follow-up care for breast cancer patients as well as the specialists. Who does your follow-up will depend on decisions made by you and the doctors who have given your treatment as well as on your health care plan. You probably have had treatment with several doctors—a surgeon for your original operation, a plastic surgeon for breast reconstruction, a radiation oncologist for radiation therapy, and a medical oncologist for chemotherapy. You need an agreement among the team as to who is your lead doctor, how you can alternate visits (so you don't have to see multiple doctors), and how the results of the tests will be shared and discussed among the different specialties.

STAGE OF CANCER TREATED	SUGGESTED CHECKUPS
In situ: **Lobular or Ductal**	Medical history and physical every 6 to 12 months for 5 years, then once every year. Yearly mammogram. If taking tamoxifen, yearly pelvic exam.
Stages I–IV	History and physical exam every 4 to 6 months for 2 years; every 6 months for next 3 years, then yearly.
After Lumpectomy	Mammogram of treated breast every 12 months after radiation treatment, then mammography of both breasts every 12 months.
After Mastectomy	Mammogram of remaining breast every 12 months.
If Taking Tamoxifen	Pelvic exam every 12 months.
If Recurrence is Suspected	Blood and chemical tests; chest x-ray; bone scan; x-rays of bones with symptoms or bones positive on bone scan; CT or MRI of areas with symptoms; biopsy of recurrence, if possible.

Is there anything special I should look for between these checkups?

Call your doctor if you have the following problems: pain in your breast, shoulder, hip, lower back or pelvis; changes in your breast or in your scar such as lumps, thickenings, redness or swelling; loss of weight or appetite; a persistent hoarseness or cough; nausea, vomiting, diarrhea, or heartburn that lasts for several days; changes in your menstrual cycle or flow; dizziness, blurred vision, severe or frequent headaches, or trouble walking; or digestive problems that seem unusual or that do not go away. Remember, that these symptoms can be caused by many other things, such as the flu, a common cold, menopause, or arthritis. They are not necessarily signs that the cancer has returned, but you need to report them to your doctor so that an accurate diagnosis can be made.

Why should I continue to do a monthly breast self exam?

Monthly breast self-examination is particularly important after you have had breast cancer because you have a greater chance of getting cancer in the other breast. You need to do breast self-examination every month no matter what kind of treatment you have had. To do it effectively, you need to learn what is normal for you now. Ask your doctor or nurse to help you learn what to expect and how to perform the examination. If you have had a breast removed, you need to understand the scar area and what to look for. If you have had breast reconstruction, you need to feel carefully around the implant and under your arm. If you have had radiation, you need to understand the different feeling of the breast tissue itself. You need to report any changes to your doctor.

Recurrence

What is meant by a local recurrence?
A local recurrence is when the cancer returns only in the breast area. If the disease returns in another part of the body, it is called metastatic breast cancer or distant disease.

Where is breast cancer most likely to spread?
The lungs, bone, and liver are the areas where breast cancer is most likely to spread. Other possible sites include the kidneys, ovaries, brain, pituitary gland, adrenal glands, and thyroid gland.

Can breast cancer that comes back be treated?
Breast cancer that recurs locally can often be treated and, in some instances, can be cured. However, if it comes back in another part of the body, it usually cannot be cured, although many women have lived for many years following their recurrence.

What will my treatment choices be?
Your choice of treatment depends on your hormone receptor levels at the time of your recurrence, the kind of treatment you had before and your response to that treatment, the length of time from first treatment to when the cancer came back, whether your recurrence is local or widespread, and whether you still have menstrual periods, and other factors. The treatments may be radiation, surgery, chemotherapy, or hormonal. You should consider going into one of the ongoing clinical trials testing newly developed chemotherapy and biologic agents, bone marrow transplants, or peripheral stem cell support in Phase II studies. (Call the Cancer Information Service at 1–800–4–CANCER to get information on these studies.) There is more information on clinical trials in Chapter 11, New Advances and Investigational Treatments.

Will I have pain with recurrent breast cancer?
It depends on where it recurs. If you have pain, there are several treatments that can be used. You may be given pain medication, or you may be given radiation therapy if the pain is due to bone metastases. One recent development

for treating pain from bone metastases is Strontium–89 (Metastron) which is given on an outpatient basis in a single intravenous injection and provides relief which usually lasts an average of six months. More information on Strontium–89 can be found in Chapter 26, When Cancers Recur or Metastasize. Further detailed information on pain is in Chapter 27, Living With Cancer.

What are the experiences of other cancer patients in dealing with recurrence?

We have been told by many cancer survivors that recurrence is their greatest fear. When recurrence does happen, most people deal with it in much the same way as they did their first bout with the disease. However, many feel more upset about their recurrence than they were with their original diagnosis. This may be because many are sicker, or feel they have less support from their families. Some also feel angry about their treatment choices. Some think that because the cancer has come back they are going to die. Some women say that they find it hard to talk about recurrence with their spouses and family members but are able to talk about it with people outside of their families. There is more information on this subject in Chapter 26, When Cancers Recur or Metastasize.

Is there any information on what recurrence means to the spouse and family of the patient?

Recurrence is very difficult on the families of patients. Some feel angry and fearful. Others talk about the injustice of the recurrence and express feelings of grief, as well as concern with coping and with the impact that this event has on the family.

Is it usual to feel that your doctor thinks you have more family support than you have?

Many patients have noted this fact. They feel that their doctors and nurses assumed they had adequate support from their families and that they were coping better than they actually were. They also felt that their doctors presumed they had more knowledge about the disease than they actually did.

If I have had breast cancer, am I at higher risk for getting other kinds of cancer?

Women who have had breast cancer are at higher risk for getting cancers of the endometrium, ovary, and colon. You are also at higher risk for getting cancer in the other breast.

**If I have had radiation therapy, am I at an even higher
risk for developing a new cancer in the opposite breast?**
Having breast cancer in the first breast puts you at higher risk for developing it in the opposite breast, compared to women without the disease. Radiation treatment for breast cancer—which can cure breast cancer—adds a little, but not very much to that risk. A study by the National Cancer Institute showed that fewer than three percent of the second primary breast cancers that occurred in women diagnosed with breast cancer between 1935 and 1982 could be attributed to radiation therapy administered five years or more previously. The small increased risk of cancer in the opposite breast due to radiation therapy occurred only in women who were treated when they were under 45 years of age. If you are under 45 years of age and having radiation treatment, talk to the radiation oncologist about what steps will be taken to minimize radiation exposure of the opposite breast during treatment.

Web Pages to Check Out

www.cancer.gov: For general up-to-date information, and for clinical trials.

www.cancer.org: For general up-to-date information and community resources.

www.breastcancer.org: Best site for general information.

www.komen.org: Breast cancer–related information.

www.y-me.org: Information and support for people with breast cancer.

www.r2tech.com/sit: To see if your facility is using ImageChecker, the computer program that gives more accurate views of suspicious areas in the breast, log on to the manufacturer's Web site.

www.cancer.org or **www.BreastDoctor.com:** Information on sentinal node biopsy.

www.healthpages.com: Information on location of mammography clinics, approved centers, costs, comparisons.

www.pregnantwithcancer.org: For pregnant breast cancer patients.

www.breastcancer.org: Lymphadema.

www.cancercare.org: Support groups.

www.youngsurvival.org: Young Survival Coalition. Phone: 1–877–YSC–1011.

Also see Chapter 2, Searching for Answers on the Web, for more information.

Books You May Want to Read

A Breast Cancer Journey, Your Personal Guidebook. American Cancer Society, 2001.

Cancer Patient's Workbook. Joanie Willis. New York: DK (DorlingKindersley Publishing, Inc.), 2001.

Dr. Susan Love's Breast Book. Susan M. Love, MD, Addison-Wesley, 2000.

Fourteen

PROSTATE CANCER AND OTHER MALE CANCERS

After getting a diagnosis of a high PSA, many men immediately decide that the only solution is to have a total prostatectomy. They want the cancer gone. But it's not as straightforward as that. First of all, the PSA test is not the simple definitive test it is sometimes advertised to be. You need to fully understand the ramifications of your PSA test, the nature of prostate cancer, as well as the consequences of each treatment before making any decisions.

YOUR PSA IS not normal. You've heard all the controversies about the blood test (prostate specific antigen, or PSA for short) for detecting prostate cancer early, but you haven't paid too much attention. Now, it's happened to you and you need some facts.

You have no symptoms, no urinary difficulties, no warnings. You went for a routine check up and were told your PSA is abnormal, which means you may have cancer. You will have to make some very critical medical decisions.

The best advice we can give is:

- **Don't be in a hurry to make a decision.**

- **Don't do anything until you understand what your PSA reading means, the implications of possible treatments, and options you might consider. Have a second PSA done to confirm the reading.**

- **Learn about all your choices.**

- **Keep in mind that some decisions are irreversible.**

You've probably been raised to believe that when it comes to health, the doctor knows best. Taking matters into your own hands may violate everything you've been taught. However, it's important in the case of a prostate cancer diagnosis, that you study the whole picture and make a decision based on the real facts (rather than the scare of the word "cancer") and your own lifestyle and beliefs. Do your homework and get comfortable with all the pros and cons before you decide.

Over the past few years, a dramatic evolution in the detection of prostate cancer has occurred because of the use of the PSA test and ultrasound techniques. That's the good news.

The bad news is that in many cases, even when these techniques are used in a competent manner, doctors are still unable to distinguish individual patients whose cancers will not progress from those whose cancers will eventually grow and spread. Furthermore, it is no secret that top experts still cannot agree on what is the best and most effective treatment for prostate cancer.

The ramifications of the PSA blood test can take you on a rollercoaster ride of decisions that can drastically change your way of life. The possible aftereffects of the various courses of treatment available are not always clear to most men. There are many ifs, ands, and buts that you need to weigh very carefully before you decide on what is right for you.

With new techniques available for detection and treatment, men have more choices than ever before, some of which are controversial. Because of the number of options, decision-making can be very difficult. Gathering information, studying and digesting the facts, and talking with doctors from different disciplines are important, intelligent, and essential steps to take before making a decision. Treat this information gathering the way you treat buying a new car—check out all the options before you make a decision.

NOTE: We often hear people mispronounce the word prostate, adding an "r" in the last syllable. The correct pronunciation is "pros-tate," without the "r" in the second syllable.

THINGS YOU SHOULD KNOW
ABOUT YOUR PROSTATE

- Prostate problems don't always mean prostate cancer. Eight out of ten times, the problems can be traced to other causes.

- Most men have at least one bout of prostatitis (inflammation of the prostate) in their lifetimes.

- Men who have acute prostatitis have an abrupt onset of fever, pain at the base of the penis, and painful urination.

- With chronic prostatitis you may have low-grade, recurring infections that cause discomfort. Bacterial and nonbacterial forms of chronic prostatitis require different treatments.

- The prostate also becomes enlarged as the result of hormonal changes associated with aging. This condition is known as benign prostatic hypertrophy or BPH. By the age of 60, prostate enlargement is found in almost all men. When this happens, it may narrow the passageway for urine flow, causing a variety of symptoms such as difficulty in starting the flow of urine, decreased force of the urinary stream, dribbling of urine and increased frequency of urination. Occasionally, it may lead to a complete stopping of urine flow.

- Early prostate cancer usually has no symptoms. Today, it is generally first detected by a PSA test—a blood test that detects prostate-specific antigen, a protein produced by prostate glands.

- Early detection also includes a digital rectal examination that the doctor performs as part of a physical examination. Men should have a digital rectal exam each year after the age of 40.

- Of 100 men 50 and over who are screened, 85 will have normal PSA levels (4 ng/ml or below). In the remaining 15 men, only three will have biopsies that show cancer.

- Work is underway, using the techniques of protein profiling and computer-based artificial intelligence, to devise a new blood test that would more accurately detect prostate cancer at an early stage with fewer false positives that lead to unnecessary biopsies. There also are several new tests being worked on to determine the aggressiveness of tumors.

- Prostate cancer requires treatment depending on the stage of the disease, the age of the patient, and a full understanding of the treatments available.

- At the time prostate cancer is diagnosed, 75 percent of prostate cancers are localized (Stages I and II), 15 percent have spread to the area near the prostate and 11 percent have metastasized to other parts of the body.

- No treatment for prostate cancer is totally free of the possibility of some sexual or incontinence problems. It is important that treatment be discussed with, and done under the guidance of a skilled, experienced urologist.

- Several new treatments are in clinical trials, including new methods of surgery and of delivering radiation and the use of neutron and proton radiation.

Has Agent Orange been associated with prostate cancer?

Agent Orange, a mixture of herbicides used during the Vietnam War mainly to defoliate forest trees, and other herbicides used during the Vietnam War have been associated with prostate cancer, but not as strongly as with some other cancers. It is classified in the second category: limited/suggestive evidence of an association. However, if you are a Vietnam veteran and have been diagnosed with prostate cancer, you should qualify for VA disability compensation and the special access to medical care that the VA has offered to Vietnam veterans for health problems from Agent Orange exposure.

What is the PSA test?

The PSA test is a blood test that measures prostate specific antigen, a protein produced by the prostate gland. First approved in 1986, the PSA test was used to monitor prostate cancer patients' response to treatments. Its success led to its use as a screening tool and the number of new cases of prostate cancer rose dramatically. This rise has now leveled off, especially in the elderly. The National Cancer Institute notes that the issue of screening men who have no symptoms for prostate cancer by using the PSA test and ultrasound in addition to the digital rectal examination is controversial, because there is currently a lack of evidence that screening will actually reduce deaths from prostate cancer. In addition, there is no agreement on which treatment is best for local disease, and treatments used have serious side effects.

Are there any other tests that measure prostate specific antigen?

At present, the PSA test is the most useful diagnostic tool in prostate cancer, but some other screening methods have been studied. One such method, sometimes used when the PSA level rises steadily, is PSA velocity. Another is PSA density, which compares the size of the prostate with the PSA readings. A man with a large prostate gland can expect to have a higher PSA than a man with a small gland. Another screening test is HK2, an enzyme in the

WHO IS AT RISK FOR PROSTATE CANCER

Age	Risk increases with age, especially after age 50. More than 80 percent of all prostate cancers are diagnosed in men over age 65.
Race	Black men in parts of the U.S. have the highest incidence of prostate cancer—70 percent more often in African-American men than Caucasians.
Genetics	Increased risk if first-degree relative has had prostate cancer.
Diet	High fat intake suspected.
Occupation	Working with cadmium, zinc, rubber, dewaxing process in oil refining indicated in studies.
Other	Obesity and previous bouts with sexually transmitted diseases. Agent Orange exposure.

PSA family that is believed to be responsible for converting free PSA to active PSA. The higher the percentage of free PSA in the bloodstream, the less likely the chance of prostate cancer. Other studies are being done with pro-PSA, B-PSA, and protein profiling, but none of these are presently in everyday use. Gene studies are also being conducted which may in the future serve as clinical markers for prostate cancer.

What are considered to be normal PSA levels?
Researchers are continuing to study this question. It appears that normal levels may differ according to age. Recent studies suggest the following age-specific PSA levels:

- Age 71–80: 6.5 ng/ml
- Age 61–70: 4.5 ng/ml
- Age 51–60: 3.5 ng/ml
- Age 41–50: 2.4 ng/ml

In addition, an annual rise in PSA level of about 0.04 ng/ml in men over age 60 is not considered abnormal. In broad terms, many physicians feel that a PSA of less than 10 in men aged 55 to 79 is considered a low risk. A 10 to 19.9 is considered an intermediate risk and a 20 or over is considered a high risk.

Important note: PSA blood tests should be done *before* cystoscopy or needle biopsy, because these procedures may *raise the PSA levels*. The digital exam by itself does not significantly increase serum PSA, but cystoscopy and needle biopsy may. Decisions about prostate cancer should never be made on the basis of one PSA reading.

How often should a man be checked to see if there are signs of prostate cancer?

A digital rectal examination should be performed every year on all males over the age of 50. The American Cancer Society is also recommending that a PSA test be performed yearly on men 50 years of age and over. The National Cancer Institute's early detection guidelines do not include routine PSA screening for men without symptoms. Those in high risk groups, such as African-Americans or those whose family members have a predisposition to prostate cancer, are advised to begin the yearly testing at 40 or 45.

What are some of the issues involved in the controversy over using the PSA test as an early detection tool?

A number of issues and a number of "unknowns" are involved. Like all medical tests, PSA is not foolproof. It can indicate a cancer when none exists. However, it is felt that it can increase the ability to find localized cancers with further testing. According to the National Cancer Institute, much remains unknown about the interpretation of PSA levels, the test's ability to discriminate cancer from benign prostate conditions, and the best course of action following a finding of elevated PSA, especially in younger men. Since in some cases, men with suspicious PSAs will receive treatment that may cause impotence and incontinence, the concern is that PSA screening may result in treatments without any benefit. It is important to remember that decisions should not be made on the basis of a single PSA reading.

What are the symptoms of cancer of the prostate?

Symptoms which should not be ignored include a weak or interrupted flow of urine, inability to urinate or difficulty in starting urination, need to urinate frequently (especially at night), blood in the urine, urine flow that is not easily stopped, painful or burning urination, and continuing pain in the back, pelvis or hips. These symptoms are often the same symptoms that indicate other prostatic problems, but they are symptoms which should be checked by the doctor who can detect the difference between a cancerous and non cancerous enlargement of the prostate. **Be aware, however, that early prostate cancer often does not cause any symptoms, which is why regular digital exams are recommended.**

SYMPTOMS OF PROSTATE CANCER

Small prostate cancers often do not cause any symptoms. When symptoms do occur, they may include:

- Frequent urination, especially at night.
- Trouble starting or holding back urinating.
- A weak or interrupted urine flow.
- Pain or burning feeling during urination.
- Blood in the urine.
- Continuing pain in lower back, pelvis, or upper thighs.

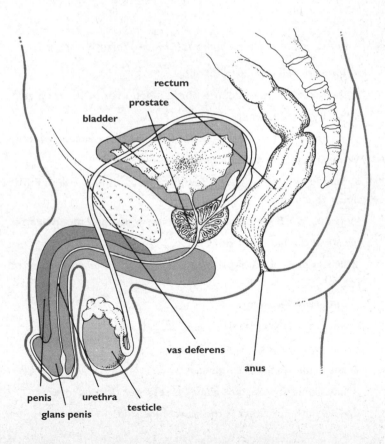

Male reproductive organs (ILLUSTRATION BY DOLORES BEGO)

What kind of doctor is best for treating prostate problems?
A urologist, a doctor who specializes in treating diseases of the urinary tract and the male reproductive system, is best qualified to determine whether symptoms are caused by prostate cancer, BPH, or some other condition such as an infection or stones in the prostate. This doctor will have the necessary skills, equipment and experience to help you make the decisions that will be facing you. **Don't leave the decisions to a general physician or even to the urologist alone.** You need to hear the pros and cons of the different treatments from doctors who deal with prostate cancer every day. A visit with a radiation oncologist will be needed for you to understand whether or not you are a candidate for radiation. If you are interested in investigating cryosurgery, you will need someone expert in that field. Ask your general physician to help you get appointments with several specialists you wish to see. If you belong to a health maintenance organization (HMO) or an other managed care plan, check to make sure which physicians you can see and what coverage you have, especially for second opinions and additional testing.

Questions to Ask If the Doctor Thinks You Have Prostate Cancer

- **What sort of lump did you feel?**
- **Is the prostate enlarged or is there a definite nodule or ridge?**
- **Where was it located?**
- **Were the PSA (prostate-specific antigen) test results elevated?**
- **What was the PSA reading?**
- **Would it be wise to wait a few months and do another PSA before doing the biopsy?**
- **Was the PSA done before or after the digital and blood exams?**
- **How will the biopsy be done??**
- **Will you be rechecking the extent of the tumor with an ultrasound probe?**
- **What is my Gleason grade?**
- **What is the DNA status?**
- **What type of cancer is it?**
- **What is the stage of the disease?**
- **What size is my prostate gland? Is it larger than normal?**
- **Where in the prostate is the cancer located?**

Questions to Ask Before Deciding on Treatment for Prostate Cancer

- What type of treatment do you suggest?

- Why do you feel this treatment is better for me than other possible treatments?

- Are there other treatments that will achieve the same results?

- Is it possible for me to have no treatment at this time, but to have you follow me closely to see if there are future changes?

- What are the benefits and drawbacks of each kind of treatment?

- What are the drawbacks to having radiation or radiation seeding instead of surgery, or surgery instead of radiation?

- Is radiation seeding or cryosurgery a possibility for my condition?

- Will radiation be prescribed following surgery?

- How often do you do this type of surgery or radiation?

- Can I have radiation (either internal or external) and later, if it doesn't work, have surgery to remove the prostate? Is it worth the risk?

- How extensive will the surgery or radiation be?

- Where will the scar be?

- How will the treatment affect my sex life?

- Can you do nerve-sparing surgery so that I will not be impotent? How successful has this surgery been in your patients to date?

- If I lose my ability to function sexually, what are my alternatives?

- Is cryosurgery a possibility?

- Do you recommend hyperthermia?

- Do you recommend having hormonal therapy before doing surgery to shrink the tumor?

- Will treatment make me incontinent? How long will incontinence continue? Will incontinence be permanent? Will exercises help me alleviate incontinence?

- Will you be doing extensive lymph node dissection to check for cancer spread? Will doing the dissection change your treatment plans? What are the side effects in your experience?

- What restrictions will there be on my activities after treatment?

- When can I return to normal activities after this treatment?

Questions You Should Ask Yourself

- Have I checked fully with the doctor about all my options and the risks involved?

- Have I considered each option with my age, my present state of health, my lifestyle and my mental attitude in mind?

- Am I prepared to accept the fact that treatment to remove my prostate may leave me incontinent, impotent or both? How will I live with these consequences?

- Do I want to get another opinion before proceeding with the treatment this doctor recommends?

- Do I want to get a second opinion from a surgeon or urologist if I originally saw a radiation oncologist or see a radiation oncologist if I saw a surgeon or urologist?

- Can I live with watchful waiting? Or do I need to have something done right now?

What does the prostate look like?

The prostate gland is about the size of a walnut. It also is designed somewhat like a walnut with sections bisected down the center by the urethra, which connects the bladder to the opening of the penis. Located below the bladder and in front of the rectum, it is divided into glandular zones—the peripheral, the central, and the transitional. The urethra, the tube that emerges from the bladder and carries urine, is surrounded by the prostate. The prostate gland is close to the front wall of the rectum, which is why it is possible for the physician to feel it with his finger during a rectal examination. Most prostate cancers are found in the peripheral zone.

What is the role of the prostate gland?

The prostate is a male sex gland, part of a man's reproductive system. Its major function is to provide the majority of the seminal fluid which nourishes the sperm. The prostate needs male hormones to function. During ejaculation, the prostate gland squeezes fluid into the urethra to aid in the transport and nourishment of sperm.

How does the prostate gland develop?

The prostate gland weighs only a few grams at birth. At puberty it undergoes further growth and reaches adult size by about age 20. A second spurt of growth starts in most men at about age 40—and this may cause problems, since the growth will sometimes compress the remaining normal gland, leading to urinary obstruction. The average size of the prostate gland is about 30 grams. Many grow to be much larger—100 to 200 grams. A prostate gland that is larger than normal may produce PSA that is higher than average.

Who usually gets cancer of the prostate?
The risk of developing cancer of the prostate increases with age. Cancer of the prostate usually occurs in men over 55 years of age. The incidence varies from country to country. African-American males have the highest incidence. Japanese-American men have the lowest. Statistics show that men with relatives who have had prostate cancer are more than three times as likely to develop the disease. There is some evidence that workers who have been exposed to cadmium and zinc, rubber, or the dewaxing process of oil refining may be at higher risk for prostate cancer. Those who have had past bouts with sexually transmitted diseases are also at increased risk.

Does prostate cancer run in families?
Scientists have confirmed the existence of a gene for prostate cancer. Their research indicates that 65 percent of men diagnosed with prostate cancer before the age of 56 develop cancer because they are carriers of the prostate cancer gene. They also estimate that 97 percent of men who carry this gene will develop prostate cancer by age 85. A test for the presence of the prostate cancer gene has not yet been found but work continues in many scientific laboratories to uncover the mysteries of the gene. In addition, men who have fathers or brothers who have had prostate cancer diagnosed before the age of 60 are more likely to develop prostate cancer, and should be tested before age 50. They are the men who have the highest incidence of prostate cancer and tend to get it earlier. It is not yet known whether all of these men carry the inherited gene or whether similar lifestyles have a role to play.

What causes prostate cancer?
It is believed that changes in the sex hormones have an influence on prostate cancer. Hormones are required for the normal growth and development of the prostate and men who have been castrated almost never develop prostate cancer. Prostate cancer can be induced in mice by prolonged administration of testosterone. Testosterone levels are higher in patients with prostate cancer than in those with other prostate problems. However, doctors cannot explain why one person gets prostate cancer and another does not. The effects of diet are being studied. Some evidence suggests that a diet high in fat increases the risk of prostate cancer, but this link has not been proven. Other studies point to an increased risk to workers exposed to the metal cadmium during welding, electroplating, or making batteries. Rubber industry workers also appear to develop prostate cancer more often than is normal. Studies are also being conducted to determine whether benign prostatic

hyperplasia or a sexually transmitted virus increases the risk for prostate cancer.

Does testosterone replacement increase the risk of prostate cancer?

There seems to be some correlation between increasing the supply of the male hormone with an increased risk of prostate cancer, heart attacks and strokes. At the present time, no clinical trials have been done to determine the safety of testosterone replacement and none are planned because of the risks involved. Testosterone gels have only been approved by the Food and Drug Administration for treatment of hypogonadism (very low levels of testosterone), a condition that can result from genetic disorders, chemotherapy, radiation therapy or tumors. Unlike women, whose levels of estrogen drop dramatically at menopause, men have a slow, steady decline in testosterone—about ½ or one percent per year—starting at age 30. Any use of testosterone should be cautiously approached because of the potential risks involved. It is important to note that hormonal therapy given for treatment of prostate cancer, is designed to **lower** levels of testosterone. (See information under Hormone Treatment in this chapter.)

Is it true that men who have had vasectomies are more likely to develop prostate cancer?

There have been some studies that appear to point to the possibility that men who have had vasectomies may be at greater risk for prostate cancer as well as other studies that questioned these findings. An expert committee convened by the National Institutes of Health has found that the association, at most, is a small one. Further studies are needed to determine whether or not vasectomy is associated with prostate cancer in any way. In the meantime, screening for prostate cancer should not be any different for men who have had a vasectomy than for those who have not.

Testing for Prostate Cancer

How is the digital rectal exam done?

The doctor is able to feel the prostate gland with a rubber-gloved finger inserted through the anus. A cancerous lump feels hard, like a marble, in what is normally a fleshy gland. Though not the most dignified of examinations, the checking of the prostate gland so that any abnormality can be detected early, is an important part of any physical. The doctor will ask you to either bend from the hips with elbows on the examining table or on your knees. Some doctors prefer to have the buttocks elevated in the knee-chest position. In either case, the doctor will ask you to "bear down" as he inserts his finger. It is normal to experience sensations of having to urinate or defecate during the examination.

Is the PSA test a substitute for the digital rectal exam?
No. Many men wish they could skip the digital rectal exam and just have what seems to be the simpler blood tests. However, used alone, the PSA test does not diagnose prostate cancer. It is important to have the digital rectal exam because it gives the doctor the chance to feel whether or not there are lumps on the part of the prostate that can be felt.

What happens if the doctor finds I have an elevated PSA?
In most cases, the doctor will want to do further testing to determine why the reading is high. An elevated PSA does not always indicate that cancer is present. Thirty six percent of patients with nonmalignant tumors have a moderately elevated PSA. The presence of cancer can sometimes be confirmed by the removal of a small piece of prostate tissue for microscopic examination. In the past, a finger guided needle biopsy was used or a surgical procedure was required . Most doctors now will obtain a needle biopsy with ultrasound probes.

Is the PAP test used in prostate cancer?
The Prostate Acid Phosphatase (PAP) test was once a routine test used to measure a protein produced by prostate cells. Results of the test can be misleading, but it is still sometimes used to confirm widespread disease.

How is an ultrasound guided needle biopsy done?
The probe is placed in the rectum and bounces high-frequency sound waves into the prostate. The different densities between normal prostate tissue and cancer show up as shadows on the ultrasound image. The ultrasound probes are often able to discover cancerous tissue that is missed by a digital examination. The biopsy is then done using the ultrasound to guide the probe. Ultrasound images allow the surgeon to guide a springloaded device that fires a needle through the wall of the rectum into the prostate to capture bits of possibly cancerous tissue. The needle is withdrawn so the sample can be analyzed.

Does it hurt to have an ultrasound directed biopsy?
The device fires the needle so rapidly that it is virtually painless. Some 5 to 10 percent of patients feel a little ache when the gun is fired. There is no anesthesia or catheter and you can usually return home when the procedure is completed.

What is a ProstaScint Scan?
A ProstaScint Scan is similar to a bone scan. It uses low-level radioactive material that attaches only to prostate cells to find cancer that has spread beyond the prostate. This test may be ordered if the PSA level begins to rise

after treatment and other tests are not able to find the exact location of the recurrent cancer.

What tests are usually recommended when the doctor finds a problem with the prostate?

If the doctor feels any abnormality when doing a digital rectal exam or when the PSA level is above normal, other tests will have to be done. Ultrasound guided needle biopsies are usually done so that samples of the tissue can be examined. Blood tests and urine studies will usually be ordered. The doctor may order other tests such as CAT scans, bone scans and chest films as well as kidney-function tests, intravenous pyelogram, and lymphography to determine the extent of disease.

Are there any new methods of detecting prostate cancer without doing a biopsy?

Dynamic contrast enhanced MRI, also called DCE-MRI, 3TP MRI, or three-time-point MRI, uses high resolution imaging, a contrast material (low molecular weight Gd-based extracellular contrast agent) and data from three strategically chosen time points (before contrast material given, two minutes and six minutes after) to produce color maps of the tumor. 3TP MRI helps doctors pinpoint exactly where the cancer is and differentiate between benign and malignant disease. It is anticipated that this new method will offer a

TESTS THAT MAY BE USED TO DIAGNOSE PROSTATE CANCER

- Complete history and physical examination.
- Digital rectal examination.
- Ultrasound guided needle biopsies (samples of tissue taken from different areas of prostate and examined microscopically) or fine needle aspiration.
- CT scan (produces detailed cross-sectional images).
- MRI scan.
- Radionuclide bone scan (helps show if cancer has spread to bones).
- ProstaScint scan (attaches only to prostate cells to find if cancer has spread beyond prostate).
- Lymph node biopsy.
- Seminal vesicle biopsy.

standardized, reproducible technique for using MRI to diagnose breast and prostate cancer. This procedure is now in clinical trials.

Is contrast enhanced MRI used in any other way?
Contrast enhanced MRI, in combination with molecular tumor markers, is also being studied in clinical trials to see whether it can predict tumor response and disease-free survival in women with breast cancer who are getting adjuvant chemotherapy.

What type of cancer are most prostate cancers?
Over 95 percent of prostate cancers confined to the prostate gland are adenocarcinomas varying in appearance and differentiation. The remainder are usually squamous cell or sarcomas. Most are found in the posterior lobe and are usually multifocal (found in more than one spot).

Does where the cancer is located in the prostate make a difference?
The prostate is divided into three zones. Next to the urethra is the transitional zone. This is surrounded by a large shell of glandular tissue called the peripheral zone, where most cancers start. Surrounding the ejaculatory ducts is the central zone. Cancers in the peripheral or outer area are considered more serious. Cancers in the transitional or inner area are at lowest risk. If the cancer has penetrated the capsule and has gone into surrounding connective tissue, it will be categorized in a higher stage than one that is contained inside the capsule.

What features help to determine whether my prostate cancer is a more or less serious disease?
A number of different criteria will determine which prostate cancers are likely to be more serious. They include the volume or size, the Gleason grade, the pattern of growth, serum PSA, and the area where the cancer is located. All of these should be taken into account when making decisions about what treatment will be used.

Does my age make a difference in determining what treatment will be used?
Yes, it does. Younger men, who have no other serious illnesses, are more likely to die from their prostate cancers. On the other hand, older men, especially those with localized tumors, are less likely to suffer any real disabilities from their prostate cancer and more likely to die of other illnesses. Doctors usually treat younger men more aggressively, although some doctors are using watchful waiting for sexually-active younger men diagnosed with early-stage prostate cancer with low Gleason grades.

FACTORS THAT HELP DETERMINE TREATMENT

FACTOR	LESS SERIOUS	MORE SERIOUS
Tumor Size or Volume	Small	Large
Grade	Well differentiated	Moderate or poorly differentiated
Growth Pattern	Confined to prostate	Extra capsular or with positive margins
PSA level	Normal	Elevated
Age 40–49	under 2.5	over 2.5
Age 50–59	under 3.5	over 3.5
Age 60–69	under 4.5	over 4.5
Age 70–79	under 6.5	over 6.5
Location of Tumor	Inner area (transitional)	Outer area (peripheral)

What is the Gleason grade?

The Gleason grade is a method used by doctors to determine how close to normal the cells look when the tissue is examined under the microscope. Though the following may be hard for the layman to translate, the system recognizes the following five patterns of cells:

1. Closely packed, single, separate, round, uniform glands; well-defined tumor margin.

2. Single, separate, round, less uniform glands separated by stroma up to one gland diameter; tumor margin less well defined.

3. Single, separate, irregular glands of variable size; enlarged masses with cribriform or papillary pattern; poorly defined tumor margin.

4. Fused glands in mass with infiltrating cords, small glands with papillary, cribriform, or solid patterns; cells small, dark or hypernephroid (clear cells).

5. Few or no glands in background of masses with comedo pattern; cords or sheets of tumor cells infiltrating stroma.

How is the Gleason grade determined?

The grade is determined by assigning one number to the most prominent pattern of your cells and another to the secondary pattern and adding the two together. The total can be anywhere from 2 (1+1) to 10 (5+5).

What do the Gleason grades mean?

The grades measure differentiation—the medical term used to describe how closely cancer cells resemble their normal counterparts. Grades 2 to 4 indicate that the tumor is well differentiated, 5 to 7 indicate that it is moderately differentiated and 8 to 10 indicate that it is poorly differentiated.

What is meant by well differentiated?

Cancer cells are described as well differentiated when they look much like normal cells of the same type and are able to carry out some functions of normal cells. Poorly differentiated and undifferentiated tumor cells are disorganized and abnormal looking. As a general rule, the more the cells look like normal cells under the microscope, the slower growing they are. The greater the difference in the appearance of the cell from what is normal, the higher the number that is assigned on the Gleason grade.

What does the Gleason grade mean in terms of deciding on treatment?

Like the PSA and digital exam, the Gleason grade can be valuable in making a decision about the type of treatment chosen.

Are there other grading systems?

There have been some 30 grading systems proposed, but most have not been universally accepted. You may hear of a system based on the slight variations in the size of the nuclear structure of the cell that uses only three grades.

Grade 1 = Low grade. Slightly enlarged nuclei.
Grade 2 = Medium grade.
Grade 3 = High grade, loss of cell cohesion, large variation in size of nuclei.

MEANING OF GLEASON GRADES

Gleason 2, 3, 4	Most like normal cells. Well differentiated. Slow growing. Low probability of metastasis. Low grade.
Gleason 5, 6, 7	Can behave like normal cells or like aggressive cells. Moderately differentiated. Moderate probability of metastasis. Moderate grade.
Gleason 8, 9, 10	Least like normal cells. Poorly differentiated. High probability of metastasis. High grade.

What are the Partin tables?

The Partin tables were originally developed by a group of urologists at Johns Hopkins University in 1997 and are used as a guide to predicting the risk for a specific patient. Using PSA figures, clinical stage and Gleason score, the Partin tables attempt to measure:

1. The probability that the patient has completely organ-confined disease
2. The probability that the prostate cancer has extended into and perhaps through the capsule of the prostate
3. The probability that it has extended into his seminal vesicles
4. The probability that the cancer has spread into lymph nodes.

Although Partin tables can help the doctor guide you in making an informed decision when contemplating treatment, remember that these tables use statistical data to predict probable outcome. As is pointed out by Dr. Partin and his colleagues, the data offered in these tables are not definitive. The different risks can have a significant impact on how a doctor will offer to treat a prostate cancer patient and how a patient may wish to be treated.

Are there any other tests for prostate cancer?

A new test to determine the need for prostate biopsies, called serum proteomic patterns, is being perfected. This test, which can give results in 30 minutes, analyzes the patterns of proteins found in blood samples. It is still being evaluated but it is hoped that it will be used to determine the need for prostate biopsies in men with PSA levels from 2.5 to 10 ng/ml or who have abnormal digital rectal exams. A clinical trial is being conducted at the University of North Carolina Lineberger Comprehensive Cancer Center.

Is the grade of cancer similar to the stage of cancer?

No. They are two different measurements. Grade is used to describe how closely cancer cells resemble their normal counterparts. Stage (see Stage and Treatment charts which follow) takes into account the various components of what is known about your cancer and how far it has progressed so that the doctor can determine what treatment is most appropriate.

How is prostate cancer staged?

There are several classifications used to stage prostate cancer, including the TNM system, and systems that use the letters A to D or the numbers I to IV. The one most commonly used is the Stage I to Stage IV system.

What is the TNM system?

The TNM method is an international system that can be used to compare the results of treatment worldwide. It uses Stages I to IV based on the assessment of three components:

T = size of tumor and level of invasion

N = lymph node involvement, size, number

M = metastases

What is the Jewett system of staging?

This system uses the letters A through D to indicate approximately the same categories as the I to IV system. So if your doctor refers to your cancer as a Stage A1, you will understand that he is using the Jewett system.

How curable is cancer of the prostate?

Cancer of the prostate may be cured when it is localized and frequently responds to treatment for long periods of time even when it has spread beyond the prostate.

Does cancer of the prostate sometimes spread?

Cancer cells can break away from the original tumor in the prostate, spread through the bloodstream and lymphatic system, and form tumors in other parts of the body. When cancer of the prostate spreads outside the prostate itself, it often shows up in nearby lymph nodes or lymph glands. Prostate cancer can also spread to the bones, liver, lung, bladder, and other organs. When cancer spreads from the prostate to other parts of the body, often to the bone, the disease is identified as metastatic prostate cancer rather than bone cancer, liver cancer, etc. Usually the PSA test is used to determine if the cancer has spread. To determine if there are other signs of cancer, the doctor may order a CT or CAT scan to check for swollen lymph nodes, or an MRI to check the prostate and nearby lymph nodes. A bone scan may be ordered since rapid growth in bones may be a sign of spreading cancer, although it can also be the result of other bone problems. A chest x-ray may also be done to check the lungs.

What is the role of testosterone in prostate cancer?

The normal prostate is dependent upon circulating androgens, principally testosterone, to function. Prostate cancer is also dependent on the male sex hormone, testosterone, which can stimulate its growth. That is the reason why hormone therapy decreasing the stimulation of testosterone is sometimes prescribed to curb the cancer.

UNDERSTANDING YOUR TREATMENT OPTIONS

What is the best treatment for prostate cancer?

Even the top physicians in urology cannot agree on which method of treatment is best for prostate cancer. The latest information from the National Cancer Institute noted that **radical prostatectomy and radiation therapy apparently were equally effective during the first ten years in treating tumors limited to the prostate.** Studies that are available do seem to indicate that after ten years there is a higher incidence of recurrent or persistent tumor as measured by PSA and local progression after radiation treatment than there is with surgery. However, there are still questions as to whether the men treated in these studies were at comparable stages of disease, since prostatectomies are often reserved for those with the smallest cancers confined to the prostate.

Results of studies comparing radical prostetectomy, internal radiation, and watchful waiting for early stage prostate cancer are just beginning to appear. The data seem to confirm that the treatments give similar results, but the follow-up period has not been long enough to make a definitive statement. Each method—as well as many of the newer and less well-tested treatments—has its advantages and disadvantages. What you need to untangle and determine is which method best suits the way you choose to live. Your quality of life is an important factor. There are advantages and disadvantages to each treatment, but at least there are treatments available to you to control your cancer, even though you may not be totally happy with some of the consequences of some of them (also see Chapter 5, Cancer Controversies).

What are the most common treatments for prostate cancer?

The most commonly used treatments are:

- **Prostatectomy:** The complete removal of the prostate in an operation. (Usually used for patients in good health who are under the age of 70.)

- **External Radiation:** A linear accelerator is used to deliver radiation to the prostate area—usually given five times a week for seven weeks.

- **Hormonal Manipulation:** Removal or suppression of the male hormone, testosterone. Either a suppressor hormone (Lupron) is injected or the testicles are removed (orchiectomy). May be used prior to other treatment for removal of prostate or as treatment when cancer has advanced.

- **Watchful waiting:** Used when cancer cannot be felt but is signaled by other testing, or for older men who have decided that quality of life is more important than the statistically short time that may be gained through aggressive therapy.

You have many more possible choices for treatment than you might have been led to believe. Some have been used for many years. Others have not been tested fully but are being explored. Many men are deciding to try some of the more experimental methods because they fear the consequences of some of the standard treatments. No method is entirely risk free. Some methods have been used longer than others, so the results cover a longer period of time. The biggest problem, if you have early stage prostate cancer, is that it is difficult for your doctor to know whether or not your cancer will progress and metastasize. This dilemma is the principal reason for the differences of opinion among doctors.

Some other treatments still considered in the testing stage include:

- **Radiation Seeding (Internal Radiation or Brachytherapy):** Radioactive seeds (palladium, iridium) are implanted in the prostate.

- **Cryosurgery:** Use of freezing techniques to destroy the prostate.

- **Chemotherapy:** Has not proven to be successful in the past, but a combination of drugs as well as chemotherapy implants are in clinical trials. Not used for early stage cancers.

- **Hyperthermia:** Use of heating techniques. Presently being studied in various parts of the world.

- **Other:** Other less conventional and more controversial and experimental approaches, including nutritional approaches which have not been clinically verified or tested, are being used.

Can the doctor tell from a biopsy whether my cancer is likely to be the type that spreads?

Prostate cancers show wide variations in terms of how likely they are to spread. If the cancer cells closely resemble normal microscopic prostate cells, the tumor is usually considered to be "low grade." If the cancer cells invade neighboring tissue structures such as nerves or blood vessels, the tumor is designated as "high grade" to indicate a more aggressive form of prostate cancer. What is most difficult about prostate cancer is that many tumors remain small and never cause any problems, but some break away from the prostate and appear in the bones. However, researchers say they do not know for certain which will spread and which can be ignored— which poses a difficult dilemma for patients and doctors. The doctor will use the biopsy findings along with other studies to reach a decision about treatment.

WHAT TREATMENT DO DOCTORS PREFER?

In 1988 a survey was done of 304 urologists, radiation oncologists, and oncologists in the United States, Canada, and Great Britain. Each one was asked what treatment he would choose if he was 67 years of age, diagnosed with cancer confined to the prostate and had moderately differentiated prostate cancer. Of the American urologists (whose specialty is surgery), 79 percent said they would have surgery, while 92 percent of the radiologists chose radiation. Among the British doctors four percent chose surgery, 44 percent chose radiation and 52 percent chose watchful waiting. This survey is dated, but it is interesting.

What type of cancer are most prostate cancers?

Over 95 percent of prostate cancers that are confined to the prostate gland are adenocarcinomas, which vary in appearance and differentiation. The remainder are usually squamous cell or sarcomas. Most are found in the posterior lobe and are usually multifocal.

If the cancer of the prostate is discovered in a very early stage should I risk the side effects of surgery or radiation or should I wait and see if the cancer progresses?

Unfortunately, there are not, at this time, foolproof guidelines, although many doctors feel it is safest to have radiation or surgery to remove the prostate. Research presently in progress assesses the benefits of various treatments. Treatment is not a guarantee against metastatic cancer, but seeks to reduce the risk, though by an uncertain amount. If cancer is discovered in the very early stages, one choice, with a full understanding of the risks, may be to wait and watch. These thoughts may be helpful:

- **If 70 to 75**, waiting and having frequent checkups is a treatment option.

- **If the cancer appears to be low-grade in appearance** when viewed under the microscope and clearly confined to the prostate, you may be advised to wait and watch. (One population-based study has shown excellent survival without any treatment in patients with well or moderately well-differentiated tumors clinically confined to the prostate, irrespective of age.)

- **If the cancer is too small to be felt with a digital rectal exam**, you may want to proceed slowly.

- **Important note:** In any of these cases, if no treatment is immediately recommended, it is important that you have frequent, regular digital examinations, PSA testing, and ultrasound follow-up to detect any changes as soon as they occur.

DECISION MAKING FACTORS

TYPE OF TREATMENT	WHAT IT MEANS	PROS AND CONS
Radical Prostatectomy. Approaches to surgery listed below are determined by physician. But it is important for you to understand what is being planned.	Removal of entire prostate including seminal vesicles and small cuff of attached bladder neck.	Considered a cure if cancer is localized to the prostate. Lymph nodes removed to determine if it has spread. If spread is detected, many surgeons do not continue with operation. High incidence of urinary incontinence and dribbling as well as erectile function loss.
Radical Retropubic Prostatectomy.	Most commonly used method. Open surgery through six-inch vertical incision in lower abdomen; often possible to preserve nerves that produce erection (see nerve-sparing prostatectomy).	Impotence (60–90 percent); incontinence (30–60 percent); difficulty urinating; best for large prostates; allows lymph node dissection for staging; fewer rectal injuries.
Radical Perineal Prostatectomy.	Surgery done through incision between anus and scrotum.	Good choice for heavier men; lymph nodes cannot be removed through same incision. Difficult to do nerve-sparing operation.
Nerve-sparing Prostatectomy.	Surgery performed with specific aim of preserving erectile function; often only nerve on side opposite cancer is spared to assure all cancer cells removed. Not always possible to spare potency.	If both nerves spared, may expose patient to risk of leaving cancer cells in area surrounding prostate. Impotence (30–60 percent). Must be done by an expert.

(continued)

DECISION MAKING FACTORS (continued)

TYPE OF TREATMENT	WHAT IT MEANS	PROS AND CONS
External Radiation.	Machine directs high-energy rays or particles at prostate for a short time each day for a period of weeks.	Possible radiation effects to rectum and bladder. Diarrhea or urinary frequency. Impotence (40–65 percent). Potency progressively may diminish. Little incontinence. Some studies show radiation comparable to surgery, without side effects of prostatectomy.
Internal Radiation (Bracytherapy).	Radiation seeds are inserted into the prostate either with or without surgery. Use of ultrasound has helped make it possible to implant more accurately. Allows higher dose of radiation directly to prostate. (Lymph node dissection may be done as separate procedure.)	Wide variability of complication rates. Less risk of impotence (25 percent). Some loss of sexual performance. Little incontinence (0–2 percent).
Watchful Waiting.	No treatment. An alternative for men over 70 with localized disease. Must have follow-up PSA, prostate exams, and urinalysis every six months.	Tumor may get larger and grow outside prostate. Can decide later to have treatment.
Cryosurgery.	Destruction of tissue by freezing; probe is inserted into tumor. Experimental treatment.	Short hospitalization and recovery period. Frequent urination, burning, pain with urination. High percentage become impotent (80 percent).
Hormonal Treatment.	Pills or monthly injections of hormones.	Hot flashes, decreased libido, some breast enlargement. Not considered curative.

DECISION MAKING FACTORS (continued)

TYPE OF TREATMENT	WHAT IT MEANS	PROS AND CONS
Orchiectomy.	Surgical removal of testicles to eliminate major source of testosterone.	Hot flashes, decreased libido. Not considered curative.
Hyperthermia.	Heating with a probe raises temperatures 20 to 40 percent above normal body temperature to destroy prostate tissue. Definitely, at this time, an experimental method.	Though various types of hyperthermia have been used over the last century without definitive results, emerging techniques are being studied.
Chemotherapy.	Variety of cancer drugs, such as cyclopho-sphamide, doxorubicin, interferon, ketacomozole, suramin, and taxol, being tested but presently not being used except in clinical trials.	Numerous drugs being tried, on metastatic or recurrent cancer in clinical trials.
Lymph node dissection.	Done for diagnostic purposes. Sometimes done with a laparoscope as separate operation (through four small incisions) to determine if cancer has spread before radiation or other treatment.	If done with prostatectomy, it is part of the operation. May impair lymphatic drainage, causing lymphedema. Lymphedema may occur years after primary treatment.
Laser surgery.	Done with laser. May be used when man has radiation and blockage needs to be opened up.	Not considered a primary treatment at this time. Does not cause bleeding; fewer risks of immediate surgical complications. Requires catheter for longer period. Longer recovery. No tissue available for biopsy.

Does age make a difference in deciding what kind of treatment option to choose for prostate cancer?

Since prostate cancer is slow-growing, many doctors feel that a 70 to 75 year-old man diagnosed with an early stage of prostate cancer should probably opt for the least invasive treatment. Watchful waiting may be the answer for some. Hormonal treatment or radiation might be recommended rather than surgery, since they have fewer side effects. In younger or more active men, the decision is less clear—surgery to remove the entire prostate is often recommended. You should be aware that there is a great deal of controversy about what treatment is best and at what age it is wise to opt for less invasive treatment. Although some early results are in, most studies are incomplete as to how the effectiveness of each of the treatments compares in long-term remission.

Prostatectomy Surgery for Prostate Cancer

What is a prostatectomy?

A prostatectomy is the surgical removal of all or part of the prostate. A radical or total prostatectomy is the removal of the **entire** prostate. A radical prostatectomy is the surgery used for treating prostate cancer.

What are the chances of my being incontinent and impotent following surgery?

Much depends on the location of the cancer and the skill of the surgeon. If the cancer has spread outside the prostate capsule, the surgeon performing the prostatectomy may have to cut the nerves that control erection. Additionally, the skill of the physician and the location of the cancer have a great deal to do with the outcome. According to the National Cancer Institute, among men over 65 years of age, 60 to 90 percent of men who have had prostate cancer surgery are impotent following surgery. All men who have had prostate surgery are incontinent for the first few weeks. The amount of time men remain incontinent varies greatly—for many it can take up to a year. About 32 percent of men have some kind of long-term incontinence. It is important to question the doctor carefully about his experience and the results he achieves with his patients, since studies show that results differ substantially from doctor to doctor.

Is hormone therapy ever used before prostate surgery?

Hormone therapy is sometimes prescribed for a number of months before surgery to reduce prostate size or, as doctors say, to "debulk" the tumor.

Are there different kinds of prostatectomy operations?

A prostatectomy is done in one of two ways. In **retropubic** prostatectomy, the prostate and nearby lymph nodes are removed through an incision in the abdomen. This is the most common method. In **perineal** prostatectomy, the incision is made between the scrotum and the anus. Nearby lymph nodes sometimes are removed through a separate incision in the abdomen. It is important to ask your doctor exactly what kind of operation is planned.

What determines which type of prostatectomy operation will be done?
The choice of approach depends on the doctor's training, surgical expertise and personal preference. But you should have this information before surgery.

What are the advantages of a retropubic prostatectomy over the perineal prostatectomy?
Doctors who perform this abdominal operation feel this approach causes fewer rectal injuries and results in lower rates of postoperative incontinence. Furthermore, it is possible to operate and check the pelvic lymph nodes without an extra operation.

What are the advantages of perineal prostatectomy?
The perineal prostatectomy is done through an incision in the scrotum, in front of the rectum. It is less traumatic for the body than an abdominal incision, with quicker recovery and less pain. It is often used in men who are obese. The two major disadvantages are that a separate operation may be needed to check the lymph nodes and it is difficult to spare the nerves that control erection.

Who are the best candidates for a prostatectomy?
Those most likely to have a successful prostatectomy are relatively young, healthy men who have small cancers confined to the prostate.

What is nerve-sparing prostate surgery?
Impotence—the inability to have an erection—is the most common long-lasting side effect of prostate cancer surgery. A nerve-sparing procedure to retain the nerves that control erections was developed in 1982 by Patrick Walsh, MD, of Johns Hopkins University. Many surgeons now use this procedure which, when done by experts in the field, preserves potency in 50 to 70 percent of patients. About 75 percent of patients can have the special procedure. The other 25 percent require more extensive surgery. However, some men, particularly if they are older, still become impotent even with nerve-sparing surgery. Many surgeons are doing the nerve-sparing procedure as long as it does not compromise the cancer treatment—something that sometimes cannot be determined until the surgery is being performed. Some are now sparing only the nerves on the side of the prostate opposite where the cancer is, rather than both nerves. It is wise to ask your surgeon about how he performs the procedure so that you can understand what the possible aftereffects of your operation will be.

STAGE AND TREATMENT CHOICES FOR PROSTATE CANCER

STAGE	DESCRIPTION	TREATMENT
Stage I T1a, N0, M0; well differentiated; Stage A1.	Cancer confined to the prostate. It cannot be felt and there are no symptoms. Found through PSA, ultrasound, or accidentally when surgery is done for other reasons. T1a involves one area of the prostate and is well differentiated.	1. Careful observation without further immediate treatment in selected patients. 2. External radiation (should be delayed four to six weeks if TURP was performed). 3. Radical prostatectomy with or without nerve-sparing technique usually with lymphadenectomy; possibly postoperative radiation if capsular penetration or PSA rises more than three weeks after surgery. 4. Implant radiation seeding (125, palladium, iridium) with ultrasound or CT guidance. 5. *Clinical trials*: external radiation using 3-D conformal treatment planning or other trials.
Stage II T1a, NO, MO; moderately differentiated; poorly differentiated; or undifferentiated. T1b, NO, MO; T1c, NO, MO; TI, NO, MO; or T2, NO, MO.	Cancer can be felt during rectal exam. Cancer cells found only in prostate gland. T2a involves half a lobe or less. T2b involves more than half a lobe but not both lobes. T2c involves both lobes of the gland.	1. Careful observation without further immediate treatment in selected cases. When disease progresses, hormonal therapy may be used, followed by radiation treatment if needed. 2. External radiation (delayed four to six weeks if TURP performed); possibly postoperative radiation. 3. Radical prostatectomy with or without nerve-sparing technique; usually with lymphadenectomy. 4. Radiation seeding with ultrasound or CT guidance. 5. *Clinical trials:* external radiation using 3-D conformal treatment planning; other clinical trials.

STAGE AND TREATMENT CHOICES FOR
PROSTATE CANCER (continued)

STAGE	DESCRIPTION	TREATMENT
Stage II T2, NO, MO; stage A2; BI; or B2.	A2 involves moderately or poorly differentiated or multiple spots on the gland. BI involves single nodule in one lobe; B2 involves more extensive involvement of one lobe or both lobes.	1. Radical prostatectomy with or without nerve-sparing technique; usually with pelvic lymphadenectomy; possibly postoperative radiation. 2. External radiation (delayed four to six weeks if TURP performed); for bulky T2b tumors, hormonal therapy may be added. 3. Careful observation without further immediate treatment. 4. Radiation seeding with ultrasound or CT guidance. 5. External radiation with tomography-based 3-D conformal treatment planning. 6. *Clinical trials*: Cryosurgery, hormonal therapy followed by radical prostatectomy.
Stage III T3, NO, MO; Stage C	Cancer cells have spread outside the covering (capsule) of the prostate to the tissues surrounding it. Seminal vesicles may have cancer in them. T3c is cancer that is in the seminal vesicles.	1. External radiation. 2. Hormonal manipulation (orchiectomy or LHRH agonist). 3. Radical prostatectomy with lymphadenectomy followed by radiation if capsular penetration or seminal vesicle invasion found during operation or if level of PSA is detectable three weeks after surgery. 4. Careful observation without further immediate treatment in selected patients. 5. Treatment for patients with urinary problems: radiation, radical surgery, TURP, hormonal manipulation. 6. *Clinical trials*: neutron/photon radiation, proton beam radiation, percutaneous cryosurgery, or other trials.

(continued)

STAGE AND TREATMENT CHOICES FOR
PROSTATE CANCER *(continued)*

STAGE	DESCRIPTION	TREATMENT
Stage IV T4, NO MO; any T, N1-3, MO; any T, any N, M1; Stage D1, D2.	Cancer cells have spread to lymph nodes or to organs and tissues far away from prostate.	1. Treatment determined by age, other illnesses, symptoms, spread to bone or lymph nodes. 2. Hormonal treatment: orchiectomy alone or with flutamide or nilutamide; LHRH agonists, leuprolide plus flutamide; estrogens. 3. External radiation (delay four to six weeks after TURP) plus hormonal therapy. 4. Radiation to reduce symptoms. 5. Surgery (TURP) to reduce symptoms. 6. Careful observation without further immediate treatment. 7. *Clinical trials*: Radical prostatectomy and orchiectomy, systemic chemotherapy.
Recurrent	Cancer has come back after it has been treated. It may come back in the prostate or in another part of the body.	1. Radiation if recurrence is in prostate area (if prior treatment was prostatectomy). 2. Prostatectomy if initial treatment with radiation. 3. Hormonal therapy. 4. Pain medication, external radiation or radioisotopes (stonium-89) or other treatments for bone pain. 5. *Clinical trials*: chemotherapy or biologic agents.

What happens if all the nerves that control erection are removed?

If all the nerves that govern an erection must be removed, then you must face the fact that you will be sexually impotent. Even though you will continue to have the same desires and you can still have an orgasm, you will not be able to become erect. This is a question that you should discuss with your partner as well as with your doctor beforehand. Whatever the outcome, it is helpful to be open about your concerns and discuss them with your partner.

Will I be sterile after a total prostatectomy?

Since the prostate gland produces most of the fluid released at the time of sexual intercourse and climax, patients are sterile—unable to father a child in the normal fashion—following this operation. Removal of the entire prostate gland, including the prostatic urethra means there is no place for the sperm to be deposited since the vas deferens are divided.

Why is a biopsy done during surgery?

The biopsy is done during surgery to determine whether the cancer has spread beyond the margins or outer edges of the prostate which may mean that further treatment will be needed.

Why is pelvic lymph node dissection (lymphadenectomy) done and why is it important?

Pelvic lymph node dissection is done to determine if the cancer has spread to the lymph nodes since prostate cancer spreads by way of the blood vessels and lymph system. If the lymph nodes are free of any signs of cancer, this is considered proof that the cancer has not spread. The determining factor when deciding whether lymph node dissection is necessary is whether the treatment will be altered if the lymph nodes are found to be cancerous. Physicians do not agree on how extensive dissection of the lymph nodes needs to be, though most physicians are using "modified" dissection. In a retropubic prostatectomy, lymph node dissection is usually done as a matter of course. Experts feel that in cases where a perineal prostatectomy is being performed, the PSA is below 10, the Gleason score is low-grade, and the tumor cannot be felt but was found with ultrasound, the lymph node dissection may be omitted. With larger, less differentiated tumors, a pelvic lymph node dissection is more important.

When is a lymphadenectomy performed?

Usually this surgery is performed at the start of the operation for retropubic prostatectomy. A pathologist examines the nodes while the patient is waiting for the operation to proceed and if no evidence of cancer is found in the lymph nodes, the prostate will be removed. If the nodes are found to be cancerous, surgery will usually be done to remove obstructive tissue, but usually the entire prostate will not be removed.

TYPE OF OPERATION FOR PROSTATE CANCER	HOW DONE	ADVANTAGES AND DISADVANTAGES
Retropubic Prostatectomy.	Vertical incision from navel to pubic bone. Prostate, seminal vesicles, and lymph nodes removed through incision in abdomen. Most common operation for prostate cancer.	Fewer rectal injuries and lower rates of incontinence. Not necessary to do separate operation on pelvic lymph nodes because they can be removed through same incision.
Perineal Prostatectomy.	Incision is made between scrotum and anus. Incision is usually an inverted "U" around inner side of anus.	Less traumatic surgery, less pain, quicker recovery. Often used on obese men. However, separate operation may be needed to check lymph nodes. May be more difficult to spare nerves that control erection.

Is lymphadenectomy ever done ahead of time to determine if there is spread of cancer?

Laparoscopic lymphadenectomy is sometimes done when other indicators, such as a high PSA level and a high Gleason grade, show a possibility of spread. A laparoscopic lymphadenectomy may also be used when a perineal prostatectomy is planned or when another type of treatment has been chosen but the man wishes to have the lymph nodes checked to determine if there has been any spread of the cancer. The laparoscopic procedure for lymph node dissection uses four cuts of about one-half inch each, rather than a single incision, and takes two to three hours to perform.

What preparation needs to be done before prostate surgery?

Preparation is similar to that for most abdominal surgery. Daily enemas and laxatives may be given to remove fecal material so there is a "clean field" for the surgery. The day before surgery you will eat no solid foods and drink only clear liquids. Your pelvic area may be shaved. It is important for you to let doctors and nurses know about any health issues, such as hypertension, heart disease, diabetes, or lung problems, as well as any drugs that you are presently taking.

Are blood transfusions needed during prostate operations?
Transfusions are sometimes needed during surgery for a radical prostatectomy, since as much as two pints of blood may be lost during surgery. Be sure to ask the doctor if there is a possibility you will need a blood transfusion. Many men bank their own blood beforehand to eliminate any risk of receiving blood that has been contaminated with hepatitis, AIDS, or other transmittable diseases.

What is involved in banking blood?
Usually, a patient can donate a pint of blood every week or ten days for the month before surgery. Many doctors recommend that you take iron pills during this time to assist the body in replacing your donated blood. Blood can be stored for about 45 days. You should have at least three days between the last donation and your surgery.

Questions to Ask Your Doctor Before Prostate Surgery

- What kind of operation will you be doing?
- What do you consider the advantages of surgery over other treatments for my prostate cancer?
- Will you do nerve-sparing surgery? How successful has it been in your experience?
- What are my chances of becoming impotent? Will this be temporary or permanent?
- What sort of limitations will the operation put on my sexual activity?
- What percentage of your patients are permanently incontinent?
- Will you be doing retropubic or perineal surgery?
- Where will the scar be?
- What kind of tests will I need before my operation?
- Would it be appropriate for me to have hormone therapy before surgery to reduce the size of the cancer?
- Should I plan to bank my blood beforehand in case a transfusion is needed?
- What kind of anesthesia will be used? Epidural? Spinal? What are the advantages of each?
- How long does the operation take?
- Will I have drains, catheters, and intravenous lines after my operation?
- Will I need a nurse for the first few days?

- How soon will I be up out of bed?

- Does the hospital have patient controlled painkiller equipment so I can control how much pain relief I need?

- Is it your practice to check the lymph nodes first with a lymphadenectomy before proceeding with the removal of the prostate?

- What happens if you find the cancer has spread?

- Is there a possibility that I will need radiation following surgery?

- How long will I be in the hospital?

What kind of anesthesia is usually used for prostate cancer surgery?

Many doctors prefer epidural anesthesia, the narcotic often used for women during labor. The potent drug is given directly around the spinal cord, blocking pain but leaving you aware. Epidural anesthesia assures a total absence of pain, normal muscle function and complete relaxation. Others use a spinal anesthetic which blocks all pain, as well as the ability to feel and use the legs. However, spinal anesthesia is usually avoided if you have had back surgery or spinal cord injuries. General anesthesia can also be used to put you into a drug-induced sleep and to allow close control of vital functions especially if you have abnormally low blood pressure or certain types of heart problems. Muscle relaxants may be given during surgery to decrease the amount of general anesthetic needed.

How long will the operation take?

Usually a radical prostatectomy will take two to four hours, including the removal and examination of the lymph nodes of the pelvis. Tissue from the prostate and lymph nodes are sent to the pathologist during the operation so that they can be analyzed to see if the cancer has spread. This analysis, called a frozen section, is a rapid procedure that freezes the tissue quickly, giving the surgeon an almost immediate reading on the status of your cancer. Since the freezing process can distort it and make the reading less accurate, the final result of the biopsy can take several days. This is called a permanent section biopsy and your doctor will report the results to you.

How does the pathologist determine whether the prostate tumor has spread beyond its margins?

When the tumor is removed and sent to the pathologist, it is painted with a substance similar to India ink. This colors the margins, or outer edges, of the prostate so that they can be examined and identified on the slides. If the cancer cells extend beyond the margins, then it is obvious that it has spread. If the cells are contained entirely within the margins, the cancer is said to be encapsulated, and usually no further treatment is recommended. If the margins are involved, additional postoperative radiation treatment will probably be recommended.

How long will it be before I know the results of the permanent section biopsy taken during the surgery?
It can be several days to a week before the final results of the biopsy are known. The tissue is put through a time-consuming multistage procedure that involves a series of solutions to remove water and fatty substances. It is then saturated with warm liquid paraffin. When it has cooled and hardened, the tissue in paraffin is cut into thin slices. The slices are placed on slides so that the tissue can be studied under the microscope.

Should I make arrangements for the doctor to talk with someone I designate as soon as the surgery is completed?
If you want someone to be able to talk to the doctor after your operation, to be involved with any decisions that might be necessary, or to be there when you come back to your room, make sure you tell your doctor who that person is, ask where the person should wait and how long the procedure will take. Some hospitals and surgicenters have a special waiting room while others will tell you to have family and friends wait in your room. Also, if you feel strongly that someone should **not** be given any information until you are alert, be sure to explain this to your doctor beforehand. These are all things you want to discuss before the operation.

Does the length of time I spend in the operating room indicate the seriousness of the operation?
It depends on the individual case. There are several situations that can make your time in the operating room longer but have no bearing on your own operation. For instance:

- You were taken from your room some time in advance of the actual operation.

- The anesthesiologist may make some additional preparations that last 30 minutes or even an hour.

- The surgeon takes longer than expected on the operation before yours, thus starting on your operation later than scheduled.

- You could spend more time than anticipated in the recovery room.

- Those people who are waiting for you should understand that they should not judge the length or seriousness of the operation by the amount of time you spend in the operating room.

Will I need to go to a recovery room after my operation?
Yes. After the operation, you will be watched and checked by the medical team until you are stable enough to move. The recovery room has equipment for monitoring your heart and respirators for assisting you in breathing if you need them. You can get intravenous fluids and blood in the recovery room. Normally the recovery room is run by a physician anesthesiologist. Respiration therapists will probably help you cough and inflate your lungs. If you have had general anesthesia, you may spend several hours in the recovery room.

Is there a possibility of a blood clot following prostate surgery?
Blood clots are one of the most common causes of sudden death after surgery and can occur days or weeks after the operation. A pulmonary embolus is a large blood clot in a vein of the leg or pelvis that breaks loose. If it is large and reaches the heart it can totally block blood flow and result in an almost instant drop of blood pressure.

What can be done to avoid the risk of blood clots?
During surgery, most doctors use special stockings that inflate and deflate to keep the blood flowing through the veins. After surgery you will probably be given support stockings to wear. You will be helped to sit up and dangle your legs over the side of the bed. The day after surgery, you will be helped to get up and walk, and you will be encouraged to increase your walking daily. This will speed your recovery and minimize the complications from surgery.

Questions to Ask Your Doctor After Prostate Surgery

- **How long will the catheter stay in place?**
- **Are bladder spasms to be expected?**
- **How long can I expect my urine to look cloudy?**
- **When will the stitches be removed?**
- **How long will the dribbling and feeling of urgency to urinate continue?**
- **How long can I expect to be incontinent?**
- **Are there exercises I can do to strengthen the muscles that control urination?**
- **When can I start driving a car, using stairs, lifting, walking, playing tennis, golf or other active sports again?**
- **How long will it be before I am fully recuperated?**

Will I be in pain following surgery?
You will have some postoperative pain that may require narcotics for relief. Many hospitals have patient controlled analgesia machines so you can administer the pain relieving medication as you feel it is needed so that pain and discomfort are minimized.

What is the purpose of the tube that's put down my throat?
There may be a slow-down in the normal intestinal contractions because organs were moved during the operation, so a tube is sometimes placed through your nose and into your stomach and connected to a suction machine. Fluids that accumulate because of lack of normal stomach and intestinal contractions are removed through the tube. It will probably be left in place for a few days until your body begins to work normally again—and you begin to pass gas, which is a sign that things are back to normal. Once the tube is removed, you'll be able to eat normally.

Will I have a drain following surgery?
A drain, which runs from the site of the surgery through a small slit in the abdomen, allows blood, urine, or other tissue fluids that would otherwise accumulate in the surgical area to be drained outside the body. Keeping the surgical areas free of these fluids promotes faster healing and lessens the possibility of infection. Drains are usually removed after there is no more drainage, usually five to six days after surgery. Removal is not painful.

Is it common for testicles to be swollen after prostate surgery?
Since prostate surgery involves the nodes and ducts which normally drain the groin, thighs, and scrotum, these areas may be swollen for several weeks after surgery. As your body heals, this condition will subside.

Why is a catheter needed during and after surgery?
A catheter (also called a urinary tube or Foley catheter) is placed into the bladder at the time of surgery. It helps to drain the bladder during recuperation and serves as a splint for healing around the area where the bladder neck is stitched to the stump of the urethra. Urine drains automatically through the catheter into a urine bag. You can keep discomfort to a minimum by keeping the end of your penis clean and softened with ointment. The catheter tube will be secured to your thigh with tape, and you may need to experiment to find the most comfortable angle for securing the catheter tube. Care must be taken to prevent accidental removal, so try to refrain from pulling on the catheter. Premature removal can interfere with recovery.

How long does the catheter remain in place?

Depending on your progress, the catheter usually remains in place for two to three weeks after radical prostatectomy. This means you will still have the catheter when you go home from the hospital. You will be taught how to care for it before you leave. You must make sure the catheter is well secured to the thigh and avoid traction and tension on it. Make sure the tube between the penis and the bag is not blocked by being crimped or pinched, especially at night. Keep the bag below the penis so that urine drains into the bag. If urine cannot flow from your bladder or flows back into the bladder, it can create bladder problems. After it is removed, there may be some dribbling and urgency to urinate for several weeks. For most individuals, this condition gradually improves as muscles heal and strengthen.

Do I have to wait until the catheter is removed before I can drive?

Most doctors suggest that you do not drive until your catheter has been removed. After the removal of the catheter (usually two to three weeks) you should limit driving to short distances for another two weeks.

Are bladder spasms common after prostatectomy surgery?

Bladder spasms may occur after a prostatectomy. These spasms come on rapidly and usually go away in a few minutes. They can be quite painful. Sometimes these spasms are caused by a blocked catheter, due to kinked tubing, mucus plugs, or blood clots. Once the spasms start, you have little choice but to relax as much as you can until they subside. If you have spasms too often, your doctor can prescribe antispasmodic drugs.

Is it normal for my urine to be cloudy?

Your urine may be cloudy for several weeks after surgery. It will clear up as the wound heals.

How long will convalescence take?

Convalescence time can vary, but most men are able to do all the things they did prior to surgery after three or four months.

What can be done if I find that I have difficulty urinating following surgery?

This should be reported to the doctor. It is a problem that sometimes follows radical prostate surgery and usually means that the bladder neck area that was stitched to the urethra has contracted resulting in a restricted urinary stream. This can be repaired by the doctor either with a dilating instrument or through the urethra.

Is incontinence to be expected following a prostatectomy?

Many men are surprised to discover that the operation causes them to lose their ability to control urine. They are embarrassed that they must use incontinence pads for the dribbling. Very often, incontinence will lessen as you heal. It should continue to improve gradually for up to six months or a year after surgery. A small percentage of men who undergo radical prostatectomy will have loss of bladder control. Many men report that they must continue to wear pads to prevent leakage. Many say they have intermittent dribbling caused by coughing or exertion. Incontinence can sometimes be overcome through the strengthening of muscles with simple exercise.

How can I strengthen muscles to improve incontinence?

Corrective exercises (one type is Kegel exercises), designed to strengthen your perineal muscles, may be helpful.

- Empty your bladder. Try to relax yourself completely. Tense your muscles by pressing your buttocks together. Hold this position and count to ten. Relax and count to ten. Do this exercise for ten minutes each time, three times a day. At the beginning, you may not be able to hold the position for the count of ten or you may tire before you have completed the entire set. If so, stop exercising and go back to it later.

- When starting to urinate, shut off the stream for a few seconds, then start voiding again. Do this exercise each time you urinate to improve urinary control.

- Remember to urinate as soon as you feel the need. Do not wait.

- It may take several weeks or months of daily exercise before you notice a difference.

When can I resume sexual activities after a prostatectomy?

If you had nerve-sparing surgery, it may take six months to a year or two before you are able to achieve an erection, but you can usually resume sexual activity within six weeks following surgery, when the operative site is healed.

What happens to the PSA after prostate surgery?

The PSA usually falls to 0.0; sometimes it will be reported as less than 0.3 or 0.5. These minor variations are meaningless. If the PSA variation is small and slow, it should be carefully watched. However, there are a substantial number of men with elevated or rising PSA level after surgery who do not have any other symptoms for many years, so a rising PSA alone is not enough to change the treatment plan. If it is decided that further treatment is necessary, it may be radiation or hormones.

Following a prostatectomy, is radiation sometimes recommended?

It depends on what has been found during surgery and whether your PSA level returns to normal. In some cases, when the surgery shows that the cancer has spread beyond the prostate capsule or into the seminal vesicles, for example, or when the PSA level remains elevated three weeks after surgery, postoperative radiation may be necessary.

What is lymphedema?

Lymphadema may occur in men who have had surgery or radiation therapy for prostate cancer. It is an accumulation of lymph fluid that may cause swelling in the legs following the removal of lymph nodes (lymphadenectomy). Unable to drain, the lymph fluid remains in the soft tissue where infections can develop. People who have had lymph node dissection are at greatest risk. Lymphedema is most commonly seen in women who have had axillary nodes removed during breast cancer surgery. Curiously enough, not everyone who has lymph node surgery has lymphedema. Lymphedema, however, can occur soon after treatment or as many as 15 years after surgery.

Does lymphedema mean my cancer has spread?

Many people fear that lymphedema indicates the cancer has spread or returned. Another fear is that the swollen, nonfunctional limb may be permanently disfigured. It is important to discuss your fears with the healthcare professionals in your life, so you can take the necessary measures to keep lymphedema under control. Positioning, massage, exercise, special garments, and pumps are all used in treating lymphedema.

How can you tell if you have lymphedema?

About half of patients who have lymphedema report a feeling of heaviness or fullness in the affected area. A slight indentation may be visible when the skin on the limb is pressed. Depending on how extensive the problem is, a deeper fingerprint may take anywhere from five to 30 seconds to return to normal. At the extreme, the limb may swell to one and a half to two times its normal size. You should always be aware of any signs of infection in the involved area—redness, pain, heat, chills, swelling, or fever. Though rare, infections can move quickly and become serious very rapidly.

How important is it to get immediate care?

Immediate care is essential. Untreated, the condition can result in a permanently swollen leg. Awareness of the possibility of lymphedema and the need for immediate medical attention may help to keep the problem from becoming chronic. Obesity, immobility, poor nutrition, prior radiation or surgery, and concurrent medical problems such as diabetes, hypertension, kidney disease, cardiac disease, or phlebitis can all be contributing factors to the onset of lymphedema. Those who have any of those problems should be extremely aware of the symptoms and the need for lifelong adherence to prevention and control of lymphedema.

Where can I get information about lymphedema?

The National Lymphedema Network provides printed information and other assistance to those who develop lymphedema as a result of lymph node surgery or radiation therapy. The address is 1611 Telegraph Avenue, Suite 1111, Oakland, CA 94612. The telephone is 1–800–541–3259, and its Web site is www.lymphnet.org. See Chapter 28, Where to Get Help, for more resource information.

Two Kinds of Radiation Therapy—External or Internal

What kinds of radiation therapy are used for prostate cancer?

Two kinds of radiation treatments are possible—external and internal. Sometimes both internal and external radiation are used.

How effective are radiation and radiation implants in treating prostate cancer?

Both kinds of radiation therapy are being used to treat some prostate cancers and the success rates indicate that these treatments are as effective as radical surgery, especially with early stage disease. There is still controversy among physicians about the circumstances under which radiation is most effective for treating prostate cancer. However, according to some authorities, it appears that when similarly staged patients are treated with surgery or radiation and carefully compared at the end of ten years, there is no difference in the outcome. In addition, again according to limited studies, there is no factual basis for the belief that younger patients should be treated with surgery because they will live longer, that radiation shows late failure or that the patient sacrifices a survival advantage when he selects radiation treatment.

After ten years, however, there is some evidence that increasing PSAs and local recurrences become more common in men who had radiation treatment than those who have had surgery. What is still not resolved is whether these differences are due to the fact that men in the studies who had prostate surgery were less advanced at the start than those who had external radiation treatment.

External Radiation Treatment for Prostate Cancer

What is involved with external radiation therapy?

The patient goes to the outpatient department of the hospital for a period of time—usually five days a week for five to eight weeks. With a machine, the rays are aimed at the tumor and the area around it. At the end of treatment, an extra "boost" of radiation is often given to a smaller area of the pelvis where most of the tumor is found.

What kinds of side effects and aftereffects can be expected from external radiation therapy?

Many men who have radiation therapy are able to continue their normal routines, although during the last weeks of therapy, many complain of feeling very tired. Some suffer from skin reactions as well as diarrhea, bleeding, difficult urination, abdominal cramping, rectal soreness, hemorrhoids, and cystitis. Some men find they have some temporary pain upon ejaculation and there may be a permanent decrease in semen volume. Like other treatments for prostate cancer, external radiation has some serious aftereffects, which may not show up for months or years after treatment. In a group of **100 men** who have had prostate radiation, it has been shown that the following side effects may be expected:

Impotence	40
Some long-term incontinence	6
Severe incontinence	7
Difficult urination	5
Rectal problems	11
Severe rectal problems	2

What are the advantages and disadvantages of radiation treatment?

Radiation is ideal for the man who cannot, or does not wish to have his prostate removed, or whose health makes surgery a higher risk. It avoids many of the risks of surgery and anesthesia, such as surgical bleeding, hospitalization, pain, or heart attacks, strokes or blood clots. There is some risk of developing some degree of bladder or rectal irritation. Some of the side effects, such as bloody urine or impotence, can appear months or years after treatment.

What is the most effective kind of radiation equipment?

An important factor to successful external radiation is the type of machinery used in your radiation treatment. A high-energy linear accelerator is the most effective for treating the pelvic area. Many radiation oncologists feel that low energy photons or cobalt-60 units can cause a higher incidence of complications. A total of 6000 to 7200 rads is usually given over the entire treatment period.

What is three-dimensional conformal radiation?
3-D conformal radiation is a new technology, presently undergoing clinical trials. It allows radiation doses to be increased significantly because its accuracy makes it possible to pinpoint prostate tumors so even closely adjacent normal tissue is spared from radiation. This computer-based system creates a very accurate picture of the prostate, enabling radiation oncologists to fashion multiple beams shaped exactly to the contour of the prostate gland. The technique makes it safer to deliver a maximum dose of high energy x-rays directly to the tumor.

Are some men at higher risk for complications after radiation treatments for their prostate cancers?
Men who are at increased risk for major complications after treatment include those who have had a number of TURPs (transurethral resection of the prostate) in their history, those with bladder infections or kidney stones, those who have autoimmune diseases such as lupus, ulcerative colitis, or enteritis, and those who have had multiple prior abdominal surgeries.

Are younger men with prostate cancer better off having prostate surgery rather than some form of radiation?
This is a question that will continue to be debated among physicians. A respected medical text, *Cancer: Principles & Practice of Oncology*, edited by Doctors Vincent T. DeVita, Jr., Samuel Hellman, and Steven A. Rosenberg states in its chapter on prostate cancer: "There is no basis in fact for the frequently made statements that younger patients should be treated with surgery because they will live longer, that radiation shows late failure, and that the patient sacrifices a survival advantage when he selects radiation treatment." So, for younger men, as for all other men with prostate cancer, the important thing to remember is that you need to study the pros and cons of each treatment and how they will affect your life. You need to understand your own case before making a decision on treatment.

Is hormone treatment sometimes prescribed before radiation is given?
Some doctors recommend that hormonal therapy be given before or during radiation to "debulk," or reduce the size of the tumor and make it more manageable for treatment. Hormonal treatment in addition to radiation is presently in clinical trials.

Does radiation treatment get rid of the cancer permanently?
As with surgery, about half of the men who have radiation may still have positive biopsy results for cancer two to three years after treatment. Some studies imply that biopsies taken within 18 to 24 months after radiation treatment may be unreliable because this slow-growing tumor also regresses slowly.

Questions to Ask Your Radiation Oncologist Before You
Have External Radiation Treatments

- Exactly what type of radiation treatment will I be getting?

- Will it be done with a high-energy linear accelerator?

- Is three-dimensional conformal radiation available anywhere in the area?

- Are you planning to do a lymph node dissection. If so, why?

- Do you advise hormone treatment to reduce the cancer before radiation? Will I continue hormone treatment after radiation?

- Who will be responsible for coordinating my radiation treatment? For giving my treatment?

- Who should I ask if I have questions about my radiation treatment?

- Can I continue to work during these treatments?

- Is there a more convenient place where my treatments can be given?

- How long will it take for each treatment? For the whole series?

- Will I be able to drive myself to and from my treatments?

- What side effects can I expect?

- What should I do if these side effects occur?

- What side effects should I report to the radiation oncologist?

- What are the long-term side effects or after effects?

- How much will it cost? Is it covered by insurance?

- How much of a risk is involved?

- Are there any alternatives to external beam radiation treatment I should consider?

- When will you be checking my PSA again? How rapidly should I expect it to drop?

- If a biopsy is suggested earlier than 18 months after radiation treatment ask, "What information do you expect to get from a biopsy at this time?"

Is it wise for me to consider having a lymphadenectomy before having radiation to determine whether the cancer has spread?

The reason for doing a lymphadenectomy is to help in the medical management and decisions involved with treating the cancer. It has no therapeutic value. Lymphadenectomy is considered by many doctors to be an imperfect procedure. If positive nodes are found and a different treatment is decided upon, then it may be worthwhile. But if the treatment will remain the same whether the nodes are found to be negative or positive, you may well decide you do not want to submit to the procedure.

Are there possible side effects to a lymphadenectomy?

One of the rare but possible side effects that can be troublesome when radiation follows a lymphadenectomy is the possibility of leg and genital lymphedema (swelling). Lymphedema is caused by impaired lymphatic drainage, sometimes appearing many years after treatment. When chronic lymphedema develops, it is a lifelong condition that requires constant monitoring and therapy. (See Chapter 8, Surgery, for additional information on lymphedema.)

What is a laparoscopic lymphadenectomy?

This procedure, which is done to determine if the cancer has already spread to the lymph nodes, uses four puncture wounds of about one-half inch each, rather than a single vertical incision. It is performed inside the intestinal or abdominal cavity. This procedure has an increased risk of bowel obstruction because of adhesions or injury. Though it sounds simple, the procedure takes two to four hours to perform, but you will usually be able to go home the next day. If your doctor suggests a laparoscopic lymphadenectomy, be sure to ask why it is being done and how the information will change or modify your planned treatment. (The standard lymphadenectomy is performed through a six-inch vertical lower abdominal incision outside the abdominal cavity without exposing the area to surgical trauma.)

Is radiation used for treating prostate cancer that has already been treated with surgery?

Radiation is often used following a prostatectomy if there are positive nodes or positive surgical margins. It is usually given soon after recovery from surgery. A lower radiation dose can be used if given soon after surgery rather than waiting until there are signs of problems. (See Chapter 4, What Is Cancer?, for information on surgical margins.)

Is radiation effective for treatment of prostate cancer that has spread to the lymph nodes?
Just as surgical removal of the prostate does not remove cancer that has spread to the lymph nodes, radiation rarely cures cancer that has already spread. It is sometimes used to treat symptoms.

If I have recently had a TURP procedure when can I start radiation?
For those who have had prior transurethral resection of the prostate (TURP), radiation is usually delayed for four to six weeks after the operation to allow for complete healing.

Will external radiation affect my blood counts?
Sometimes it may. The radiation oncologist may find you have low white blood cell counts or low levels of platelets, which can affect your body's ability to fight infection and to prevent bleeding. If your blood tests show these problems, you may have to go off treatment for a week or so to allow your blood counts to come back up.

What kind of doctor will I go to for my radiation treatments?
Radiation is a very specialized field, requiring treatment from a team especially trained in therapeutic radiology. The radiation oncologist, sometimes called a therapeutic radiologist, heads the team and plans the treatment. The radiation oncologist will decide what specific treatments should be used, supervise its administration and evaluate you at intervals during the course of the treatment to see whether it is working.

Will I have a choice as to where I have my radiation treatments?
Have a frank discussion with your doctor about why a specific radiation oncologist or radiotherapy department is being recommended. You may want to explore whether or not it would be advantageous for you to use a larger medical center rather than a small hospital or private office closer to home. A large radiation center will have several types of equipment and beams to use for treatment, whereas a smaller general hospital or private office may have less sophisticated equipment. You must weigh for yourself the advantages of convenience versus the technology and expertise a larger medical center may have to offer. Of course, your type of health insurance may limit where you can receive your treatment. Radiation treatment is a science in which many advances have been made, both in technology and in application. The radiation team and their equipment will be playing an important part in your treatment. **Look for a center near you using computers to achieve three-dimensional planning and treatment.**

Will I have my first treatment at my first appointment with the radiation oncologist?

Probably not, although it depends on how complex your case is. It is highly unlikely that you will have your first treatment during your first appointment, because your treatment plan and necessary casts and shields need to be made. Treatment plans are different for each patient, so it may take more than one visit before your treatment actually begins.

How will I be shielded from unnecessary radiation?

There are many safeguards to protect you from unnecessary radiation to the parts of your body that do not need treatment. All the machines are shielded so that the large amounts of radiation are given only to a specific area. The treatment field is usually lit with a light that outlines the surface through which the radiation will pass. A series of safeguards in the machine limits the radiation to this lighted area of your body. Shields, usually made out of lead blocks, are used to protect small areas of your body not needing treatment.

How are the casts made?

You will be put in the position you will assume during treatment. The cast is made right on your body, using a material such as plaster or plastic. Small windows are cut into the mold to allow the beam to be directed to the precise area to be treated. The radiation oncologist can use the body mold on you over and over again so the beam is always directed to the proper area.

How will the spot be marked where the radiation is to be given?

Once the location has been decided, the radiation oncologist or the radiation therapist will draw marks on your skin. Marking pens, indelible ink, or silver nitrate may be used. You will be asked not to wash away these markings. After your first week of treatment, you may have permanent markings put on your skin. Usually a small pinpoint tattoo is placed on the corners of the treatment field.

Is the treatment plan ever changed?

Your original radiation treatment plan may be added to, subtracted from or changed, as the radiation oncologist feels is appropriate. There are a number of reasons for making changes as the treatment goes along. Do not be alarmed if the plan is changed. It does not mean that the disease is getting worse or that the disease has progressed.

Why is the radiation treatment sometimes given from different angles?

One way of giving the maximum amount of radiation to the tumor—and the minimum amount to normal tissue—is by aiming radiation beams at the tumor from two or more directions. The patient, or the machine, is rotated. The patient and the machine are placed so that the beams meet each other where the tumor is located. The tumor thus gets a high enough dose of radiation to be destroyed but normal tissues escape with minimum radiation effects since the beams take different pathways to reach the tumor.

Why is the radiation given over a period of time instead of all at once?

The radiation must be strong enough to kill the tumor and still allow the normal tissues to heal. The radiation oncologist determines the total radiation dose necessary and divides it into the number of single-treatment doses that will add up to this total dose by the time of the last treatment. This process, dividing the doses of radiation, is known as *fractionation*. Fractionation is a very important part of planning and delivering radiation since it affects both the tumor and the normal tissues.

What happens to the PSA after radiation treatment?

Don't be upset if your PSA level does not immediately drop to zero. The PSA level should drop below 1.0 over a period of several months. Some doctors think that the slower the PSA drops, the more successful the treatment. If, after a period of time, the PSA level starts to rise above 3 or 4, hormonal therapy may be recommended.

Is it wise to have a biopsy after radiation to see if the treatment was effective?

As with the PSA, biopsies done shortly after radiation are believed to be less accurate than those done between 18 and 24 months after treatment. It is generally believed that the results of biopsies done within the first 18 months after external radiation treatment may be unreliable and should be avoided.

How long do the treatments take?

The actual treatment lasts from one to five minutes. You are usually in the treatment room for five to fifteen minutes for each treatment. The most usual schedule is to have a treatment each day for five days, with weekends off. Usually you will not have treatments on holidays.

What is the actual treatment like?

Most people say that they feel nothing while the treatment is being given. A few say that they feel warmth or a mild tingling sensation. You will feel no pain or discomfort and it will be unusual if you have any kind of sensation. If, by any chance, you do feel ill or very uncomfortable during the treatment, tell the radiation oncologist. The machine can be stopped at any time. You need to remain very still during treatment, but you can breathe normally. Try to relax. Some people bring their headsets and soothing music into the treatment room with them. You may feel cold in the treatment room, since the temperature is kept cool for the proper operation of the machine.

Will the radiation I am getting make me radioactive?

No. External beam radiation does not cause your body to become radioactive. There is no need to avoid being with other people because of your treatment. You can hug, kiss, and have sexual relations with others.

Will I have tests each time when I go for my radiation treatments?

There may be some tests during the course of the treatment, but not each time. It will depend on your treatment plan. Usually tests such as blood counts are taken so the radiation oncologist can determine if the radiation is doing damage to other parts of your body. Sometimes x-rays and other tests are needed to determine if the radiation oncologist should change the treatment plan.

What kinds of side effects can be expected from external radiation therapy?

Many men are able to continue their normal routines while having radiation therapy, although many complain of feeling very tired during the last weeks of therapy. But most men find they are back to normal about three months after treatment. Mild diarrhea is commonly reported as are rectal soreness, skin reactions, abdominal cramping, hemorrhoids, and cystitis. Many of the complications are temporary and usually clear up after a few weeks.

Other possible aftereffects include:

- Some temporary pain upon ejaculation and a permanent decrease in semen volume.

- Impotence (usually occurs in 40 percent of men who have radiation treatment for prostate cancer).

- Rectal bleeding (common due to ulceration of the rectal wall, where the radiation dosage is concentrated). This can usually be treated with enemas containing steroids or by laser.

- In rare cases, it may be necessary to have a temporary colostomy to allow time for healing.

- Incontinence and swelling of the legs and genital area (lymphedema) are less frequent side effects.

Will I lose my hair as a result of radiation?

The hair on your head will not fall out because of radiation for prostate cancer, but there may be changes in the hair on your lower abdomen or pubic area. Usually the hair in those areas will thin out because of the radiation.

Why would I have rectal soreness as the result of radiation?

Rectal soreness (referred to as proctitis) can be the result of radiation damage to the intestinal tract. A diet that is low in fibrous foods often will help to allow healing. Some doctors will suggest the use of steroid enemas or suppositories to help alleviate symptoms. Antidiarrhea medication is sometimes prescribed.

What can be done about cystitis caused by radiation?

Cystitis, the inflammation of the urinary bladder that causes pain on urination, usually occurs during the first few weeks of therapy. You should try to drink at least two quarts of fluid each day. The doctor may also prescribe antispasmodics and analgesics to help alleviate some of the symptoms.

What can be done if I experience diarrhea?

Diarrhea can be one of the side effects. It can cause you to lose fluids and become dehydrated. So be sure to drink plenty of clear liquids. Discuss the problem with your doctor if the diarrhea persists. You can get more information about diet and radiation by looking at Chapter 27, Living with Cancer or by calling the Cancer Information Service, 1–800–4–CANCER and asking for the booklet "Eating Hints."

What happens when there is damage to the bladder due to radiation?

Bladder damage can result from radiation treatment, causing frequent urination. Bleeding from the bladder is another possible side effect. If bleeding occurs, call your doctor.

What are the long-term side effects of external radiation therapy?

There is a chance, with external beam radiation, that serious injury to the bowel and bladder may result. For this reason, it is essential that your radiation treatment be done by a qualified radiation oncologist who understands sophisticated radiation techniques,

Will I become incontinent as a result of external radiation therapy?

Although you may have some difficulty in urination, including pain and increased frequency, incontinence is not usually a major side effect of external radiation. Acute, temporary reactions may occur, but chronic problems or late reactions are unusual.

Will I become impotent after radiation treatment?

Radiation can affect erections by damaging the arteries that carry blood to the penis. As the radiated area heals, internal tissues may become scarred. The walls of the arteries may lose their elasticity so they can no longer expand enough to let blood in to create a firm erection. Although potency is preserved at the start, it may diminish over time. See Chapter 27, Living with Cancer, for more information on sexual side effects.

May I go swimming while I am having my radiation treatments?

You probably can, as long as it does not cause your skin to become too dry. You need to rinse your skin well with fresh water if you have been swimming in saltwater or in a chlorinated pool.

Can I continue my usual activities during treatment?

Continue doing as much as you can without feeling tired and strained. Many people find they can continue to work during the treatment period. This is a time to listen to your body and to take good care of yourself. In addition, your radiation oncologist may suggest that you limit some activities, such as sports. There also is more information about radiation in Chapter 9, Radiation Treatment.

Do Medicare and Medicaid pay for radiation treatments?

Both Medicare and Medicaid cover the major portion of the cost of treatment. For Medicare, if the radiation oncologist is a participating physician (one who has agreed to accept the charges established by Medicare), the physician will be paid 80 percent of the recognized charge. You will pay the other 20 percent. If you have a Medigap insurance policy, it will usually cover the 20 percent copayment. Be sure you are not confused by the "billing balance" that some radiation oncologists who are not participating physicians, add to your copayment bill. For instance, if Medicare pays $100 as the "reasonable" charge, a nonparticipating radiation oncologist may charge $120 for the procedure. Medicare would pay the patient or physician $80. If you pay the $20 copayment, $20 will remain as the billing balance. You should be aware that some states have legislated against the practice of balance billing.

Radiation Seeding for Prostate Cancer

What is radiation seeding?

Radiation seeding, sometimes called internal radiation, interstitital implantation, or brachytherapy, selectively places radioactive particles or seeds into the prostate. A number of years ago, the only way to do this was with abdominal surgery. Now the seed is implanted with the help of ultrasound into the prostate through the perineum (the area between the rectum and scrotum). It is usually done in the hospital as an outpatient procedure.

Why was radiation seeding unsuccessful when first used?

Radiation seeding was used extensively in the 1970s, being done with abdominal surgery and freehand implantation of gold or iodine seeds. Studies showed that this method was not as successful as external radiation over the long term because there was no way to check where the seeds were placed and was discontinued. New techniques—using ultrasound to place the seed in a precise location, plus the use of faster-acting iodine or palladium seeds—have enabled doctors to reevaluate this treatment. Studies of various radioactive sources with ultrasound imaging are in progress. Since the new methods have been in use about five years, the long-term results of these implant treatments are not yet available, although the short-term results are promising.

Are there after effects with radiation seeding?

Like prostate surgery and external beam radiation, internal radiation seeding has some serious after effects. Not as many studies have been conducted on this treatment, but there is some information about side effects. The following side effects developed in a group of **100 men** who have had internal seeding:

Impotence	25
Incontinence	0–2
with TURP	15
Serious rectal problems	20

Who is the best candidate for radiation seeding?

Radiation seeding implants are most appropriate in men with small, well- or moderately-differentiated cancers, or men for whom surgery is considered a high risk for other reasons.

What are the advantages of radiation seeding?

This treatment has fewer side effects, takes less time to do, requires less time in the hospital and costs less than radiation or surgery.

How is radiation seeding done?

Radiation seeding is usually done with the help of ultrasound and computer. The doctor implants radioactive material directly into the tumor with long needles passed through the perineum. Radioactive iodine and palladium are most commonly used. The procedure and results are presently under clinical evaluation. Doctors feel the use of ultrasound imaging techniques for guiding implantation directly to the cancer is a big step forward in perfecting this technique. Be sure to ask if there will be lymph node dissection (pelvic lymphadenectomy), if your treatment plan includes internal radiation therapy.

Is hormonal treatment ever used before seed implantation?

The use of hormonal therapy for a period of up to six months prior to treatment can help to decrease the tumor volume and size of the prostate and may make the radiation seeding treatment more effective.

How is radiation seeding planned?

Using ultrasound scans, your physician will create a map of your prostate. This will be used to calculate the exact number of seeds needed for complete coverage and accurate placement. Usually 40 to 100 seeds are implanted in the prostate gland. A treatment-planning computer constructs the implant model to optimize radiation distribution.

What does the treatment involve?

After spinal or general anesthesia, an ultrasound probe is positioned in the rectum to accurately reproduce the treatment plan and to allow needle alignment. A template guidance device, which is attached to the ultrasound probe, has holes that correspond to the grid on the ultrasound computer screen. Implant needles are put through the appropriate template holes. These needles may be preloaded with the seeds or may attach to an applicator that dispenses the radioactive seeds through the needle and into the prostate. Each needle is guided through the template, then through the perineum (the area between the rectum and scrotum) to its predetermined position. The ultrasound unit's screen allows the physician to see the needle's exact position in the prostate. A predetermined number of seeds are then implanted as the needle is withdrawn from the prostate. When all seeds have been inserted, the ultrasound image is reviewed to verify seed placement.

How long does this procedure take to complete?

The actual procedure takes about an hour or two to complete. Often it is done as an outpatient or overnight procedure under spinal or general anesthesia. You will be in the recovery room until the effects of anesthesia have disappeared. An antibiotic will usually be prescribed. Pain medication is not usually necessary.

What are the possible after effects of radiation seeding?

There may be bruising and swelling between the legs which disappears in a few days. Urinary discomfort—a sense of urgency, burning during urination, slight bleeding or blood in the urine—is to be expected one to two weeks after the seeding, but will diminish as the seeds lose their radioactivity. Rectal irritation and occasional rectal bleeding may occur, but should subside in less than three months.

Will I be impotent after radiation seeding treatments?

You may experience erection problems immediately following your treatment, but a large percentage of men who have had this treatment report they are still able to have erections, although they may not be as firm as they were before treatment. Various studies show that 75 percent of men who had strong erections before treatment will continue to be able to achieve a full erection. The other 25 percent will experience some decrease in their ability, but will still be able to have intercourse.

Can seed implantation cause long- or short-term incontinence?

Right after the treatment and until the seeds lose their energy, some patients experience a sense of urgency and slight dribbling. The risk of long-term incontinence is extremely low, probably less than one percent.

Can I have radiation seeding if I previously had a TURP?

If you previously had a TURP (transurethral resection of the prostate) the changes in your prostate gland make it difficult to distribute seeds uniformly. There is a greater risk of urinary incontinence, so radiation seeding is usually not recommended.

Does the PSA usually fall after radiation seeding?

PSA values usually fall back to the normal range within three to six months after implantation. However, there have been some cases where PSAs rise following radiation seeding and early biopsies have shown that cancer is still present in the prostate. Some doctors think that cancer cells take time to die off, and although some may look like cancer, they appear to have stopped dividing. These doctors feel that prostate cancer patients who have had radiation seeding should not be biopsied for 12 to 18 months after treatment, even if their PSA rises. Some physicians theorize that the PSA rises after radiation seeding because of the regrowth of normal prostate cells which can continue to reflect on the PSA reading. The stability of the PSA level is the most important factor.

Can radiation seeding be done a second time if there appears to be further cancer in the prostate?

If the cancer is confined to the prostate, it is possible to have another seed implant performed in the area that was not treated previously.

Is radiation seeding sometimes combined with external radiation?
Sometimes when the cancer is locally advanced, external radiation will be used before or following the implant procedure.

**Is lymph node dissection (lymphadenectomy)
done before radiation seeding?**
Sometimes lymph node dissection is done to determine if the cancer has spread to the lymph nodes. The dissection is usually not done if the cancer is low grade and the PSA level is low. Generally, the laparoscopic method of lymph node dissection is used instead of an abdominal lymph node operation. Some physicians feel that lapraoscopic lymphadenectomy is not as accurate as an abdominally performed lymph node dissection. It is possible to do the laparoscopic lymph node dissection at the same time as the seeding, but the two procedures are most often done separately. Before agreeing to lymph node dissection be sure to ask what type of procedure is being planned, the expected results and whether or not the surgery is necessary. (See Chapter 8, Surgery, for more information on this procedure.)

*Questions to Ask Your Radiation Oncologist
About Radiation Seeding*

- **Do you think internal radiation seeding will work for me?**

- **How many of these procedures have you done? What are the results?**

- **What kind of radioactive material will you be using?**

- **How will the radioactive material be put in my body?**

- **Are you planning a lymph node dissection? How will it be done? Why is it being done? Is it necessary?**

- **Will I need anesthesia? Will it be local or general?**

- **How long will I need to be in the hospital for this procedure?**

- **Will I have to stay in bed during this time?**

- **Will I be able to have visitors? Will there be any restrictions on the visitors?**

- **Will the implant be permanent?**

- **Will I be radioactive while the implant is inside me? For how long?**

- **What side effects should I expect?**

- **When will it be safe to have intercourse?**

- **When will I be able to get back to my normal routine?**

- How much will it cost?
- Will my health insurance cover the treatment?

Will the radiation seeds be left in permanently?
Yes. The seeds lose some energy each day. You do not have to take any special precautions after you leave the hospital.

What is the difference between iodine and palladium seeds?
The half-life of Iodine 125 seeds is approximately 60 days. After two months, the activity is reduced by 50 percent. Palladium has a half life of 17 days. Within two months it has given up 90 percent of its energy and has lost almost all of it by the end of six months. The seed dosages of iodine and palladium are prescribed to produce the same effect. However, some doctors feel that iodine is more effective for slower growing cancers and palladium better for faster growing cancers.

Will the radiation seeds spread radiation to others?
The Nuclear Regulatory Commission has determined that no radiation precautions need to be taken with internal seeding for prostate because seeds lose their activity very quickly at short distances from the seeds. The radioactive seeds in your implant do not transmit rays outside your body. However, some doctors recommend that children not sit on the patient's lap for the first two months after the procedure. Pregnant women should avoid prolonged close contact for the first two months after the procedure. At a six foot distance from the patient there is no limit to the length of time a pregnant woman can remain in the same room with the patient.

Will I have any side effects immediately after this treatment?
If you have had general anesthesia, you may feel drowsy, weak or nauseated for a short time after your operation. There may be signs of blood or blood clots in the urine immediately after the procedure. If blood in the urine persists you should report it to your doctor. Also report any burning, sweating, or other unusual symptoms.

Will I be in pain as a result of my radiation seeding treatment?
Most of the time you will not have severe pain, although you might be uncomfortable. You may be given sleeping pills or other medication to relax you. If you feel you need medicine for pain, tell the radiation oncologist or urologist. You may have a catheter in your bladder for a short time after the procedure, but will probably be able to urinate the next day without a problem.

How long after the radiation seeding treatment will I be able to go back to work and my normal activities?

You can usually go back to work and to your normal activities, such as exercising or walking, within a few days. Doctors advise that you not resume sexual activities for about four to six weeks.

What is high-dose rate brachytherapy?

High-dose rate brachytherapy, also called high-dose rate remote radiation therapy or remote brachytherapy, is a newer type of internal radiation seeding in which the radioactive source is removed between treatments. In prostate cancer, high-dose rate brachytherapy may be used for early-stage tumors as the only treatment; in combination with external radiation; or when cancer has come back after treatment with radical prostatectomy, external radiation, or radiation seeding. Thin hollow tubes, called treatment catheters, are precisely positioned around and through the prostate. When treatment is to begin, the ends of the tubes are attached to a computer-guided treatment unit, called an afterloader, which delivers the radioactive source, usually Iridium-192, precisely to the tumor, minimizing harm to nearby organs and lessening side effects. The treatments, after the catheters are positioned and checked by CT scan, take about 15 minutes. Depending on the stage of the cancer, three or four treatments are usually needed.

Cryotherapy for Prostate Cancer

Is cryosurgery being used in treating prostate cancer?

Some men have chosen cryotherapy after considering other possible alternatives because of the relative simplicity of the treatment and the reduced costs and side effects.

What kinds of after effects have been reported following cryosurgery?

Long term problems that can be expected after cryosurgery in a group of 100 men who had the procedure include:

Impotence	70–80
Incontinence	1–2
Incontinence with prior radiation	50
Blocked urethra	5–20

What is cryosurgery?

Cryosurgery, sometimes referred to as cryotherapy or cryoablation, is the use of extreme cold to destroy cancer cells. Liquid nitrogen is circulated through cryoprobes, which are placed in contact with the tumor.

Who are the best candidates for cryosurgery?

Cryosurgery is used to treat men with early stage cancer confined to the prostate gland and the surrounding area, particularly when standard treatments such as surgery and radiation are unsuccessful or cannot be used. There are two groups of men in which clinical trials are being conducted:

- Men with Stage II prostate cancer who prefer not to have a radical prostatectomy or radiation therapy or who have risk factors that make other treatments infeasible.
- Men diagnosed with Stage III prostate cancer.

Are there cases where cryotherapy should not be used?

Cryosurgery is not considered an effective treatment for prostate cancer that has spread to the lymph nodes or other parts of the body.

How is cryotherapy performed?

The liquid nitrogen or carbon dioxide is placed in a hollow metal probe used to freeze and destroy unwanted or diseased tissue, which is then absorbed by the body over time. Probes are positioned directly into the prostate through the area between the anus and the base of scrotum.

Does cryotherapy involve surgery?

The treatment is considered a surgical procedure. A small incision is made for insertion of the cryoprobe through the skin. It takes two to three hours to perform under general or spinal anesthesia. After a catheter is put in place to drain the bladder through the lower abdominal wall, probes are positioned directly into the prostate through the perineum. Once the freezing process is completed, the probes are removed and the insertion sites are closed with stitches that dissolve. Most men are able to leave the hospital on the second day after surgery.

Questions to Ask Your Doctor Before You Have Cryosurgery

- Do you think I am a good candidate for this procedure? Why?
- What are the side effects?
- How many cryosurgeries have you done?
- What is your rate of complications?
- What are possible complications in my case?
- How will you manage these complications if I have them?

- **Do you prescribe hormone therapy prior to cryosurgery?**

- **How long will I be in the hospital?**

- **When will I be able to resume normal activities?**

- **What percentage of your patients become incontinent? Is it temporary or permanent?**

- **Will I be impotent? Will this be temporary or permanent?**

- **Do you require your patients to have a biopsy after six months to check results? Why?**

- **How many biopsies do you do?**

- **How often will I need to see you after the operation?**

- **If you live in a different city than where you have the cryosurgery done? Can my regular urologist follow my case and will you forward information to him? Can he remove the catheter for me?**

- **What can you advise me about insurance and Medicare coverage?**

What happens to the destroyed tissue after cryosurgery?

During the cryosurgery process the cells become severely dehydrated and shrink. Once engulfed by ice, they break down and are frozen intracellularly. As melting occurs, the destruction continues and the capillaries supplying oxygen and other nutrients to the tumor are damaged beyond repair. Clotting and local tissue swelling and the invasion of the immune system's scavenger cells cause the destroyed tissue to be absorbed by the body. During the next weeks, the body's white blood cells engulf the dead cellular material, leaving behind normal fibrous tissue. When examined on followup, what remains will be a shrunken, prostatic capsule, relatively free of glandular tissue.

How do I prepare for cryotherapy?

Before cryosurgery you will be given specific instructions regarding diet and enemas. The enema will help clear your bowels so that the ultrasound will be clear.

What are the risks and side effects of cryotherapy?

The risks associated with cryosurgery are the same as those for any surgical procedure. There are sideeffects, although they may be less severe than those associated with prostate surgery or radiation therapy. The urinary system may be affected. Incontinence can also result from cryosurgery, although these side effects may be temporary.

What are the advantages of cryotherapy?

The advantages include a decrease in the incidence of serious complications, a short hospital stay and the ability to repeat the procedure if needed. There is no abdominal incision and bleeding complications are minimal. Cryotherapy is usually less expensive than other treatments and requires a shorter recovery time and a shorter hospital stay.

What are the disadvantages of cryotherapy?

The major disadvantage is the uncertainty regarding the long-term effectiveness of the treatment. If freezing is not carefully controlled, tissue near the rectal wall may be damaged causing a fistula to develop between the rectum and urethra. Men who have undergone radiation therapy for prostate cancer are at greatest risk for this complication. In addition, because the effectiveness of the technique is still being assessed, insurance coverage problems may arise.

Will I still be able to have erections after cryotherapy?

Because the experience with cryotherapy is still limited, the results are not fully known. Some men report that they are able to continue to have erections. About 20 to 30 percent of men who had erections prior to cryosurgery have regained this ability within six months to a year after treatment. It is possible that this rate may increase over time since nerves can regenerate following freezing.

Will I be incontinent after cryotherapy?

Incontinence has been reported in only 1.5 percent of men who had cryosurgery and who had not had prior radiation. Those who had prior radiation had about a 50 percent chance of having some degree of incontinence following the procedure. Urinary control may improve over time for most of these men, but may not return completely.

What other problems can occur following cryotherapy?

Tissue sloughing may occur when pieces of prostate tissue break off and fall into the bladder or urethra, blocking the flow of urine. Tissue sloughing usually corrects itself without the need for further treatment. Fistulas, or holes, can develop between the urinary and gastrointestinal tract, which may require a surgical operation later to repair. Irritation to the bladder or urethra is another common side effect that causes problems with urination such as need to urinate with little warning, pain with urination, and burning sensations.

Should men with large prostates consider cryotherapy?
Cryotherapy works best when the prostate gland is about 40 grams or less in size. At some centers, physicians prescribe three to four months of total hormone blockage, using both the monthly shots of LHRH and flutamide to shrink the gland before doing the cryotherapy.

How long will I be in the hospital?
Usually one or two days. Most men can get up and move about the afternoon after cryotherapy, eat their evening meal and leave the next day. A small tube just below the navel will be left in place for about ten to 14 days. (You may find sweat pants are more comfortable than regular trousers while the tube is in place.) This suprapubic tube is placed in the bladder as a safety release valve for the first time you urinate through the penis. Antibiotics are usually prescribed.

When can I go back to doing my regular activities?
You can usually resume your regular activities within a week or two.

Is there pain involved with the procedure?
There is tenderness in the area between the anus and the testicles at the point where the cryoprobes are inserted. There usually is some swelling of the testicles. As with all such treatments, there is some discomfort, but most men do not require pain medication. Healing is usually complete within three months.

Does it hurt to have the suprapubic catheter removed?
Usually there is no pain involved when the catheter is removed.

Can the cryotherapy procedure be repeated if I have a recurrence?
One of the benefits of cryotherapy is that it can be repeated if the first procedure does not eliminate the cancer. The physician may selectively freeze areas where recurrence occurs.

Is cryosurgery covered by insurance or Medicare?
Many insurance companies cover cryosurgery; in others it appears that reimbursement is made on a case-by-case basis. Insurers who pay for the procedure have cited shortened length of hospitalization and lower costs as reasons for coverage. Medicare covers cryosurgery for stages T1–T3. It does not cover cryotherapy if used for salvage therapy after radical prostatectomy, external radiation or seed implants.

Hormonal Treatments for Prostate Cancer

How does hormonal treatment work?

Hormone therapy is one of the standard options for treating prostate cancer. You may hear several different terms used to describe hormone treatment—combination hormone therapy, androgens, complete hormone blockage, complete androgen blockage, and ablation. Because prostate cancer is sensitive to hormones, it has been found that eliminating testosterone from the body deprives the cancer of this hormone and usually prevents it from growing. Testosterone is controlled by a pituitary hormone called luetinizing hormone. Two drugs, goserelin acetate and leuprolide, affect the pituitary gland's response to the chemical signal to make testosterone, and lower the testosterone to the same low levels as if your testicles had been taken out in an operation. However, some testosterone may be produced from adrenal hormones. Flutamide has been found to block the effects of remaining hormone.

How is hormonal treatment used in treating prostate cancer?

Hormonal manipulation—either with hormone drugs or with the surgical removal of the testicles—is being used in different ways in treating prostate cancer.

- It may be used when the cancer is localized but in an advanced stage.
- It may be the primary treatment in older men when it is felt that radiation or surgery is too much or inappropriate.
- It is sometimes used before cryosurgery or radiation seeding or before or after surgery or radiation to reduce the prostate size or to keep the cancer from growing.
- It may be the treatment of choice if the cancer has spread or returned after previous treatment.

What are the different types of hormonal treatments used for prostate cancer?

A number of different therapies are available. These include:

- leutinizing hormone-releasing hormone agonist (LH-RH)
- antiandrogen
- orchiectomy (removal of testicles)
- estrogen (DES)

Questions to Ask Your Doctor About Hormonal Treatment

- **What kind of hormonal treatment do you suggest for me?**
- **Why are you suggesting this type of hormonal treatment?**
- **How long will it be before we know if this treatment works for me?**
- **How often will you check my PSA level to see how well it is working?**
- **What are the possible side effects?**
- **Will I get hot flashes?**
- **What is the cost of the treatment?**
- **Is it covered by insurance?**
- **Do you ever advise your patients to have an orchiectomy? Do you do the surgery? What are the risks? What are the advantages and disadvantages?**
- **Do you advise having hormone therapy before or after surgery or radiation? Before radiation seeding or cryosurgery?**
- **How do you usually treat bone metastases?**
- **How much does it cost? Is it covered by insurance or Medicare?**

What are luteinizing hormone-releasing hormone agonists, often referred to as LHRH (Lupron, Depo Lupron, Zoladex)?

LHRH, the normal brain hormone controlling the secretion of luteinizing hormone from the pituitary gland, suppresses testicular androgen and is responsible for stimulating the secretion of male hormones by the testes. The natural hormone LHRH is secreted by the brain in minute amounts and successive pulses of the hormone are released approximately once every 90 minutes. When first discovered, doctors hoped LHRH would increase fertility and gonadal functions. When copied in the laboratory and made 100 to 300 times more potent than the natural hormone, though, it was found to have the opposite effect, blocking the effects of the natural hormones. Therefore, LHRH is now used to inhibit testicular functions. Several forms made in the laboratory are used, including the leuprolides (Lupron and Depo Lupron) and goserelin (Zoladex).

How is the LHRH treatment given?

Lupron is usually given by injection in the muscle of the buttock. **Zoladex** is a pellet injected under the skin's surface somewhere on the abdominal wall. Longer–acting versions of these medications are now available which allow injections lasting several months. The shot stimulates a short burst of testosterone which your body interprets as having too much testosterone, causing the body to shut down the hormone production. In some cases, during the

For years, scientists have known that prostate cancer cells depend on male sex hormones for their growth. Like breast cancer, prostate cancer is sensitive to hormones. These hormones stimulate the growth of prostate cancer cells. When certain hormones are eliminated from the body, the cancer may stop growing and become inactive for a period of time—from one to ten years. The purpose of hormone therapy is to lower levels of testosterone. Although it is not a curative treatment, hormone therapy is often used to treat prostate cancer that has spread because it can affect cancer cells throughout the body. The treatment may be given before or after prostatectomy or radiation therapy and sometimes before and/or after radiation seeding or cryotherapy.

period when the flare–up of testosterone levels occurs there can be problems, such as increased bone pain. The addition of antiandrogen helps block tumor flare in the first few weeks or months of treatment, after which the antiandrogen is often discontinued. This treatment is expensive and causes loss of libido and thus potency.

How are antiandrogens used?

Androgens are hormones secreted by the testes and adrenal glands, which are necessary for the development and functioning of the male sexual organs and characteristics. Antiandrogens reduce or eliminate the activity of these androgens. There is some evidence that this male hormone also plays a role in stimulating prostate cancer. **Flutamide**, which is sold under the brand name **Eulexin**, is a synthetic nonsteroidal antiandrogen which blocks the cells' ability to absorb any hormone, producing what is called total androgen blockage and thus blocking any androgens from the adrenal not suppressed by LHRH treatment. Another nonsteroidal antiandrogen **bicalutamide**, is sold under the brand name **Casodex**.

How is flutamide used as a treatment for prostate cancer?

This drug has been used alone as well as in combination with LHRH or immunotherapy in an attempt to suppress tumor growth in prostate cancer. In many cases, when used alone, sexual potency can be preserved. It is effective, but less so than LHRH. Flutamide and nilutamide are sometimes used together or in combination with an orchiectomy in Stage IV cancers to produce bone pain relief and slow the progression of the cancer.

What are the side effects of flutamide?

Side effects are generally limited to mild diarrhea and breast enlargement, but liver poisoning can sometimes occur. The patient usually recovers when the drug is stopped. Usually radiation is given to the breasts before treatment is started to alleviate the side effect of breast enlargement. Your PSA levels may drop if you stop taking flutamide after a prolonged period of time taking it.

What is Casodex (bicalutamide)?

Casodex is a newer drug, similar to flutamide, but it only has to be taken once a day, either morning or evening. It is a nonsteroidal antiandrogen often used with a luteinizing hormone-releasing hormone (LHRH) analogue. When given with an LHRH analogue, it achieves maximal androgen blockage by preventing any remaining testosterone from binding to receptor sites in prostate cancer cells.

What are the side effects of Casodex?

Hot flashes are experienced by about half of those taking the pill. Constipation, back pain, lack of strength, pelvic pain, nausea, and diarrhea have also been reported.

How does estrogen therapy (DES) work?

Estrogen is a synthetic female hormone that reduces or eliminates the body's production of testosterone. Diethylstilbestrol (DES) is sometimes prescribed in the form of a daily pill, though this treatment is used less often now that alternative treatments are available. There are side effects to this treatment, such as breast enlargement or tenderness, nausea, vomiting, loss of libido, impotence, and blood clots. This form of treatment is not appropriate for men who have a history of heart disease or embolism.

What is intermittent therapy?

Hormone therapy is sometimes used on an intermittent basis. It is first used until your PSA drops down to its lowest level and stabilizes. Then it is withdrawn. When the PSA level starts to climb again, the hormone therapy is started again. Therapy is then continued until the PSA drops down again. This intermittent treatment is being studied in clinical trial.

When is an orchiectomy used for prostate cancer?

Most men are appalled at the thought of an operation on their testicles. Castration is a difficult issue emotionally. Yet, orchiectomy, the technical name for removal of the testicles, has been used for many years to control prostate cancers. The spread of prostate cancer can often be controlled by removing the testicles—man's natural source of the male sex hormone. Removal of both testicles is called a bilateral orchiectomy. This procedure, which is considered a low-risk operation, eliminates the major source of testosterone.

Without these hormones, the growth of prostate cancer cells slows down. Men who have had the operation report there is little or no pain except for some possible swelling, bruising, or soreness that lasts a few days.

How is the orchiectomy operation done?
The operation consists of the removal of both testicles through a small incision, leaving the scrotum intact. It is usually performed as an outpatient procedure, done under anesthesia with absorbable stitches.

Is an orchiectomy the same as castration?
Orchiectomy and castration both mean that the testicles are removed.

How effective is an orchiectomy?
As a treatment for dropping the testosterone level, an orchiectomy achieves the desired goal quickly and efficiently. The testosterone level drops to zero within the first 12 hours after the operation. If there is pain caused by cancer in the bone, it usually disappears. In terms of cost, the one-time cost of the operation makes it much less expensive than the cost of the other alternatives and it is usually covered by insurance. On the other hand, the permanence of an orchiectomy concerns some men since other effective treatments may be discovered for which they would no longer be eligible.

Treating Bone Metastases

How are bone metastases caused by prostate cancer treated?
Eighty to 85 percent of metastases from prostate cancer are found in the bone. The other ten to 15 percent are in soft tissue including lymph nodes, liver and lung. For those with bone metastases, the treatment recommended is usually orchiectomy with or without antiandrogens or LHRH with or without flutamide or estrogens. Orchiectomy shows a remarkable, an almost immediate, improvement in bone pain. There are clinical trials underway for nutron/photon radiation, chemotherapy, and other hormonal treatments.

What other kinds of treatment are available for bone metastases?
External beam radiation may be used if the metastatic cancer is confined to one area. Where there are more widespread problems, investigation is underway with bone-seeking radioisotopes and radioactive monoclonal antibodies. Strontium-89, sometimes referred to as Metastron, is an injectable form of radiation sometimes used for treatment of multiple painful bone metastases. Zoledronic acid and parmidronate, part of a family of drugs called bisphosphonates, are also being used to treat osteoporosis and bone pain. They

HORMONAL TREATMENTS

TYPE OF TREATMENT	PROS AND CONS	POSSIBLE SIDE EFFECTS
LHRH (Lupron/Depo Lupron/ Zoladex).	Monthly injection. Achieves same effect as orchiectomy surgery. Sometimes used with flutamide.	May cause hot flashes, breast tenderness, reduced sex drive, possible flareup immediately after start of treatment.
Antiandrogens Flutamide (Eulexin), Nilutamide, Casodex, total androgen blockage.	Given in pill form, three times a day. Radiation usually given to breasts. Can be added to other treatment if PSA levels rise. (Casodex is given in pill form, once a day.)	Diarrhea, hot flashes, reduced sex drive. Occasional liver problems.
Orchiectomy (Removal of testicles).	Simple, outpatient surgery, immediate drop in testosterone levels. Is considered emasculating by many men. Not reversible.	Hot flashes, breast tenderness, impotence.
Estrogen (DES).	Given in daily pill form. Low cost but high risk. There are other safer options. Testosterone levels drop in 30–60 days.	Higher doses can cause strokes or blood clots.

have been approved by the FDA and are being studied, in conjunction with chemotherapy, for reducing bone pain in prostate cancer patients. They may be able to prevent fractures by increasing bone mineral density.

How does Strontium-89 (Metastron) work?

Strontium-89 is injected and goes directly to the sites of metastatic bone disease where it is absorbed in the bones like calcium. The injection contains small amounts of a specially selected form of radioactive strontium, chosen because almost all of its radiation is given to the area where it is absorbed— precisely where it is needed. A single injection generally provides pain relief for an average of six months, and has minimal effect on normal bone and surrounding tissues. The effects of Strontium-89 are confined within your body. Other people cannot receive the effects of radiation through contact with you. However, for the first week after injection, Strontium-89 will be present in your blood and urine and your doctor will discuss simple precautions that should be taken. S-89 is not recommended for patients with cancer that does not involve bone.

What are the side effects of Strontium-89 (Metastron)?
Some people experience a mild facial flushing immediately after injection. This may happen when the medication is administered too quickly (in 30 seconds rather than in a one or two minute time frame). Some people have a mild, but temporary, increase in pain several days after the injection that may last for two or three days. Doctors usually prescribe an increase in pain killers until the pain is under control. After one or two weeks, or sometimes a little longer, the pain begins to diminish and continues to diminish, with effects lasting for up to six months. You may be advised to reduce the dose of other pain medications gradually. Eventually, you may not need painkillers at all. You can eat and drink normally. There may be a slight fall in your blood cell count. Your doctor will probably take routine periodic blood tests. Repeated dosages can be given if the doctor feels this is the most appropriate treatment.

Are there any new treatments for prostate cancer that has metastasized and cannot be treated with standard therapy?
Immune system cells (called dendrictic cells) that identify harmful cells—are removed from the body, activated in the laboratory, and infused back into the body as a vaccine. The treatment consists of three leukapheresis procedures (collection of white blood cells) and three infusions of the vaccine over a 30 day period. This treatment is presently undergoing clinical trials to determine its effectiveness.

Sex, Incontinence, and Other Side Effects

When treatment makes the patient impotent is there any way that he can regain sexual functioning?
If the nerves were not removed during surgery, sexual function may return— though it may take a considerable period of time, often as long as a year or

more, before it returns to normal. For those where function is no longer possible, there is another alternative. A number of prostheses have been invented which can be implanted so that normal sex can be resumed. However, most experts suggest that it is important to wait at least six months to a year to see if function will return before deciding upon implant surgery. You may want to discuss your sexual concerns with an oncology clinical nurse specialist, a sex therapist or sex counselor.

Why do I still have problems having an erection even though the doctor says my prostate surgery or radiation therapy was successful?

There are many reasons for a man to lose his ability to have an erection. It happens to everyone at times—even to those who don't have cancer. Emotional stress—worry about cancer, depression, being tired, trying too hard, worry, alcohol—all can result in erection problems. Any signs of an erection give you proof that your body is cooperating, but the psyche is so sensitive that it may take quite a long time for you to feel certain enough of your masculinity for you to resume normal intercourse. A number of men report that they had their first orgasm after cancer treatment while asleep, during a sexual dream. If you have such an experience, it is proof that you can achieve erection, since sleep erections are not affected by psychological factors. Perhaps this is a good time for you to experiment with other pleasuring techniques. If the doctor says there is no physical reason for the problem, perhaps the cause is psychological, due to pressure you yourself feel about getting an erection. The pace of sexual adjustment after treatment often depends upon your feelings about yourself. An appointment with a sex therapist or a self-help book on sexuality may help you to gain a better understanding of the problem.

What methods are used to allow men who have had surgery or radiation that has resulted in impotence to have intercourse?

There are a number of nonsurgical and surgical approaches now available. A most successful method is Viagra, a simple pill that delivers an enzyme which promotes erections.

Is the Viagra pill effective for men with sexual problems following prostate cancer treatment?

Viagra and several similar new products—tadalafil (Cialis) and vardenafil (Nuviva)—have proven to be extremely successful for men with prostate problems. These products increase the flow of the blood to the penis. The newer products may be even more potent than Viagra.

Does testosterone topical cream work in enhancing erections?

A testosterone topical cream, AndroGel, is being prescribed for men with low testosterone levels. However, since hormonal therapy given for prostate cancer is designed to lower levels of testosterone, other methods of enhancing erections should be used by men with prostate cancer.

What injectable drugs are available to help produce erections?

Highly effective drugs such as alprostadil (Caverject), papaverine, phentolamine, and prostaglandin E1 produce erections in many men when injected with a very fine needle into the side of the penis. This usually painless injection is reported to be effective in 75 to 85 percent of men. Frequent use can cause a buildup of scar tissue where the needle is injected.

How do the impotence drug injections work?

The newest drug, alprostadil (Caverject), is a synthetic version of a naturally occurring form of prostaglandin E1, which is found in human tissues and fluids and plays a role in erection by widening blood vessels. The drug is injected into the penis shortly before intercourse. It relaxes and widens the muscles in the arteries that supply blood to the penis. The increased blood flow compresses the veins against a rigid fibrous sheath. It usually induces erection within five to 20 minutes. Possible side effects include mild-to-moderate pain at the site of injection, and scarring of penile tissue. A few men may have an abnormally prolonged erection. If the erection lasts more than a few hours, you will need to go to the emergency room for an injection to reverse the effects of the drug.

Who gives the injection?

The doctor in the doctor's office usually gives the first injection so that the dose can be adjusted as needed. You will be shown how to prepare the medication, get the correct dosage, and inject the needle. Your partner may wish to learn the technique and incorporate it as part of your sexual ritual. Most men are surprised at how easy and painless it is to use this method to encourage erections.

How do vacuum erection devices work?

There are external, noninvasive systems which use vacuum devices that are quite effective. One such device is made of a semi-rigid material and worn like a condom. The sheath is put on and a vacuum is applied to draw the penis out to fill it. The device is left in place for intercourse. Another device requires putting the penis in a vacuum that draws blood into the organ. When an adequate erection has been produced, it can be maintained by putting a constricting band around the base of the penis which helps maintain the erection for about 30 minutes. These devices work in most cases, whether or not nerves have been preserved, since they do not depend on the body to produce the erection. The vacuum forces the blood to flow into the penis. Two companies that make such devices are: Osbon Medical Systems of Augusta, Georgia which makes ErecAid; and Mission Pharmacal Company maker of the VED pump (1–800–531–3333).

Are there disadvantages to using the vacuum erection device?
One disadvantage is the loss of spontaneity involved in making preparations, since three to five minutes are required to produce an erection. However, some couples use the device as part of the foreplay ritual and find that this turns the disadvantage into a plus. In addition, because the rigidity of a normal erection depends on the engorgement of internal tissue, and since only the part of the penile shaft beyond the constricting ring is engorged, the result may be a less firm erection. (NOTE: Many companies offer a money-back guarantee, so before purchasing, it would be wise to ask if a full refund is possible.)

Are there side effects to using the vacuum erection device?
Reported possible side effects are extremely minor—a reddish rash on the penis and bruising if the vacuum pressure is maintained for too long.

How do surgically implanted devices work?
There are a number of prosthetic designs that can help a man achieve a controlled erection. Some are simply malleable, semi-rigid rods implanted inside the penis. Newer types of inflatable penile prostheses operate hydraulically to harden or soften the penis. A plastic reservoir about the size of a tangerine is implanted inside the body beneath muscles near the bladder. The implanted reservoir serves as a permanent storehouse for water. Two thin plastic tubes connect the reservoir to a hydraulic pump planted in the scrotal sac, which in turn is attached to two hollow cylinders, much like balloons, that are implanted in the penis. To achieve an erection, the small pump is gently squeezed. This releases the salt water that fills the reservoir, which flows down into the cylinders and causes the erection. The fluid returns to the reservoir when a release valve implanted inside the scrotum is pressed.

Does the body sometimes reject these implants?
Prophylactic antibiotics are used and most times the implants are successful. Only about one percent of implants are rejected or create infections. In those

cases the prosthesis is removed and the infection is treated. Many times the prosthesis can be reimplanted.

How long does penile implant surgery take?

Implant surgery takes from about 30 minutes to two hours. Many patients spend two to five days recuperating in the hospital. Full recovery requires four to six weeks. The usual complications of surgery are possible—infection, bleeding, and abnormal scarring. Complication rates are low on the whole. Although no mechanical device is a perfect replacement, most men who have had the surgery say they are satisfied with the implant results.

Dealing with Urinary Problems

Once I am past the initial recovery period will I still have to deal with dribbling of urine?

Unfortunately, for some men it may take some time following treatment before the muscles are strengthened enough to control urination. However, doing the daily corrective exercises, described in this chapter, the problem should lessen and in many cases will eventually disappear.

Is incontinence sometimes temporary?

In many cases, incontinence is temporary. It may be helped with corrective exercises, known as Kegel exercises, described earlier, or through behavior modification, which adds the scheduling of bathroom visits to train the bladder to hold urine longer. These techniques can hasten the recovery from temporary incontinence after surgery. Sometimes, however, the incontinence persists and may become a permanent condition.

What are some practical ways of dealing with incontinence after a prostetectomy?

Many men find that incontinence can be managed with the use of incontinence pads, available at most drugstores, which can be slipped into undershorts or shorts with additional padding to catch any dribbles. There are also external collection devices made of rubber, similar to a condom. These are pulled over the penis and held in place by a band around the waist. A drainage tube connects to the collection bag, which is secured to the leg by a band. A penile clamp can be used to control the flow of urine. You must be careful not to apply too much pressure because the clamp can restrict blood flow through the penis. On a less sophisticated, but very practical basis, one support group told us they use small baggies, filled with either a pad or tissues and secured with a twistie wire.

How does the doctor decide what is causing my long-term incontinence?

There are several main causes of incontinence in men who have been treated for prostate cancer: damage to the bladder neck, to the sphincter muscles, or to other muscles around the prostate gland. The doctor will do a physical examination and take a detailed history of your problem. Keep a diary that tracks how often you urinate, when you leak, what activities (such as exercise, walking, sneezing) you were doing when you leak, and how many pads you use. This will help the doctor diagnose your specific problem. You may also have a urodynamic test to reproduce your specific symptoms, a cystoscopy (bladder exam), or an ultrasound.

What are the most common treatments for long-term incontinence?

Doctors often suggest behavioral techniques or prescribe drugs. Learning behavior modification techniques is time consuming, usually requiring one hour-long session per week for eight to 12 weeks. Although behavior modification is effective in more than 50 percent of patients, it may not be covered by insurance.

What drugs are used for long-term incontinence?

Several drugs, including oxybutynin, imipramine and hyoscyomine, are used to treat severe incontinence. These drugs relax bladder muscles and inhibit spasms. You may have some side effects, such as dry mouth and constipation.

Is electrical stimulation used to treat incontinence?

Electrical stimulation is being studied. It includes a probe that delivers electrical stimulation for a few seconds several times a day for several weeks. Early results show promise for this treatment.

What do collagen implants do for incontinence?

Collagen is injected into the body of the urethra to reinforce the sphincter muscle by adding tissue to prevent leakage. (The collagen is made from a protein extract of connective tissue from cows and purified for human use). A skin test is done before to make certain that you are not allergic to the substance. The FDA requires doctors to receive special training before performing the procedure. The collagen is injected though a flexible needle into the tissues at the bladder neck. Doctors perform collagen injections with either local or general anesthetic. A number of treatments are usually required to achieve results and the treatment can be repeated.

Are there any devices to cope with long-term urinary problems following prostate surgery?

There are devices that are similar to the penile implant that are sometimes used to solve the problems of urine control. A reservoir is implanted which is controlled by a small pump implanted in the scrotum. A cuff is implanted around the urethra. When the cuff relaxes as the control pump is squeezed, the urine gathered in the bladder is released. The cuff closes on its own in about two minutes. The system automatically repressurizes until the man feels the need to urinate again.

Can the same patient have a prosthesis for both impotence and incontinence?

A patient can have two prostheses implanted—one to restore potency and the other to control incontinence.

Are there clinical trials being done for preventing prostate cancer?

The Prostate Cancer Prevention Trial was designed to test whether finasteride (Proscar), a drug used to treat benign prostatic hypertrophy, could prevent prostate cancer. Over 18,000 men were enrolled in the trial. In June 2003 it was stopped early when analysis found that finasteride was clearly effective in reducing the incidence of prostate cancer—18 percent of finasteride group developed prostate cancer compared with 24 percent of the control group—a reduction of nearly 25 percent. A newer trial called SELECT (Selinium and Vitamin E Cancer Trial) is enrolling 32,000 men for a seven-year trial to determine the effectiveness of selinium and Vitamin E in preventing prostate cancer.

Questions to Ask Your Doctor About Follow-up

- **Will you be doing my main follow-up?**
- **Will I also need to see any of my other doctors?**
- **How often will I need to see you?**
- **What tests will you be doing during my follow-up exam?**
- **What will you be looking for?**
- **What should I be watching for between my visits with you?**
- **What symptoms should I report? To whom?**

What kind of follow-up is needed for prostate cancer?

During the first year, checkups should be scheduled every three months; the second to fifth year every six months and thereafter, every 12 months. Blood and urine tests will be done at each checkup, acid and alkaline phosphatase and PSA tests should be done every six months for the first five years.

What happens if my PSA starts to rise after I've been treated?

When the PSA level starts to increase after treatment, most doctors begin treatment with female hormones. Sometimes this treatment can lower the

PSA to an acceptable level for a number of years. Female hormones (estrogens) suppress the production of testosterone and lead to the death or weakening of many, but not necessarily all, prostate cancer cells. Cycling this treatment—that is, giving it and then withholding it—while checking to see if the PSA has decreased, is the usual method of dealing with this problem. If a significant drop occurs, the drug is withheld until the PSA rises again. This treatment can be repeated a number of times. This intermittent hormone therapy, where LHRH (Lupron, Zoladex or Precis) is cycled on and off, either on a timed cycle, or based on PSA response, is being used although there is no long-term data available to statistically determine the effectiveness of this treatment. After several years of hormonal therapy, sometimes the testes turn off and the medication may be discontinued for a period of time with or without very delayed return of testosterone levels. When the cancer cells become resistant to hormonal treatment, cycling the hormonal treatment on and off over several months may induce positive responses. Hormonal treatment can be expensive.

What evidence is there that Vitamin D may stop prostate cancer?
A study funded by the National Institutes of Health found that giving patients with recurring cancer high doses of Vitamin D (Calcitriol or Rocaltrol) each week appears to slow or even stop the growth of cancer. Previous research had found that vitamin D, given in high levels, inhibited the growth of cancer in the laboratory. Further research is being done to see if the vitamin can keep the disease under control over the long term. The new studies will focus on patients with recurrent prostate cancer. These men suffer from serious side effects. The hope is that the Vitamin D will delay the need for aggressive treatment. If the study proves the long-term use of Vitamin D poses no risk, patients possibly could stay on this treatment the rest of their lives to keep the cancer from progressing.

Support Groups

How do I find appropriate support groups?
There are two general kinds of support groups available—support groups led by health professionals and self-help groups run by people who have prostate cancer. Some groups offer support, some education, some are for patients alone, some for family members and some for both. There are groups including people with different kinds of cancer and some that are made up only of men with prostate cancer. Man-to-Man and US Too are two support groups set up especially for prostate cancer patients. Online support groups can be found at www.acor.org. You will find that some groups are less traditional and focus on alternative techniques such as visualization, relaxation,

and meditation. All offer encouragement, information, strategies for coping, and a wonderful place to form friendships with others. Many of these groups are run by local hospitals. The American Cancer Society offices often sponsor Man-to-Man support groups in local communities, and provide information about support groups in your area either by telephone or through its Web site. In addition, the I Can Cope program addresses the educational and psychological needs of cancer patients and their families. A series of eight classes are set up to discuss cancer, how to cope with daily health problems, how to express feelings, living with limitations and available local resources. You also can check with your doctor, the social services department of your hospital, or the Prostate Cancer Survivors' Network, or look on the Web for Cancer Care's nationwide directory of support groups (www.cancercare.org).

What is PAACT?

The organization, Patient Advocates for Advanced Cancer Treatments (PAACT), is a clearinghouse for information on prostate cancer treatments. Its focus is on nonsurgical treatments, primarily combination hormonal therapy, cryotherapy, and suramin. Material is not always medically accurate, but it is an important advocacy group. Membership includes a subscription to the Cancer Communication Newsletter. See Web site information at end of chapter for how to read the newsletter on the Web.

CANCER OF THE TESTICLE

Discovering you have testicular cancer is devastating and frightening—especially since it usually occurs at the prime of a young man's life. Cancer of the testicle is one of the most common cancers in white males between 15 and 35 years of age. Men with undescended testicles are at greater risk for developing testicular cancer. It most commonly occurs in only one testicle. Though it was once considered to be incurable, the many advances in treatment make this a highly curable form of cancer, especially when discovered in an early stage.

WHAT YOU NEED TO KNOW ABOUT CANCER OF THE TESTICLE

- It occurs mostly in younger men, aged 25–35.
- It is highly treatable, usually curable.
- If localized, both fertility and sexual potency can usually be maintained.

Do I need a special kind of doctor for treatment?

Since this is an unusual type of cancer, the patient with suspected testicular cancer would be well advised to seek out a urologist in one of the large medical centers who specializes in testicular cancer. Close cooperation among surgical oncologist, radiation oncologist, and medical oncologist will help ensure the most successful outcome.

Questions to Ask Your Doctor Before Deciding on Treatment for Cancer of the Testicle

- **Are you planning to do a needle or simple biopsy? (If the answer is yes, get a second opinion before allowing the procedure.)**
- **Will only one testicle be removed?**
- **Is the tumor confined to one testicle?**
- **What is the cell type—seminoma or nonseminoma?**
- **Will this operation make me sterile?**
- **As insurance, will you make arrangements for sperm banking in case I become sterile?**
- **Will my sex life change?**
- **Are you planning any follow-up treatment?**

What are the testes and how do they function?

The testes are egg-shaped glands situated in the scrotum. They produce spermatozoa. The sperm is collected at the back of the testicles in a maze of coiled tubes called the epididymis. It then travels up toward the seminal vesicles and prostate through a long tube known as the vas deferens.

Who is most likely to get testicular cancer?

Most testicular cancers are found in young men. It is more common in white men than in blacks. Many cancers of the testicle appear to have some relation to undescended testicles. Damage to testicular tissue from viral infections that may appear at the same time as mumps may increase the risk of testicular cancer, but this has not been confirmed. Low birth weight (below five pounds) seems to increase the risk of testicular cancer. Sons of women with a history of unusual bleeding or spotting during pregnancy, those who used sedatives, alcohol, or were exposed to x-rays while pregnant may be at higher risk. It is not contagious.

Are men with undescended testicles at greater risk for testicular cancer?

Testicular cancer is most often found in young men who have undescended testicles. In the male fetus, the testes are formed near the kidneys and, in normal

SYMPTOMS OF TESTICULAR CANCER

- Lump in either testicle
- Painless enlargement of testicle
- Dull ache in lower abdomen or groin
- Heaviness in scrotum
- Sudden collection of fluid in scrotum
- Dragging feeling in scrotum
- Tenderness or enlargement of breasts

development, descend to the scrotum shortly after birth. If they never make this descent or descend after the age of six, the chances of having testicular cancer are three to 14 times more than in men with normally developed testicles. Surgery is sometimes done before the age of six to place the testicle in the appropriate place in the scrotum. However, the risk, even when this is done, appears to be greater in men who were born with undescended testicles.

Is testicular cancer a common type of cancer?
Testicular cancer accounts for only one to two percent of cancer in American men. The peak age is 20 to 40, then it declines until age 60 when there is a slight increase. It is more common among white men than blacks. Scandinavian men have the highest incidence. In Denmark it accounts for 6.7 percent of all cancers. Asian and African countries have the lowest rate.

How is testicular cancer usually discovered?
Most are discovered accidentally by the patient. Most are found on the sides of the testicle, but some appear on the front. Young men should get into the habit of practicing a simple exam known as TSE or testicular self exam. It is easily accomplished and should be done each month, during or soon after a warm bath or shower. While standing, the man gently rolls one testicle between his thumb and fingers, checking for lumps, swelling, or other changes. The process is repeated for the other testicle. Any hard, firm, or fixed area should be checked by a physician.

What are the symptoms of testicular cancer?
Painless enlargement of the testicle is the most common symptom. The first sign might also be a small, hard lump, about the size of a pea, which is painless when touched. There may be a dull ache in the lower abdomen and groin,

TESTS FOR DIAGNOSING AND STAGING TESTICULAR CANCER

- **Testicular Ultrasound** to help distinguish between epidiymitis and tumor.

- **CT Scans** of various sections of the body.

- **Orchiectomy,** after determining that the mass is not caused by infection or other underlying problem, to remove the entire testicle for biopsy. The surgery constitutes the diagnostic step and the first phase of treatment.

- **IMPORTANT: Biopsy of the Testicle Prior to Removal of the Affected Testicle is not Recommended. A SECOND OPINION SHOULD BE SOUGHT.**

- **Intravenous Pyelogram**

- **Lymphangiogram**

- **Blood Tests** (tumor markers—AFP and HCG) to help in proper planning for treatment.

- **Surgery** may be recommended to remove lymph nodes.

or a heaviness in the scrotum. Some men complain of a dragging sensation. The breasts may feel tender or be enlarged. In some rare cases there may be a painful mass which can indicate bleeding within the testicle.

How is cancer of the testicle diagnosed?
Ultrasound will usually be used to evaluate the tumor. A CT scan of the chest, abdomen, and pelvis is usually done to determine if there is any spread. After ruling out infection and other diseases that can mimic testicular cancer through careful physical examination and medical tests, the standard procedure for a suspicious lump in the scrotum is surgical removal of the entire affected testicle, done through an incision in the groin. The operation is performed to establish the diagnosis, as well as to remove the tumor.

Are tumor markers used in diagnosing, staging, and monitoring cancer of the testicle?
These tumors produce marker proteins that are used in diagnosis, staging and monitoring cancer of the testicle. AFP and HCG, are two that are most commonly used. LDH (lactate dehhydrogenase) may also be used to determine tumor bulk.

Why isn't a biopsy of the lump done without removing the whole testicle?
If the problem is cancer—and most tumors in the testicles are cancerous— cutting through the outer layer of the testicle may cause the disease to spread

STAGES OF CANCER OF THE TESTICLE

STAGE	DESCRIPTION
Stage I	Cancer found only in testicle.
Stage II	Cancer found in lymph nodes in abdomen as well as in testicle.
Stage III	Cancer spread beyond lymph nodes in abdomen to other parts of body such as lungs or liver.
Recurrent	Cancer has returned after being treated—either in the testicles or in another part of body.

locally. If the doctor suggests a simple biopsy, you should seek another opinion before surgery.

What are the implications of having a testicle removed?
Many men assume that the removal of the testicle will affect their ability to have sexual intercourse or make them sterile. A man with one healthy testicle can still have a normal erection and produce sperm. A gel-filled implant, which has the weight, shape, and texture of a normal testicle, can be inserted surgically to restore normal appearance. If part of the scrotal skin must be removed, it may be more difficult to restore the scrotum to a normal appearance.

Is it a good idea to bank sperm when you have testicular cancer?
You will want to ask your doctor if this is necessary or advisable. Recent studies have shown that the majority of men with testicular cancer recover fertility, although this might take two to three years after treatment has been completed. Some men with testicular cancer have impaired sperm production and could be ineligible for sperm banking.

What are the differences between seminoma and nonseminoma cancer of the testicles?
There are many different kinds of testicular cancer, but they are generally placed in two broad categories of germ cell tumors: seminoma and nonseminoma. Seminomas account for 40 percent of all testicular germ cell tumors. Nonseminomas are actually a group of cancers that include choriocarcinoma, embryonal carcinoma, teratoma, and yolk sac tumors. Each of these two major types of testicular cancer grows and spreads differently and each is treated differently. It is important to find out the extent or stage of the disease so that proper treatment can be planned.

TREATMENTS FOR CANCER OF THE TESTICLE

STAGE	TREATMENT
Stage I: Seminoma	1. Removal of testicle (radical inguinal orchiectomy) followed by external beam radiation to lymph nodes in abdomen. *Clinical Trials:* Removal of testicle with careful follow-up.
Stage I: Nonseminoma	1. Removal of testicle (radical inguinal orchiectomy) and removal of some lymph nodes in abdomen (lymph node dissection). If possible, surgery is done to preserve fertility. Monthly blood tests and chest x-rays first year and every 2 months second year. Chemotherapy at any signs of recurrence. 2. Removal of testicle (radical inguinal orchiectomy followed by careful testing). CT scan every two to four months during first year.
Stage II: Seminoma	1. If tumor is nonbulky: Removal of testicle and external beam radiation. If tumor is bulky: Removal of testicle followed by chemotherapy or external beam radiation to lymph nodes in abdomen and pelvis.
Stage II: Nonseminoma	1. Removal of testicle and lymph nodes in abdomen (lymph node dissection). Monthly checkups with chemotherapy if test results are not satisfactory. 2. Removal of testicle and lymph nodes in abdomen (lymph node dissection) followed by chemotherapy. 3. Removal of testicle and lymph nodes in abdomen (lymph node dissection) followed by chemotherapy. If cancer remains, further surgery may be done to remove the cancer. *Clinical trials:* Chemotherapy instead of lymph node dissection.
Stage III: Seminoma	1. Removal of testicle followed by chemotherapy. *Clinical trials:* Removal of testicle followed by chemotherapy

(continued)

TREATMENTS FOR CANCER OF THE TESTICLE *(continued)*

STAGE	TREATMENT
Stage III: Nonseminoma	1. Chemotherapy
	2. Chemotherapy followed by surgery to remove any cancer masses. Further chemotherapy if cancer cells remain.
	Clinical trials: New chemotherapy drugs; high-dose chemotherapy with autologous bone marrow transplant (in some patients).
Recurrent	1. Systemic chemotherapy; high-dose systemic chemotherapy with autologous bone marrow transplant, surgery.
	Clinical trials: New chemotherapy drugs.

What does lymph node dissection do?

This operation, referred to as lymphadenectomy, is sometimes done to determine if the cancer has spread so that the disease can be treated properly. Since cancer of the testicle spreads first to the retroperitoneal lymph nodes (the nodes deep in the abdomen below the diaphragm), this surgery may also help control the disease by taking out any nodes that are involved. You should understand that this diagnostic procedure, since it removes many nerves necessary for erection and ejaculation, may alter sexual ability and function. Statistics show that 90 percent of men who had undergone this surgery had a reduction in or total loss of ejaculate. Some patients may recover their ability to ejaculate as a result of the healing of nerve tissue or regeneration of nerve fibers.

How often should I see a doctor for checkups after being treated for cancer of the testicles?

Generally, patients are checked and have blood tests to measure their tumor marker levels every month for the first two years after treatment. Regular x-rays or scans may be ordered. After that, checkups may be needed just once or twice a year. Testicular cancer seldom recurs after a patient has been free of the disease for three years. Follow-up may vary for different types and stages of testicular cancer.

CANCER OF THE PENIS

This is a very rare cancer that sometimes occurs at the tip of the penis and is almost exclusively found in uncircumcised males between the ages of 50 and 70. In men who have been circumcised early in infancy, penile cancer is almost nonexistent. When diagnosed early, cancer of the penis is highly curable. Sometimes cancers from the bladder, prostate, lung, pancreas, kidney, testicle, or ureter can spread to the penis. Since it is an unusual and rare type of cancer, it should be treated by an oncologist at a large medical center who has expertise in this type of cancer.

What causes cancer of the penis?
The most common factor is the presence of a foreskin since this cancer is extremely rare in circumcised men. Human papillomavirus (HPV) is suspected as a cause. 31 to 63 percent of patients with penile cancer test positive for HPV. Data shows that wives or ex-wives of men with penile cancer had a threefold higher risk of cervical cancer. Men with psoriasis who are treated with ultraviolet A phototherapy are also at increased risk for cancer of the penis. Cigarette smoking has been linked to penile cancer.

What are the symptoms of cancer of the penis?
A pimple or sore on the penis, a small nodule, white thickened patches, raised, velvety patch, wart, or ulcer, especially one that is painless, can all be symptoms. In addition, bleeding associated with erection or intercourse, persistent abnormal erection without sexual desire, foul-smelling discharge, or a lump in the groin should all be carefully investigated.

What is the usual treatment for cancer of the penis?
The usual treatment is surgery. Approximately 90 percent of patients with cancer of the penis, if it is found in the early stages, will be cured through the surgical removal of the tumor. If the cancer has spread to the groin, nodes in the groin usually will be removed. Radiation therapy and chemotherapy are also sometimes used in these cases.

What are the treatments for penile cancer?
There are different types of surgery used for operating on cancers of the penis. Any one of these methods may be used:

- **Wide local excision:** removing the cancer and some normal tissue on either side.
- **Microsurgery:** removing the cancer and as little normal tissue as possible.

STAGES OF CANCER OF THE PENIS

STAGE	DESCRIPTION
Stage I	Limited to glans and foreskin.
Stage II	Found in deeper tissue of glans and spread to shaft of penis. Not spread to lymph nodes.
Stage III	Found in penis and lymph nodes in groin.
Stage IV	Found throughout penis, has invaded lymph nodes in groin and/or spread to other parts of the body.

- **Radiation:** either external or internal seeding.
- **Laser surgery:** using a narrow beam of light to remove cancer cells.
- **Circumcision:** removing the foreskin.
- **Partial penectomy:** removing part of the penis.
- **Total penectomy:** removing the entire penis.
- **Lymph nodes:** may also be removed during surgery or at another time.

Will I have sexual problems as a result of surgery on the penis?

If only part of the penis has been removed, you may still be able to achieve erection and have the ability to perform penile-vaginal intercourse to the point of ejaculation.

Are prosthetic devices available?

There are several kinds of penile prostheses. Your doctor can advise you where to get information.

What is the treatment for a metastatic tumor that appears on the penis?

Usually if the tumor has metastasized from another part of the body, the doctor will remove the tumor surgically and use radiation to help relieve any pain or side effects.

What kind of followup is necessary for cancer of the penis?

The doctor will teach you how to check yourself to detect any changes in the penis area, and this self-examination should be done monthly. The first year, checkups will usually be scheduled every three months, the second year, every six months and yearly thereafter. Urine and blood stool tests will be done at

TREATMENTS FOR CANCER OF THE PENIS

STAGE	TREATMENT
Stage I	*If cancer is limited to the foreskin:*
	1. Wide local excision and circumcision
	If cancer begins in glans and does not involve other tissues:
	1. Flruroruracil cream; OR microsurgery.
	If tumor begins in glans and involves other tissues:
	1. Partial penectomy with or without removal of lymph nodes in groin.
	2. External or internal radiation.
	3. Microsurgery.
	Clinical trials: YAG or CO2 laser therapy.
Stage II	1. Partial, total, or radical penectomy; OR
	2. Radiation therapy followed by penectomy.
	Clinical trials: YAG laser treatment.
Stage III	1. Penectomy and removal of lymph nodes on both sides of groin.
	2. Penectomy followed by radiation therapy.
	Clinical trials: chemotherapy or chemotherapy with radiation.
Stage IV	1. Wide local surgery or microsurgery to reduce symptoms.
	2. Penectomy or radiation therapy.
	Clinical trials: chemotherapy plus surgery or radiation therapy.
Recurrent	1. Surgery.
	2. Radiation.
	Clinical trials: chemotherapy or biological therapy.

each visit; chest x-rays every six months for the first year, then yearly; and CBC, IVP and CT scan of the pelvis yearly.

Web Pages to Check Out

www.cancer.gov: For general up-to-date information, and for clinical trials.

www.cancer.org: For general up-to-date information and community resources.

www.acor.org: Online support groups.

www.oncology.com: Patient information Web site of the American Society of Clinical Oncology. Includes information on 50 types of cancer, treatments, coping, side effects, as well as live chats, message boards, a drug database, and a medical dictionary.

www.HopeLink.com: Lists clinical trials.

www.cancer.gov/cancerinfo/pdf: Lists clinical trials.

www.Prostate pointers.org: Support groups and other information.

www.UsToo.com: Glossary, support groups.

www.auanet.org: Web site of American Urological Association, with information for patients.

www.usa.org: Patient advocate organization for prostate.

www.phoenix5.org: Regarding Partin tables.

www.etrac.com: High-dose rate brachytherapy.

Also see Chapter 2, Searching for Answers on the Web, for more information.

You May Want to Read

Marks, Sheldon, MD, urologist, *Prostate & Cancer*, Tucson, AZ: Perseus Pub, 1999.

LUNG CANCER

Everyone knows about lung cancer and its relationship to smoking. It is estimated that about 80 percent of all lung cancers could be eliminated if everyone stopped smoking tomorrow. But if you already have lung cancer that statistic is of little help to you. What you need to know now is how to deal with the fact that you have lung cancer.

NEW SCREENING TECHNIQUES are being studied for lung cancer. Researchers are finding that a low-dose CT scan, called a spiral, or helical scan, can be a successful tool in finding lung cancers early. This is good news because up until now most lung cancers were found at an advanced stage when they had already spread outside the lung. Studies are underway to determine whether or not the CT screening saves lives. There also is work being done to identify molecular and genetic changes in cells that would allow doctors to find the cancer earlier. Clinical trials using new drugs, including antiangiogenesis drugs, are showing promise. A many-pronged effort continues with surgical, medical and radiation oncologists as well as pathologists, molecular biologists, and immunologists attempting to answer the very basic questions of how to find, treat, and cure lung cancer.

What you need to know about lung cancer

- Symptoms of lung cancer are elusive. Many of them are like symptoms of other common ailments. Usually they vary depending on where in the lung the cancer is located and the nature of its growth pattern.

- A cough is a common symptom of lung cancer. It occurs when a tumor irritates the lining of the airways or blocks passage of air.

- Many lung cancers are discovered during routine annual checkups, while doctors are taking chest x-rays. However, spiral CT, a new kind of x-ray and positron emission tomography (PET) are now finding lung cancers earlier.

- There are two main types of lung cancer—small cell and nonsmall cell. About 80 percent of lung cancers are nonsmall cell.

- No matter what the stage of your lung cancer, there are treatment choices you can make.

What's new in the treatment of lung cancer?

There are several new treatments that are being studied for lung cancer:

- Antiangiogenesis drugs, such as the experimental anti-VEGF which prevents the endothelial cells from reproducing new cells to form new blood vessels, are being used in patients with nonsmall cell lung cancer.

- Novel antifolates, a class of drugs that targets the folic acid metabolic pathways and affects the availability of certain B-complex vitamins, are being tested in clinical trials in patients with mesothelioma, a relatively rare type of lung cancer.

- Taxanes, which affect cell structures that play an important role in cell function, are being added to other chemotherapy drugs in treating patients with nonsmall cell lung cancer.

- New radiation treatment procedures—3-D conformal radiation therapy, high-dose-rate brachytherapy, and intensity modulated radiation therapy—allow the shape and intensity of radiation beams to be changed so that they are more focused on cancer cells and away from the normal tissue and organs. Timing radiation to the patient's breathing cycles, called respiratory gating which allows the doctor to treat less of the normal lung tissue, is another innovation in lung cancer treatment.

- Vaccine therapy is being used with patients who have completed treatment for limited stage small-cell lung cancer but are still at risk for cancer recurrence.

- Drugs, known as signal transduction inhibitors that block signals that make cancer cells grow and spread, are being tested.

- Photodynamic therapy is being used in lung cancer treatment. A special light-sensitive drug is injected. The doctor, using a bronchoscope, shines a laser light on the lung. The light activates the drug, which collects in the cancer tissue and kills the cancer cells.

What causes lung cancer?

Scientific research indicates that 80 to 90 percent of lung cancers are caused by smoking.

Do people who have never smoked ever get lung cancer?

Yes. A small proportion of lung cancer cases are due to other causes. People who have been exposed for many years to smoking, or irritating substances in the air, including second-hand smoke and pollution, are more likely to have lung cancer than people who have breathed unpolluted air all their lives. It is also possible that the tendency to get lung cancer may be inherited. Clinical studies suggest that blood relatives of lung cancer patients are more likely to have lung cancer than people who do not have a family history.

Has Agent Orange been associated with cancers of the lung, bronchus, larynx, or trachea?

Agent Orange, a mixture of herbicides used mainly to defoliate forest trees, and other herbicides used during the Vietnam War have been associated with cancers of the lung, bronchus, larynx, and trachea, but not as strongly as some other cancers. They are classified in the second category: limited or suggestive evidence of an association. However, if you are a Vietnam veteran and have been diagnosed with any of these identified cancers, you should qualify for VA disability compensation and the special access to medical care that the VA has offered to Vietnam veterans for health problems from Agent Orange exposure. You do not need to prove that your illness is related to your military service. It is presumed to be service-connected. For more information, see Chapter 4, What Is Cancer?

What is a spiral CT scan?

A low-dose spiral CT scan, sometimes called a helical scan, is a test that is being used to screen smokers and former smokers to see if lung cancer can be found earlier. The spiral CT scan can show smaller tumors than can a chest x-ray. However, it is not covered by many health plans. At the present time, only about 15 percent of lung cancers are found before they have spread and most of those are found when doctors are doing tests for other health reasons. This new scanning technique may be helpful to find lung cancers when they are more curable.

WHO IS MOST LIKELY TO GET LUNG CANCER?

- Men and women who smoke cigarettes. This is by far the most important risk factor, causing 80 to 90 percent of all lung cancers.

- Cigar and pipe smokers, although the risk for these smokers is not as high as for cigarette smokers.

- People who smoke marijuana and crack-cocaine.

- People who are exposed to other people's smoke, either at work or at home.

- People between 50 and 75 years of age.

- People whose lungs have been scarred due to past lung infections or tuberculosis and those with chronic pulmonary disease.

- Asbestos workers, especially those who also smoke.

- Persons exposed to radon.

- Uranium and hard rock miners and those who work with coal tars, petroleum, chromium, vinyl chloride, nickel, and arsenic.

- People with certain genetic factors or hereditary conditions that may predispose them to cancer. A slight increase has been seen in the incidence of lung cancer among siblings and children of those with lung cancer.

- People who are deficient in Vitamin A.

- Persons who live in polluted urban areas.

- Persons who have been exposed to Agent Orange.

Is positron emission tomography used in finding lung cancer?
Positron emission tomography, or PET, can be used in finding lung cancer. A radioactive substance is injected into the body. The substance is attracted to the cancerous areas and makes the lung cancer easier to detect.

What do the lungs look like?
The lungs are two spongy, pinkish-gray organs that take up much of the room inside the chest. They enfold the other organs of the chest such as the heart, the large blood vessels entering and leaving the heart, and the esophagus (the tube which carries food from mouth to stomach.) The left lung has two lobes or sections. It is smaller than the right lung because the heart takes up some of the space on the left side of the chest. The right lung has three lobes and is a little bigger than the left one. Tubes called bronchi make up the inside of the lungs.

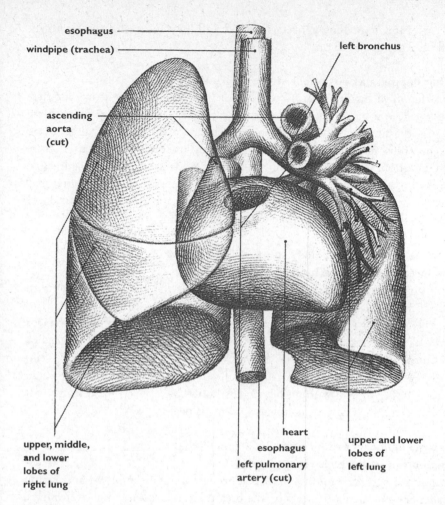

esophagus

windpipe (trachea)

left bronchus

ascending
aorta
(cut)

upper, middle,
and lower
lobes of
right lung

heart

esophagus

left pulmonary
artery (cut)

upper and lower
lobes of
left lung

Lungs

Where does lung cancer start?

Most lung cancers begin in the bronchi (the larger air tubes) or the bronchi-oles (the smaller tubes branching off the bronchi) in the moist mucous layer of the breathing tubes. Most cancer researchers believe that 20 or more years may pass between the time someone is first exposed to a cancer-producing substance, such as tobacco smoke, and the time cancer actually develops. There are usually no symptoms of early stage lung cancer.

What are the major types of lung cancers?

Lung cancers fall into two broad categories—nonsmall cell lung cancer and small cell lung cancer. 70 to 85 percent of people who have lung cancer have nonsmall cell. There are, in all, more than a dozen different cell types of lung cancers. How your lung cancer is treated and how successful the treatment will be depends partly on the cell type.

What happens when cancer starts to grow in the lung?

As a tumor on the lining of a bronchus or bronchiole grows, it may interfere with the flow of air through the breathing tube and cause a wheeze or whistling noise as the air passes through the narrowed part of the bronchus. The tumor also may cause a cough as it obstructs the upward movement of mucus. If there is an infection, the mucus you cough up could be dark or rusty. Sometimes an already existing cough will seem to become more persistent, or bleeding may occur due to small ulcers that may appear on the tumor. You may see streaks of blood in the mucus that you cough up. Heavy bleeding is rare.

What symptoms am I likely to have if the cancer has spread outside the lung?

Sometimes fluid accumulates in the lining outside the lungs, causing fluid to collect in the pleural cavity. This can cause chest pain and make it hard to breathe. A tumor growing between the two lungs may press on the esophagus and make it hard to swallow. It may affect the nerves that go to the voice box and make you hoarse or affect the nerves of your eye and make an eyelid droop. When it grows in one of the smallest bronchial tubes, it may grow to the size of a golf ball without having any noticeable effects—and it may not be discovered for many years unless an x-ray is taken.

Can my lung cancer be caused by a cancer that started somewhere else in my body?

Cancer can spread from one place to another through the blood and lymph nodes. Several, such as cancers of the breast, kidney, colon stomach, testicles, bladder, and reproductive organs, may spread to the lungs. However, lung cancer that starts in your lung is different from cancer that has spread or metastasized to the lung and is treated differently. For information on cancers that have metastasized, see Chapter 26, When Cancers Recur or Metastasize.

What kind of doctor should be treating me if I have lung cancer?

Usually your internist or general physician will refer you to a specialist. Specialists who treat lung cancer include thoracic surgeons, radiation oncologists, and medical oncologists. Before the start of any treatment, a review of the biopsy should be done by an experienced lung cancer pathologist.

In what type of lung cancer is arm and shoulder pain a symptom?

One type of lung cancer, known as a superior sulcus tumor, is sometimes incorrectly diagnosed as cervical arthritis or bursitis because of arm and

SYMPTOMS OF LUNG CANCER

- Cough is the most common symptom. Almost 75 percent of lung cancer patients report having a cough before they are diagnosed. Any change in a smoker's cough is a significant symptom and should not be ignored.

- Wheezing.

- Constant chest pain.

- Shortness of breath during routine, everyday activities that have not caused breathing difficulty in the past. (Don't worry about the shortness of breath that develops after rapidly running up several flights of stairs, since even the healthiest person will feel short of breath under those conditions.)

- Spitting up sputum, even a small amount, especially in the early morning.

- Flecks or streaks of blood, coughed up or in the sputum (may look rusty rather than red).

- Persistent hoarseness.

- Drooping eyelid.

- Fever.

- Neck enlargement.

- Repeated pneumonia or bronchitis.

- Loss of appetite. Weight loss.

- Clubbing of the fingers.

- Arm, upper back, and shoulder pain.

shoulder pain symptoms. The tumor is located in the upper part of the chest and usually extends into the adjoining ribs and spine, producing shoulder and arm pain, sometimes extending to the forearm and the fourth and fifth fingers. An x-ray of the chest, with special attention to the superior sulcus area, helps to diagnose this tumor.

Are lung tumors ever benign?

Benign tumors (adenomas) occur, but they are rare. Prior to surgery they are difficult to distinguish from cancerous tumors and therefore are treated in the same manner.

What is histoplasmosis?

Histoplasmosis is a disease caused by a fungus which grows in soil and material contaminated with bat or bird droppings. You need to be aware

TESTS THAT MAY BE USED TO DIAGNOSE LUNG CANCER

- Sputum cytology (studying the mucus for signs of cancer)
- Chest x-rays
- CT scan, spiral CT or helical scan
- PET scan
- Spirometry (measures breathing efficiency of lungs)
- Bronchoscopy exam (to look into breathing passages)
- Ultrasound (sonogram)
- Needle aspiration (to remove cells that are hard to reach with bronchoscope)
- Mediastinoscopy (surgery to check for diagnosis)
- Thoracentesis (to check fluid from pleura)
- Thoracoscopy (to look at surface of lungs and spaces between them)
- Thoroscopy (to look at the chest wall lining and lung surface)
- Paracentesis (to check fluid from the abdomen)
- Pulmonary function tests
- For small cell lung cancers, a bone marrow biopsy may be done.

NOTE: Not all of the tests are done on all patients. However, it is important to have thorough testing and staging before starting any treatment. More detailed information on these tests can be found in Chapter 6, How Cancers Are Diagnosed.

that past infections can leave spots on the lung, which show up in scans and may be mistaken for lung cancer. Antifungal medications are used to treat severe, chronic, and disseminated cases. Mild disease usually resolves without treatment and past infection results in partial protection against reinfection.

What tests are usually recommended to diagnose lung cancer?
First, the doctor will ask you about your history, if you smoke, and how long you have been smoking, whether or not any close relatives have had lung cancer, and what symptoms you are having. Then the doctor will do a physical examination and will listen to your lungs. You may need to have chest x-rays, CT or PET scans, or other tests. A sputum test (taking a sample of your mucus and examining the cells under a microscope) may be ordered.

Will a biopsy be done?

A biopsy is needed to confirm whether or not you have lung cancer. There are several ways of getting tissue from your lungs, including needle aspiration, thoracoscopy, bronchoscopy, thorancentesis, and thoracotomy. See Chapter 6, How Cancers Are Diagnosed, for a description of these tests.

Is a biopsy always necessary?

A biopsy is essential because it gives the pathologist a specimen to study so the cell type and the degree of malignancy can be identified.

Why is it important to have my biopsy reviewed?

It is important before allowing any treatment to begin to make certain that your diagnosis is correct. Some cases of small cell lung cancer, which respond well to chemotherapy, can be confused on microscopic examination with nonsmall cell carcinoma, which has a different treatment.

What is a CT scan guided biopsy of the lung?

This is a biopsy done using a CT scan. You are placed on a table, given a sedation intravenously and a preliminary scan will be done. After local anesthesia, the biopsy needle will be put into the tumor. Additional CT scans are done to confirm that the needle is in the right location and the biopsy sample will be taken. You will be watched for a few hours and sent home.

How does lung cancer spread?

Lung cancer usually begins as a tiny spot, most often on the inner lining of a bronchial tube. Lungs have a rich supply of blood and lymph vessels close to the cancer cells. If these cells get into the bloodstream or the lymph system, they can spread to other parts of the body.

Where does lung cancer usually spread?

Lung cancer most commonly spreads, or metastasizes, to the brain, liver, and bone, although it may spread to any organ of the body. See Chapter 26, When Cancers Recur or Metastasize, for additional information.

What tests will be used to determine if the cancer has spread?

There are several and your doctor may use one or a combination of the following, depending on your type of cancer and what previous tests showed: CT scan, PET scan, magnetic resonance imaging (MRI), radionuclide scanning of the liver and or the bone, mediastonocopy, and mediastinotomy.

What are the stages of lung cancer?

The stages are different depending on whether you have small cell or non-small cell lung cancer. Nonsmall cell cancer is staged using the TNM system, which defines the size of tumor, involvement of lymph nodes, and whether cancer has spread. For small cell lung cancer, there are three stages: limited, extensive, and recurrent.

Why is staging so important?

Staging plays a critical role in the selection of treatment, so careful initial evaluation to define the location and extent of your cancer is essential. Staging depends on the combination of clinical examination, x-rays and laboratory information, and an understanding of the pathology determined by the biopsy of lymph nodes, bronchoscopy, and any surgical biopsy procedures. The doctor will determine as accurately as possible through thorough testing the full extent of your cancer and whether it has started to spread.

What should lung cancer patients know about treatment?

There are choices for treatment for each stage of lung cancer. When you are diagnosed with lung cancer you should consult specialists in medical, radiation, and surgical oncology to decide on a specific treatment plan that is right for you.

Are all kinds of lung cancer treated the same way?

No. There are different treatments depending on the cell type, the extent of the disease, and the way the disease responds to treatment. Surgery, radiation therapy, and chemotherapy may be used. Surgery is done when it is likely that all of the tumor can be removed. Radiation is used to damage cancer cells and stop them from growing and dividing. Chemotherapy is used, especially in small cell lung cancer, which spreads quickly, to try to kill cancer cells not only in the lung but also in other parts of the body. Many times the different treatments are combined.

Questions to Ask Your Doctor About Treatment

- **What kind of lung cancer do I have?**
- **Is it small cell or nonsmall cell lung cancer?**
- **Has the cancer spread outside the lung?**
- **What is the stage of the disease?**
- **What are my treatment choices?**
- **Is surgery a choice for me?**
- **Will the remaining lung work well enough so that I can be active after the operation?**

- Is the operation considered a risk?

- In my condition, will anesthesia be a problem?

- How long will the operation last?

- How will I feel after the operation?

- How long must I stay in the hospital?

- Would you suggest that I get involved in a clinical trial?

- If I am not operated on, what other treatment do you suggest?

- Will I need radiation therapy?

- Will chemotherapy be used?

- Is laser surgery an option?

- Can cryosurgery be used?

- Am I a candidate for photodynamic therapy?

- What are the risks and side effects of each treatment?

- What will treatment cost?

- Where can I find someone before surgery to help me work on my breathing and coughing to keep my airways clear?

Nonsmall Cell Lung Cancer

What are the different cell types of nonsmall cell cancers?
The three main kinds are:

- **Squamous cell**, also called **epidermoid**. It is most common in men and in older people. It starts in one of the larger breathing tubes and usually does not grow or spread as quickly as other types of lung cancer.

- **Adenocarcinoma** is the most common type in women. It usually begins along the outer edges of the lungs and under the lining of the bronchi. Bronchoalveolar adenocarcinoma develops in the air sacs and is more common in women and in people who do not smoke.

- **Large cell lung cancers** have large, abnormal-looking cells. These tumors usually begin in the smaller breathing tubes but may be in any part of the lung.

Are there other cell types of nonsmall cell lung cancer?
There are several other cell types, including: spindle cell variant, acinar, papillary, solid tumor with mucin, giant cell, clear cell, adenosquamous carcinoma, and undifferentiated carcinoma.

How is nonsmall cell lung cancer staged?

Staging of nonsmall cell lung cancer depends on the size of the tumor (T), any involvement of lymph nodes (N) and whether or not the cancer has spread (M). The staging groups for nonsmall cell lung cancer are 0 to IV. Stages I, II and III are subdivided into groups A and B.

What are the treatments for nonsmall cell cancer?

At the time of diagnosis, patients are usually placed in one of three treatment groups:

- cancer that can be treated with surgery. You will have an operation or, if you cannot have surgery, radiation treatment will be given.

- cancer that has spread to nearby lymph nodes. You could have radiation alone, radiation with chemotherapy, or surgery alone.

- cancer that has spread to other parts of the body or to another lobe of the lungs. You may have radiation therapy to shrink the cancer and to relieve pain or other symptoms or you may have chemotherapy. Radiation may be external or internal. Internal radiation involves putting materials that produce radiation (radioisotopes) through thick plastic tubes into the cancerous area. Chemotherapy or radiation therapy may be used before or after surgery.

TREATMENT CHOICES FOR NONSMALL CELL LUNG CANCER

STAGE	TREATMENT
Occult	Evaluation (x-ray, bronchoscopy, computed tomographic scan) to find site and nature of primary tumor. Treatment determined by establishing stage of disease and is same as patients with similar stage disease.
Stage 0 or **Carcinoma *in situ***	Surgery, to remove small portion of lung where cancer cells are found (segmentectomy or wedge resection) **or** Endoscopic photodynamic therapy.
Stage I	Surgery to remove small portion of lung or lobe of lung **or** Radiation, if patient cannot be operated **or** *Clinical trials:* chemotherapy following surgery **or** chemoprevention after surgery **or** Endoscopic photodynamic therapy.
Stage II	Surgery to remove small portion of lung or lobe of lung **or** Radiation, if patient cannot have surgery.

TREATMENT CHOICES FOR NONSMALL
CELL LUNG CANCER (continued)

STAGE	TREATMENT
	Clinical trials: chemotherapy after surgery with or without other treatments **or** radiation therapy after surgery.
Stage III-A	Surgery **or** Surgery with lymphadenopathy **or** radiation (for patients who cannot have chemotherapy plus surgery **or** Chemotherapy with or without surgery or radiation **or** Clinical trials of combined treatments. **Superior Sulcus Tumor:** Radiation and surgery or radiation therapy or surgery alone (selected cases) **or** Chemotherapy combined with radiation and surgery or clinical trials of combined treatments. **Chest Wall Tumors:** Surgery **or** Surgery and radiation therapy **or** Radiation therapy **or** Chemotherapy combined with surgery or radiation.
Stage III-B	Radiation **or** Chemotherapy and radiation therapy **or** Chemotherapy and radiation therapy followed by surgery **or** Chemotherapy **or** Radiation for relief of pain or symptoms. *Clinical trials:* new fractionation schedules, radiosensitizers, combined treatments.
Stage IV	Radiation **or** Chemotherapy and radiation **or** Chemotherapy and radiation followed by surgery **or** Chemotherapy. *Clinical trials:* new chemotherapy regimens and drugs.
Recurrent	Radiation therapy for relief of pain and symptoms **or** Chemotherapy **or** Surgery for brain metastases **or** Laser therapy **or** Internal radiation for endobrochial lesions **or** Stereotactic radiosurgery for highly selected patients.

What are some of the new treatments being tested for lung cancer?

There are clinical trials underway that combine surgery, radiation and chemotherapy, or immunotherapy. Several new chemotherapy drugs also are being tested.

When is radiation used to treat patients with nonsmall cell lung cancers?

Traditionally, radiation has been used for two purposes. It can be an effective treatment for nonsmall cell cancer that cannot be operated on but has not spread. It also can be used to reduce pain or obstruction in cases where a cancer cannot be operated on, since radiation can be pinpointed to small areas. Doctors may use radiation therapy following surgery or to treat patients whose cancer has spread from the lung to other parts of the body. Some radiation treatments may be given in two slightly smaller doses in one day to allow a higher daily dose to be delivered in smaller, but more frequent dosages. Neutron or particle beam radiation is sometimes used in lung cancer in place of photons, the classic form of radiation.

Is chemotherapy ever used before surgery?

Yes, either chemotherapy or chemotherapy and radiation can be used before surgery to shrink the tumor in nonsmall cell lung cancer.

Small Cell Lung Cancer

What is small cell lung cancer?

Small cell lung cancer, also called oat cell, is usually found in the cells that line the major breathing tubes. Less common than nonsmall cell lung cancer, it tends to grow quickly and is more likely to spread to other organs in the body.

What are the stages of small cell lung cancer?

There are three main stages: limited, where the cancer is found only in one lung and not in the lymph nodes; extensive, where the cancer has spread outside of the lung, either to other tissues of the chest or to other parts of the body; or recurrent, where the cancer that has been treated comes back, either in the lungs or in another part of the body.

How is small cell lung cancer treated?

Small cell cancer has usually spread beyond the lung by the time it is found. Because it can spread quickly, it is usually treated with chemotherapy. In many cases, treatment also includes radiation therapy to shrink or destroy the primary tumor in the lung or tumors elsewhere in the body.

STAGES OF NONSMALL CELL LUNG CANCER

STAGE	DESCRIPTION
Occult TX, N0, M	Cancer cells in sputum (mucus coughed up from lungs); no tumor found in lung.
Stage 0 TIS, N0, M0	Also called carcinoma *in situ*, it is found in lung, in a few layers of cells. The cancer has not grown through top lining of lungs.
Stage I T1, N0, M0 T2, N0, M0	Found only in the lung; divided into IA and IB depending on size of tumor.
Stage II T1, N1, M0 T2, N1, M0 T3, N0, M0	Spread to nearby lymph nodes or to chest wall, the diaphragm, the mediastinal pleura. Divided into stages IA and IB, based on size of tumor and spread to lymph nodes.
Stage IIIA T1, N2, M0, T3, N2, M0 T3, N1, M0 T3, N2, M0	Cancer has either spread to lymph nodes in mediastinum, to lymph nodes on opposite side of chest or in lower neck.
Stage IIIB Any T, N3, M0 T4, any N, M0	Same as above but the cancer usually cannot be operated on.
Stage IV Any T, Any N, M1	The cancer has spread to other parts of body or to another lobe of the lungs.
Recurrent	The cancer has returned after previous treatment.

When is surgery usually used in treating lung cancer?

Surgery is used when there is a good chance that the tumor is confined to only one lung. The affected part, or possibly the whole lung, may be removed. If the cancer has spread to the lymph nodes in or near the affected lung, the surgeon still may be able to remove all of the cancer. Sometimes it is possible for the surgeon to remove a cancer that has grown outward from the lung into a small part of the chest wall. This operation will include the removal of the lung and the cancerous tissue on the chest wall.

STAGES OF SMALL CELL LUNG CANCER

STAGE	DESCRIPTION
Limited	Cancer is found only in one lung and in nearby lymph nodes.
Extensive	Cancer has spread outside of the lung, where it began, to other tissues in the chest or to other parts of the body.
Recurrent	Lung cancer that has been treated has come back, either in the lungs or in another part of the body.

What tests will the doctor do to decide whether or not my body can endure having part of my lung taken out?

Before doing lung surgery, the doctor will do pulmonary function tests to measure your breathing and how much air is going into your lungs. You also may have other tests to measure how well your lungs are adding oxygen to your blood and taking out carbon dioxide, how well the tiny blood vessels are working, and how well the blood flows between your lungs.

Should I begin exercises to strengthen my lung before I have my surgery?

If you are going to have any part of your lung removed, it is useful to have counseling on several issues before surgery. You may speed your recovery if you learn how to cough correctly, to bring up sputum from your lungs, and to keep your breathing passages open. It's easier to learn ways to develop the remaining lung and to fill it completely with air before you are operated on and have stitches in that area.

What is a segmental or wedge resection?

This operation removes only a small part of the lung.

What is a lobectomy?

A lobectomy is the removal of an entire lobe of the lung.

What is a pneumonectomy?

A pneumonectomy is the removal of an entire lung.

What is video-assisted thorascopic surgery?

Video-assisted thorascopic surgery (VATS) is done through a small incision, with the aid of a video camera and a television screen. The doctor can

TREATMENT CHOICES FOR SMALL CELL LUNG CANCER

STAGE	TREATMENT
Limited stage	Chemotherapy and radiation to chest with or without radiation to brain (prophylactic cranial irradiation) **or** Chemotherapy with or without cranial irradiation **or** Surgery followed by chemotherapy with or without cranial irradiation.
Extensive stage	Chemotherapy with or without radiation to brain **or** Chemotherapy and radiation to chest with or without radiation to brain **or** Radiation to parts of body where cancer has spread, such as bone or spine. *Clinical trials:* New drugs and new ways of giving all of above treatments.
Recurrent	Radiation to reduce discomfort. *Clinical trials:* new drugs.

perform a resection or a lobectomy, using the camera and screen to look at the details. Also called "keyhole" surgery, it allows for faster recovery and less time in the hospital.

Are any lymph nodes removed during surgery?
The doctor will remove some lymph nodes in the area where the cancer cells have been found so that they can be looked at under the microscope.

When is surgery not used in treating lung cancer?
Surgery will not usually be used when the cancer has spread to the other lung or if a tumor has grown from the lung into organs in the chest, such as the heart, esophagus, trachea, or large blood vessels. Also, surgery may not be used if the cancer has spread to the lymph nodes in the neck, or to other organs such as the liver, kidneys or brain. See Chapter 26, When Cancers Recur or Metastasize. Surgery is also seldom recommended for small cell lung cancer because it is faster growing and often not as confined as nonsmall cell lung cancer.

Does the surgeon sometimes operate and not remove the lung?
If the surgeon finds that the cancer has spread too far to remove it all, or is in an area where removal is impossible, the lung may be left untouched and the

operation ended. Radiation and chemotherapy will be used to help shrink the tumor growth.

Will the surgeon sometimes remove a lung even though the cancer cannot be totally removed?

This is the surgeon's judgment call—and this is the reason why you want to have the most experienced and knowledgeable doctor you can find. If, for example, the tumor is causing serious bleeding and you are coughing up blood, or if there is an infection with abscess formation, it may be necessary to remove the lung. Radiation with or without chemotherapy may then be used to help reduce the remaining cancer.

How do I breathe during a lung operation?

Special equipment is used to assist you in breathing. Your other lung continues to function while the surgeon is working on the diseased lung.

After a lung is removed, what happens to the space that's left in the chest?

Like an empty closet, space left after surgery manages to get filled up. Body fluid and scar tissue help to fill the void. Structures from the opposite side may shift toward the side of the operation. The other lung usually expands. Until this happens, there may be a feeling of one-sidedness or emptiness on the side of the operation. During your recovery period, you will be encouraged to lie on the unoperated side so that the operated lung can heal unrestricted.

Where are the incisions made for a lung operation?

Usually they are made beneath and behind the shoulder blade, parallel to the ribs. They are visible when the back is exposed.

How long do most lung cancer operations take to perform?

Approximately two to five hours, depending on what is being done.

Will I have tubes in my chest when I wake up from the operation?

The doctor may put in tubes to drain any fluid or air from inside the chest. They will be taken out in a few days.

When can I get out of bed?

You will probably be up in about 24 hours, depending upon the extent of the operation and your physical condition.

TYPES OF SURGERY USED IN LUNG CANCER

PROCEDURE	MEANING
Thoracoscopy	Exploratory chest operation, used as a diagnostic tool. Small incisions made. Allows visual examination of lung surfaces and space through a viewing tube. May be used to decide if thoracotomy needed.
Thoracotomy	Exploratory chest operation, used as diagnostic tool. Major surgery. Allows examination of lung and surrounding areas. If tumor is found to be operable, may be combined with one of procedures below.
Segmentectomy or **wedge resection**	Removal of small portion of lung.
Limited pulmonary resection	Any surgery that is less than the removal of the entire lobe of the lung.
Lobectomy	Removal of entire lobe of one lung.
Bilobectomy	Removal of two of the right lung's three lobes.
Pneumonectomy	Removal of entire lung.
Sleeve pneumonectomy	Removal of entire lung as well as lower trachea. Airway is reconstructed.
Extended resection	Part of chest wall, left atrium, diaphragm, etc. are removed. Reconstruction usually done with prosthetic material.
Sternotomy	Midline splitting of sternum, sometimes used so doctor can see both sides of chest to locate undetected cancer; possible removal of small portion of each lung.
Mediastinotomy or **Mediastinoscopy**	Surgical procedure to allow doctor to check whether lung cancer has spread to lymph nodes behind breastbone.

Will it be painful to lift my arms or take a deep breath?

For a week or so after lung surgery, you may find it painful. However, you need to breathe deeply. Your nurse, doctor or respiratory therapist will teach you breathing exercises. They can give you medication to help control the pain.

Can I breathe and live normally if I have a lung removed?

You can breathe and live normally after the removal of one or two lobes of the lung, except that there might be restrictions placed on doing strenuous physical exercise. If your entire lung is removed, you may tend to get short of breath when you exert yourself. However, at rest, you will breathe normally.

What if I decide I don't want my lung removed?

If your general health is good and the cancer is confined to one lobe or one lung, the doctor will probably recommend removal of the entire tumor. If all the cancer is removed, statistics show there is an excellent chance for recovery. Talk to your doctor before making this kind of decision. Explain your concerns and reservations and let the doctor give you the rationale for why the surgery is necessary. This is not a decision to be made lightly or without being fully informed of the risks involved in postponing or rejecting surgery.

Can the doctor do anything for my cough?

If you do have a cough, especially if there is a change in pattern of the cough during your illness, you need to tell your doctor about it. The doctor will want to check to see what is causing it. Depending on where you are in your treatment, there are different ways of treating a cough.

What can be done if I feel like I can't breathe?

If you find it difficult to breathe, have a feeling of tightness in your chest, are breathing fast, or have shortness of breath, you need to check with your doctor so that the cause can be found. It may be that you have anemia, that your muscles are weak, or that you have fluid in your lungs. If you have asthma, emphysema, heart disease or any other lung disease, that may be the cause of your difficulty in breathing. Or it may be that the tumor is blocking a part of your airway. It is important to find out why you have the breathing problem and how it can be taken care of, because difficulty in breathing can make you feel tired.

Can I do breathing exercises to help?

The Alliance for Lung Cancer suggests some exercises you can try:

- Take in a normal breath of air through your nose, counting the seconds it takes to breathe in. Then exhale through your slightly opened lips in a normal way, but for twice as many counts as when you inhaled. Thus, if you counted to six when you inhaled, count to twelve when you exhale. This is called controlled breathing and will make you feel like you are getting enough air.

- Lie down, with a pillow under your knees. Place one hand on your chest and the other on your stomach, at the end of your breastbone. Exhale slowly through your slightly opened lips while squeezing your stomach muscles upward and inward, pressing your stomach down toward the floor. When you take in a breath of air, your stomach should rise. What you are trying to do is to use all of your lungs instead of just the upper part. This will take practice to do, but it can make a great difference in your breathing.

- Try some relaxation techniques several times a day. Concentrate especially on relaxing your shoulders and arms. Relaxed muscles use less oxygen than do tense ones. Some people find that listening to music helps them relax. See Chapter 27, Living with Cancer, for other relaxation suggestions.

Should I do other kinds of exercise to help me feel better?
When you don't use your muscles, you find that you will have muscle loss. So it's important that you not spend all your time in bed and that you try to exercise every day to build up your strength. If you can, take a walk, even if it's just a short one at the beginning.

When will other treatments start after surgery?
It depends on what other treatments you will have. Any additional treatment usually does not start until you have recuperated from your surgery.

Will I need special treatment if I have
chronic bronchitis or emphysema in addition to lung cancer?
Many patients with lung cancer also have other lung problems. These conditions, along with the cancer, may make you more susceptible to lung infections. Your total condition will be assessed before treatment is started. The assessment will take into consideration whether your preexisting condition prevents you from lung surgery and whether it is possible for you to have radiation treatment. If you have one of these conditions, your doctor may treat it along with the lung cancer and will take it into account in making treatment choices.

What else can help my breathing problems?

If you are having trouble breathing, the doctor may prescribe medication to help open up your breathing tubes. An expectorant may be given to you to make it easier to cough up the mucus in your lungs that can plug up the breathing passages. If shortness of breath becomes a difficult problem, the doctor will probably prescribe oxygen. Influenza and other infections can be difficult for you if you have lung cancer. Your doctor will probably suggest an appropriate flu shot for you in the fall. If you have other infections, you will be given antibiotics. Being alert to the possible problems means you can report them to your doctor so that they can be dealt with at an early stage.

What is high dose rate brachytherapy?

High-dose rate brachytherapy, also called high-dose rate remote radiation therapy or remote brachytherapy, may be used for lung cancers that are located in the major bronchi (breathing passages) to give additional radiation to people with lung cancer. It also may be used to improve breathing, reduce bleeding or improve physical status, and to treat recurrent tumors when it is no longer possible to operate or to use external radiation. A bronchoscope is used to locate the tumor. Two or three thin catheters are placed between the tumor. The bronchoscope is removed, leaving the catheters in place. Special x-ray films are taken to assure the correct placement of the catheters. When treatment is to begin, the ends of the catheters are attached to a computer-guided treatment unit, called an afterloader, which delivers the radioactive source precisely to the tumor. Three to four treatments are usually needed.

Questions to Ask Your Doctor About Follow-up

- Will you be doing my main follow-up?
- Will I also need to see any of my other doctors?
- How often will I need to see you?
- What tests will you be doing during my follow-up exam?
- What will you be looking for?
- What should I be watching for between my visits with you?
- What symptoms should I report? To whom?

How often do I need to see the doctor after being treated for lung cancer?

It's important that you see the doctor so that your condition can be monitored. The first year you will need to see the doctor every three months, the second to fifth year, every four months, and twice a year thereafter. Chest x-rays will be done at each visit. Blood, urine and CEA (and sputum cytology, if needed) will probably be done every six months during the first year, and yearly thereafter. You should be sure to report any bone pain, appetite loss, cough, suspicious mucus, chest pain, wheezing, hoarseness, or swelling of the face and arms to the doctor.

Mesothelioma

What is mesothelioma?

Mesothelioma is a relatively rare cancer that affects the membrane lining the chest cavity, the membrane lining the cavity of the abdomen, or the membrane lining the cavity around the heart. There are three main types of malignant mesothelioma: epitheloid, sarcomatoid, and mixed/biphasic. The most common first symptoms are shortness of breath, pain in the wall of the chest, which is aggravated by deep breathing, or abdominal pain that may vary from vague discomfort to severe spasms. Most mesotheliomas are found in people who have worked with asbestos and are smokers.

NOTE: Although most tumors of mesothelial tissue are malignant, benign tumors can occur. They may grow to be quite large, but surgery can usually cure them.

How is malignant mesothelioma staged?

You may hear different names for staging. There are three staging methods used—the Butchart system, TNM system, and the Brigham system. Each system uses different variables. The Brigham System stages mesothelioma according to whether or not it can be surgically removed and whether there is lymph node involvement. The Butchart Staging System is based on how far the disease has spread to other organs. The TNM system considers the size and spread of the tumor, involvement of lymph nodes, and metastasis. The TNM system divides its four stages into two main ones: localized, which includes Stage I, and advanced, which includes Stages II, III, and IV.

How is malignant mesothelioma treated?

Surgery is a common treatment. The doctor may take out part of the lining of the chest or abdomen and some of the tissue around it. If your mesothelioma is in the chest area, a lung may be removed. Sometimes parts of the diaphragm, the muscle below the lungs that helps with breathing, is also removed. External radiation, radiation seeds, or chemotherapy may also be used. Chemotherapy may be given directly into the chest or abdomen. Sometimes the treatments are combined.

STAGES OF MALIGNANT MESOTHELIOMA

STAGE	TNM SYSTEM	BUTCHART SYSTEM	BRIGHAM SYSTEM
Stage I	Cancer is found in the lining of the chest cavity near the lung and heart, in the diaphragm, or the lung.	Cancer is found in lining of left or right chest cavity. May also be found in diaphragm on same side.	Cancer is operable. Has not spread to lymph nodes.
Stage II	Cancer has spread beyond the lining of the chest wall to lymph nodes in the chest.	Cancer has spread into the chest wall or esophagus, or both sides of chest lining. In some cases it may have spread to lymph nodes in chest.	Cancer is operable. Has spread to lymph nodes.
Stage III	Cancer has spread into the chest wall, center of chest, heart, through the diaphragm or abdominal lining, and, in some cases, into nearby lymph nodes.	Cancer has spread through the diaphragm into the lining of the abdomen, the abdomen, or lymph nodes beyond the chest.	Cancer cannot be operated on. Cancer has spread to chest wall, heart, or through the diaphragm or abdominal lining, and, in some cases, into nearby lymph nodes.
Stage IV	Cancer has spread to distant organs or tissues.	Cancer has spread to distant organs or tissues.	Cancer has spread to distant organs or tissues.
Recurrent	Cancer has come back after it has been treated.		

What are carcinoid tumors?

Carcinoid tumors appear in many parts of the body. They appear in the lungs, but rarely. The majority of people who have them have no symptoms when they are diagnosed. They are low-grade malignant tumors, often found in young people, who are considered to have an excellent long-term prognosis. If they have not spread, carcinoid tumors can be treated by surgery.

What about the patient who continues to smoke even after lung cancer is discovered?

This is a difficult question to deal with, but a judgmental approach only increases the person's anxiety and makes it difficult to have an open discussion. There is no question that cigarette smoking, in the face of lung cancer treatment, makes it more difficult to recover since it cuts back on breathing capacity and increases the risk of pulmonary infections. Studies show that stopping smoking, even after lung cancer is discovered, is beneficial to healing. However, it is helpful to remember that compulsive cigarette smoking is an addictive behavior, not one that results from a lack of willpower. The strongest argument for stopping is the increased feeling of good health that will result once the cravings have started to diminish. It all must ultimately be left up to the patient to make the decision. Interestingly enough, experience shows that 95 percent of those who quit smoking do so on their own without the help of an organized program. If you are the patient and would like to talk with someone about the steps you might take to quit, you can call 1–800–4–CANCER. A trained person will talk with you and help you think through what you may do that can help you to stop smoking. The whole process can be accomplished on the telephone without leaving your home or hospital.

Can the damage from smoking be undone?

Once a person stops smoking, the body starts to clean the lungs and protect them from further damage as well as to decrease the risk for lung cancer. It takes a significant amount of time for the lungs to get rid of tars and other substances and a number of years—some researchers say as long as 25 years, depending on how long the person has smoked—to reduce the risk of cancer to the level of someone who has never smoked. However, the lungs are able to repair themselves and physicians report that they start to "pink up" and recover shortly after smoking is stopped.

Is marijuana smoking harmful to the lungs?

There is some evidence and no surprise that marijuana may have the same harmful effects as cigarette smoke. Since marijuana cigarettes contain much more tar than do tobacco cigarettes, they may be more harmful. Marijuana smokers inhale very deeply and hold the smoke for a long time in their lungs and smoke the cigarette down to the very end where tar concentrations are the highest. Crack-cocaine users also have a greater risk for lung cancer.

TREATMENT FOR MALIGNANT MESOTHELIOMA

STAGE	TREATMENT
Localized (Stage I)	If found only in one place in the chest or abdomen, surgery to remove part of pleura (lining) and some of tissue around it. If found in larger part of the lining, surgery to remove lining and tissue near it, with or without radiation **or** External radiation **or** Surgery with or without chemotherapy **or** Surgery to remove sections of pleura, lung, part of diaphragm, and part of lining around heart. *Clinical trials*: surgery followed by chemotherapy given inside the chest **or** Surgery, radiation and chemotherapy **or** New chemotherapy drugs.
Advanced (Stages II, III, IV)	Draining of fluid in chest or abdomen. Drugs may be put into chest or abdomen to prevent further fluid buildup **or** Surgery or radiation to relieve symptoms **or** Single-drug chemotherapy. *Clinical trials*: combined drug chemotherapy, chemotherapy given inside the chest, **or** Surgery, radiation and chemotherapy combined.
Recurrent	Depends on many factors, including where cancer returned and what treatment was used before. *Clinical trials:* biologicals, new chemotherapy drugs or physical approaches.

Does lung cancer come back after it has been treated?

Unfortunately, there is a high risk of the lung cancer coming back even after it has been treated. It may be in the same place as before or as a metastasis. There also is a risk of getting a new primary lung cancer that may be of the same cell type or a different cell type as the original cancer.

Web Pages to Check Out

www.cancer.gov: For general up-to-date information, and for clinical trials.

www.cancer.org: For general up-to-date information and community resources.

www.alcase.org: Alliance for Lung Cancer. Offers advocacy, support and publications.

www.lungcanceronline.org: Excellent resource compiled by Karen Parles, lung cancer survivor.

www.mesotheliomaweb.com: Patient support and clinical trials.

Also see Chapter 2, Searching for Answers on the Web, for more information.

Sixteen

GASTROINTESTINAL AND URINARY CANCERS

We take the digestive and urinary systems of our bodies for granted. After all, without thinking about it, our insides have been working without instruction from us for years. Furthermore, most of us consider our digestive system and bowels an unpleasant topic for conversation. This may explain why it's easy to ignore warning signals and put off seeking help when early symptoms occur.

STATISTICS SHOW THAT cancers in the colon and rectum are the second most common form of cancer among American men and women in the over 40 age group—so this chapter will focus on colon and rectal cancers, in addition to stomach, liver, pancreatic, and esophageal cancers. Urinary tract cancers, which include the bladder and kidney, are also covered.

The gastrointestinal system is also called the digestive tract, or it may be referred to as the colorectal system, the intestines, or the bowels. We will refer to it as the GI tract or system, since that is what it is commonly called. You go to a GI doctor (a gastroenterologist) to be treated for problems in this part of the body. Cancers of the bladder and kidney, on the other hand, are part of the urinary tract and are the specialty of the urologist.

The GI tract consists of a large and complex series of twists and turns and is vulnerable to what we eat and to our daily stresses. It can become inflamed and irritable for no known reason, can contract in spasms, develop pouches that become infected, or can develop engorged veins that can cause pain and bleeding. And, of course, it is a prime area for cancers to develop and hide. Although cancer is only one of many possible causes of GI problems, an awareness of the warning signs and appropriate cancer-related checkups can help to catch symptoms at an early stage. When detected early and treated promptly, 75 percent of these digestive tract cancers can be cured.

The biggest fear of those who are facing surgery in the GI tract is that they will end up with an artificial opening, called an ostomy. This is commonly described as having a "bag." In the majority of cases today, the doctor will usually rejoin the healthy parts—so you can function normally. **It is reassuring to know that about 85 percent of patients will not need to have an artificial opening.** In many cases, the doctor may do a temporary artificial opening to allow healing, which is later reversed with a second procedure to close the opening. Thanks to new techniques and new surgical materials, the number of patients who require permanent ostomies has been greatly reduced.

What tests are usually done to diagnose cancers in the intestinal tract?

A number of tests are usually ordered, depending upon symptoms. They could include:

- Health history and physical examination.
- Digital rectal examination.
- Stool blood test (fecal occult blood test).
- Direct visual inspection (sigmoidoscopy and/or colonoscopy).
- X-ray examination of large bowel called lower GI series.
- CEA blood test.

What kind of doctor should I see if I have symptoms of gastrointestinal cancer?

Gastroenterologists specialize in diseases of the GI tract from mouth to anus, including the small and large intestines, stomach, esophagus, liver, and pancreas.

Questions to Ask Your Doctor If You Are Diagnosed with Gastrointestinal or Urinary Cancer

- **Where is the cancer located?**
- **Is there any sign that it has spread?**

SYMPTOMS OF GASTROINTESTINAL CANCER

- Changes in bowel habits, such as constipation or diarrhea.
- Very dark, mahogany red or bright red blood in or on the stool. (See the doctor immediately.)
- Abdominal discomfort.
- Gas pains or cramps.
- Constant indigestion or heartburn.
- Persistent narrowing of the stools.
- Urgent, painful need to have a bowel movement.
- Feeling of incomplete emptying following bowel movement.
- Unexplained weight loss, anemia, unusual paleness, fatigue.

- **What kind of operation will be performed?**
- **Am I a candidate for keyhole surgery?**
- **Will I need blood transfusions during the operation? Should I bank my own blood before going to the hospital?**
- **How long will I have to be in the hospital?**
- **How long will the operation take?**
- **Should I plan on having a nurse with me following the operation?**
- **Will the operation require that I have a colostomy?**
- **Will the colostomy be temporary or permanent?**
- **If permanent ask: Can you show me exactly where the opening will be? Can I try on the appliance so that I can be sure the opening will be comfortable? What kind of long-term supervision do you give to colostomy patients?**
- **Will the operation change my eating habits?**
- **Will there be sexual side effects?**
- **Will I be scheduled for radiation before or following surgery? If yes, be sure to read Chapter 9, Radiation Treatment.**
- **Will I be scheduled for chemotherapy? If yes, be sure to read Chapter 10, Chemotherapy.**
- **Who will be performing the surgery? How often does he do this type of operation?**

- **Is there a patient who has had this operation who could talk with me about it?**

- **Is there a wound ostomy continence nurse you recommend?**

- **Is there a local United Ostomy Association chapter?**

- **After the operation: What type and stage of cancer do I have?**

- **Were lymph nodes removed? Am I likely to have lymphedema as a result of the lymph node removal?**

- **Do you suggest additional treatment? Can I enroll in a clinical trial?**

- **How soon will I be able to resume my normal activities?**

- **When can I start to play golf, or tennis, or resume exercising?**

COLON AND RECTAL CANCERS

Where are the colon and rectum situated?

The colon and rectum are different segments of the same organ. The colon, also called the large intestine or bowel, is the first five to seven feet of the large intestine. It starts at the right lower part of the abdomen and, defying the laws of gravity, continues upward on the right side of the abdomen, close to the liver under the ribs. This section is known as the ascending colon. It makes a left turn and crosses to the left side of the abdomen. This two to two and a half foot portion is known as the transverse colon. The next portion, called the descending colon, heads down the left side of the abdomen to the pelvis. The final section, which is s-shaped and referred to as the sigmoid colon, along with the final eight or 10 inches located in the pelvis behind the urinary bladder, are known as the rectum. The final two inches are referred to as the anal region. The colon joins the small intestines to the rectum. The colon and rectum form the lower end of the digestive tract.

What is the difference between colon and rectal cancer?

Cancer affecting either the colon or rectum is many times referred to as colorectal cancer. Technically, cancers that begin in the colon are colon cancers, and cancers that begin in the rectum are rectal cancers.

Where is the small intestine (bowel) located?

The small intestine, which is also called the small bowel, is part of the digestive tract and consists of three parts. The area where it joins the lower end of the stomach is called the duodenum. The jejunum is the portion between the duodenum and the ileum. The ileum joins the large intestine in the lower right side of the abdomen, just above the appendix. The small intestine is

WHO IS MOST LIKELY TO GET COLON AND RECTAL CANCERS

- Men and women who are 50 and over.
- Those with someone in immediate family with colon or rectal cancer or adenomas.
- Those who eat a high fat diet from animal sources, who are not active physically, who are obese or who smoke.
- Those with a personal history of ulcerative colitis, pancolitis, or Crohn's colitis.
- Those who have previously had colon or rectal cancers.
- Those who have had noncancerous growths (adenomas) in the colon.
- Those whose parent, brother, or sister have had familial adenomatous polyposis (FAP) or hereditary nonpolyposis colon cancer (HNCC). Only about 5 percent of people with colorectal cancer have an inherited gene.
- In women, those who have had ovarian, endometrial, or breast cancer are more likely to develop colon or rectal cancers.

longer than the large intestine—about 20 feet in length—but is narrower in width, which is why it is referred to as the "small" intestine.

What kinds of tumors develop in the intestinal tract?
There are two kinds of tumors, primarily—benign growths such as adenomas or polyps—and malignant growths, which are cancerous. Most colon and rectal cancers are adenocarcinomas, which are usually found in the lining of the large bowel. Other less common types of cancers of the intestinal tract include sarcomas that begin in the connective tissues, lymphomas that arise in the lymphatic tissues, and rarer cancers such as carcinoid tumors.

What tests should I have to assure that cancers in the intestinal tract are discovered early?
There are several tests that can be useful in detecting colon and rectal cancer early in people without symptoms.

- Digital rectal examination.
- Fecal occult blood test (stool-blood test).
- Flexible sigmoidoscopy.
- Colonoscopy. Virtual colonoscopy is being studied.
- Double contrast barium enema, also called a barium enema with air contrast.

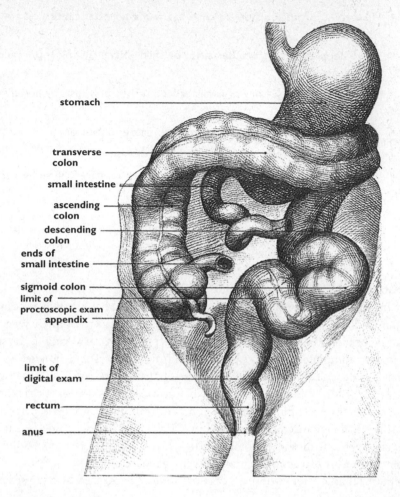

Colon-rectal area

How often should I have these tests?
The American Cancer Society suggests that men and women without symptoms, beginning at age 50, have:

- Flexible sigmoidoscopy every five years **or**
- A fecal occult blood test every year **or**
- Colonoscopy every ten years **or**
- Double-contrast barium enema every five years.

Who is at higher risk for getting colorectal cancer?
You are at a higher risk for getting colorectal cancer if:

- A parent, brother, sister, or child has had colorectal cancer or polyps before 60 **or**
- Two people—parent, brother, sister or child—have had colorectal cancer at any age **or**
- There is a family history of familial adenomatous polyposis or hereditary nonpolyposis colon cancer **or**
- You have had colorectal cancer or adenomatous polyps **or**
- You have had chronic inflammatory bowel disease.
- You are not physically active, are obese, smoke, have unhealthy eating habits or are over 50 years of age.

If you are at higher risk, you need to be seen regularly by a gastroenterologist, who will determine the schedule of testing depending on your history.

What kind of warning signs should I watch for?

The most common warning signs are changes in bowel habits, such as constipation or diarrhea, feeling that your bowel does not empty completely, rectal bleeding or blood in the stool, changes such as persistent narrowing in the size of stools, cramping or steady stomach pain or weakness and fatigue. Some symptoms depend on the location and size of the tumor. Tumors in the right side of the colon sometimes grow large before causing discomfort because the contents of the ascending colon are fluid and can pass through a narrowed intestine area. Any discomfort caused by a tumor on the right side is usually dull and vague. A tumor on the left side, where fecal matter is more solid, is likely to cause obstruction symptoms, gas pains, cramps, or bleeding. Any symptoms that last for two weeks or more should be checked by a physician.

What is a polyp?

A polyp is a growth originating from the mucous membranes of the intestine. It grows from the wall into the inner space of the bowel. (Polyps also occur in the bladder, rectum, uterus, nose, etc.) They are very common, occurring in ten to 15 percent of all adults. Benign polyps may cause intermittent bleeding, the passage of mucus with bowel movements, or, if they are large, obstruct the passage of bowel movements. However, they do not spread to other parts of the body and are most often found during routine intestinal examinations. Cure, through removal, entails little surgical risk. However, some types of polyps that develop in the colon and rectum have the potential to become cancerous as they grow larger. For this reason, it is important to have regular checkups and to be aware of changes in bowel functions so that polyps can be removed when they are in a pre-cancerous stage.

Are there different kinds of polyps?

Yes. The most common colon and rectal polyps, called hyperplastic polyps or hyperplastic mucosal tags, are harmless. Small adenomas, less than one centimeter in size, rarely contain invasive cancer cells. Half of those greater than two centimeters will prove to be cancers. Polyps are described as pedunculated when they grow on a stalk that connects the head of the polyp to the bowel wall. Flatter types of polyps that grow directly on the wall of the bowel, are known as sessile polyps. Polyps differ in their structure, texture, and microscopic characteristics, as well as in their potential for cancerous change. About 85 percent of adenomas are tubular, which means that they grow in tubelike patterns. Only about five percent of these are likely to develop into cancerous tumors. A very small percentage of adenomas are villous, which means that when observed under the microscope they form fingerlike projections. Of these, about 40 percent are likely to develop into cancer. Of the ten percent of polyps that are classified as a combination of tubular and villous cells (referred to as tubulovillous), about 22 percent will develop into cancer. The greater the number of polyps, the greater the risk of cancer, particularly when there are three or more polyps. The doctor will make recommendations about treatment and follow-up treatment based upon the type and number of polyps found.

How does the doctor remove a polyp?

It depends on where the polyp is located, what type it is and how large. Polyps that are discovered during a colonoscopy usually can be removed at that time without any additional procedure. They are usually burned or clipped off and removed through the rectum. Others will require surgery if they are large or flat. The incision, in such a case, is made at the area of the polyp, the colon is opened, and the polyp is removed. The polyp will be examined under a microscope to see if there are cancer cells. If cancer is found, the segment of the intestine where it grew must be removed.

Can aspirin reduce the risk of colon polyps?

Two clinical trials have reported results of their studies. One involved over a thousand people who had had at least one precancerous polyp (adenoma) removed within the last three months. They were randomly assigned to take one baby aspirin (80 milligrams) or one standard aspirin (325 milligrams) or a placebo (dummy pill). Three years later, the group that took baby aspirin had the best preventive effect—38 percent of patients taking baby aspirin had polyps compared to 45 percent of those who took the standard aspirin and 47 percent of those who took the placebo. The second trial involved 635 patients who had colon or rectal cancer. Half took a standard aspirin and half a placebo. The study was ended early because results were so definitive. After 31 months, 17 percent of those who took the aspirin had new polyps compared to 27 percent in the placebo group.

What are the kinds of intestinal cancers that are considered inherited conditions?

Two types of colorectal cancers are commonly recognized as having a hereditary basis—familial adenomatous polyposis and hereditary nonpolyposis colon cancer. (Very often they are referred to by their abbreviated names FAP and HNCC.) Familial polyposis is an inherited condition with hundreds of polyps in the intestine. Such polyps grow in the mucous membrane and almost always become cancerous between the ages of 30 and 50 if they are not removed. Hereditary nonpolyposis colon cancer also is found in young people, but only a few polyps develop. Women with this condition also have a higher risk of cancer of the endometrium.

How will I know if I am at high risk?

There are some guidelines for determining whether or not you are at high risk for either of these inherited conditions. You are at high risk if you have at least three relatives with colorectal cancer and at least one had cancer before age 50 (at least two of the relatives are your mother, father, sister or brother) and more than two generations are involved in a row. If you are in this high risk category, you might want to see a genetic counselor. In addition, you will need to have regular checkups starting at an early age and see a doctor immediately if you have any symptoms of bowel problems.

Can I be tested to see if I have this genetic problem?

These genetic problems are well defined and you can be tested. There is additional information about genetics and cancer and genetic counseling in Chapter 11, New Advances and Investigational Treatments.

Am I at higher risk if I am of Eastern European Jewish extraction?

About 6 percent of American Jews of Eastern European origin, also identified as Ashkenazi Jews, have been found to have a change in their DNA, called I1307K APC, which puts them at a higher risk for colorectal cancer.

Are there organizations for families with inherited colon cancer?

Intestinal Multiple Polyposis and Colorectal Cancer (IMPACC) is an organization specifically designed to provide support for families with either of the forms of hereditary colon cancer. Their address is PO Box 11, Conyngham, PA 18219, telephone 570–788–1818, email: impacc@epix.net.

Is there any screening test that can detect changes in the colon gene?

There is research underway on a test that can find changes in the APC gene, a tumor suppressor-type gene that is associated with colorectal cancers. The test would detect abnormal APC gene changes in stool samples. If successful, this simple test would identify colorectal cancer at the earliest stages. Those in whom the changes are identified could be followed with additional tests, such as colonoscopy.

Do hemorrhoids (piles) turn into cancer?

No. However, do not make the mistake of assuming that rectal bleeding is always caused by hemorrhoids, because one of the symptoms of cancer of the colon or rectum is bright red blood in stools. Rectal bleeding should be checked by a doctor to determine its cause.

How is the digital rectal examination done?

The doctor, wearing thin gloves, puts a greased finger into the rectum and gently feels for lumps. This examination will detect the presence of any abnormalities in the lowest four inches of the rectum. Any stool on the gloved finger will also be checked for blood.

What is the fecal occult blood test (FOBT)?

The fecal occult blood test, also called the guaiac test (pronounced gwi-yak), is a simple, inexpensive method of testing stools for traces of blood. Usually you will take stool samples from three consecutive bowel movements to check for intermittent bleeding. To increase the accuracy of the stool analysis, the doctor may ask you to start a meat-free, high-fiber diet (avoiding such vegetables as radishes and red peppers) 48 hours before the collection of the first stool specimen and continuing through the next three days. Vitamin C, iron, and aspirin also should be avoided during this time to ensure that the test is accurate.

What is a flexible sigmoidoscopy?

A flexible sigmoidoscopy is the primary test done to examine the inside of the lower part of the colon. The doctor uses a special instrument, a lighted, flexible, hollow tube called a sigmoidoscope which is inserted into the anus. The flexible fiberoptic sigmoidoscope allows viewing higher into the colon, about a third of the way. At the time of the sigmoidoscopy, a biopsy forceps may be inserted through the inside of the instrument to remove a small piece of tissue for examination. The sigmoidoscopy test is usually done in the doctor's office. To prepare for this examination, the doctor will usually instruct you to have an enema the night before or the morning of the examination. If bleeding, obstruction, or diarrhea is present, the doctor will suggest a less vigorous bowel cleansing. This procedure is best done by a gastroenterologist or a physician who is especially trained to do this test. Complications from this examination are rare, but an inexperienced doctor could perforate the bowel, causing serious problems. The procedure may be a bit uncomfortable and you may feel pressure, but in most instances, there is no pain.

What is a colonoscopy?

A colonoscopy is an examination of the colon by means of a flexible, lighted tube, slightly larger in diameter than an enema tube. Aided by a video monitor, the doctor is able to view the entire colon as well as the rectum and remove any polyps or to take a biopsy from any part of the colon. Before undergoing a colonoscopy, your colon needs to be cleansed. Your doctor will give you instructions on how to do this. The colonoscopy is done under local anesthesia, along with medication to relax you during the procedure. The doctor will insert some air into the colon. Occasionally, the air will cause a feeling of pressure or the same kind of discomfort as gas pain. It is important that you check the doctor's credentials before having a fiberoptic colonoscopy to be certain that the doctor is skilled in its use, since in the hands of an unskilled physician, perforation and other complications may occur.

What is virtual colonoscopy?

Virtual colonoscopy is a new method, presently under study, that looks at the inside of the colon by taking a series of x-rays (spiral CT scans). You will prepare for this test the same as if you were having a regular colonoscopy. The doctor inserts some air into the colon. Using a high power computer, 2-D and 3-D pictures are reconstructed, letting the doctor see the inside of the colon on a computer monitor. The pictures can be turned for better views, saved, and looked at after the test, even years later. It is anticipated that the test can be done more quickly, without anesthesia and probably at lower cost than the colonoscopy.

Is a lower GI series the same as a barium enema?

The barium enema is done in order to make it possible to take the x-rays of the lower GI or gastrointestinal tract. For this test, a white liquid called barium, that appears white on the x-ray film, is inserted as an enema into the colon. The barium coats the inside of the large intestine and x-rays reveal any polyps, growths or constricted or displaced areas. Air may be pumped into the colon during the test to expand the bowel and make small tumors easier to see. This technique is called an air contrast or double-contrast barium enema. The barium enema feels much like an ordinary enema, causing a feeling of fullness.

What preparation should be made before these tests?
The doctor will provide you with exact instructions, which usually include a liquid diet and laxatives to help clear the colon of waste so that all areas of the colon can be inspected.

Is one of these tests better than another?
Each of the tests has its advantages and disadvantages.

- The fecal occult blood test is easy to do at home, is the least expensive (about $20) and presents the fewest risks. On the other hand, it misses most polyps and some cancers, and must be done every year. It is most effective if it is done in combination with a flexible sigmoidoscopy every five years.

- The flexible sigmoidoscopy can be done fairly quickly, has few complications and only needs to be done every five years. However, it sees only about a third of the colon. If problems are found, you will need to undergo another procedure to have them taken care of.

- The double-contrast barium enema, a more complex test to do, can usually see the entire colon and needs to be done every five years. But it can miss some small polyps and cancers. You will need to cleanse your bowel before you have the test, and if problems are found, you will need to undergo another procedure to have them taken out.

- The colonoscopy, the most complex test, allows the doctor to examine the entire colon. The doctor can biopsy and take out polyps and diagnose other diseases while doing this test. Colonoscopy needs to be done only every ten years. However, it can miss small polyps. You will need to cleanse your bowel and take medication before you have the test. It takes longer to do and is more risky.

You need to discuss which test is best for you with your doctor. The choice usually depends upon several factors, such as the availability of the tests, the preference of the doctor, what your insurance company will cover and your own decision on which is better for your lifestyle.

If tumors are found, must they always be removed?
Yes. Most doctors agree that even benign tumors such as polyps and adenomas should be removed because they may eventually develop into cancer.

Can cancers of the colon and rectum recur?
Cancer of the colon and rectum can recur at or near the site of the original tumor, and can spread to other parts of the body. Patients treated for large bowel cancer have a two to ten percent chance of developing a new cancer that

is not a recurrence of the original tumor in the colon or rectum. Regular follow-up by the doctor is important to detect any recurrences at an early stage.

How serious is surgery for tumors of the colon and rectum?

The surgery varies depending on the location, kind, and size of the tumor. Polyps near the rectum can often be removed through the rectum without anesthesia in a surgeon's office, or on an outpatient basis in a hospital, or during an overnight hospital stay. For any benign tumor, the procedure is simple removal of the tumor at its base. If the tumor is cancerous, the tumor, as well as a generous portion of the colon above and below, must be removed.

What are the stages of colon and rectal cancers?

Once cancer is diagnosed, the doctor needs to know the stage of your disease to plan treatment. Several different methods of staging are used for colon and rectal cancer and you should ask your doctor what stage of cancer you have. Both colon and rectal cancer are usually staged by a system approved by the American Joint Committee on Cancer and the International Union Against Cancer, which uses Stage 0, I, II, III, and IV to describe the extent of colon and rectal cancers. Stage 0 indicates early cancer that hasn't spread beyond the limiting membrane of the first layer of colorectal tissue. Stage IV means that the cancer has spread to other parts of the body—usually the liver or the lungs. You also might hear the term Duke's or the modified Astler Coller staging system. Both use letters (A, B, C, D) to designate stages. (Chapter 4, What Is Cancer?, gives further information on the meaning of staging descriptions.)

What kind of treatment is used for colon and rectal cancers?

Cancers of the colon and rectum differ in their patterns of growth and their response to various treatments. Many factors are involved in determining treatment, such as the location of the tumor, the stage of the cancer, the type of cancer cells, and your age and general health. The doctor may recommend one, or a combination of treatments. The charts include separate information for colon and for rectal cancers.

What operations are performed for colon cancer?

The doctor may do one of several surgeries:

- **Polypectomy:** taking out polyp.
- **Local incision:** doctor puts tube through rectum to colon and takes out cancer without cutting through the wall of the abdomen. Used for very early stage cancer.

STAGING FOR COLON AND RECTAL CANCER

STAGE	DESCRIPTION
Stage 0 (Carcinoma *in situ*)	Very early cancer, found only in top lining of colon or rectum.
Stage I (Duke's A or modified Astler-Coller A and B1)	Tumor extends to second or third layers beyond top lining and involves inside wall of colon or rectum but has not spread to outer wall or outside.
Stage II (Duke's B or Modified Astler-Coller B2 and B3)	Tumor penetrates outside colon or rectum to nearby tissue, but has not gone into lymph nodes.
Stage III (Duke's C or Modified Astler-Coller C1–C3)	Cancer has spread to nearby lymph nodes but has not spread to other parts of the body.
Stage IV (Duke's D)	Cancer has spread to other parts of the body.
Recurrent	Cancer has recurred after being treated. Recurrence may be in colon or other parts of body—often liver or lungs.

- **Colectomy:** removing cancer and small amount of healthy tissue around it.

- **Anastomosis:** removing the cancer and sewing back together the healthy cut ends of the colon (anastomosis also can be used to bypass the tumor).

- **Colostomy:** Putting an opening (stoma) on the outside of the body for waste to pass through. Used if doctor cannot sew two ends of colon back together. Sometimes done temporarily and when colon heals, operation can be reversed.

Can "keyhole" surgery be used for colon cancer?

Keyhole surgery, known in the medical world as laparoscopic or minimally invasive surgery, is being used for colon cancer, mostly at major centers or through clinical trials. The doctor makes several small incisions, each about one-half inch long. Surgical tools and a miniature camera are inserted. The video camera lets the doctors "see" inside the body while doing the surgery. Another incision about two to three inches long is made to bring the intestine out so that the doctor can take out the part with cancer and sew the two ends back together. Early studies are showing that this method shortens the time a person spends in the hospital, makes for a quicker recovery, and produces fewer side effects. However, this method of doing surgery for colon cancer has not yet been tested in clinical trials. One recent study cautioned against using this method until larger scale, longer term trials have been conducted.

How are doctors using radiation therapy in treating cancer of the rectum?

Radiation is used in a number of ways in treating rectal cancer. Because rectal cancers sometimes recur at their original site, many doctors are recommending the use of radiation therapy shortly after the surgery as a precaution. Recent research indicates that treatment with radiation before and/or after surgery reduces the risk of the cancer recurring locally. In order to preserve the sphincter muscle, which controls bowel evacuation, one approach is to use high doses of radiation before surgery. Also being evaluated is the use of radiation at the time of surgery, when the tumor is exposed and the surrounding normal tissues can be shielded. This technique is sometimes used in treating tumors that have penetrated the bowel wall and invaded nearby tissue. Another procedure, called endocavitary irradiation, uses a tubular device that is fitted into a special proctoscope. With this technique the radiation can be aimed directly at the tumor. Endocavitary irradiation can be used to cure small, early stage rectal cancers. It is also used for larger tumors, when the patient cannot have surgery, and for the control of pain and bleeding in large tumors that cannot be removed surgically.

Are chemotherapy and radiation used together for cancer of the rectum?

Research has shown that using chemotherapy (5–FU) and radiation therapy together after surgery, for people with Stage II and III cancer of the rectum, has lengthened both disease-free and overall survival time. Clinical trials are studying the effectiveness of presurgery chemotherapy and radiation for cancer of the rectum.

Are blood transfusions recommended during surgery for patients with colon and rectal cancers?

Some studies indicate that packed red blood cells are better than whole blood during surgery for patients with colon and rectal cancers. Many doctors limit the transfusion of blood whenever medically feasible. Some medical centers are now performing bloodless surgery by using laser and harmonic scalpels, argon beam, and drugs that help to reduce the loss of blood.

What is a stoma?

A stoma is an opening in the skin that allows the end of the small or large intestine to be brought through the abdominal wall and fastened at the skin level. It provides a new way for waste to leave the body. The diameter of the

TREATMENT CHOICES FOR COLON CANCER

STAGE	DESCRIPTION
Stage 0	Local excision or simple polypectomy or colectomy with anastomosis.
Stage I (Duke's A or Modified Astler-Coller A and B1)	Colectomy with anastomosis.
Stage II (Duke's B or Modified Astler-Coller B2–B3)	Colectomy with anastomosis **or** *Clinical trials* of chemotherapy, radiation therapy or biological therapy after surgery.
Stage III (Duke's C or Modified Astler-Coller C1–C3)	Colectomy with anastomosis; if spread to nearby tissue, possible chemotherapy or radiation following surgery. *Clinical trials:* New combinations of chemotherapy **or** biological agents; radiation therapy after surgery with or without chemotherapy or biological agents.
Stage IV	Colectomy or colostomy; surgery to remove parts of other organs such as liver, lungs and ovaries, where cancer may have spread or chemotherapy **or** radiation therapy to relieve symptoms. *Clinical trials:* new combinations of chemotherapy or biological therapy.
Recurrent	If recurs In only one part of body, operation to remove cancer. If has spread to several parts of body, chemotherapy or radiation therapy. *Clinical trials:* New chemotherapy drugs or biological therapy.

opening may vary from 1/2 inch to 3 inches or more. After a colostomy, the patient wears a special bag to collect body waste.

What is the operation used to create a stoma called?
The operation is called an *ostomy*. Whether permanent or temporary, it takes the name of the area where it is performed. If in the colon, it is called a colostomy and usually means that a portion of the colon and the rectum has been removed. If in the ileum (the lowest part of the small intestine) it is called an ileostomy and means that a portion of the small intestine has been removed. A total colectomy means that the entire large intestine and rectum have been removed.

TREATMENT CHOICES FOR RECTAL CANCER

STAGE	DESCRIPTION
Stage 0	Local excision **or** Simple polypectomy **or** If cancer too large, resection **or** Internal or external radiation therapy.
Stage I	Surgical resection with or without anastomosis **or** Surgical resection with or without radiation therapy and chemotherapy **or** Internal and/or external radiation therapy. *Clinical trials:* Radiation and chemotherapy at time of surgery.
Stage II	Resection with or without anastomosis, followed by chemotherapy or radiation therapy **or** Partial or total pelvic exenteration followed by radiation and chemotherapy **or** Radiation with or without chemotherapy followed by surgery and chemotherapy **or** Radiation during surgery followed by external radiation and chemotherapy **or** *Clinical trials*
Stage III	Resection with or without anastomosis followed by radiation therapy and chemotherapy **or** Partial or total pelvic exenteration followed by radiation and chemotherapy **or** Radiation therapy with or without chemotherapy followed by surgery followed by chemotherapy **or** Radiation therapy during surgery followed by external radiation therapy and chemotherapy **or** Chemotherapy and radiation to relieve symptoms **or** *Clinical trials*
Stage IV	Resection and anastomosis to relieve symptoms **or** If spread to liver, lungs or ovaries, surgery to remove cancer **or** Radiation therapy or chemotherapy for symptoms **or**

TREATMENT CHOICES FOR RECTAL CANCER *(continued)*

STAGE	DESCRIPTION
Stage IV *(continued)*	Chemotherapy following surgery.
	Clinical trials: New chemotherapy drugs and biological therapy.
Recurrent	Surgery to remove tumor or to relieve symptoms **or**
	If cancer recurs in one part of body, operation to remove cancer **or**
	Radiation and/or chemotherapy to reduce size of tumor and relieve symptoms **or**
	Clinical trials: New chemotherapy drugs or biological therapy.

Is a stoma uncomfortable?

A well-cared-for, healthy stoma is comfortable and painless and does not interfere with physical activity. However, much of the success with which a patient is able to handle the stoma is determined by the way in which the surgery is carried out, as well as by the attitude of the patient.

How can I insure a stoma that works well for me?

Many factors contribute to a "good" stoma. First of all, make certain that your surgeon is someone who specializes in this particular type of operation. Some surgeons undertake these operations without the benefit of repeated experience, and though they provide a stoma that is surgically correct, the stoma may not function well from the patient's point of view. Be sure to ask how often the doctor has performed the surgery and what kind of long-term routine supervision he gives or suggests. You might ask the doctor if there is a patient who has had the operation who would be willing to talk with you. Be absolutely certain that before the operation the doctor has marked the site for the stoma so that you know exactly where it will be. It should be located in an area that is free of wrinkles, is slightly convex, away from old scars and creases and can be easily seen by you. Stomas situated in scars, in the navel, or where you wear your belt can be quite unmanageable. Prominent bones, the waistline, or fat can all interfere with the use of ostomy appliances. Of course, the type of ostomy you have determines to some extent where the stoma will be and the nature of the discharge you will have. Your doctor can show you a diagram of the portion of your colon to be removed and where the stoma will be. It also would be useful to ask to speak to a wound ostomy continence nurse (WOCN) before you have your operation.

What does a wound ostomy continence nurse do?

The wound ostomy continence nurse, who used to be called an enterostomal therapy (ET) nurse, is a specialist in ostomy care and rehabilitation. WOCN nurses coordinate patient care, teach nursing personnel in hospital and clinics and work closely with the nursing and medical professions to improve the quality of ostomy rehabilitation programs. You should try to speak with a WOCN nurse before your operation. Your doctor or The United Ostomy Association and its chapters can refer you to a WOCN nurse in your area.

How long is the hospital stay for colon or rectal surgery?

The time varies according to the extent of the surgery. Your doctor will be able to tell you what to expect. A simple operation for the removal of polyps is sometimes done on an outpatient basis or may require one or two days of hospitalization. A tumor removed through the abdomen may require four to ten days. As with any surgery, complications can extend this time. In the case of operations that are done in several stages, the patient may have to plan on several hospitalizations, each requiring a varying amount of time in the hospital.

How long does it take to get adjusted to a colostomy appliance?

A great deal depends upon your attitude. There will be mental as well as physical adjustments to be made. You will wear a pouch, but they are odor-free. You can get disposable or reusable ones. You can bathe and shower, either with or without the pouch. There usually are no restrictions on what you can eat. The colostomy or ileostomy should not interfere with your work, except if you do heavy lifting. You should be able to wear the same clothing as before, including a bathing suit. You can travel but should not carry heavy suitcases. You also will be able to participate in sports unless they include heavy body contact. After a few months' time, most people become accustomed to the routine and it becomes a normal part of life.

Will Medicare cover any of my ostomy supplies?

Medicare covers some of the supplies that you will need, including pouches and special pouch features, skin barriers, tape and paste, and absorbent flakes.

How does the body function without a large portion of the intestines?

The removal of a portion of the small intestine or even all of the colon and rectum sounds as though it would be impossible for the body to function.

The fact is that after successful surgery, the body adjusts with very little difficulty—and people report that they feel better than they ever did. The problem area has been removed and the intestine that remains is perfectly capable of performing its functions. You have about 20 feet of small intestine and five feet of large intestine. You can live quite normally without a portion of the small intestine and without your entire large intestine. Most digestion actually takes place before food reaches the colon. The colon's function is to absorb the water from the already digested material and to transport waste through its length and store it until it is ready to be expelled from the body. The remaining portions of the colon learn to assume some of the water absorption role of the intestine that was removed.

What common problems signal that a person with a colostomy should call the doctor?

You should call the doctor if you have:

- Cramps lasting more than two or three hours.
- Severe, unusual odor lasting more than a week.
- Unusual change in stoma size or appearance.
- Obstruction at the stoma or slipping out of place of stoma.
- Excessive bleeding from stoma opening, or moderate amount in pouch in several emptyings. (Eating beets can lead to red discoloration.)
- Injury or cut in stoma.
- Continuous bleeding at junction between stoma and skin.
- Severe watery discharge lasting more than five or six hours.

Where can I get information about living with an ostomy?

A remarkable organization, United Ostomy Association, exists with the sole purpose of helping people who have had ostomies. Any questions you have are certain to be covered in its publications or on its useful Web site. The UOA offers a journal, visitors either before or after the operation (call its toll free number), seminars, a youth camp, support groups along with a variety of information compiled from the experiences of many hundreds of patients, nurses and doctors. Local chapters are located across the country and are listed in the yellow pages under "Associations" or "Social Service Organizations." The American Cancer Society in your area can tell you where the nearest chapter of UOA is located and has literature on this subject and often sponsors ostomy meetings.

Are there any sexual side effects from colon cancer surgery?

The sexual side effects depend upon the extent of your surgery as well as your treatment. Most people with colon cancer return to normal after surgery. Those who have colostomies that are reversed after a period of time may have a longer recovery period, but once the final surgery is done, life can return to normal. If it is necessary to have a total pelvic exenteration, usually for a large, advanced tumor of the colon, both a urostomy and colostomy may be needed. In men, nerves involved with erection will probably be damaged; in women the vagina may be reconstructed so that sexual adjustments must be made. Both men and women, however, find that, with patience and understanding, they can make changes in their sexual lives that allow them to find pleasure in less conventional ways. See Chapter 27, Living with Cancer, for more information on sexuality problems. The United Ostomy Association Web site also has useful information on this topic.

What kind of periodic checkups should someone with cancer of the colon or rectum have?

It is important for anyone who has been treated for cancer of the colon or rectum to be carefully rechecked on a regular basis by a physician. Follow-up studies may include:

- Complete physical exam
- Stool blood test
- Colonoscopy
- CT, MRI, and other scans
- CEA tumor marker testing (not necessary for rectal cancer)
- PET scans

What is a CEA test?

The CEA test measures the level of carcinoembroyonic antigen that may be found in greater amounts in the blood of patients with colon cancer. This protein is present in the human embryo but is normally found only in minute amounts in healthy adults. *This test is not a conclusive cancer test because CEA values are not elevated in all people with the disease.* Furthermore, the level of this protein can be abnormally high in the blood of people who do not have cancer, including smokers and those with noncancerous growths or inflammation of the gastrointestinal tract. Because of these facts, the CEA test, if used, is used only in addition to other tests in making a definitive diagnosis. Although it does not by itself determine whether or not cancer is present, it may signal the need for further diagnostic tests.

When are PET scans used?
PET scans with immunoscintigraphy (a radioactive isotope scan using an antibody against CEA) are usually used to find the site of recurrence when the CEA blood level is rising. It is proving to be more effective than either CT or MRI.

What is the outlook for patients whose colorectal cancers have spread to the liver, lung, or ovary?
There are several treatments that can be used. In some patients, surgery is done to remove secondary tumors in the liver or chemotherapy may be delivered directly into the liver. Surgery is also often successful in treating solitary metastases in the lung or ovary. It may be combined with chemotherapy. Radiofrequency ablation—killing cancer cells by heating them with microwaves delivered through a needle inserted directly into the tumor—may be used. A number of new chemotherapy drugs are under investigation, including irinotecan in combination with 5-FU and luecovorin, oxaliplantin, and IMC-C225 (a monoclonal antibody). Additional investigational agents include antiangiogenesis factors, novel tumor receptor targets, and chemotherapy enhancers. It is useful to enroll in a clinical trial that is testing new methods of treatment. See Chapter 11, New Advances and Investigational Treatments, and Chapter 26, When Cancers Recur or Metastasize, for more information.

Will my family members need to be monitored closely?
Your immediate family—mother, father, brothers, sisters, and children—need to have special follow-up because they are at a higher risk for the disease. Colonoscopy will probably be used to look for polyps in the colon and to remove them if they are found. If polyps are taken out, they cannot develop into cancer. If you have FAP or HNCCP, your relatives will require special screening. See Chapter 27, Living with Cancer, for more information.

STOMACH OR GASTRIC CANCER

The stomach makes up a relatively small part of the digestive system. It lies under the ribs in the left upper part of the abdomen, crossing over to the right below the liver. It hangs completely free in the abdominal cavity. The upper part of the stomach connects to the esophagus, and the lower part connects to the small intestine. Food comes through your mouth, into your throat to your esophagus and into the stomach where it is partly digested. It then passes into the small intestine to the large intestine. Unfortunately, because there may be no symptoms or only vague symptoms, cancer of the stomach can be present for a long period of time and become quite large before it is detected.

WHO IS MOST LIKELY TO GET CANCER OF THE STOMACH

- People over 55.
- Males.
- Blacks.
- People who eat foods that have been preserved by drying, smoking, salting or pickling dry, salted foods.
- People with helicobacter pylori, the bacteria that causes some stomach ulcers and inflammation.
- People who have pernicious anemia.
- Cigarette smokers.
- People who have had stomach surgery.
- People who have Menetrier's disease or atrophic gastritis.
- People who have familial polyposis.

SYMPTOMS OF STOMACH CANCER

- Indigestion.
- A sense of discomfort or vague pain.
- Fullness or bloating or burping.
- Slight nausea, heartburn, indigestion, or loss of appetite. (These are all signs we find easy to ignore. However, if they persist—even intermittently—for a period of two weeks or more, you should consult your doctor.)

Later signs can include:

- Dark stool which may signal blood in the stools.
- Vomiting; it may be bloody.
- Rapid weight loss.
- Severe abdominal pain.
- Weakness and fatigue.

(These symptoms may also indicate the presence of an ulcer.)

What You Need to Know About Cancer of the Stomach

- The number of cases of stomach, or gastric cancer, has gone down dramatically in the United States in the past 60 years, although it is still common in other parts of the world such as Japan, Korea, and Latin America.

- It can develop in any part of the stomach and may spread to other organs.

- Stomach cancer is treated by surgery. Sometimes chemotherapy and radiation are used before or after the operation.

- A drug known as imatinib mesylate or by its trade name, Gleevec, which interferes with the growth of cancer, is being tested for a type of stomach cancer known as GIST.

- You can live quite comfortably with part of your stomach or even no stomach at all.

How is the diagnosis of stomach cancer made?

A careful history and physical and rectal examination come first. Laboratory tests, such as red and white blood cell counts and plasma tumor markers will be checked. An upper GI series and gastroscopy, with multiple biopsy and brush cytology, in which the stomach lining is gently scraped to give the pathologist material for study, will be done to determine if cancer cells are present. If cancer cells are found, a CT scan, ultrasound, or other tests may be needed.

Do doctors sometimes suspect cancer of the stomach and find a benign tumor?

It is not always easy to distinguish a malignant tumor from a harmless benign tumor even with today's most advanced techniques. It is possible for surgery to uncover an ulcer, a benign tumor or a cancerous tumor.

Does having an ulcer make me more likely to get stomach cancer?

Having stomach ulcers won't necessarily increase your chance of getting stomach cancer. However, some studies show that if you have had an infection of the stomach that causes ulcers (helicobacter pylori) you may be more likely to get the disease.

How is cancer of the stomach usually treated?

The usual treatment for cancer of the stomach is prompt surgical removal of the malignant tumor. The operation involves the removal of a part (subtotal or partial gastrectomy) or all of the stomach (total gastrectomy), depending on the location of the malignancy. After a total gastrectomy, the doctor connects the part of the stomach that remains to the esophagus or the small intestine. If

STAGES OF CANCER OF THE STOMACH (GASTRIC CANCER)

STAGE	DESCRIPTION
Stage 0	Found only in innermost layer of stomach wall.
Stage I	In second and/or third layers of stomach wall but not in lymph nodes or in second layer of stomach wall, and spread to lymph nodes very close to tumor.
Stage II	In second and/or third layer (muscle layer) of stomach wall, and spread to lymph nodes away from tumor, or in third layer and spread to lymph nodes close to tumor, or in all four layers of stomach wall but not spread to lymph nodes or nearby organs.
Stage III	In third layer of stomach wall and spread to lymph nodes away from tumor, or in all four layers of stomach wall and spread to lymph nodes or nearby tissues; may or may not have spread to lymph nodes very close to tumor.
Stage IV	Spread to nearby tissues and to distant lymph nodes, or spread to other parts of body.
Recurrent	After treatment, cancer recurs in stomach, or in other part of body such as liver, bones or lymph nodes.

a total gastrectomy has been done, the esophagus will be connected to the small intestine. Sometimes other abdominal organs, such as the esophagus, spleen, and pancreas, are removed if they are in the area of the tumor and are believed to be affected. Chemotherapy may be used after surgery in treating stomach cancer. It might be given directly into the abdomen (intraperitoneal chemotherapy). Radiation may also be used during—intraoperative radiation—or after, surgery. Biological therapy in combination with chemotherapy and/or radiation is being tested in clinical trials.

When will I be able to eat normally again?
Right after the operation you will be fed intravenously. Then you will be given liquids by mouth, then soft and finally solid foods. You may have some temporary problems with eating certain foods. If you have chemotherapy or radiation therapy, you may also have side effects from them. You need to talk with your doctor about what side effects you might expect, as well as about special diets and how long you will need to be on them.

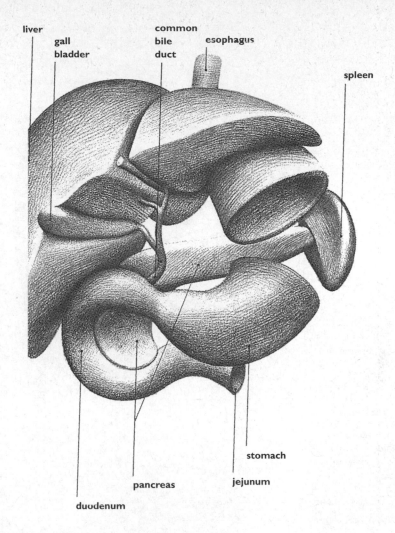

liver

gall
bladder

common
bile
duct

esophagus

spleen

stomach

jejunum

pancreas

duodenum

Front view, major internal organs

How can a person live without a stomach?

People who have had all of their stomachs or part of their stomachs removed lead quite normal lives. They usually find it more comfortable to eat smaller, more frequent meals and adjust to this way of life quite easily. If the whole stomach has been taken out, a diet that is low in sugar and high in fat and protein will be suggested.

What is the dumping syndrome?

Following the removal of the stomach, some people develop what is referred to as the "dumping syndrome"—nausea, weakness, dizziness, sweating,

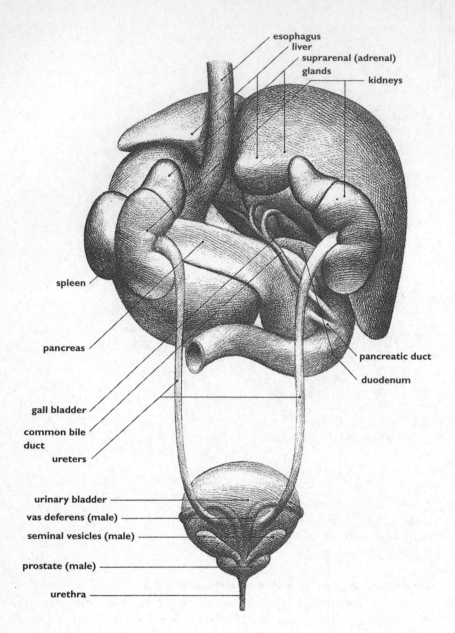

esophagus
liver
suprarenal (adrenal)
glands
kidneys

spleen

pancreas

pancreatic duct

duodenum

gall bladder

common bile
duct

ureters

urinary bladder

vas deferens (male)

seminal vesicles (male)

prostate (male)

urethra

Rear view, major internal organs

TREATMENT OF CANCER OF THE STOMACH (GASTRIC CANCER)

STAGE	DESCRIPTION
Stage 0	Subtotal gastrectomy. Lymph nodes removed **or** Total gastrectomy. Lymph nodes removed.
Stage I	Subtotal gastrectomy or total gastrectomy. Lymph nodes removed. Surgery followed by chemotherapy plus radiation **or** *Clinical trials:* Chemotherapy and/or radiation therapy followed by surgery.
Stage II	Subtotal gastrectomy or total gastrectomy. Lymph nodes removed **or** Surgery followed by radiation and/or chemotherapy **or** *Clinical trials:* Chemotherapy and/or radiation therapy followed by surgery.
Stage III	Total gastrectomy. Lymph nodes removed **or** Surgery followed by radiation and/or chemotherapy **or** *Clinical trials:* Chemotherapy and/or radiation followed by surgery.
Stage IV	Total gastrectomy. Lymph nodes removed **or** Surgery to relieve symptoms, reduce bleeding or remove tumor blocking stomach **or** Radiation to relieve symptoms, reduce bleeding or shrink a tumor blocking the stomach **or** Chemotherapy to relieve symptoms. *Clinical trials:* New chemotherapy drugs and chemotherapy followed by surgery.
Recurrent	Chemotherapy to relieve symptoms **or** Surgery to relieve symptoms, reduce bleeding or remove a tumor blocking the stomach **or** Radiation to relieve symptoms, reduce bleeding or shrink a tumor blocking the stomach **or** *Clinical trials:* New chemotherapy drugs and biological therapy.

palpitations—which occurs when the remnant of the stomach empties itself of food too quickly. This can usually be controlled by frequent, small feedings and by following a high-protein diet with the addition of dry foods and fluids between meals. Some people also have problems with upset stomach, which may be because the bile is backing up either into your esophagus or your smaller stomach. Tell the doctor if you are having these symptoms.

Where does stomach cancer spread?

Stomach cancer can spread to the liver, pancreas, or colon. It might also spread to places further away from the stomach, such as the lungs and ovaries. If it spreads to the ovaries, it is called Krukenberg tumor.

What kind of continuing checkups are needed following stomach cancer?

The first and second year, you will probably see your doctor every three months; the third through fifth year, every six months and yearly thereafter. Stool tests are usually done at each visit. Follow-up CT scans, x-rays, CEA, CBC, panendoscopy, and liver function tests are usually done every six months for the first two years and yearly after that. The GI series is usually done yearly.

ESOPHAGUS

There are two cell types of cancer of the esophagus—squamous and adeno-carcinoma. While the number of cases of squamous cell has been decreasing in the past 20 years, the number of cases of adenomacarcinoma of the esophagus has grown faster than any other kind of cancer.

What is the esophagus?

The esophagus is the foodpipe. It is a long, hollow muscular tube, about ten inches long, that goes from the back of the throat down to the stomach, carrying food and liquids.

Are most tumors of the esophagus cancerous?

Most tumors in this area are malignant. More men than women have esophageal cancer, and it occurs most often between the ages of 50 and 70.

What are the symptoms of cancer of the esophagus?

The most common symptom is difficulty in swallowing, sometimes called *dysphasia* by those in the medical profession. Your food may seem not to be going down properly, feeling as though it sticks behind the breastbone. There may be sensations of pressure and burning or pain in the upper middle part of the chest, hoarseness, cough, fever or choking. The sensation may seem to get worse and then to get better. Sometimes it comes and goes.

How is cancer of the esophagus diagnosed?

The doctor will take a careful history and do a physical exam. You will probably have a chest x-ray and other tests. You may have a barium swallow— you will drink a liquid that has barium in it that will coat the inside of the

SYMPTOMS OF CANCER OF THE ESOPHAGUS

- Pain or difficulty in swallowing solids or liquids
- Severe loss of weight
- Pain in throat or back, behind breastbone or shoulder blades
- Hoarseness
- Cough
- Vomiting
- Coughing up blood
- Indigestion and heartburn
- Pain in the chest not related to eating

WHO IS MOST LIKELY TO GET CANCER OF THE ESOPHAGUS

- Smokers, both cigarette and smokeless tobacco.
- People who drink alcohol often or who drink heavily.
- People who both smoke and drink.
- People with Barrett's esophagus.
- People over 60.
- Men.
- People who have had damage to the lining of the esophagus.
- People who have had other head and neck cancer.

esophagus. An x-ray will be done to see if there are changes in the shape of your esophagus. The doctor may also order an esophagoscopy. The doctor will insert a lighted tube into your esophagus to collect cells and tissues that will be looked at under the microscope to see if there are cancer cells.

If cancer cells are found, what other tests will I need?
If cancer cells are found, you will need tests to see if the cancer has spread. These might include a bronchoscopy to look at your lungs and a laryngoscopy to look at your voice box. You might also have an endoscopic ultrasound (endosonograph), thoracoscopy, and a laparoscopy. Scans such as MRI, or a CT or PET scan may be done to determine the stage of your cancer.

TREATMENT OF CANCER OF THE ESOPHAGUS

STAGE	DESCRIPTION
Stage I Cancer is found only in top layers of cells lining esophagus.	Surgery (esophagectomy) **or** Clinical trials of chemotherapy plus radiation, with or without surgery **or** Clinical trials of new therapies before or after surgery.
Stage IIA, IIB Cancer involves deeper layers of lining of esophagus or has spread to nearby lymph nodes.	Surgery (esophagectomy) **or** Clinical trials of chemotherapy plus radiation, with or without surgery **or** Clinical trials of new therapies before or after surgery.
Stage III Cancer more deeply in wall of esophagus or spread to nearby tissues or lymph nodes.	Surgery (esophagectomy) **or** Clinical trials of chemotherapy plus radiation, with or without surgery **or** Clinical trials of new therapies before or after surgery.
Stage IV Cancer has spread to other parts of body.	External or internal radiation to relieve symptoms and improve quality of life **or** Laser surgery or electrocoagulation to relieve symptoms **or** Chemotherapy **or** Clinical trials of chemotherapy.
Recurrent Cancer has come back after treatment.	Relief of symptoms **or** Clinical trials or new therapies.

How is cancer of the esophagus treated?

If the cancer is found to be in Stages I, II or III, surgery is usually the treatment, although chemotherapy and radiation are also sometimes used. Surgery involves the removal of the esophagus in an operation called an esophagectomy. Any remaining part of the esophagus that is healthy is reconnected to the stomach. A plastic tube or part of the intestine is sometimes used to connect the two parts, so that you can still swallow. Stage IV cancers are usually treated with radiation. Sometimes a tube is inserted to keep the esophagus open. Being studied in clinical studies are the use of surgery with or without radiation as well as the use of chemotherapy plus radiation or chemotherapy with or without surgery.

Will I have side effects from the surgery?
You will be taught special breathing and coughing exercises to keep your lungs clear after the operation. This is a short-term side effect. You will need to be sure that you eat well. This may be hard for you because you might have problems with swallowing. Rather than eating three meals a day, try to eat several small meals and snacks during the day. If you have problems, be sure to talk with a dietitian.

How often should you see your doctor after treatment for cancer of the esophagus?
The first year, every three months; the second to fifth year, every four months, and after that, every six months.

What is Barrett's esophagus?
A syndrome called Barrett's esophagus often occurs in people who suffer persistent heartburn or whose stomach contents back up (reflux). This can irritate the esophagus and, over time, can cause Barrett's. The cells lining the lower part of the esophagus either change or are replaced with cells that could become cancerous. Instead of the white, skin-like tissue that normally coats the area, these cells are salmon-colored, and look more like the inside of the stomach. Although most cases appear to remain benign, scientists say a large majority of patients with esophageal cancer begin with Barrett's syndrome. The syndrome is seen mainly in white men. Women and African-American men appear to be less susceptible.

LIVER CANCER

The liver performs many complex functions. It breaks down worn-out red blood cells and converts them into bile, regulates the level of many hormones, stores sugar and regulates the amount which circulates in the blood. It controls the metabolism of cholesterol and stores vitamins A,D,E, and K. Cancer that starts in the liver is uncommon in the United States and Europe, though it is the most common cancer in other parts of the world. There is some scientific evidence to show that aflatoxin (a fungal poison that contaminates grain and other foods improperly stored in warm, moist places) and hepatitis B and C virus may trigger a P53 gene mutation. In addition, a small percentage of those who are diagnosed as having cirrhosis of the liver may eventually develop liver cancer. Many cancers spread or metastasize to the liver, but these are not considered liver cancer. For information on cancers which have metastasized to the liver, see Chapter 26, When Cancers Recur or Metastasize.

WHO IS MOST LIKELY TO GET CANCER OF THE LIVER?

- People who have a chronic infection from hepatitis B or hepatitis C.
- Men (twice as likely as women).
- People who have family members with liver cancer.
- People over age 60.
- People who have cirrhosis of the liver.
- People who have been exposed to aflatoxin.

SYMPTOMS OF LIVER CANCER

- Discomfort in the upper abdomen on the right side, which becomes more acute with deep breathing.
- A hard lump just below the rib cage on the right side.
- Lack of appetite.
- Pain around right shoulder blade.
- Abdominal swelling.
- Feeling full or bloated.
- Episodes of unexplained fever and nausea.
- Jaundice, which means that the skin and eyes have a yellow cast and urine is dark.

What You Need to Know About Cancer of the Liver

- Those with history of chronic liver disease (hepatitis B or C viruses) are more likely to get cancer of the liver.
- The only cancer classified as liver cancer is one which starts in the liver. It is usually treated differently than cancer in the liver that has spread or metastasized to the liver from another organ.
- Liver cancer is difficult to treat. You should be seen by a doctor who specializes in this disease.

Where is the liver located?

The liver, the largest organ in our body, is behind the ribs to the right side of your stomach. The liver has two parts, a large right lobe and a smaller left lobe.

Are there different kinds of liver cancer?
There are primary liver cancers which start in the liver, and there are cancers that spread from another part of the body (or metastasize) to the liver. Primary liver cancer is different from cancer that has spread from another part of the body to the liver and is treated differently. For information about cancers that have metastasized to the liver, see Chapter 26, When Cancers Recur or Metastasize. For information about childhood liver cancer, see Chapter 24, When a Child Has Cancer. Most primary liver cancers are adenocarcinomas—either hepatocellular or cholangiocellular. Those that have a fibrolamellar variant have proven to be the most curable.

What kind of doctor treats liver cancer?
Primary cancer of the liver is a very rare kind of cancer in the United States. It is important for you to seek out a surgical or medical oncologist who treats this type of cancer.

What kind of testing is done to diagnose liver cancer?
A battery of tests will be done to determine the diagnosis. You may have CT scans, ultrasound tests, and an MRI of the area. If a lump is detected, the doctor may use a needle biopsy or a laparoscopy to obtain a tissue biopsy. An angiography may be needed to determine whether you have a primary liver cancer or whether it is a cancer that has spread from another part of your body. Blood tests such as AFP and liver function tests are also prescribed.

How is the AFP test used in diagnosing liver cancer?
Alpha-fetoprotein, known as AFP, is a biologic marker that is helpful in diagnosis. Fifty to 70 percent of American patients with hepatocellular cancer have elevated levels of AFP, so this test is significant in making a diagnosis. However, people who have some germ cell cancers and on rare occasions, pancreatic and stomach cancers, have high levels of AFP, so this test should be used with other testing to make a definitive diagnosis.

What are the stages of liver cancer?
There are three main stages: localized resectable, localized unresectable, and advanced. If you have localized resectable liver cancer, the cancer is in one place, and it can be taken out leaving some parts of normal liver. It has not spread and your liver still works well. If you have localized unresectable liver cancer, it has not spread either to the lymph nodes or to other parts of the body, yet it cannot be removed for various reasons, such as the location of the tumor, poor liver function, or other health problems. If your liver cancer is advanced, it means that the cancer is found in both lobes of the liver or it has spread to other parts of the body.

STAGES AND TREATMENT OF LIVER CANCER

STAGE	TREATMENT
Localized resectable Cancer is found in only one place in the liver and can be removed.	Surgery to remove cancer from liver **or** Liver transplant in selected patients **or** *Clinical trials:* Regional arterial infusion of chemotherapy **or** systemic chemotherapy **or** new anticancer agents.
Localized unresectable Cancer is found in only one part of the liver but cannot be totally removed.	Chemo embolization **or** Cryosurgery **or** Percutaneous ethanol injection **or** Radiofrequency ablation **or** Liver transplant **or** Chemotherapy either regional or systemic. *Clinical trials:* Surgery, radiation and chemotherapy **or** Surgery followed by chemotherapy **or** Radiation with radiosensitizers.
Advanced Cancer has spread through much of the liver or to other parts of the body.	*Clinical trials:* Biological therapy **or** chemotherapy **or** Combination chemotherapy, radiosensitizers, radiation therapy **or** Chemoembolization.
Recurrent Cancer has come back after it has been treated.	Depends on prior treatment, where located, whether there is cirrhosis of the liver.

What operations are used to remove localized resectable liver cancer?

If you have localized resectable liver cancer, you may have a hepatectomy—an operation that takes out part of the liver. It might be a small piece with the tumor, a lobe or a larger part of your liver. A healthy piece of the liver is left which will take over the work of the liver. Some patients might have a liver transplant, called a total hepatectomy, where the whole liver is taken out and another liver is transplanted. Liver transplants are very rare.

What kind of treatment will I have if I have unresectable liver cancer?

There are several treatments that might be used: radiofrequency ablation, percutaneous ethanol injection, cryosurgery, hepatic arterial infusion, chemoembolization or liver transplant.

What is radiofrequency ablation?

Heat is used to kill the cancer cells. A probe with tiny electrodes is inserted, either directly through the skin or through a small or large cut in the stomach. Other ways of using heat include using a laser (an intense beam of light) or microwave therapy.

What is percutaneous ethanol injection?

Using a small needle, the doctor will put alcohol (ethanol) directly into your liver to kill the cancer cells. This may need to be done once or twice a week, either outpatient or in the hospital. You may have fever and pain after having this injection.

Are chemotherapy drugs put directly into the liver?

Chemotherapy drugs can be delivered directly into the liver. If you have hepatic arterial infusion, the doctor will put a tube, or catheter, into the artery that brings blood to the liver. The chemotherapy will be inserted through this tube. Another option is having a small pump implanted into your liver, then the chemotherapy can be sent continuously through the pump.

What does the technique called chemoembolization involve?

A small tube, or catheter, is inserted into a blood vessel in the leg and guided to the artery that supplies blood to the liver. Chemotherapy is injected into the artery. Small particles are used to block the blood from flowing through the artery, keeping the drug in the liver longer. You will need to be in the hospital for this procedure.

Is cryosurgery ever used in liver cancer?

Some doctors have found that cryosurgery, which uses an ultrasound-guided metal probe to freeze small cancerous tumors with liquid nitrogen, can be useful for some patients. Cryosurgery is used when cancer is caught before it affects the entire liver or where there are too many tumors to be taken out surgically. People who have cryosurgery usually recover more quickly and have less pain, fewer infections and bleeding.

What treatments are used if the liver cancer is advanced?

If the cancer is found in both lobes of the liver, or if it has spread to other parts of the body, you might be treated with chemotherapy, radiation therapy, or both. The chemotherapy may be injected in the vein or through chemoembolization or hepatic arterial infusion. Radiation is given externally.

Are there other new techniques being tried for liver cancer?

Researchers around the world have been experimenting with ways of selectively delivering drugs or radioactive isotopes directly to the liver. Different techniques include the use of polymer beads to deliver antibodies directly to the tumor site.

Questions to Ask Your Doctor About Follow-up

- **Will you be doing my main follow-up?**
- **Will I also need to see any of my other doctors?**
- **How often will I need to see you?**
- **What tests will you be doing during my follow-up exam?**
- **What will you be looking for?**
- **What should I be watching for between my visits with you?**
- **What symptoms should I report? To whom?**

What kind of checkup schedule should I expect to be on following liver cancer?

You will probably be seeing the doctor for checkups every two to three months for the first two years, then every three to six months for the third through fifth year, and yearly thereafter. CT scans and ultrasound tests will probably be done every six months for the first two years and yearly thereafter. Alpha-fetoprotein, bilirubin, and alkaline phosphatase testing will usually be done every two to three months for the first two years, every six months in the third through fifth years, and yearly after that.

PANCREATIC CANCER

The pancreas is a key organ in the body and has two important, basic functions. It produces gastric juices that break down your food and it produces insulin and other hormones that regulate the storage and use of food. Pancreatic cancer is known as a "silent" disease because it occurs without presenting any real symptoms, usually until it is in a very advanced stage, which cannot be cured. Recurrence of cancer of the pancreas is the rule rather than the exception.

What You Need to Know About Cancer of the Pancreas

- Because it is hidden deep in the body behind other organs and has few early symptoms, cancer of the pancreas is usually found at an advanced stage.

- About 95 percent of pancreatic cancers begin in the exocrine pancreas, the area of the pancreas that produces the juices that break down our food.

- About five percent begin in the endocrine pancreas, the area that produces hormones.

- The symptoms for the two types of pancreatic cancer are different, as are the treatments and the results.

Where is the pancreas?

The pancreas is located behind the stomach, inside a loop formed by part of the small intestine. It is surrounded by the liver, intestine, and other organs. About six inches long, the pancreas has a wide head, a narrower body, and a thin tail.

What tests are usually done to diagnose pancreatic cancer?

There are many tests that may be used to diagnose cancer of the pancreas. They include: blood urine and stool samples to check for bilirubin, ultrasound, CT scan, endoscopic retrograde cholangiopancreatography (ERCP), percutaneous transhepatic cholangiography (PTC), and needle biopsy.

Are most doctors qualified to diagnose and operate on pancreatic cancer?

Pancreatic cancer is relatively rare. It requires the expertise of a doctor who has experience in dealing with such cases. Major medical centers, especially those specializing in cancer treatment, have had more experience than most smaller facilities. You should at least get a second opinion at a major center. Ask your doctor to check if there are clinical trials being done, or call the Cancer Information Service or check the Web for information on clinical trials.

Why is cancer of the pancreas difficult to diagnose?

Because the pancreas is hidden behind other organs, it cannot be examined physically, except with surgery. Furthermore, because discomfort at first is vague, and comes and goes, early signs may be ignored. The pain may manifest itself as a backache, making it difficult for the doctor to make a diagnosis. Even when the symptoms become more pronounced, physical examination, routine x-rays of the gastrointestinal system and blood tests may fail to indicate the cause of the problem. The upper GI test, or barium swallow, that outlines the upper digestive tract rarely reveals early pancreatic cancer.

WHO IS MOST LIKELY TO GET CANCER OF THE PANCREAS?

- People over age 60.
- Cigarette smokers.
- People who have diabetes.
- Men.
- African-Americans.
- People who have a family history of pancreatic, colon, or ovarian cancer.
- People who have chronic pancreatitis.

Is ultrasound helpful in detecting pancreatic cancer?

Ultrasound is highly accurate in detecting small tumors at the head of the pancreas but is less accurate in identifying those in the body and tail. It may also help distinguish cancer from pancreatitis but can sometimes suggest the presence of a tumor when there is none. For this reason, ultrasound is usually used in addition to other diagnostic methods.

How are CT scans used in diagnosing pancreatic cancer?

CT scans are more accurate than ultrasound, though they may miss small and early tumors but are excellent for locating those cancers that have changed the shape of the pancreas and those that have spread beyond its borders.

What does endoscopic retrograde cholangiopancreatography (ERCP) do?

This examination uses a flexible fiberoptic tube that the doctor passes down through the stomach and into the pancreatic ducts. A dye is injected through the tube into the pancreas and x-rays are taken. It can also be used to obtain a sample of pancreatic cells for examination.

What does percutaneous transhepatic cholangiography (PTC) do?

A fine needle is inserted into the liver and a dye is injected. This substance spreads through the gallbladder and bile ducts to reveal blockages caused by a tumor at the head of the pancreas. Samples of pancreatic cells can also be taken.

Are tumor markers used to diagnose cancer of the pancreas?

There are no tumor specific markers for cancer of the pancreas. Most patients with pancreatic cancer will have an elevated serum CA 19–9, but it is not a good enough test to use alone in making a diagnosis. The increase of

SYMPTOMS OF PANCREATIC CANCER (EXOCRINE)

- Vague discomfort that comes and goes.
- Upper abdominal or lumbar back pain that gradually worsens, often most severe at night.
- Back pain that is aggravated by lying flat and relieved by sitting up or lying in a fetal position.
- Pain that radiates to the back or is limited to the back.
- Pain in the back that is relieved by bending forward or by standing.
- Pain that occurs several hours after meals and is more severe at night.
- Weight loss.
- Yellow skin and eyes and dark urine from jaundice.

SYMPTOMS OF PANCREATIC CANCER (ENDOCRINE)

- Pain in the abdomen.
- Diarrhea.
- Stomach pain.
- Tired feeling all the time.
- Fainting.
- Weight gain not caused by overeating.

CA 19–9 may indicate recurrence, but a normal CA 19–9 does not mean that there is no recurrence.

Are all tumors and growths in the pancreas cancerous?
It is important to remember that all cysts, tumors, and inflammations of the pancreas do not indicate the presence of cancer. Any growth, whether benign or cancerous, may cause the cells that produce insulin to overproduce, resulting in symptoms that include intense hunger, trembling, fainting, confusion, or convulsions. The operation to remove a cyst is a low-risk one. However, if cancer is found, it may be necessary to operate so as to bypass the obstruction or to remove the entire gland.

What kinds of cancers of the pancreas are there?
There are two major kinds: islet cell cancer of the endocrine pancreas and adenocarcinoma of the exocrine pancreas. Cancers of the endocrine and exocrine pancreas differ in many ways. Cancer of the endocrine pancreas is a highly treatable and often curable collection of tumors. Cancer of the exocrine pancreas, on the other hand, is much more difficult to treat and is not often curable.

What is the most common type of cancer of the pancreas?
The largest percentage of pancreatic cancers are cancers of the exocrine pancreas, and of these, about 90 percent are duct cell cancers that are found in the lining of pancreatic ducts. About three-fourths of exocrine cancers start in the head and neck of the pancreas. Most of the rest begin in the main body of the pancreas and fewer than ten percent start in the tail. In some patients, cancer is found throughout the pancreas.

What kind of surgery is done to remove cancers of the pancreas?
The surgery depends on where the tumor is, the stage of disease, as well as personal factors, such as age and overall condition. An operation, called the Whipple procedure, removes the head of the pancreas, a small part of the small intestine, bile duct, stomach, and some of the tissues around it. Enough of the pancreas is left to continue making digestive juices and insulin. Distal pancreatectomy takes out only the head or the tail of the pancreas, along with the spleen. A total pancreatectomy is a more complex procedure which removes the whole pancreas, part of the small intestine, part of the stomach, the bile duct, the gallbladder, spleen, and lymph nodes in the area.

When are bypass operations done for pancreatic cancer?
When the duodenum is blocked, the surgeon may bypass the duodenum and connect the common bile duct with the jejunum, which is below the duodenum. Or, instead of an operation, a stent (a tiny plastic or metal mesh tube) might be used to keep the duct or duodenum open. If the cancer is blocking the flow of food from the stomach, the stomach may be sewn directly to the small intestine so that you can eat normally.

Is radiation being used during surgery as a treatment for exocrine pancreatic cancer?
Radiation therapy, given before or after the operation, is being studied as a treatment for pancreatic cancer.

Are biological therapies being used for pancreatic cancer?
Alpha interferon, recombinant IL–2 and combinations of these and other drugs such as 5–FU, cyclophosphamide, leucovorin, and granulocyte macrophage

STAGES OF PANCREATIC CANCER (EXOCRINE PANCREAS)

STAGE	DESCRIPTION
Stage I	Cancer is found only in pancreas and has not spread to other organs.
Stage II	Cancer has spread to nearby organs such as the duodenum or bile duct but not to lymph nodes.
Stage III	Cancer has spread to lymph nodes; may or may not have spread to nearby organs.
Stage IV	Cancer has spread to other nearby organs, such as stomach, spleen or colon or to distant organs such as liver or lungs.
Recurrent	Return of cancer after treatment either in pancreas or other part of body.

PANCREATIC CANCER (ENDOCRINE OR ISLET CELL)

TYPE	DESCRIPTION
Gastrinoma	Increased gastrin may cause ulcers in stomach.
Insulinoma	Increased insulin, body stores sugar instead of burning it, causing hypoglycemia (often benign).
Miscellaneous VIPoma, somatostatinoma, pancreatic polypeptide, glucagonoma	Different hormones affected.
Recurrent	Return of cancer after treatment, either in pancreas or other part of body.

colony-stimulating factor are being tried for patients with pancreatic cancer. Studies also are being conducted to explore the effectiveness of monoclonal antibodies for inoperable pancreatic cancer.

How is endocrine or islet cell cancer of the pancreas staged?
Islet cell cancers of the pancreas are not staged in the same manner as other cancers. Rather they are divided into three groups: those occurring in one

TREATMENT FOR PANCREATIC CANCER (EXOCRINE)

STAGE	TREATMENT
Stage I	Surgery to remove head of pancreas, part of small intestine and some of surrounding tissue (Whipple procedure) **or** Total pancreatectomy **or** Surgery to remove tail of pancreas (distal pancreatectomy) if in tail of pancreas **or** Surgery followed by chemotherapy and radiation therapy **or** *Clinical trials*: Radiation after surgery combined chemotherapy given before or after radiation.
Stage II	Pancreatectomy with or without chemotherapy and radiation therapy **or** Radiation therapy with chemotherapy **or** Surgery or other treatments to reduce symptoms **or** *Clinical trials*: radiation therapy plus radiosensitizing drugs; radiation and chemotherapy before surgery; internal radiation, radiation during surgery; new types of radiation therapy; chemotherapy.
Stage III	Pancreatectomy with or without chemotherapy **or** Radiation with chemotherapy **or** Surgery or other treatment to reduce symptoms **or** External radiation and chemotherapy to reduce symptoms **or** *Clinical trials*: Surgery plus radiation plus radiosensitizing drugs; radiation during surgery with or without removal of cancer; radiation with chemotherapy after surgery; radiosensitizers; chemotherapy; implanted radiation.
Stage IV	Pancreatectomy with or without chemotherapy and radiation **or** Radiation with chemotherapy **or** Chemotherapy alone **or** Surgery or other treatment to reduce symptoms **or** Treatments for pain. *Clinical trials*: Postoperative radiation, radiation combined with chemotherapy, Chemotherapy; intraoperative radiation or radiation implants
Recurrent	Chemotherapy **or** Surgery to reduce symptoms **or** External radiation to reduce symptoms **or** Treatments for pain. *Clinical trials:* Chemotherapy; biological therapy.

TREATMENT FOR PANCREATIC CANCER
(ENDOCRINE OR ISLET CELL)

TYPE	TREATMENT
Gastrinoma	Surgery to remove cancer **or** Surgery to remove stomach (gastrectomy) **or** Surgery to cut nerve that stimulates pancreas **or** Chemotherapy **or** Hormone therapy **or** Hepatic arterial occlusion or embolization **or** *Clinical trials.*
Insulinoma	Surgery to remove cancer **or** Chemotherapy **or** Hormone therapy **or** Drugs to relieve symptoms **or** Hepatic arterial occlusion or embolization **or** *Clinical trials.*
Miscellaneous	Surgery to remove cancer **or** Chemotherapy **or** Hormone therapy **or** Hepatic arterial occlusion or embolization **or** *Clinical trials.*
Recurrent	Treatment depends on prior treatment and where it has reappeared.

site, those occurring in several sites, and those metastatic to regional lymph nodes or distant sites.

Are there different types of islet cell cancers of the pancreas?

There are three main types: gastrinoma, insulinoma, and miscellaneous. Gastrinoma makes large amounts of gastrin, a hormone that causes too much acid to be made in the stomach. Insulinoma makes too much insulin and allows the body to store sugar instead of using it for energy. Insulinomas are far more likely to be benign than malignant. They are slow-growing and can be cured by surgery. In the miscellaneous category are VIPoma, somatostatinoma, glucagonoma, and pancreatic polypeptide.

How is islet cell cancer treated?

Most often, islet cell cancer is treated with surgery. The doctor may take out the cancer and most or part of the pancreas. Sometimes, if there are ulcers, the stomach (gastrectomy) is taken out. Chemotherapy, hormone therapy, hepatic arterial occlusion, or embolization may be used.

What are the aftereffects when the pancreas is removed?
The recovery period is a long one. The side effects of treatment also may make it difficult for you to eat, to digest food, and to keep your blood sugar level. The doctor may need to give you medicine to replace the enzymes and hormones made by the pancreas. You will need to be followed closely by your health care team.

How often should checkups be scheduled following pancreatic cancer?
Since pancreatic cancer can recur within one to three years, the doctor will usually schedule frequent checkups—every three months for the first and second year, every six months for the third to fifth year and every year thereafter. Ultrasounds and CT scans will usually be done every six months for the first five years, then yearly. Any signs of bile or gastrointestinal obstruction should be reported immediately.

OTHER DIGESTIVE SYSTEM CANCERS

There is a group of other, less often seen cancers that invade other parts of the digestive system. These include cancers of the gallbladder, bile duct adrenal gland, and anus. All are uncommon, even rare, cancers and require the services of physicians who are experienced in treating them.

How is cancer of the gallbladder treated?
Surgery is usually done to remove the gallbladder if the cancer has not spread to surrounding tissues, or to relieve symptoms of cancer if it is blocking the ducts. The operation to remove the gallbladder is called a cholecystectomy. If needed, part of the liver around the gallbladder and nearby lymph nodes may also be taken out. If the cancer has spread and the bile ducts are blocked, an operation, called a biliary bypass, allows the doctor to do surgery to bypass the blocked ducts by cutting the gallbladder or bile duct and attaching it to the small intestine. If bile has built up in the area, the doctor may drain the bile through a tube to the outside of your body or may have the tube go around the blocked area and drain to the small intestine. External radiation, with or without surgery, may be used to kill the cancer cells and shrink the tumor. Chemotherapy is also used to relieve symptoms. The use of radiosensitizers is being studied.

How is bile duct cancer treated?
When bile duct cancer is only in the duct, which connects the gallbladder to the first part of the small intestine, the doctor will take out the whole bile

duct and construct a new duct. Lymph nodes will also be removed. If all of the cancer cannot be removed because it has spread, surgery will be done to bypass the blockage and radiation, either external or internal, may be given. Being studied are the use of radiation therapy with the addition of radiosensitizing drugs and chemotherapy or biological therapy.

What is cancer of the anus?

The anus is the opening at the end of the rectum through which body waste passes. Cancer of the anus, often a curable disease, is more likely to occur in the outer part of the anus in men and in the inner part of the rectum, the anal canal, in women. Cases of this cancer are uncommon but have been rising. Scientists believe that people with papilloma virus and male homosexuals have increased risk.

How is cancer of the anus treated?

There was a time when most of these cancers were treated with surgery that resulted in the removal of the anus and vulva in women and the anus and scrotum in men. The patient would need to dispose of waste through a colostomy bag. Today, many of these cancers can be treated with radiation, internal or external, with or without chemotherapy. The operation now most often used leaves the ring of muscle around the anus so that body wastes can be passed as before. Internal radiation therapy is used for some patients.

URINARY TRACT CANCERS

The bladder system, or urinary system, includes a number of organs—the bladder, urethra, ureters, and kidneys—and is responsible for eliminating waste products and maintaining stable chemical conditions in the body.

The Bladder

The bladder, which is a muscular, hollow organ in the lower abdomen, stores urine and increases in size as the urine accumulates. The urine enters the bladder from the kidneys through two tubes called ureters. Urine leaves the bladder through another tube, the urethra. In women, the urethra is a short tube that opens just forward of the vagina. In men, it is longer, passing through the prostate gland and then through the penis. The bladder is the seat of many disorders, including bladder stones, tumors, infections such as cystitis, as well as obstruction and paralysis.

What You Need to Know About Cancer of the Bladder

- Bladder cancer begins in the cells lining the bladder.
- They are named after the cells that become cancer: transitional (divided into papillary and nonpapillary), squamous, and adenocarcinoma.
- Surgery is one of the main treatments for cancer of the bladder.
- Chemotherapy, radiation therapy and biological therapy may also be used, before and after surgery.
- There are several different operations that might be done for this cancer.
- You need to understand the stage of your disease and exactly what surgery will be done so you will be prepared for the side effects.

Is blood in the urine always a sign of bladder cancer?
No. Bloody urine may be a first sign, but it can also be a sign of other urinary problems. However, any sign of blood in the urine, even if it happens only once, is a warning to see your doctor immediately. Bloody urine can also be a sign of conditions such as tumors, infections, or bladder stones. Other symptoms of bladder cancer include a change in bladder habits with an increase in the frequency of urination and, rarely, retention of urine, or incontinence.

What kind of doctor treats bladder cancer?
Urologists and medical oncologists are the specialists who treat bladder cancers.

What kind of testing is done to diagnose bladder cancer?
The doctor will do a complete physical examination. A bladder tumor can sometimes be felt during a rectal or vaginal exam. Urinary cytology, the examination of urine samples under the microscope, is often done using a saline solution that is inserted and collected through a catheter. Samples of suspicious tissue are obtained with a cystoscope. The doctor inserts the cystoscope through the urethra, visually observing the inside surface of the bladder, and, if needed, taking small samples of the tissue. Sometimes you will need anesthesia to have a cystoscopy. An intravenous pyelogram is usually done, in which an opaque dye visible on x-ray film is injected into a vein before x-rays are taken. The x-ray shows an outline of kidneys, ureters and bladder. Tumors larger than one centimeter (about one-half inch in diameter) can sometimes be seen. Other methods of scanning this area of the body such as CT scans and ultrasound are also used to help determine the extent of the cancer. Once bladder cancer is diagnosed, other tests may be performed such as chest x-rays, liver function tests, and radioactive liver and bone scans.

SYMPTOMS OF BLADDER CANCER

- Blood in the urine.
- Pain during urination.
- Need to urinate often or urgently.
- Lower back pain.

WHO IS MOST LIKELY TO GET BLADDER CANCER

- People between the ages of 50 and 80.
- Cigarette smokers are two to three times as likely as others to have bladder cancer. Pipe and cigar smokers are also more likely to have it.
- Caucasians have twice as much bladder cancer as Hispanics and African-Americans. Asians have the lowest rates.
- Men are two to three times as susceptible as women.
- Workers in rubber and leather industries, and printers, painters, chemical and metal workers, pesticide applicators, hairdressers, textile workers, machinists, and truck drivers.
- Those who eat a diet high in fried meats and fat.
- People who have been treated with cyclophosphamide, arsenic, or have had radiation therapy for cancer of the cervix.
- Family or personal history of bladder cancer.
- People who live in the northern states. (Incidence is 40 percent higher in the northern states than in southern states.)

What are the major types of bladder cancer?
More than 90 percent of bladder cancer is transitional cell, which is divided into papillary and nonpapillary cancer. A very small percentage are squamous cell carcinomas or adenocarcinomas.

What is papillary cancer of the bladder?
Papillary cancer is the most common type of bladder cancer, is usually not invasive and the most easily cured. It starts on the bladder wall but grows into the bladder cavity and remains attached to the bladder wall by a mushroom-like

TREATMENT CHOICES FOR BLADDER CANCER

STAGE	DESCRIPTION
Stage 0 or **0CIS** Found only on surface of the lining of bladder.	Transurethral resection (TUR) with fulguration **or** TUR with fulguration followed by intravesical biologic therapy or chemotherapy **or** Segmental cystectomony **or** Radical cystectomy. *Clinical trials*: Photodynamic therapy, biological therapy or chemoprevention.
Stage I Cancer is found deep in the inner lining of bladder, but not to muscle	Transurethral resection (TUR) with fulguration **or** TUR with fulguration followed by intravesical chemotherapy (injected into bladder) or intravesical biological therapy **or** Radium implants with or without external beam radiation therapy **or** Segmental cystectomy **or** Radical cystectomy. *Clinical trials*: Chemoprevention, intravesical therapy.
Stage II Cancer has spread to the muscle of bladder.	Transurethral resection with fulguration **or** Segmental cystectomy **or** Radical cystectomy with or without node dissection **or** External beam radiation alone **or** Internal radiation before or after external radiation. *Clinical trials*: Chemotherapy before or after cystectomy; chemotherapy plus radiation.
Stage III Cancer has spread throughout muscular wall to layer of tissue surrounding bladder. May have spread to prostate in men and uterus or vagina in women.	Radical cystectomy **or** External radiation with or without radiation implants **or** Segmental cystectomy **or** External radiation therapy plus chemotherapy. *Clinical trials*: Chemotherapy before or after cystectomy **or** Chemotherapy and external radiation.

TREATMENT CHOICES FOR BLADDER CANCER *(continued)*

STAGE	DESCRIPTION
Stage IV Extends to wall of abdomen or pelvis. May have spread to nearby lymph nodes and other parts of body.	Radical cystectomy **or** External radiation **or** Urinary diversion to reduce symptoms **or** Cystectomy to relieve symptoms **or** Chemotherapy. *Clinical trials:* Chemotherapy before or after cystectomy **or** Chemotherapy and radiation without operation.
Recurrent	Surgery, chemotherapy or radiation **or** *Clinical trials.*

stem. This type of tumor may be single or multiple, pea-sized, or large enough to occupy the entire bladder. The tumor cells, though they are cancerous, often appear to be almost normal.

What is non-papillary cancer of the bladder?
Non-papillary cancers are believed to develop from carcinoma *in situ*, a flat lesion that can progress and become invasive.

What is superficial bladder cancer?
Cancer that is only in the cells in the lining of the bladder, is called superficial bladder cancer. It is also called cancer *in situ*. After treatment, this cancer may come back as another superficial bladder cancer.

What is invasive bladder cancer?
Invasive bladder cancer is cancer that grows through the lining of the bladder and goes into the muscle wall.

How is bladder cancer treated?
Treatment depends on the stage of bladder cancer, the pathologic grade of the tumor, and the age and health of the patient. It may involve surgery, chemotherapy, immunotherapy, radiation therapy, or a combination of these.

Questions to Ask Your Doctor Before Bladder Surgery

In addition to those at the beginning of the chapter, consider the following:

- **What sort of operation are you planning?**
- **Will I be a candidate for continent urinary diversion?**
- **How often do you perform this kind of surgery?**
- **Will you use radiation prior to surgery?**
- **What kind of problems do people you've operated on have after this type of surgery?**
- **What other options are there for my stage of cancer?**
- **For men: Do you do nerve-sparing surgery so that I will still be able to have erections after surgery?**
- **For women: Are you planning to remove part of the vagina? What sort of operation will it be? How will this affect me sexually?**

What are the different types of treatments and operations used for bladder cancer?

A number of different methods are used depending on where the cancer is located and how far it is advanced. A transurethral resection (TUR), segmental cystectomy, cystectomy, radical cystectomy, and/or urinary diversion may be performed to remove the cancer.

Is laser therapy ever used?

Laser treatment is sometimes used for superficial tumors. Treatment of these small, superficial tumors of the bladder is usually performed on an outpatient basis, with the patient under local anesthesia. There is a possibility of side effects, including inflammation of the bladder mucosa.

What is photodynamic therapy?

Photodynamic therapy is a newer type of treatment being tried for early stages of bladder cancer. A special drug that makes cancer cells more sensitive to light is injected into the bladder, and a special light is used to eradicate tumors.

What is transurethral resection (TUR)?

This is the removal of a bladder growth with a cystoscope inserted into the bladder through the urethra. The doctor then uses electrical current to remove superficial bladder tumors and to destroy any cancer cells remaining in the bladder. This treatment is used only on small growths where only the superficial layer of the bladder has been affected. (This treatment is sometimes referred to as "fulguration," which means the destruction of living tissue with electrical current.) After this treatment, you will see the doctor regularly every three or four months, because in about one-quarter of all cases, tumors recur in the same vicinity.

What is a segmental resection or partial or segmental cystectomy?
This is an operation in which a section of the bladder is removed. A segmental resection is performed only if a tumor is localized in one area of the bladder and is in an area where there is an adequate margin of tissue that can be removed from around the tumor, or with a localized tumor where the area is difficult to reach and cannot adequately be removed with a TUR. Most often, since bladder cancer usually appears on various parts of the bladder at once, more extensive surgery may be necessary. After a segmental cystectomy, you should be able to urinate normally, although you may not be able to hold as much urine in your bladder as you did before and thus may need to urinate more often. These problems may lessen as you recover.

What is a radical cystectomy?
A radical cystectomy removes the bladder as well as the tissue around it. It is used for invasive bladder cancer or for superficial cancer that is in a large part of the bladder. For males, it means the removal of all of the bladder, the prostate, the seminal vesicles, the vas deferens, and pelvic lymph nodes. In women, the entire bladder, the uterus, the ovaries, fallopian tubes, and part of the vagina are usually removed. The rectum is most often left in place, though it is sometimes necessary, more frequently in men than in women, to remove the rectum if the tumor has grown into that area. Because it can be a complicated operation, it is important to seek out a doctor who is experienced in this type of surgery. Be sure to discuss and understand beforehand exactly how extensive the surgery will be, what other options you might have, and what all the consequences of the surgery are. At the start, when surgery is first being discussed, you may be anxious just to get the surgery over with, and you may not even focus on the sexual and other side effects because you feel your life is so threatened by the fact that you have cancer. Understanding the consequences of your surgery will help you to plan for your future. Frank discussion with your partner throughout the diagnosis, treatment and recovery process will help to make it possible for you both to learn to deal with the new changes in a pleasurable manner.

What are the sexual side effects of a radical cystectomy?
Since the surgery is very radical, there usually are sexual adjustments to be made. In women, the operation usually removes half of the vagina and the urethra. Usually the surgeon uses the remaining back wall of the vagina to rebuild the vaginal tube. When reconstructed, this means that the vagina is narrower

than normal. Another method used is the separation of the back wall of the vagina from the rectum behind it, creating a vaginal tube that may be normal in width but more shallow than normal. Men should ask their doctors if nerve-sparing surgery is possible. As explained in Chapter 14, Prostate Cancer and Other Male Cancers, the surgery may be done so that nerves surrounding the prostate can be spared so normal erection is still possible. However, men who wish to have children, need to consider sperm-banking before the operation. Both men and women should discuss the pros and cons of each type of surgery with their physician or other health professional. Talk to your healthcare team about what changes the operation will make in your particular case, since many new methods are being used for dealing with living without a bladder.

Can a person live without a bladder?

Many people live without a bladder. And there are new techniques being used to remove urine when the bladder has been eliminated. One method uses a part of the small intestine to make a new urine storage pouch inside the body (continent reservoir) that is connected to the remaining part of the urethra. Urine then passes out of the body through the urethra making it unnecessary to have an opening outside the body. When this solution is not possible, the surgeon may use part of the small intestine to make a tube through which urine can pass out of the body through an opening (stoma). This procedure is called a urostomy. Ask your doctor for a referral to a wound ostomy continence nurse before the operation so that you can be prepared for the changes that will occur. (See information on wound ostomy continence nurses under colon cancer in this chapter.)

What other side effects do women have?

If you have a radical cystectomy with your uterus and ovaries removed, you will have instant menopause and you will not be able to become pregnant.

Do bladder tumors tend to recur?

Bladder tumors have a tendency to recur either in the same location or in some other part of the bladder. Most of these growths are noninvasive. Most recurrences can be treated successfully if they are found in an early stage.

Does bladder cancer metastasize to other parts of the body?

Many bladder cancers are slow growing and do not spread to other parts of the body. Metastases, when they do occur, usually are found in the pelvic nodes and usually remain localized initially. Early detection and removal is the surest cure, since cancers which are not removed can spread to the lung, bones, and liver.

Where can I get information about living with bladder surgery?
There are over 500 United Ostomy Association chapters in the United States and Canada. They offer a tremendous amount of very specific information about urostomy surgery and dealing with life after a urostomy. There is an ostomy visitor service which provides preoperative and postoperative visits. Its Web site (www.uoa.org) gives ample information about specialty groups, chat rooms, publications, and support group chapters near you. Please be sure to contact the United Ostomy Association, Inc., 19772 MacArthur Boulevard, Suite 200, Irvine, CA 92612–2405; telephone 1–800–826–0826.

Is it usual for a patient to be depressed after this kind of operation?
It is not unusual to feel depressed. It is important for everyone to understand that this is a temporary but normal feeling. An inability to cope with the new way the body functions may make you feel that you'll never be able to cope with anything again. The depression usually subsides once you learn the new patterns of life. Again, we cannot stress strongly enough the wisdom of contacting the United Ostomy Association. Their material is very specific covering care of the stoma, helpful ideas and practical tips, complications, types of appliances, social and sexual questions, as well as coping with skin problems, odor, and injury.

What other kinds of treatments are used besides surgery?
Chemotherapy, either intravesical (putting the drugs directly into the bladder through a tube in the urethra) or intravenous, may be prescribed to try to improve results or to preserve the bladder. Chemotherapy may be given alone, combined with surgery, radiation or both. Internal or external radiation, biological therapy and photodynamic therapy are all used depending upon the stage of your cancer, your age, and your overall condition. Chemoprevention—using drugs or vitamins to delay recurrence—is being studied. There are a number of treatment options for each stage of bladder cancer. You would be wise to study them and discuss the pros and cons of each with a well-qualified doctor.

What is intravesical biological therapy?
Doctors are using BCG (Bacillus Calmette-Guerin) to stimulate the immune system to kill cancer cells in the bladder. It is used after TUR for superficial bladder cancer. The doctor puts the BCG into the bladder by catheter where it is held by the patient for two hours. You may need to urinate often and may have some pain when urinating after this treatment. Also you may see blood in your urine, feel nauseated, or have chills and a fever.

How often should I see my doctor after treatment for bladder cancer?

It is important to see your doctor regularly—every three months for the first year, every six months for the second year and every year thereafter. If your bladder was not removed, the doctor will do a cystoscopy to look for superficial tumors that can be taken out. Your urine will be tested and you may have blood tests and x-rays.

KIDNEY CANCER

Kidneys come in pairs—one on each side of the back portion of the abdomen. They are located on each side of your body, toward the back, just above the waist on either side of the spine. An adrenal gland is located on the top of each kidney. The kidney is encased in a membrane called a capsule. Inside each kidney are tiny tubules that filter and clean the blood, take out waste products and make urine. The kidneys are best known for producing urine, filtering waste products from the blood, and returning to the circulating blood those substances that are necessary for normal chemical balance. They also make an important hormone that helps regulate the formation of new red cells in the bone marrow. Overall, the role of the kidney is to monitor the body's internal environment—keeping fluids and chemicals in balance. The central part of each kidney is hollow and receives the body fluids. The urine leaves the kidney and passes down the ureter—a long tube—that connects with the bladder.

What You Need to Know about Kidney Cancer

- Not all tumors that are found in the kidney are cancer.
- Kidney cancer is difficult to diagnose.
- The most common kind of kidney cancer in adults is renal cell cancer.
- Renal cell cancer can often be cured if found only in the kidney.
- Transitional cell cancer, which affects the renal pelvis is a less common form of kidney cancer. It is similar to cancer that occurs in the bladder and is often treated like bladder cancer.
- In children, the most common kind of kidney cancer is called Wilm's tumor. Its treatment is different from adult kidney cancer (see Chapter 24, When a Child Has Cancer).
- Kidney cancer is usually treated by surgery. Treatment may also include biological therapy, radiation, hormones or chemotherapy.
- There is research underway that suggests that some kidney cancers may be genetic.

WHO IS MOST LIKELY TO GET CANCER OF THE KIDNEY?

- Smokers.
- People who are overweight.
- Coke oven workers. People who work with asbestos.
- Women treated with radiation for disorders of the uterus.
- Long-term dialysis users.
- People with von Hippel-Lindau disease.

What kind of doctor should be used for kidney cancer?

It is important to choose a board-certified urologic surgeon to treat kidney cancer and a hospital or medical center that is experienced in dealing with kidney cancer.

What tests are done to diagnose kidney cancer?

The doctor will order a blood test, a urine test, and a variety of imaging tests to look at the kidney and other nearby organs, such as intravenous pyelogram (IVP), CT scan and ultrasound imaging. Additional tests may include a selective renal arteriography or inferior venacavagram. Kidney cancer is difficult to diagnose and requires careful and thorough testing and because of this has been labeled the "internist's tumor."

Will I need a biopsy?

If the test results show that you may have kidney cancer, you will need to have a biopsy. That is the only sure way to diagnose cancer. A thin needle will be put into the tumor and a piece of tissue will be taken out. It will then be checked by a pathologist for cancer cells. Before you have a biopsy, be sure that you understand how and where it will be done, whether you will be awake, whether you'll be able to drive yourself home and how soon you will get the results.

Do abnormal liver function tests before an operation mean the cancer has spread to the liver?

Abnormal liver function tests before surgery may be due to a paraneoplastic syndrome that is reversible with the removal of the tumor.

Are all kidney tumors cancerous?

No. Many are benign. The benign growths often are filled with fluid and can be classified as cysts. They vary in size. However, whether the tumor is cancer cannot always be determined without surgery.

SYMPTOMS OF KIDNEY CANCER

- Blood in the urine.
- A feeling of a lump or mass in the kidney region.
- Weight loss.
- Fatigue.
- Recurrent fevers.
- A pain in the side that does not go away.
- Anemia.
- A general feeling of poor health.

There are usually no symptoms of early kidney cancer.

What are the different types of kidney cancers?
There are several kinds of kidney tumors. Over eight out of ten are renal adenocarcinomas or renal cell cancers. These tumors start in the lining of the tubules of the kidney. The remaining 20 percent of kidney cancers begin in cells in other parts of the kidney. Transitional cell cancers, oncocytomas, papillary adenocarcinomas, fibrosarcomas or other sarcomas, and Wilms' tumors are other, rarer kinds of kidney cancers. For more information on Wilms' tumor, which is a childhood kidney tumor, please see Chapter 24, When a Child Has Cancer.

What is the von Hippel-Lindau disease gene?
The discovery of the von Hippel-Lindau disease gene has been a major step in the understanding of kidney cancer. When this gene is defective, it can cause not only von Hippel-Lindau disease but also tumors in other parts of the body including clear cell renal carcinoma, the most common form of kidney cancer. Von Hippel-Lindau disease is an inherited disorder.

Questions to Ask Your Doctor Before You Have Treatment for Kidney Cancer

- **What kind of kidney cancer do I have?**
- **What is its stage?**
- **What kinds of treatments are available to me? How are they done?**
- **What are the side effects of the different treatments?**
- **Where will I have the treatments? How long will they last?**
- **Will I need to be in the hospital? If I have pain, how will that be treated?**

TESTS THAT MAY BE USED TO DIAGNOSE CANCER OF THE KIDNEY

- Complete history and physical exam
- Blood and urine tests
- IVP (intravenous pylogram)
- Arteriogram
- CT scan
- MRI
- Ultrasound

- **Will my insurance cover the treatments?**
- **Is there a clinical trial for my type and stage of cancer?**

Do kidney cancers ever disappear spontaneously?
Kidney cancer is one of the few tumors in which the unexplained disappearance of tumors is well documented. This occurs very rarely and tumors sometimes reappear.

What is a nephrectomy?
A nephrectomy is the removal of the kidney. Thousands of such operations are performed each year for cancer as well as for other reasons. A simple nephrectomy means that only the kidney is removed, leaving the surrounding area intact. There are few complications unless the tumor has spread beyond the kidney. In most cases a radical nephrectomy removes the kidney, the adrenal gland above the kidney, the surrounding fatty tissue, and the lymph nodes adjacent to the kidney. A partial nephrectomy means that only the part of the kidney around the cancer is removed. This type of operation is usually performed when the other kidney has poor function or has previously been removed.

Can one live normally if a kidney is removed?
Fortunately, people can live perfectly normal lives with only one good kidney.

What is arterial embolization?
This is a procedure that is designed to block the flow of blood to the tumor in the kidney. The doctor injects small pieces of a special gelatin sponge or alcohol into the artery that provides the blood supply to the tumor. This method

TREATMENT CHOICES FOR RENAL CELL CANCER

STAGE	DESCRIPTION
Stage I Cancer is found only in the kidney.	Radical nephrectomy **or** Simple nephrectomy **or** Partial nephrectomy **or** If surgery is inadvisable: external radiation **or** Arterial embolization **or** *Clinical trials.*
Stage II Cancer has spread to fat around kidney but not beyond capsule that contains kidney.	Radical nephrectomy **or** External radiation before or after operation **or** Partial nephrectomy **or** *Clinical Trials* **or** If surgery is inadvisable: external radiation or arterial embolization.
Stage III Cancer has spread to renal vein or to inferior vena cava (vein that carries blood from lower part of body to heart) or to lymph nodes around kidney.	Radical nephrectomy with possible removal of lymph nodes and/or renal vein or vena cava **or** Arterial embolization followed by radical nephrectomy **or** External radiation to relieve symptoms **or** Simple or radical nephrectomy to relieve symptoms **or** Pre- or post-operative external radiation and radical nephrectomy. *Clinical trials*: adjuvant alpha interferon.
Stage IV Cancer has spread to nearby organs such as bowel or pancreas or to distant parts such as lungs, bone or skin.	Interleukin-2 **or** Alpha interferon **or** External radiation to relieve symptoms **or** Simple nephrectomy to relieve symptoms **or** If spread to area around kidney: radical nephrectomy **or** If spread further: nephrectomy plus limited surgery where it has spread **or** *Clinical trials*: Chemotherapy and biological therapy.
Recurrent Either in original area or other parts of body.	Interleukin-2 **or** Alpha interferon **or** Radiation therapy to relieve symptoms **or** Vinblastine **or** *Clinical trials*: Chemotherapy and biological therapy.

usually is used only in patients who cannot have surgery or to relieve symptoms. Sometimes it is used before the operation to make the surgery easier.

Is it important for me to donate blood before my operation?
Check with your doctor. If you are going to have a blood transfusion during the operation, your surgeon may want three or four units of blood on hand. Because you may not be able to delay the operation, and there may not be time for you to donate your own blood (the process takes several weeks), you may want to ask family members or friends to donate blood on your behalf. You should discuss this with your doctor.

Will I have side effects from my operation?
If your kidney is removed, your other kidney will be taking over for both organs. You will need to be checked on how much liquid you take in and put out. You may need intravenous feedings. You may find it difficult to breathe and may need to do special breathing exercises. You will probably be tired and weak. If you have arterial embolization you might have fever, nausea, pain or vomiting, and need to have intravenous fluids.

Are any other treatments used for cancer of the kidney?
Biological therapy, chemotherapy, hormone therapy and radiation therapy sometimes are used, most of which are part of clinical trials. These treatments may also be used to relieve pain.

What is transitional cell cancer of the renal pelvis and ureter?
This cancer of the kidney affects the tissues (transitional cells) that collect urine (renal pelvis) and in the tube that connects the kidney to the bladder (ureter). It is staged and treated differently from renal cell cancer of the kidney.

What is a uretoroscopy?
This is a narrow lighted tube, a ureteroscope, that the doctor can put in through your bladder to look inside the ureter and the renal pelvis. With the ureteroscope, the doctor can take out a small piece of tissue for testing. The doctor may also ask you to have a CT scan or an MRI.

How is transitional cell cancer of the renal pelvis and ureter treated?
If you have cancer that has not spread outside the kidney or ureter, you will probably have surgery. You might have a nephroureterectomy where the kidney, ureter, and top part of the bladder are taken out. If only part of your ureter or kidney is taken out, it is known as a segmental resection. Sometimes if the cancer is on the surface of the renal pelvis or ureter the doctor will use electrosurgery, which burns away the tumor and the area around it with electric

TREATMENT CHOICES FOR TRANSITIONAL CELL CANCER OF THE RENAL PELVIS AND URETER

STAGE	DESCRIPTION
Localized Cancer has not spread outside the kidney or ureter.	Surgery to take out the kidney, ureter and top of bladder (nephroureterectomy) **or** Surgery to take out part of ureter or kidney (segmental resection) **or** *Clinical trials*: electrosurgery or laser therapy **or** intrapelvic or intraureteral chemotherapy or biological therapy.
Regional Cancer has spread to tissues around kidney or to lymph nodes in pelvis.	*Clinical trials*: of radiation therapy **or** chemotherapy.
Metastatic Cancer has spread to other parts of body.	Chemotherapy **or** *Clinical trials*
Recurrent Cancer has come back after it has been treated.	*Clinical trials*: combination chemotherapy **or** Other clinical trial

current and then removes it. Laser therapy might be used with a narrow beam of light removing the cancer cells.

Will chemotherapy, biological therapy, or radiation therapy be used?
Sometimes these are used, depending on the stage of the disease. Chemotherapy may be injected directly into the ureter (intraureteral) or pelvis (intrapelvic).

Is there an organization that acts specifically on behalf of kidney cancer patients?
The National Kidney Cancer Association provides information to patients and physicians, sponsors research on kidney cancer, and acts as an advocate on behalf of patients. It also will give you referrals to doctors who are doing advanced work in the treatment of kidney cancer. You can receive information by calling

or writing them: National Kidney Cancer Association, 320 North Michigan Avenue, Suite 2100, Chicago, IL, 60601; telephone 1–800–850–9132. You can also get information on kidney cancer from the Cancer Information Service and from the American Cancer Society. See Chapter 28, Where to Get Help.

How long will it take before I can return to work?
It depends on what kind of treatment you have had. If you have had an operation, many patients return to work about three weeks after surgery. It is wise to "baby" yourself a bit. It usually takes about three full months for your muscles to heal completely. After about two months, you should be ready to build up your level of exercise to help restore your muscle tone.

What kind of continuing checkup schedule should I follow?
After diagnosis and a nephrectomy, you should receive regular medical followup and supervision. The doctor will usually schedule you for checkups every three months for the first year; every four months for the second to fifth year, and yearly thereafter. Recurrences have been found most often within the first three years after surgery at the original site or in the lung, bone, liver and sometimes in the brain. Usually, when discovered early before further spread, surgery will be done to remove the new cancer. If you experience problems with weight loss, loss of appetite, weakness, headache, changes in your mental status, fevers or high temperatures, abdominal pain or skeletal pain, cough, shortness of breath, enlarged lymph glands or blood in your urine, you should be sure to let your doctor know. The symptoms may not have anything to do with your past history, but it is wise to have them checked out immediately for your own peace of mind.

ADRENAL GLAND CANCER

Does cancer occur in the adrenal glands?
A rare cancer sometimes occurs on the outer layer of the adrenal glands, which are located above the kidneys. Known as adrenocortical cancer, and sometimes diagnosed through hormone testing, a cancer on this gland may result in hormonal changes such as feminizing changes in men and masculinizing changes in women. Cushing's syndrome, which is usually observed in a rapidly developing fattening of the face and neck, may be caused by either a benign or malignant tumor in the adrenal gland.

How is cancer of the adrenal cortex treated?
You might have an adrenalectomy that will take out the adrenal gland, tissue around it and lymph nodes. Radiation and chemotherapy may also be used.

Web Pages to Check Out

www.cancer.gov: For general up-to-date information, and for clinical trials.
www.cancer.org: For general up-to-date information and community resources.
www.cancer.gov: The genetics of colorectal cancer.
www.uoa.org: United Ostomy Association.
www.kidneycancerassociation.org: Kidney Cancer Association.

Also see Chapter 2, Searching for Answers on the Web, for more information.

Seventeen

SKIN CANCER

Most skin cancers are very visible so they are easier to identify early than many other kinds of cancer. Many people have a number of small, colored spots on their bodies—moles, freckles, birthmarks, or liver spots. Some are present at birth. Others develop at different times throughout life. Almost all of these spots are normal and remain that way. But when there are changes in existing moles and other skin spots or when new spots appear, it is time to take action.

CANCER OF THE skin is the most common kind of cancer—and, because it is easy to see, it can be diagnosed and treated at an early stage. Over a million cases of skin cancers are reported annually. Most of these are categorized as basal cell or squamous cell cancers or nonmelanoma cancers. However, about 54,000 of the skin cancers are cutaneous melanomas—serious skin cancers that arise in moles or in the tanning cells of the skin and which, in later stages, can spread or metastasize to other parts of the body.

What You Should Know About Skin Cancer

- Skin cancer has a better prognosis than most other types of cancer. It is curable in over 95 percent of cases.

- There are three major types of skin cancer. The two most common types, basal cell and squamous cell rarely spread. Melanoma, the third type, is a serious condition. It has a greater tendency to metastasize to other parts of the body.

- One in five Americans will develop a skin cancer during their lifetimes. 97 percent of these cancers are nonmelanoma cancers.

- All skin cancers do not look the same. Some are small, smooth, shiny, pale, or waxy lumps. Others are rough, red or brown scaly patches. Still others look like flat or raised moles.

- Most true moles tend to be symmetrical. Suspicious moles usually are uneven—with one half not matching the other.

- Most true moles have a clear-cut border. Suspicious moles have a notched, scalloped, or indistinct border.

- True moles may be dark or light—but they are usually uniform in color. Suspicious moles have uneven or variegated color. Shades of black, brown and tan, white, gray, red or blue may be seen.

- Most moles are smaller than the size of a pencil eraser. Suspicious moles tend to be larger and may change in size.

- If caught early and surgically removed, melanoma has a cure rate of more than 96 percent.

- Even if caught later, when the melanoma is invading nearby tissue, the cure rate is nearly 90 percent.

- The cure rate for skin cancer could be 100 percent if all skin cancers were brought to a doctor's attention before they spread.

- Melanoma can occur on any skin surface.

- Melanoma occurs most commonly on the lower extremities in women and on the trunk in men.

- Melanoma is rare in black people and others with dark skin. When it does develop in dark-skinned people, it tends to occur under the fingernails or toenails or on the palms or soles.

- Any sore, blister, patch, pimple, mole or other skin blemish that does not heal within two or three weeks should be examined by a doctor.

Questions to Ask Your Doctor

- **What kind of skin cancer do I have?**
- **What kind of treatment will you prescribe for me?**
- **What are the pros and cons of this treatment?**
- **What other alternatives are there to this treatment?**

SKIN CANCER RISK FACTORS

Ultraviolet radiation	Exposure to ultraviolet radiation from the sun and other sources.
Skin color	People with light skin and blue eyes who sunburn easily are more susceptible than those with naturally dark skin.
Sun exposure	People who were severely sunburned as children. People who have intense sun exposure once in a while as opposed to outdoor workers who are constantly exposed.
Occupational	Exposure to coal tar, pitch, creosote, arsenic compounds or radium.
Moles	A very large number of very large moles present from birth.
Genetics	For melanoma: Two or more first-degree relatives—parents, children, brothers, or sisters—who have had melanoma.

- **What are the chances that this treatment will be successful?**
- **Will I have a scar? How large will it be?**
- **Will I need a skin graft or plastic surgery?**
- **Who will do it?**
- **Will I need any other treatments after surgery? How often will I need to return for checkups?**

How do skin cancers grow?

Skin cell growth begins deep below the surface of the skin, in the epidermis, where basal cells divide to produce new cells. New cells push mature cells upward to the skin's surface, where they die and flake off. In this way, the skin constantly repairs itself, as new cells grow and multiply in a controlled, orderly manner to replace dying cells. The outermost layer of the skin is made up mostly of flat, scalelike cells called squamous cells. The deepest part of the epidermis also contains melanocytes, the cells that produce the pigment called melanin. Sometimes any of these cells may begin to grow in an uncontrolled manner, leading to an overgrowth of tissue, or a tumor. The tumors may be either benign or malignant.

What are the different kinds of skin cancer?

There are a number of different kinds of skin cancers that behave in different ways. The most common type is basal cell cancer. Squamous cell cancers are the next most common. These two types of skin cancer are referred to as nonmelanoma skin cancers and account for 97 percent of all skin cancers. Melanoma (sometimes called cutaneous melanoma or malignant melanoma) is not as common as basal cell and squamous cell cancers, but it is much more serious.

What is hyperkeratosis?
This is a precancerous condition that appears as a scaly patch or small scab of skin in a sharply limited, usually small area. Hyperkeratoses are usually caused by exposure to direct strong sunlight and hot drying wind. They are nearly always found on the face, neck, and hands.

What is keratoacanthoma?
This is an unusual skin lesion that appears in a sun-exposed area and may grow rapidly to substantial size over a short period of time. It is usually a smooth, red nodule, sometimes with a central umbilical spot, which is often difficult to distinguish from other skin cancers. Keratoacanthomas do not metastasize, but careful diagnosis is important because they are similar in appearance to squamous cell carcinoma, which, in some cases, can metastasize. A biopsy is needed to determine the cell type.

What is sweat-gland cancer?
This is a very rare kind of cancer that may metastasize to the lymph nodes or to distant sites. It can originate from any gland but usually occurs near the anus, eyelids, ears, armpits, and scrotum.

What is xeroderma?
Xeroderma is an inherited condition. It is thought to be a precancerous disease. The skin is irregularly pigmented and scaly and later becomes thin, ulcerated, and scarred. It is strongly sensitized to sunlight, and cancer occurs on the areas that have been exposed to it, even briefly.

What is a limpoma?
A limpoma is a soft, fatty, noncancerous tumor that lies directly beneath the skin. It can be as small as a pea or as large as a grapefruit. Limpomas feel soft and move freely under the skin. If they are in a visible spot, or if they show signs of growth, they should be removed.

Do warts ever become cancerous?
Warts do not turn into cancer.

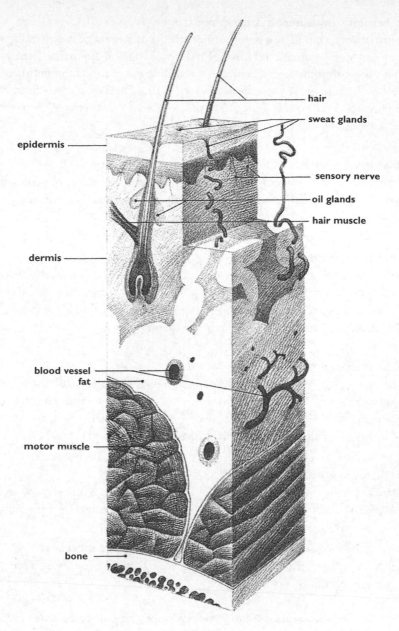

hair

sweat glands

epidermis

sensory nerve

oil glands

hair muscle

dermis

blood vessel
fat

motor muscle

bone

Cross-section of skin (enlarged)

Do hemangiomas become cancerous?

Hemangiomas, blood vessel tumors of the skin, are usually not malignant. They may appear at any time from birth to old age on any part of the body. They range from the size of a pinhead to the size of a nickel. Sometimes they bleed if they are in area that becomes irritated, such as on a man's face. Most are harmless and do not grow. Doctors usually do not remove them unless they are unsightly.

What is a ganglion?

A ganglion is a thin-walled cyst, which appears in the tendons or joints, filled with a colorless, jellylike substance and is not cancerous. Ganglions are usually seen on the inside wrists of children and young adults.

What is a sebaceous cyst?

Sebaceous cysts, also known as wens, occur when sebaceous glands become clogged and develop into cysts. These rarely turn into cancer. When they increase in size over a period of weeks or months, they should be checked by a dermatologist who will usually remove them.

What is a fibroma?

Skin fibromas very rarely become cancerous. They are small, hard lumps about the size of a cherry pit. They are not usually removed. Another type, pediculated fibromas, little tags that dangle on stalks from the skin, are common on necks and armpits and are fully treated by electrocutery.

Do tattoos cause skin cancer?

Tattoos usually do not cause cancer. However, if there is any sign of itching or bubbling around the edges, the tattoo should be checked by a physician.

What other skin conditions are there that are not cancerous?

There are a number of other skin conditions that may look suspicious, but are usually harmless. These include:

- **Seborrheic keratoses:** raised, warty-looking, appear to be stuck onto the skin's surface, easy to scrape off with a fingernail.
- **Skin tags or papillomas:** little outpatchings of skin.
- **Syringomas:** benign tumors caused by an enlarged sweat gland; different from a rare kind of sweat gland cancer that is known to metastasize.
- **Histiocytomas:** solitary, well-rounded firm nodules.

- **Senile lentigo:** also known as liver spots.
- **Sebaceous hyperplasia:** shiny, yellow, waxy-oily tumors.

How can I tell whether or not a growth is cancerous?

You cannot. You should bring any skin change to the attention of your doctor. Only a trained physician can determine the nature of an abnormal skin
growth—whether it is benign, precancerous, or malignant. If you have any
questions or doubts, seek out the opinion of a qualified dermatologist who
has had experience dealing with skin cancers. Some plastic surgeons, general
surgeons, oncologists, internists, and family doctors also have a special interest and training in dealing with skin cancers.

NONMELANOMA SKIN CANCERS

What is basal cell cancer?

Basal cell cancer is the most common and the least lethal form of skin cancer.
It accounts for 90 percent of all skin cancers in the southern states and 47 percent in the northern states. It usually occurs on areas of the skin that have been
in the sun—the face, head, neck, arms, hands, and back. Often it will appear as
a small, raised bump that has a smooth, pearly appearance. Another type looks
like a scar, and it is firm to the touch. Basal cell cancer is very slow growing, may
spread to the tissue around the cancer, but seldom spreads to other parts of the
body. If not treated properly, however, it can invade and destroy nearby bone
and cartilage. Following treatment for basal cell cancer, you should have a clinical
examination every six months for five years. It has been found that 36 percent of
those with basal cell cancers will develop a second basal cell cancer within five
years. Thereafter, yearly examinations should be done.

What is squamous cell cancer?

Squamous cell skin cancer is the second most common type of skin cancer,
after basal cell cancer. It rarely spreads, but it does so more often than basal
cell cancer. Most of the epidermis is composed of squamous cells, which are
flat. Squamous cell cancers are faster growing than basal cell. Overall, only
about two percent of squamous cell cancers spread to other parts of the
body. However, about 20 percent of squamous cell cancers that develop on
the lips or in burn scars or x-ray scars are known to metastasize. Squamous
cell cancer is two to three times more common in men than in women. Studies indicate that the risk of developing this type of skin cancer is related to
the cumulative amount of sun exposure and the degree of skin pigmentation.
Since squamous cell cancers can metastasize, if you have squamous cell cancer,

you should be reexamined every three months for the first several years and then followed indefinitely at six month intervals.

What are precancers?

Precancers are abnormal skin conditions that tend to become cancerous at a later date. The most common are senile or actinic keratosis, actinic cheilitis, and hyperkeratosis. Actinic cheilitis is a related condition that usually appears on the lower lips. These are skin conditions that appear as rough, red or brown, scaly patches. These often develop in older persons whose skin has been exposed for many years to the sun's ultraviolet rays, although some types occur on unexposed parts of the body, such as the chest, back, or arms. These different types of keratosis are not considered to be cancer, but can change into basal cell or squamous cell skin cancer. Since keratoses can become malignant, these precancerous conditions should be checked regularly. Premalignant conditions may be treated with topical agents, cryosurgery, electrosurgery, dermabrasion, shave excision, or carbon dioxide laser.

What is leukoplakia?

Leukoplakia is a condition resembling keratosis, which occurs as a white thickening on the lip, tongue, or mouth. It frequently occurs in heavy pipe smokers and tobacco chewers.

What is Bowen's disease?

Bowen's disease is a rare form of squamous cell skin cancer, sometimes referred to as precancerous dermatitis. It often occurs in several primary sites. The growth is reddish-pink and raised, with scaling. It usually occurs on the unexposed areas of the skin. Sometimes it is associated with internal malignancies.

What type of doctor should I see if I have suspicious skin spots?

Although your family doctor usually will check your skin during regular physical exams, especially if you ask that it be done, it is wise to see a dermatologist if you have suspicious skin spots. If you have malignant melanoma, it is important that you are taken care of by a team who specialize in melanoma treatment. If you need reconstructive work done as a result of skin cancer, a plastic surgeon, dermatologist, otolaryngologist, or maxillofacial surgeon would be the doctor of choice.

Can a doctor tell the difference between the different kinds of skin cancers by looking at them?

A skilled dermatologist or a doctor experienced in detecting skin cancer can usually tell the difference by looking at the spot in question. However,

TREATMENT CHOICES FOR NONMELANOMA CANCER

TYPE	TREATMENT
Basal Cell	Mohs micrographic surgery, simple excision with margin evaluation, electrodessication and curettage, cryosurgery, radiation therapy, carbon dioxide laser, topical fluorouracil (5–FU), systemic retinoids, alfa interferon chemotherapy, photodynamic therapy.
Squamous Cell	Mohs micrographic surgery, simple excision, electrodesiccation and curettage, cryosurgery, radiation therapy, topical 5–FU, carbon dioxide laser, alpha interferon, chemotherapy.
Actinic keratosis	Topical agents, cryosurgery, electrodesiccation and curettage, dermabrasion (removing top layer of skin with special machine) shave excision (shaving the very top layer of skin) or carbon dioxide laser.

dermatologists say that what sometimes looks like a benign growth can prove to be cancerous when biopsied. The only way to really know is to have the biopsy.

What kind of treatment is used in treating skin cancers?
There are a number of ways to treat skin cancer. The most common one is surgery. Others include cryosurgery, radiation therapy, electrodesiccation and curettage, carbon dioxide laser, and topical fluorouracil.

What is Mohs surgery?
Mohs micrographic surgery, is a surgical technique for skin tumor removal. Local anesthesia is first used to numb the tumor site. Thin slices of skin at the tumor site are removed and each slice is examined under the microscope. If evidence of tumor cells is found at the edges of the sample, the doctor will remove and examine another skin sample. These steps are repeated until no tumor is detected under the microscope. Depending on the extent of the tumor, this process may be repeated several times. The actual surgery involved in each sampling takes about 20 minutes, but the process may take more than an hour per sample. When preparing to have Mohs surgery, you will probably be advised to set aside a day for the necessary number of procedures. The advantage of Mohs surgery is that only the tissue that has been invaded by the tumor is removed, preserving healthy skin and allowing for the best possible cosmetic effect. Small or superficial wounds may be left to heal

by themselves. Larger wounds may need to be stitched closed. Even larger wounds may require a flap or a graft from elsewhere on your body to repair the surgical procedure. Mohs surgery has a high cure rate because the tumor is seen microscopically and can be completely removed.

When is surgery used for nonmelanoma skin cancers?

Surgery is used to remove many nonmelanoma skin cancers. Usually, surgery is performed under local anesthesia and the cancer is taken out completely at the time of biopsy with no further therapy required. In some cases, cancers are larger than they appear on the skin's surface and more tissue must be removed than might seem necessary. Many surgeons use margins of 3 to 5 millimeters for small, well-defined tumors and margins of at least 1 centimeter for large or more aggressive types of tumors.

When is cryosurgery used for skin cancers?

Cryosurgery, which uses extreme cold to freeze off the lesions, is sometimes considered for actinic keratoses, small basal cell, and squamous cell tumors. Liquid nitrogen is applied with a special spray device or a cotton-tipped applicator. The treatments can be done without anesthesia and can be performed efficiently during a routine office visit. There may be some swelling of the area following treatment and it may take about four weeks before the area treated with cryosurgery heals. Cryosurgery can result in permanent pigment loss—the area may appear pink or white when healed. Cryosurgery should not be used for sclerosing basal cell cancers or for tumors of the scalp, nose, lip, eyelid margins or lower legs, cancers fixed to the underlying bone or cartilage, at the margins of the fingers, the elbow, or for cancers previously treated with surgery.

Is electrosurgery used for skin cancer?

This method, which the doctors call electrodessication and curettage, dehydrates the tumor with high frequency electrical current and removes the tumor. You will usually have an anesthetic injected to numb the area and the cancer is scooped out with a sharp instrument with a spoon-shaped end called a curette. It is the most common method of removing basal cell cancers. In treating squamous cell tumors, the doctors use this method for very small cancers. Though it is a quick method for destroying the cancer, this method is not totally satisfactory since the adequacy of treatment cannot be assessed immediately because the doctor cannot visually detect the depth of micrscopic tumor invasion. Usually it is necessary to repeat the procedure two to three times, or more, if the tumor is large. Since distortion can occur on healing with electrosurgery, it is not recommended for use around the eyes and mouth. The treatment may leave a white scar.

Is simple surgery with biopsy examination of the margins of the skin cancer a safe method?

This is a traditional surgical treatment sometimes used for basal cell and squamous cell cancers. However, this method allows only a small fraction of the total tumor margin to be examined pathologically, and studies show that recurrence is more likely with this method.

When is radiation therapy used for skin cancers?

Radiation therapy is sometimes used to treat skin cancer that occurs in areas such as eyelids, nose or ears, which are hard to treat with surgery. Radiation may also be used for people who cannot tolerate surgery. It is sometimes used for cancers that have grown deep into tissue, are too large to be removed completely by other means, or have recurred. Several treatments may be needed. Changes in skin color and texture may occur and may become more noticeable many years after treatment.

Is topical fluorouracil (5–FU) used in skin cancer treatment?

This simple treatment, in which 5–FU cream or solution is applied for four to six weeks, is effectively used for actinic keratoses. Superficial basal cell carcinomas and squamous cell cancers *in situ* are also sometimes treated with topical 5–FU as well. However, careful and prolonged follow-up is essential, since deeply imbedded portions of the cancer may escape treatment and result in future recurrences. Swelling is common especially the first week after treatment is begun, often becoming marked and progressing to oozing, crusting, or ulceration. Itching and burning often occur, and healing usually takes three to six weeks once treatment is stopped. You usually do not have a scar as a result of this treatment.

Is carbon dioxide laser used to treat skin cancers?

Carbon dioxide laser is sometimes used for superficial types of basal cell cancers, as well as for selected squamous cell *in situ* cancers, especially if bleeding is present. The laser light beam, which produces a powerful, narrow beam of light at one wavelength, can be used to vaporize the abnormal growth. It is sometimes used in conjunction with curettage.

Will the doctor use chemotherapy?

If squamous cell or Merkel cell cancers have spread to other organs, chemotherapy may be given, either alone or with radiation.

Is alpha interferon used in treating skin cancers?

Studies are being done to determine if this treatment is appropriate for basal cell cancers.

Is photodynamic therapy being used?
Photodynamic therapy with photosensitizers is sometimes effectively used for treating superficial epithelial skin tumors.

Is Accutane being tested as a cancer preventer?
Accutane (isotretinoin), a derivative of Vitamin A is being tested for mild, nonmelanoma forms of skin cancer—from basal cell nevus syndrome (an inherited type of basal cell cancer) to multiple keratoacanthoma (a squamous cell type). Moderate doses of Accutane appear to normalize cells, making abnormal cells behave like normal cells. It is important that any use of this drug be undertaken under the direction of a physician since there are serious side effects that must be fully understood.

MELANOMA

What is melanoma?
Melanoma (referred to medically as cutaneous melanoma or malignant melanoma) is the most serious type of skin cancer. It occurs most frequently in white women and men over the age of 40 who have light complexions, red or blond hair, lots of moles on their bodies, and skin that freckles and burns easily. Women most often get melanoma on the arms and legs. In men, it is most often seen on the trunk, head, or neck. There are a number of different types of melanoma—superficial spreading melanoma, nodular melanoma, acral-lentiginous melanoma, and lentigo maligna melanoma. Intraocular melanoma is a type of melanoma affecting the eye.

What are the early signs of melanoma?
Often the first sign is a change in the size, shape, or color of an existing mole. Or it may appear as a new, abnormal lump in normal skin or as a new, ugly-looking mole. Early signs of a change in the mole, such as a darkening or a change in color, an increase in size, or an itching sensation, should be immediately checked by a doctor. Bleeding and ulceration of the mole are later signs of possible problems. Melanoma is best treated when it is found early, as it can spread quickly to other parts of the body through the lymph system or through the blood.

How do melanomas start?
Melanomas develop when a melanocyte, which is a cell that produces melanin, begins to behave abnormally. Melanin is the pigment that gives our skin its natural color. Healthy cells normally grow, divide, and replace themselves in an orderly fashion. Sometimes melanocytes grow in a cluster. These benign clus-

ters of melanocytes are called moles. (Doctors sometimes refer to them as *nevi*; one mole is called a *nevus*.) Half of all melanomas begin in a previously benign mole. Moles are very common. They may be present at birth or may appear later on—usually before age 40. They generally grow or change only slightly over time. When they are taken off, they normally do not return. Melanomas occur when the melanocytes become malignant. If a melanoma is not removed early, cancer cells may grow downward from the skin surface, invading healthy tissue. When a melanoma becomes thick and deep, the disease often spreads to other parts of the body and is difficult to control.

What are atypical moles?

Some people have certain abnormal looking moles (sometimes called *dysplastic nevi*) that may be more likely than normal moles to develop into melanoma. Most people with atypical moles have just a few of these abnormal moles; others have many. Atypical moles often look very much like melanoma.

Should all moles be removed?

Moles are very common. Since melanoma is relatively rare—about one to two percent of all human cancers—the odds that any one mole will become malignant melanoma are less than one in several million. Moles on the palms of the hands, the soles of the feet, or the genitalia are more apt to turn into malignant melanoma than are moles elsewhere. In addition, if you have a mole in a location that is likely to be irritated, such as where a bra strap rubs, or where it might be nicked in shaving, it is wise to have it removed. It should be examined to make certain it is not cancerous.

Do moles get darker during pregnancy?

Moles on a woman's body may become darker than usual during pregnancy. This is normal and not a sign of melanoma, but it is wise to have them checked.

Is melanoma inherited?

About 10 percent of all people who have melanoma have family members who also have had melanoma. There appears to be a predisposition to melanoma in some families. Genetic studies are learning more about the location of abnormalities in the DNA that make some people predisposed to melanoma cancers. Defects in the P16 gene have been identified as being related to an inherited tendency to melanoma. The same gene may also play a role in non-inherited melanoma.

Are there different kinds of melanoma?

There are four fairly distinct forms of primary melanoma. They are:

- **Superficial spreading melanoma,** which starts from a preexisting or new mole. This is the most common type. The first sign is the appearance of a flat or slightly raised, discolored patch that has irregular borders. The color varies with areas of tan, brown, black, red, blue or white. It is most likely to occur on the trunk in men, the legs in women and the upper back in both men and women.

- **Nodular melanoma** is usually invasive at the time it is first diagnosed. The color is most often black, but may be blue, gray, white, brown, tan, red, or skin tone.

- **Lentigo maligna melanoma,** also known as Hutchinson's melanotic freckle, tends to occur on the face, or in areas of the body exposed to the sun. Similar to the superficial spreading type, it remains close to the skin surface for quite a while and usually appears as a flat, or slightly elevated, mottled tan, brown, or dark brown discoloration.

- **Acral lentiginous melanoma** appears as a black or brown discoloration under the nails, on the palms of the hands or soles of the feet. It is the most common melanoma in dark-skinned people and least common among Caucasians. It usually spreads superficially before penetrating more deeply.

In addition, there are some miscellaneous unusual types: mucosal lentiginous melanomas that appear on the mouth and genitals; desmoplastic melanomas that cause fibrous adhesions; and verrucous melanomas that are rough and warty.

What do physicians look for when determining whether a mole is a melanoma?

Physicians refer to the ABCD of melanoma: Asymmetry, Borders that are irregular, Color variability, and Diameter (greater than six millimeters).

How should the biopsy for melanoma be done?

A properly performed biopsy is critical in diagnosing melanoma. Ideally, the biopsy should be performed in such a way that the complete melanoma is removed and examined for cancer.

Is sentinel lymph node biopsy ever used for melanoma?

This is a relatively new procedure in which the surgeon finds and removes only the sentinel node—the first lymph node into which a tumor drains, and the one most likely to contain cancer cells. If no cancer cells are found in the sentinel node, there probably are no tumor cells in the remaining nodes. Sentinel node biopsies, which need a specialist to perform them, are usually done on an outpatient basis.

How is the sentinel lymph node biopsy done?

A blue dye and a radioactive tracer are injected around the tumor. A hand-held radioactive detector is used to pinpoint the location of the node. The doctor makes a small incision and removes the node. The node is examined by a pathologist to see whether or not it contains cancer. If it does not, no further lymph nodes are removed. This biopsy will help the doctor decide what treatment should be done.

Is it easy to diagnose melanoma?

Diagnosis of melanoma requires the services of physicians and pathologists who are experienced in this type of cancer diagnosis. In a recent study it was found that there were differing opinions by experienced dermatopathogists (pathologists who specialize in skin diseases) in 38 percent of the diagnoses for melanoma. So there is no question that distinguishing between benign moles and early melanoma is a difficult task. If there is any doubt at all about the diagnosis, the biopsy should be reviewed by several experienced pathologists before any decisions about treatment are made.

What tests are done once melanoma is diagnosed?

Your doctor will prescribe a series of tests to stage the disease. Staging considers how deeply the cancer has penetrated the skin and subcutaneous tissue, how widely it has grown, and whether it has spread to other parts of the body. Staging procedures include a thorough physical examination, chest x-rays, blood tests, and liver function tests. In addition, lymphatic mapping and sentinel lymphadenectomy is now being used for patients with T2, T3 and T4 melanomas to accurately determine the status of the disease.

How is staging determined for malignant melanoma?

Staging is determined either by the vertical thickness in millimeters (called Breslow's classification) or by the anatomic level of the tumor (known as Clark's classification). Stages are further categorized by other classifications that indicate the thickness of the tumor and the level of invasion. Since staging is of primary importance in determining the treatment to be used, these classifications are very specific. Accurate staging of the original melanoma requires careful inspection of the entire specimen by an experienced pathologist. For further information on staging and classifications, please refer to Chapter 6, How Cancers Are Diagnosed.

What treatments are used for malignant melanoma?

The treatment for malignant melanoma depends upon the location, extent, and stage of the disease. The depth to which the skin has been invaded determines the extent of the treatment. Some melanomas that have spread to nearby lymph nodes may be curable with wide surgery of the tumor and removal of the affected lymph nodes. Melanoma that has spread to other areas, such as the liver, lungs, bone, brain and internal organs is more difficult to cure, although surgical removal of the metastasized cancer is sometimes successful. When a large amount of skin is removed, grafting may be necessary. Skin may be taken from another part of the body and grafted to the area where the cancer was removed. Malignant melanoma is the single most common tumor reported to spontaneously regress, although this occurs in less than one percent of cases.

Is chemotherapy used for treating melanoma?

Chemotherapy using isolated arterial perfusion may be used, especially if the cancer occurs on an arm or leg. In this method, in order to allow the drug to reach the tumor directly, chemotherapy drugs are put into the bloodstream of the arm or leg where the melanoma is found. Chemotherapy may also be prescribed after surgery to kill any undetectable cancer cells that might still remain in the body.

How does isolated arterial perfusion work?

Isolated arterial perfusion, sometimes called hypothermic isolated limb perfusion (ILP), is a method of administering high doses of chemotherapy directly to an affected limb. As a result, many of the side effects that are common with systemic chemotherapy are avoided. Blood circulation to and from the arm or leg is temporarily stopped with a tourniquet. Blood is withdrawn from the patient and pumped through a machine that adds oxygen and anticancer drugs. The blood is then pumped back into the major artery supplying the limb being treated. Often the blood is heated to enhance the effects of the drugs. Another technique, known as intraarterial regional infusion, is sometimes used when the cancer is limited to an arm or a leg. Again, normal blood circulation to and from the limb is stopped. Anticancer drugs are infused directly into the main artery of the limb. This treatment is sometimes used when melanoma reappears.

Are some of the newer biological treatments being used for melanoma?

A number of different types of biological therapies are being tested in clinical trials for melanoma in Stages II, III, IV and for recurrent melanoma. These include alpha interferon and interleukin-2 (IL-2). Some trials are using these in combination with chemotherapy drugs.

How do biological treatments work?

Biological treatments, also called biological response modifiers, are substances that can improve the body's natural response to infections and other disease. Both interferon and interleukin are biological response modifiers. The body normally produces these substances. Those used in cancer treatment are produced in the laboratory. There are several types of interferons, such as alpha interferon, beta interferon, and gamma interferon, which interfere with the division of cancer cells and can slow tumor growth. Interleukin-2 is a biological response modifier that stimulates the growth of certain disease-fighting blood cells in the immune system.

Is adoptive transfer used to treat melanoma?
Adoptive transfer, immune cells produced in the laboratory specifically for the patient, have shown promising results in patients with metastatic melanoma. This experimental technique, in which researchers use a small fragment of the patient's melanoma tumor to grow T cells in the laboratory using the patient's own T cells, has been pioneered by Steven A. Rosenberg, MD, of the National Cancer Institute. Exposure to the tumor activates the immune cells so that they recognize and attack the cancer cells. The immune cells multiply rapidly and attack tumor tissue and destroy metastases throughout the body. The treatment is at present highly experimental, but it is hoped that in the future it will be available to treat melanoma and other types of cancer.

Is radiation used for melanoma?
Radiation is sometimes used to treat local recurrences of melanoma that cannot be removed surgically. In cases in which the disease has spread to the lung, gastrointestinal tract, bone, or brain, radiation may provide relief from symptoms.

Is autologous bone marrow transplantation used to treat melanoma?
Though this has been tried, it has not been shown to improve survival.

Are skin grafts common following surgical removal of malignant melanoma?
Skin grafts may be necessary following the removal of skin cancers, depending upon the location and extent of the surgery. A portion of healthy skin is taken from one area of the body and moved to another area. In skin cancer, such grafts cover the areas that have been left bare by the surgical removal of portions of the skin. The replacement skin is usually taken from the back or thigh or other part of the body and stitched to the wound.

Is it painful to have a skin graft?
There is usually only a little pain and a burning sensation in the area from which the skin was removed and little or no pain at the site where it is applied.

TREATMENT CHOICES FOR MALIGNANT MELANOMA

STAGE	TREATMENT
Stage 0 TIS, N0, M0	Excision with minimal, but microscopically-free margins.
Stage I TIA, N0, M0 or T1b, N0, M0 or T2a, N0, M0	Surgical excision to remove all of tumor including as much as 2 centimeters of surrounding tissue. Skin grafting may be done to cover wound **or** *Clinical Trials:* Lymphatic mapping.
Stage II T2b, N0, M0, T3a or b, N0, M0, T4a or b, N0, M0	Surgical excision to remove all of tumor including two centimeters of surrounding tissue. Skin grafting may be done to cover wound and removal of nearby lymph nodes. *Clinical trials:* Surgical excision of tumor followed by biological therapy **or** Surgery to remove tumor plus removal of regional lymph nodes followed by chemotherapy, biological therapy, or immunological therapy.
Stage III Any T, any N, M0	Wide surgical excision with one to three centimeter margins. Skin grafting if needed. Nearby lymph nodes removed if they are cancerous. *Clinical trials:* Wide surgical excision (up to 3 centimeters), followed by biological therapy **or** Wide surgical excision, followed by adjuvant chemotherapy, immunological or biological therapy. Removal of regional lymph nodes.
Stage IV Any T, any N, any M	Surgery to remove lymph nodes that are cancerous or tumors that have spread to other areas of the body **or** Radiation therapy to relieve symptoms. *Clinical trials:* newer types of systemic chemotherapy, biological therapy, vaccines **or** radiation therapy to relieve bone, spinal cord or brain metastases **or** surgery to remove all known cancer.
Recurrent	Dependent on many factors, including prior treatment and site of recurrence. Treatment may be: Surgery to remove tumor **or** Radiation therapy to relieve symptoms. *Clinical trials:* Systemic chemotherapy **and/or** biological therapy or heated chemotherapy drugs injected into cancer.

Will the grafted skin look like normal skin?

The match of normal and grafted skin depends upon where the graft comes from. The doctor will try to match it as closely as possible—in color and texture. In a few months, the graft develops sensation. It is wise to protect the skin from the sun as the new skin can become sunburned, but will probably not darken as much as surrounding skin. The new skin will grow hair only if it came from a location where hair was originally growing.

What kind of doctor should I use for a skin graft?

This will depend upon the location of the graft, the size, and the type being done. Facial procedures are done by dermatologists, otolaryngologists, maxillofacial surgeons, and plastic surgeons.

Questions To Ask Your Doctor About Follow-up

- **Will you be doing my main follow-up?**
- **Will I also need to see any of my other doctors?**
- **How often will I need to see you?**
- **What tests will you be doing during my follow-up exam?**
- **What will you be looking for?**
- **What should I be watching for between my visits with you?**
- **What symptoms should I report? To whom?**

How often should someone who has had melanoma have a checkup?

Since anyone who has had melanoma is at increased risk for developing new melanomas as well as for a recurrence of the original melanoma, they should be checked regularly. The chance of recurrence is greater for those whose melanoma was thick or had spread to nearby tissue than for someone with a very thin melanoma. In general, recurrences of melanoma may occur within 18 to 24 months after treatment. You should see your doctor every three months for the first year; every four months until the fifth year; and every six months thereafter. Depending on your stage of disease, you may have yearly chest x-rays or CT scans of the chest and liver. It is especially important for all who have had melanoma to regularly examine their own skin on a monthly basis, if not more often.

UNUSUAL SKIN CANCERS

What is ocular melanoma?

Ocular melanoma, like melanoma of the skin, originates in melanocytes, the pigmented cells that give the eye its color. Ocular melanoma may grow in any of the uveal structures of the eye (the iris, ciliary body or choroid.) Melanoma that develops in the iris may produce a pigmented spot, changing to translucent or pink. Other signs include distortion of the pupil, presence of new blood vessels, curling of the iris near the pupil, and cataract formation. If tumors reach a large size, you may have symptoms such as loss or deterioration of vision and floating spots. Cataracts, secondary glaucoma, and inflammation also may occur.

What tests are used to diagnose ocular melanoma?

The doctor will look at your eye, may photograph it, and may order one or more of several tests, such as CT scan, MRI, ultrasound, fluorescein angiography (dye injected into blood vessel to highlight details), a chest x-ray and blood tests of your liver.

Should I go to a specialized center for treatment for ocular melanoma?

Yes. Since this is a very rare cancer and side effects accompany each form of treatment, it is important to have an open and complete discussion with well-qualified doctors, including an ophthalmologist and oncologist. Before making any decisions about treatment, anyone with this unusual type of cancer should seek out second opinions and consider the possibility of having treatment at one of the leading cancer or medical centers.

How is ocular melanoma treated?

Only a dozen years ago, melanoma of the eye meant taking out the eye and a diminished chance for long-term survival. Today, treated in a well-equipped radiotherapy center, melanoma patients are keeping not only their eyes, but also their vision to such an extent that they can continue to drive a car. Ocular melanomas can be treated with internal or external radiation, tiny laser beams, or with surgery. Usually if the melanoma is small or medium, surgery can remove it and still preserve a functioning eye. If the melanoma is large, enucleation, the removal of the entire eye, may be the treatment. In cases of choroid and ciliary body melanomas, there are more treatment options available, including localized radiation using a method where radioactive pellets are enclosed in a plastic disk covered on one side with a gold plate. The radiation released by the plaque is directed to the tumor, while the gold plate protects the surrounding tissues and the brain from receiving radiation. A few specialized radiation treatment centers are treating ocular melanomas with charged particle beam radiation with excellent results.

Are there any ocular melanomas that do not need treatment?

Small ocular melanomas that are not growing and do not interfere with vision don't have to be treated, but they do require close observation.

What is Merkel cell carcinoma?

This is an unusual type of skin cancer that often spreads to the lymph nodes in the area of the tumor. High powered electron microscopes make it possible to identify this cell type, which is most commonly found on the scalp, neck, face, and fingertips. It occurs most often in older patients, generally between the ages of 50 and 90. Unlike some skin cancers that appear as a sore that does not heal, Merkel cell cancers begin as painless, shiny lumps on the surface of the skin. Merkel cell cancers (even small ones) grow rapidly and often spread to other parts of the body. If you have such a lump, it should be seen by a dermatologist and treated. Treatment includes removal of the tumor and a wide margin of healthy tissue. Radiation therapy is usually prescribed to be directed at the site of the surgery and at adjacent lymph nodes or removal of lymph nodes is sometimes recommended.

SKIN CANCER PREVENTION HINTS

Sensible precautions can help protect you from skin cancers and help you find skin cancers early, before they have a chance of doing permanent damage. Since we know that the sun is a contributing factor in over 90 percent of skin cancers, it is wise to take precautions against the damaging rays of the sun on a year-round basis.

- Do a monthly skin exam. Become familiar with your skin and the pattern of moles, freckles, and beauty marks.
- If you detect any changes in your skin, see your doctor right away.
- Find a doctor with experience in dealing with skin cancer, one who understands the importance of family history and who is willing to remove any changing skin lesions early.
- Spend as little time in the sun as you can. Ultraviolet rays of the sun are the most frequent cause of cancer. Deliberate, repeated suntanning increases the incidence of skin cancer. Sun exposure has a cumulative effect. Infants should always be kept out of the sun, and young children should be taught sun protection early.
- Use a sunscreen, at least 15 SPF, especially between 10 A.M. and 3 P.M. Reapply the sunscreen after swimming or sweating. Remember that UV rays can pass through clouds or be reflected by snow or water. Wear tightly woven protective clothing such as sun hats, long sleeves, pants and gloves, which help reduce the penetration of ultraviolet rays.
- Do not use indoor sunlamps or tanning parlors.

KNOW THE SIGNS OF SKIN CANCER

- A skin growth that increases in size and appears pearly, translucent, tan, brown, black, or multicolored.

- A mole, birthmark, or beauty mark that changes color, increases in size or thickness, changes in texture, is irregular in outline.

- A spot or growth that continues to itch, hurt, crust, scab, erode, or bleed.

- An open sore or wound on the skin that does not heal or persists for more than four weeks, or heals and then reopens.

If you have any of these symptoms, see your doctor immediately.

Is it possible that sometime in the future we will be able to protect against skin cancers after sun damage occurs?

Scientists are working on a number of strategies that hold promise for the future in chemoprevention. Both oral and topical treatments are being studied. Included are: Vitamin A and its derivatives, isoflavones and polyphenolic antioxidants (plant-derived compounds), genistein (a soybean isoflavone), a bacterial DNA repair enzyme called T4 endonuclease V, and topical 2-(difluoromethyl)-di-ornithine.

Are sunlamps and suntanning booths safe?

All tanning devices produce ultraviolet radiation that, like ultraviolet rays from the sun, can cause eye injuries, skin burns, and may help to promote cancer. Those who tan poorly or have an increased risk of skin cancer such as persons with freckles, previous severe sunburns, multiple nevi, malignant skin lesions, or a history of immunosuppression should never use suntanning devices.

Are skin lightener creams dangerous?

The ingredient hydroquinine, suppresses production of melanin, which produces skin pigmentation. Skin bleaches are linked to skin problems like abnormal darkening. Animal studies suggest a possible cancer risk.

Do some medications increase the effects of sunlight and ultraviolet radiation?

There are some substances that are photosensitizing—that is, the substances make you more sensitive to the sun. Among them are birth-control pills, diuretics (used for high blood pressure), oral hypoglycemics (antidiabetic drugs), and phenothiazines (tranquilizers such as Thorazine), sulfa drugs (used for bacterial infections), and antibiotics ending with the suffix "-cycline." Saccharin, halogenated silcylanilides, oil of bergamot, and essences of lemon and lime also have been implicated. People taking many of the chemotherapy drugs or who have had radiation must also be aware of the effects of sunlight.

Web Pages to Check Out

www.cancer.gov: For general up-to-date information, and for clinical trials.
www.cancer.org: For general up-to-date information and community resources.
www.skincancer.org: General information.
www.jhu.edu/wctb/coms.html: Ocular (Choroidal) melanoma.

Also see Chapter 2, Searching for Answers on the Web, for more information.

Eighteen

ADULT LEUKEMIA

Many people think that leukemia is a children's disease. In fact, many more adults have leukemia than children. Of the more than 31,500 new cases of leukemia that occur each year, fewer than ten percent affect children. The rest occur in adults, many of them over the age of 60. There are two cell types—myelogenous and lymphocytic. Each of these cell types comes in an active (AML or ALL) and a chronic form (CML or CLL). We will focus on these four categories in this chapter. You will be learning a whole new vocabulary as you start dealing with the testing and treatment of your leukemia. For information on childhood leukemias, see Chapter 24, When a Child Has Cancer.

LEUKEMIAS IN ADULTS are approximately evenly divided between acute and chronic. They strike both sexes and all ages. Although the causes of leukemia are not fully understood, certain factors are known to increase the risk of developing the disease. They include genetic factors such as Down's syndrome, as well as exposure to high or repeated doses of radiation, genetic changes, exposure to some chemicals, and infections from certain viruses. Over the last thirty years, there has been a dramatic improvement in survival of patients with acute lymphocytic leukemia. In the early 1960s the five-year survival rate was four percent, in the mid-1970s it was up to 38 percent and now the five-year survival rate is 64 percent. New drugs are being tested for the treatment of several types of leukemia. A drug known as imatinib mesylate, or by its trade name, Gleevec, interferes with the growth of cancer. It has been approved by the FDA as first-line therapy for chronic myologic leukemia and a form of acute lymphocytic leukemia.

What You Need to Know About Leukemia

- Leukemia is a cancer of the organs that make blood—the lymph system and the bone marrow. The number of cells produced, the rate at which they are produced, and their ability to function are altered.

- There are four major types of leukemia, each with its own individual characteristics, abnormalities, and treatments—acute lymphocytic, acute myelogenous, chronic lymphocytic, and chronic myelogenous.

- Improvements in treatments over the last decades have made it possible for physicians to treat the disease aggressively—and in some cases to cure it.

- More than half of all leukemias occur in people over 60 years of age.

- Acute leukemia means it is a rapidly progressing type.

- Chronic leukemia usually progresses more slowly, but can be unpredictable. Many times there are no symptoms for many years. Other times it may progress more rapidly.

- The terms melogenous or lymphocytic tell you which cell type is involved.

Has Agent Orange been associated with leukemia?

Agent Orange is a mixture of herbicides used during the Vietnam War mainly to defoliate forest trees. Chronic lymphocytic leukemia (CLL) has been associated with Agent Orange and other herbicides used during the Vietnam War. If you are a Vietnam veteran and have been diagnosed with CLL, you should qualify for VA disability compensation and the special access to medical care that the VA has offered to Vietnam veterans for health problems from Agent Orange exposure. You do not need to prove that your illness is related to your military service. It is presumed to be service-connected. The association between other forms of leukemia and herbicide exposure is now being studied. For more information, see Chapter 4, What Is Cancer?

What kind of doctor is best for treating someone who has leukemia?

Leukemia can be a very difficult disease to treat, so it is essential that a qualified hematologist or oncologist who is experienced in dealing with leukemia is involved in making your treatment plans. Another important factor to be

WHO IS MOST LIKELY TO GET LEUKEMIA

- White people more often than blacks.

- People of Jewish ancestry more often than other whites.

- Males more often than females.

- Those exposed to high or repeated doses of ionizing radiation.

- Patients who received at least two grays (a measure of radiation) as treatment for a spinal condition called ankylosing spondylitis.

- Some patients with Hodgkin's disease who received radiation and chemotherapy.

- Those with some genetic abnormalities, such as Down's and Bloom's syndromes, Fanconi's anemia, neurofibromatosis, and Philadelphia chromosome.

- Those who have been exposed to Agent Orange (CLL only).

- Those who have had long-term exposure to certain chemicals and drugs, such as benzene, chloramphenicol and phylbutazone, and chemotherapy drugs such as alkylating agents.

- If one identical twin develops acute leukemia before six years of age, there is a 20 percent chance the other twin will develop it within a few months. Fraternal twins and siblings of those with leukemia are at greater risk than the normal population.

- Though not confirmed by studies, there is suggestive evidence that those living near high-voltage transmission lines (especially children) may be at risk.

considered is the hospital where you plan to be treated. Facilities with extensive supportive care capabilities that have access to blood products and a multi-disciplinary team of physicians, nurses and pharmacists help assure that the patient receives the best treatment possible.

What is leukemia?
Leukemia is cancer of the blood-forming cells. It occurs when immature or mature cells multiply in an uncontrolled manner in the bone marrow.

How do the blood-forming cells work?
The three major types of cells in the blood are red blood cells (erythrocytes), white blood cells (leukocytes), and platelets (thrombocytes). All of these cells are produced by the stem cells in the bone marrow. Most blood cells mature in the bone marrow, but some also mature in the thymus, spleen, lymph nodes, and tonsils. After maturing, the adult cells slowly seep into the blood vessels and become part of the blood.

What is the function of red blood cells?

Red blood cells act as a transportation system. They carry oxygen from the lungs to the other cells of the body and bring back waste products or carbon dioxide. If there are too few red blood cells, it is difficult for cells to get enough oxygen. This condition is called anemia and results in weakness, lack of energy, dizziness, headache, and irritability. Red blood cell counts are part of the blood counts monitored in blood tests.

What do white blood cells do?

White blood cells are the main components of the immune system. Their primary role is to fight infection. There is normally only about one white blood cell for every five hundred red blood cells. If a bacterial infection is present, the number may increase dramatically. If the white blood cell count is abnormally low, a person's chance of developing an infection increases.

Are there different kinds of white blood cells?

There are several major types, each with a specific function. **Granulocytes** fight infections. It takes nine to ten days for immature cells formed in the bone marrow to become mature granulocytes. Because granulocytes circulate for only six to ten hours, any interruption in their production quickly places you at risk for developing an infection. There are three different kinds of granulocytes: neutrophils, basophils, and eosinophils.

Mononuclear cells destroy invading antigens, particularly viruses. There are two different kinds of mononuclear cells: lymphocytes and monocytes (macrophages). In doing blood counts, laboratory tests measure the levels of these different types of white blood cells. You may hear some of these cell types referred to by other names:

- Neutrophils are also called polymorphonucleacytes, PMN, or polys. Immature neutrophils are sometimes called bands or stabs.
- Eosinophils may be referred to as "eos."
- Lymphocytes are also known as lymphs.
- Monocytes are also called monos.

What are blasts?

Blasts, or leukemic cells, are immature white blood cells. In normal marrow, less than five percent of these abnormal cells are present.

What do platelets do?

Platelets are essential in clotting of blood. Checking the platelet count is part of the testing done for those who are suspected of having, or who have, leukemia. An abnormally low platelet count (called thrombocytopenia) may result in excessive bleeding from wounds or in mucous membranes, skin, or other tissues.

What are petechiae?

Petechiae (pronounced pe-te-ke-eye) is the medical jargon for small red and/or brown spots on the skin, which are actually tiny hemorrhages. They can look like a rash. They are caused by a low blood count and decreased clotting function and are often seen in conjunction with leukemia.

What is a peripheral blood smear?

This is a blood test in which a drop of blood is smeared on a glass slide, fixed, stained, and examined under a high-power microscope. The size and shape of a large number of red blood cells, the numbers of the different types of white blood cells and the number of platelets are examined and recorded.

Why is there so much emphasis on blood tests?

When you have leukemia, blood tests become a part of your life. Since leukemia means that there is an abnormality in the production of blood, the blood counts tell the doctor about the state of your health. Blood checks help to determine how you are progressing.

What is the total white blood cell count?

The total white blood cell, or leukocyte, count measures the total number of circulating leukocytes. It is used along with the differential white blood cell count.

What is the differential white blood cell count?

The differential white blood cell count gives the percentage of the total number of the different types of white cells. Alone, this count has limited value—it must always be interpreted in relation to the total leukocyte count. If the percentage of one type of cell is increased, it can be inferred that cells of that type are relatively more numerous than normal. This is not always the case, because it is not known if this reflects an absolute decrease in cells of another type or an actual absolute increase in the number of cells that are relatively increased. If the relative percentages of the differential are known and if the total leukocyte count is known, it is possible to calculate absolute values that are not subject to misinterpretation.

What is the hematocrit count?

The hematocrit count gives the percentage of red cells in a volume of whole blood. The test separates the plasma and blood cells.

TESTS THAT MAY BE USED TO DIAGNOSE ADULT LEUKEMIA

- Physical examination.
- Laboratory tests that include blood counts, chemistries and urine tests.
- Immunophenotyping, flow cytometry and cytogenetic analysis.
- Diagnostic x-rays.
- Bone marrow aspiration and biopsy.
- Spinal tap (lumbar puncture).

How is a bone marrow biopsy done?
A bone marrow biopsy takes a small sample of bone marrow through a needle inserted into a bone—either the hip, or less frequently, the breastbone. (In a bone marrow aspiration, a fluid specimen is drawn out.) A local anesthetic is injected to numb the tissue over the biopsy site. The biopsy needle is inserted into the bone. The core of the needle is removed and the needle is advanced and rotated in both directions, forcing a tiny core of bone into the needle. Each test takes about 10 to 20 minutes. You will feel a dull to sharp pain that will last as long as the needle is being advanced and removed. The local anesthetic does not affect the deeper bone pain, but the pain lasts only a minute or less. There may be soreness at the biopsy site for several days. Test results are usually available in several days. Be sure to contact your doctor if there is bleeding that is more than just spotting.

What is immunophenotyping?
This is a way of telling whether or not a certain cell type is present in your blood, marrow, or lymph nodes. A tag is attached to antibodies that respond to specific antigens in the cell. This test can tell, for instance, the difference between myelogenous leukemic cells and lymphocytic leukemic cells.

What is a cytogenetics analysis?
This test looks at the chromosomes to see if the number and shape are normal. This analysis and immunophenotyping are important to determine what kind of treatment will be given.

What are spicules?
When doing a bone marrow test, the doctor wants to be certain to retrieve bone marrow. Spicules are bits of bone marrow with fat in them, which give a representative sample of marrow cells. Without enough spicules, it is impossible to make an accurate diagnosis of the bone marrow cells.

BLOOD COUNTS

NOTE: Values may vary according to age and individual laboratory standards.

CELL TYPE	NORMAL VALUES
Red blood cell count	*Males:* 4.5–6.0 million cells per microliter
	Females: 4.0–4.5 million cells per microliter
White blood cell count	4.5–11 thousand cells per microliter

DIFFERENTIAL WHITE BLOOD CELL COUNT (LEUKOCYTE COUNT)

Neutrophils	50–60 percent
Eosinophils	1–4 percent
Basophils	0.5–2 percent
Lymphocytes	20–40 percent
Monocytes	2–9 percent
Platelets	150,000–450,000 per microliter

HEMATOCRIT (PERCENT OF BLOOD COMPOSED OF RED CELLS)

Males	42–50 percent
Females	36–45 percent

HEMOGLOBIN

NOTE: If blood-drawing tourniquet is left on too long, may produce abnormally high values

Males	14–17 grams per 100 milliliters
Females	12–15 grams per 100 milliliters

Questions to Ask Your Doctor Before
Agreeing to Start Treatment

- **What kind of leukemia do I have?**
- **Is it a chronic or acute type of leukemia?**
- **Which cells are affected?**
- **Is this a very unusual type of leukemia?**

- **Can you explain the blood counts and tell me what is normal for me?**
- **Has the diagnosis been checked by a hematopathologist?**
- **Do you suggest that this diagnosis be confirmed by getting a second opinion at one of the large centers that specializes in this type of cancer?**
- **Would it be wise for me to get my treatment at one of the major cancer centers?**
- **How many cases like mine do you treat each year?**
- **What kind of treatment are you planning for me?**
- **Is a bone marrow transplant a choice for me after initial treatment?**

How are leukemias classified and what is the difference between acute and chronic leukemia?

Broadly, acute and chronic leukemias are classified as lymphocytic or myelogenous, according to the type of cell that is multiplying abnormally. Acute means that it is progressing rapidly with a large number of highly immature cells that cannot carry out their normal jobs in the body. Chronic means that it is progressing slowly with greater numbers of more mature cells that can carry out some of their normal functions.

Why is supportive care during treatment so essential for leukemia patients?

Supportive care, the treatment given to help with side effects and other complications, is essential for people with leukemia. You could have very low platelet and white blood cell counts and are thus at risk of life-threatening infection and bleeding. The purpose of supportive care is to prevent or reduce the effects of anemia, bleeding, and infection.

ACUTE LEUKEMIAS

Acute leukemia is a rapidly progressing type of this disease. The abnormal cells, called blasts, do not grow into normal cells. Rather they stay as immature cells that cannot carry out their specific job in the body. Many people with acute leukemia can be cured.

What are the two types of acute leukemias?

In adults, the most common type of acute leukemia is acute **myelogenous** leukemia or **AML**, which accounts for more than half of all adult leukemias. The other type of acute leukemia is acute **lymphocytic** leukemia or **ALL**. This is the adult version of the most common childhood leukemia. It accounts for only a small percentage of adult leukemias. It is more difficult to control in

TYPES OF LEUKEMIA

TYPE	DESCRIPTION
Acute Lymphocytic Leukemia (ALL)	Begins in immature B or T lymphocytes. Accounts for only 6 percent of adult leukemias. (75 percent of childhood leukemias are ALL. Treatments for children are different than for adults. See Chapter 24, When a Child Has Cancer.)
Acute Myelogenous Leukemia (AML), also called **Acute Nonlymphocytic Leukemia (ANLL)**. There are also a number of subtypes of AML	Begins in immature myeloid cells. Accounts for 54 percent of adult leukemias and 20 percent of childhood leukemias. (See Chapter 24 for more information on childhood AML.)
Chronic Lymphocytic Leukemia (CLL)	Begins in the B lymphocytes, rarely in T lymphocytes. 25 percent of adult leukemias are this type and fewer than 1 percent of childhood cancers fall into this category.
Chronic Myelogenous Leukemia (CML). Also called chronic granulocytic leukemia.	Begins in immature myeloid cells that would normally develop into granulocytes. Accounts for 15 percent of adult leukemia.
Polycythemia Vera (not a true leukemia)	Too many red blood cells made in bone marrow.
Agnogenic Myeloid Metaplasia	Improper maturing of red blood cells and white blood cells called granulocytes.
Essential Thrombocythemia (not a true leukemia)	Number of platelets in blood much higher than normal, but other blood cells are normal. Extra platelets make it hard for blood to flow normally.
Hairy Cell (HCL), also called leukemic reticuloendotheliosis	Involves blood and bone marrow, affects mostly middle-aged and older men.
Pre-leukemia or **Smoldering Leukemia** (myelodysplastic syndrome); may progress to acute nonlymphocytic leukemia (ANLL)	Bone marrow does not function normally and not enough normal blood cells are made. Occurs most often in older people, but sometimes seen in younger people.

adults than in children. These two types of acute leukemias start in different types of white blood cells. Myelogenous begins in the myelocyte cell while lymphocytic begins in the lymphocytes. Some leukemias, classified as biphenotypic, have both lymphoid and myeloid features. Some show no differentiation of either cell type and are classified as undifferentiated. It is sometimes difficult to distinguish between the two types of acute leukemias, so it is essential that proper laboratory studies be done and confirmed so that the correct diagnosis is made before any treatment is started.

How is the diagnosis made for the acute types of leukemia?

Often blood tests will show a low hemoglobin count, a low level of normal white blood cells or platelets, or the presence of leukemic blasts. As many as 10 percent of patients, however, have normal blood counts at the time of diagnosis. In such cases, the diagnosis can be confirmed with a bone marrow biopsy. Many laboratory tests are conducted using the bone marrow sample. The cell's origin is identified so that the leukemia can be properly classified. Tests using stains and dyes help identify types of cells, certain cell surface markers and other cell characteristics. If leukemia cells are found in the bone marrow, additional tests will be done, including a spinal tap (lumbar puncture) to see if the cancer is in the fluid around the spinal cord and brain and x-rays to look at the chest area.

ACUTE MYELOGENOUS LEUKEMIA (AML OR ANLL)

What is acute myelogenous leukemia?

Acute myelogenous leukemia (AML), which is also known as acute myeloid leukemia and acute nonlymphocytic leukemia (ANLL), is leukemia in which abnormal, immature white blood cells are produced in the bone marrow. Normally, the bone marrow makes cells called blasts that mature into several different types of blood cells that have specific jobs to do in the body. In AML the blasts do not mature, but continue to reproduce and become too numerous. AML is the most common form of adult leukemia and affects people aged 40 and over. There are a number of subtypes of AML that are treated in a similar manner. If left untreated, death can occur within a few months due to infection or uncontrolled bleeding.

How is the diagnosis made?

Blood and marrow cells are studied to see if the red cell and platelet counts are low and if there are leukemic blast cells. The number and shape of chromosomes are examined. Immunophenotyping and other special tests will be done to make an accurate diagnosis. In some instances, an analysis of spinal fluid may be necessary. Treatment of AML is different from treatment for

SYMPTOMS OF ACUTE LEUKEMIAS (AML AND ALL)

- Fever and flu-like symptoms.

- Changes in energy level, appetite and temperament.

- Joint and bone pain.

- Joint tenderness or swelling.

- Paleness, dizziness, weakness.

- Tiredness, shortness of breath.

- Tendency to bruise or bleed easily.

- Slow healing of cuts.

- Unexplained bleeding.

- Recurrent infections in skin, gums, lung, and urinary tract.

- Tiny red, or brown spots on skin.

- If central nervous system is affected: headache, blurred vision, confusion, unexplained fever.

Symptoms may be vague, so it is often difficult to make an early diagnosis of acute leukemia. Sometimes symptoms may be present for less than three months, sometimes for only a few days.

ALL. Therefore, laboratory diagnostic tests must be carefully done to distinguish between the two before any treatment is begun.

How are the different leukemic cells of AML classified?
The different types are classified by an M designation. The classification is important because different kinds of treatment may be used, depending on which cell type you have.

M0, M1: Myeloblastic leukemia without maturation

M2: Acute myeloblastic with maturation

M3: Acute promyelocytic leukemia

M3V: Acute promyelocytic leukemia with variant

M4: Acute myelomonocytic leukemia

M4E: Acute myelomonocytic leukemia with variant

M5: Acute monocytic leukemia

M6: Erythroleukemia

M7: Acute megakaryocytic leukemia

How is adult acute myelogenous leukemia staged?

Staging systems are not used for acute myelogenous leukemia. Treatment depends upon whether the leukemia is untreated, in remission, or relapsed.

What kind of treatment is used for AML?

If you have AML you need treatment as soon after diagnosis as possible. Most people need intensive combination chemotherapy to bring about complete remission. This means that after treatment, there will be no leukemic blast cells in your blood or bone marrow and your blood counts will be back to their normal levels. A two-drug therapy, daunorubicin and cytarabine, given during this induction therapy period has resulted in remission for approximately 65 percent of patients. No one combination chemotherapy treatment is considered standard. Postremission treatment, to maintain the remission, may also be used.

How will the drugs be given?

The drugs will probably be given through the vein (IV). A thin, flexible tube, called a catheter, will be placed in a large vein, usually in your upper chest. The chemotherapy drugs and blood cells can be put into this tube. Blood samples can be taken out through the catheter. (See Chapter 7, Treatment, for more information on how drugs are given intravenously.)

What problems might I have during induction therapy?

During this period, the two major potential complications are infection and bleeding. Frequent transfusions may be needed and broad-spectrum antimicrobial therapy is used to treat these problems. Additional treatment following the achievement of induction therapy is necessary. Other side effects of chemotherapy are discussed in Chapter 10, Chemotherapy.

What are growth factors?

Growth factors, called G-CSF (granuloctye-colony stimulating factor), or GM-CSF (granulocyte-macrophase-colony stimulating factor) may be given to increase the production of blood cells when your white blood cell count is low.

How is acute promyelocytic leukemia treated?

Two treatments, retinoic acid, a form of Vitamin A, or arsenic trioxide, are given, followed by chemotherapy. Studies are underway to determine how immature cells develop.

What treatment is used if there is a relapse after the original treatments?

Clinical trials are testing the use of new chemotherapy agents. Bone marrow transplants, which replace diseased bone marrow with healthy marrow, may be done. Either the patient's own bone marrow (removed and stored before any treatment) or bone marrow from a donor may be used. If the patient's marrow is used it is called autologous bone marrow transplant. If a donor's marrow is used, it is called allogeneic transplant. Allogeneic stem cell transplants also are being evaluated. Bone marrow transplantation is discussed in Chapter 11, New Advances and Investigational Treatments.

What does refractory disease mean?

Refractory disease means the leukemia has not responded to treatment and therefore, has not gone into remission. It means that there are still leukemic cells in the bone marrow.

Do most acute myelogenous leukemias go into remission?

Advances in the treatment of AML have resulted in substantially improved remission rates. With the aggressive treatments now prescribed, about 60 to 70 percent of adults with AML can expect a complete remission. The results are even better for those under age 60.

Does AML affect the central nervous system?

Central nervous system relapse occurs in only a small percentage of patients, although certain types of AML and patients with high white blood cell counts are at greatest risk. An analysis of a spinal fluid sample may be taken for evaluation in these cases. Central nervous system relapse is treated with chemotherapy.

What does relapse mean?

Relapse means that you have had a remission but that the leukemia cells have returned in the marrow and you have a decrease in normal blood cells. You may be treated with drugs different from your first treatment or you may have a stem cell transplant.

What are myelodysplastic syndromes (MDL)?

This is a group of blood disorders that have an increased risk of becoming AML. About half of patients diagnosed with AML initially were diagnosed as having one of these myelodysplastic syndromes—also known as preleukemia anemia or smoldering anemia. In the final analysis, these syndromes may be different stages of the same disease, since often one type of MDLS will change to another type before finally becoming AML. Even when the final evolution to AML does not occur, there may be life-threatening anemia, a drop in platelet levels, infections and ulceration of the mucous membranes. While most often seen in older people, these syndromes can occur in younger people as well. They may develop following treatment with drugs or radiation therapy for other diseases (called secondary myelodysplastic syndromes), or may develop without any known cause (called de novo myelodysplastic syndromes). Treatment may be prescribed for relief of anemia or bleeding. Allogeneic bone marrow transplant or clinical trials of chemotherapy or biological therapy are the recommended treatments.

ACUTE LYMPHOCYTIC LEUKEMIA (ALL)

What is acute lymphocytic leukemia?
Acute lymphocytic leukemia, also called acute lymphoblastic leukemia, or acute lymphoid leukemia is a disease in which too many white blood cells (lymphocytes) are found in the blood and bone marrow. Since ALL can be confused with AML, hairy-cell leukemia and malignant lymphoma, an experienced hematologist, oncologist, hematopathologist or general pathologist should be involved in the diagnosis.

How are acute lymphocytic leukemias staged?
Acute lymphocytic leukemias are not staged. The treatment depends on whether or not you have been treated before.

What kind of treatment is used for ALL?
Treatment for adult ALL uses chemotherapy. This treatment is divided into three phases: induction therapy, central nervous system prophylaxis, and postremission treatment. Great strides have been made in the treatment of childhood ALL, which is now considered one of the most curable forms of cancer. Although the advances in treatment of adult ALL have been more difficult, about 60 to 80 percent of adults go into complete remission after their induction therapy.

What is induction therapy?
Induction therapy attempts to destroy all detectable leukemic cells to control the disease in the bone marrow and to prevent the disease from spreading, especially to the central nervous system. The drugs will probably be given through the vein (IV). Usually several drugs are used.

Will there be side effects from the treatment?
You will need to be very carefully monitored to prevent or reduce the effects of anemia, bleeding, and infection and may need periodic transfusions with red blood cells to control anemia. Transfusions of platelets reduce the rate of hemorrhage, allowing treatment with anticancer drugs to continue even when the platelet count has been very low. Supportive care is an important component during this stage of treatment.

What is central nervous system prophylaxis?

A small percentage of adults with ALL have evidence of leukemia in their spinal fluid and brain (central nervous system). If so, drugs and/or radiation therapy may be used. The drugs will be put directly into the fluid surrounding your brain and spinal cord, usually by injecting them in the lower part of the spinal column. This is called intrathecal chemotherapy. Sometimes a catheter, called an ommaya reservoir, is placed under the scalp, and the chemotherapy is injected into the reservoir instead of into the spinal column. The ommaya reservoir can be used to monitor pressure, as well as to administer antibiotics and chemotherapy.

What is postremission treatment?

After remission has been achieved, further treatment is essential to make sure that a relapse doesn't happen. These treatments may be called continuation or maintenance therapy. Maintenance programs for adults use a variety of drug combinations and schedules. They are intensive and must be given by a doctor who is well experienced in this disease. Bone marrow transplantation continues to be investigated as a treatment in clinical trials. Patients at high risk of relapse may be considered for either allogeneic or autologous bone marrow transplant either during the first remission or a subsequent one. More information on bone marrow transplants can be found in Chapter 11, New Advances and Investigational Treatments.

What treatments are used when an ALL patient has a relapse?

Treatment for relapsed ALL depends on many factors, including the length of the previous remission and the site of the relapse. Clinical trials are underway testing the use of high-dose combination chemotherapy, with or without radiation, followed by stem cell or bone marrow transplant; use of new anticancer drugs and drug combinations; and biological therapy with monoclonal antibodies.

CHRONIC LEUKEMIAS

What are chronic leukemias?

In chronic leukemia, too many mature white blood cells are produced and build up in the body. They develop slowly, often with no symptoms at first, and may remain undetected for a long time. There are two types of chronic leukemias, classified by the type of cell in which they begin. Chronic lymphocytic leukemia, known as CLL, is twice as common in men as in women. The average age of diagnosis is 60. CLL is rare before age 45 and it almost never occurs in children. Chronic myelogenous leukemia, known as CML and chronic myelocytic leukemia, is slightly more common in men than in women. The average age of diagnosis is 45. CML accounts for only about 5 percent of children's leukemias.

CHRONIC LYMPHOCYTIC LEUKEMIA (CLL)

What is chronic lymphocytic leukemia (CLL)?

Chronic lymphocytic leukemia is a cancer in which lymphocytes multiply very slowly but in a poorly regulated manner, live much longer than normal, and are unable to perform their proper function. About one quarter of all CLL patients have no symptoms and the disease often is diagnosed as a result of a routine blood test. Some patients may have enlarged lymph nodes in the neck or groin or show signs of anemia. The average age at diagnosis is 60. The course of the disease varies a great deal from person to person. Some people remain without symptoms for many years. In other people, CLL may progress more rapidly.

How is CLL diagnosed?

Blood tests are used, as well as bone marrow biopsy and more sophisticated chromosomal tests. CLL is suspected when blood tests reveal an increase in the number of lymphocytes in the blood to more than 15,000 per cubic millimeter as well as the presence of certain identifying characteristics on the lymphocyte's outside surface. CLL may be confused with other related diseases, especially non-Hodgkin's lymphoma.

What kind of treatment is used for CLL?

Treatment for CLL can range from periodic observation for patients who have no symptoms to treatment of complications such as infections or to a variety of investigational treatments. Because CLL often progresses slowly and cannot currently be cured with standard chemotherapy, it is generally treated in a conservative manner. Corticosteroids are used for many patients, sometimes in combination with chemotherapy. In later stages, if the spleen is very enlarged and is destroying large numbers of normal blood cells, the spleen may be removed. Removal of the spleen does not interfere with normal living. Its functions are taken over by other components of the body.

What is leukapheresis?

Leukapheresis is a procedure that transfuses white blood cells from healthy donors into patients whose low white blood count puts them at risk for infections.

How is CLL staged?

There is no standard staging system but two are being used. The Rai Staging System uses Stages 0 to 4 and the Binet classification uses clinical stages A to

SYMPTOMS OF CHRONIC LEUKEMIA—CLL, CML AND HCL

- General feeling of ill health.
- Fatigue.
- Lack of energy.
- Fever.
- Loss of appetite.
- Night sweats.
- Enlarged lymph nodes in neck or groin.
- Enlarged spleen.
- Anemia.

CML: Pain in the left upper quadrant, vague feeling of abdominal fullness.

C. The Binet system integrates the number of nodel groups involved with the disease with bone marrow failure. An International Workshop on Chronic Lymphocytic Leukemia has recommended integrating the systems.

What is hairy-cell leukemia?

Hairy-cell leukemia is a form of chronic leukemia that involves an unusual type of B lymphocyte that has hairlike projections. It is five times more common in males than in females. The average age at diagnosis is 54. It usually begins slowly, with undramatic symptoms that may include weakness caused by anemia, development of infections and pain or discomfort due to enlargement of the spleen. Hairy-cell leukemia is easily controlled and may be cured in most patients. About one-tenth of patients require no treatment. Your doctor's decision, whether or not treatment is necessary, is based on blood counts, spleen enlargement, indications that the disease is progressive, or other complications. Surgical removal of the spleen may be recommended as the initial treatment. About half of the patients who have their spleens removed need no additional treatment. Interferon therapy may be used, but many patients relapse when it is stopped. New drugs are being tested, as is bone marrow transplantation for young patients who are in good health but have not responded to other treatments.

Are there other types of lymphocytic leukemias?

There are other diseases that look like lymphocytic leukemia. They include large granular lymphocytic leukemia, macroglobulinemia, prolymphocytic leukemia, and lymphoma cell leukemia.

STAGES AND TREATMENT FOR
CHRONIC LYMPHOCYTIC LEUKEMIA (CLL)

STAGE	TREATMENT
Stage 0, Binet Stage A More than 15,000 lymphocytes per cubic millimeter (absolute lymphocytosis). No other symptoms.	No treatment needed in most cases. Doctor will follow you closely to initiate treatment when needed. Chemotherapy may be used.
Stage I, Binet Stage A or B Absolute lymphocytosis and enlarged lymph nodes. No other symptoms.	If no other symptoms, may not need treatment. Close followup **or** Chemotherapy with or without steriods **or** External radiation to swollen lymph nodes **or** Combination chemotherapy. *Clinical trials:* monoclonal antibodies, bone marrow or stem cell transplant.
Stage II, Binet Stage A or B Absolute lymphocytosis, enlarged lymph nodes, as well as enlarged liver or spleen.	If few or no symptoms, may not need treatment. Close follow-up **or** Chemotherapy with or without steroids **or** External radiation to swollen lymph nodes **or** Radiation therapy to spleen. *Clinical trials:* monoclonal antibodies, bone marrow or stem cell transplant.
Stage III, Binet Stage C Absolute lymphocytosis and anemia. Lymph nodes, liver or spleen may or may not be swollen.	If few or no symptoms, may not need treatment. Close followup **or** Chemotherapy with or without steroids **or** Removal of spleen **or** External radiation to spleen for symptoms. *Clinical trials:* monoclonal antibodies, bone marrow or peripheral stem cell transplant.
Stage IV, Binet Stage C Absolute lymphocytosis and fewer than 100,000 platelets per cubic millimeter with or without enlarged lymph nodes, liver or spleen or anemia.	Same as Stage III.

(continued)

STAGES AND TREATMENT FOR CHRONIC LYMPHOCYTIC LEUKEMIA (CLL) (continued)

STAGE	TREATMENT
Refractory Not responsive to treatment.	Treatment will depend on numerous factors. *Clinical trials:* new chemotherapy drugs, monoclonal antibodies, bone marrow or peripheral stem cell transplant.

CHRONIC MYELOGENOUS LEUKEMIA (CML)

What is chronic myelogenous leukemia (CML)?

Chronic myelogenous leukemia is one of the four major types of leukemia, and accounts for about 20 percent of leukemia cases. It affects the cells that are developing into white blood cells, called granulocytes. It is associated with a unique chromosomal abnormality called the Philadelphia chromosome. It is one of the types that eventually progresses to a more acute form. It is very difficult to treat since present treatments do not cure the disease or prevent blastic crisis.

What is the Philadelphia chromosome?

The Philadelphia chromosome, sometimes referred to as the Ph chromosome, is an abnormal chromosome that is found in more than 90 percent of people who have chronic myelogenous leukemia (CML). This chromosome was the first to be identified for a specific cancer. The cause of the chromosomal defect and its influence in the course of the disease is not known. But it has been seen in all phases of the disease and is rarely affected by treatment. It may sometimes be seen in the acute leukemias and other diseases, but much less commonly. (Incidentally, this abnormality is an acquired genetic defect, present only in the blood cells and cannot be transmitted to offspring.)

How is CML diagnosed?

CML is usually diagnosed with the help of a complete blood count and bone marrow biopsy. Cytogenetic analysis, which measures the number of chromosomes and their shape, polymerase chain reaction, a test that can detect changes in the DNA, and FISH (fluorescence *in situ* hybridization), a test that uses chemicals to stain the cells, may also be used.

What are the symptoms of CML?

Symptoms develop gradually. About 90 percent of patients complain of fullness in the upper abdomen. This is caused by a swollen spleen that may fill most of the abdomen. Fatigue, lack of energy, fever, shortness of breath, excessive sweating, weight loss, and inability to endure warm temperatures are other symptoms.

What are the phases of CML?

CML has three distinct phases: chronic, accelerated, and blast. In the chronic phase, the most common at diagnosis, there are few blast cells in the blood and bone marrow, and there may be no symptoms of leukemia. This phase can last from several months to several years. In the accelerated phase, more blast cells and fewer normal cells are found in the bone marrow and blood. In the blast phase, 30 percent of the cells in the blood or bone marrow are blast cells and these collections of cells may form tumors in the bones or lymph nodes. Transition from phase to phase may occur gradually over a year or more, or it may occur abruptly. The blast phase or blast crisis, as it is sometimes called, usually occurs three to five years after diagnosis and is very similar to aggressive acute leukemia but is more difficult to treat.

What treatment is used for CML?

Those who have blood counts that are nearly normal may receive no treatment. They will be checked often so that treatment may be given if the disease begins to progress. Surgery to remove the spleen is sometimes done to relieve physical discomfort or other problems resulting from a severely enlarged spleen. Many people in the chronic phase of CML respond well to treatment (which may include the use of alpha interferon) and live normal lives. Patients with newly diagnosed CML are urged to consider participating in clinical trials exploring the new therapeutic approaches using bone marrow transplants, biological response modifiers, and combination chemotherapy.

What is imatinib mesylate?

This is a drug also known as STI157 or its trade name, Gleevec. It interferes with the growth of cancer. In studies it has achieved complete remission for CML patients and has been especially effective for patients who could not use interferon. It has been approved by the FDA as primary therapy. Since it is a relatively new drug, long-term effects are not yet well known. Taken by mouth, imatinib mesylate seems to have fewer side effects, most of which can be managed without stopping treatment.

STAGES AND TREATMENTS FOR CHRONIC MYELOGENOUS LEUKEMIA (CML)

STAGE	TREATMENT
Chronic Fewer than 5 percent blast and promyelocytes in blood and bone marrow, no symptoms.	High-dose chemotherapy with radiation therapy followed by stem cell transplant **or** Biological treatment (alpha interferon) **or** Imatinib mesylate **or** Chemotherapy to lower white cell count **or** Surgery to remove spleen. *Clinical trials:* biological therapy with or without chemotherapy or after stem cell transplant.
Accelerated More than 5 percent or fewer than 30 percent blast and promyelocytes in blood and bone marrow.	Stem cell transplant **or** Imatinib mesylate **or** Biologic therapy (alpha interferon) **or** High-dose chemotherapy **or** Chemotherapy to lower white cell count **or** Other chemotherapy drugs **or** transfusions of blood or blood products to relieve symptoms. *Clinical trials*
Blast: More than 30 percent of cells are blast cells. Tumors in bone or lymph nodes	Imatinib mesylate **or** Chemotherapy (new drugs) Stem cell transplant **or** Chemotherapy to relieve symptoms **or** High-dose chemotherapy **or** *Clinical trials*
Relapsing chronic myelogenous leukemia	Imatinib mesylate **or** Stem cell transplant for selected patients Biologic therapy (alpha interferon) **or** Combination chemotherapy.

What are myeloproliferative disorders?

This is a group of diseases in which too many of certain types of blood cells are made in the bone marrow. Myeloproliferative disorders include polycythemia vera, agnogenic myeloid metaplasia, and essential thrombocythemia.

What is polycythemia vera?

This disorder is characterized by the uncontrolled production of red blood cells. The spleen may swell because the extra blood cells collect there. Itchiness all over the body is one of the symptoms of polycythemia vera. In order to lower the amount of blood in the body, a needle may be placed in a vein to remove blood. This is called phlebotomy. Chemotherapy or radiation is also sometimes used to lower the number of red blood cells. New chemotherapy drugs are being studied for use in treating polycythemia vera. With treatment, many patients live with this condition for years. There is a possibility that polycythemia vera can progress to a more acute form of leukemia, so close follow-up is necessary.

What is agnogenic myeloid metaplasia?

In this disorder, red blood cells and certain white blood cells called granulocytes do not mature properly. The spleen may swell and there may be too few mature red blood cells to carry oxygen, causing anemia, which may require red cell transfusions. Usually, if there are no serious symptoms, the doctor will follow your case closely so you can be treated if symptoms develop. Treatments include: external radiation to the spleen or chemotherapy to reduce swelling of the spleen, or hormone therapy to increase the number of red blood cells, or surgery to remove the spleen. Clinical trials of biological therapy are being tested.

What is essential thrombocythemia?

In essential thrombocythemia, the number of platelets in the blood is much higher than normal, although the other blood cells are normal. The extra platelets make it hard for blood to flow normally. Treatment for this condition includes platelet pheresis, in which a special machine is used to filter platelets from the blood. Chemotherapy may be used to lower the number of platelets in the blood. New drugs and biological therapy are being studied in clinical trials.

Web Pages to Check Out

www.cancer.gov: For general up-to-date information, and for clinical trials.
www.cancer.org: For general up-to-date information and community resources.
www.leukemia-lymphoma.org: Patient information from Leukemia and Lymphoma Society.
www.bloodbank.com: Information about blood tests.

Also, see Chapter 2, Searching for Answers on the Web, for more information.

Nineteen

HODGKIN'S DISEASE, NON-HODGKIN'S LYMPHOMA, AND MULTIPLE MYELOMA

The term lymphoma is a general term for a group of cancers that develop in the lymph system, a part of the body's immune defense system. Lymphoma can start almost anywhere in the body—in a single lymph node or in a group of lymph nodes and can spread to any part of the body, including the liver, bone marrow, and spleen. Usually, the first thing a person notices is a painless swelling of lymph nodes in the neck, under the arms, or in the groin. Lymphomas occur when there is an error in the way a lymphocyte is produced. The lymphocytes may duplicate faster than normal cells or they can live longer than normal cells. Lymphomas are among the most difficult cancers to understand and to categorize. Lymphomas are divided into two major types: Hodgkin's disease and non-Hodgkin's lymphoma. Some lymphomas remain dormant with few symptoms for many years, while others are extremely aggressive. Multiple myeloma involves the plasma cells and other white blood cells that are part of the immune system.

LYMPHOMAS

Although Hodgkin's disease and non-Hodgkin's lymphoma are both lymph system diseases with some similarities, they differ widely in cell origin, how they spread, and how they are treated. The most common type of lymphoma is called Hodgkin's disease. All other lymphomas are grouped together and are called non-Hodgkin's lymphomas. In diagnosing lymphoma, the doctor will need to know the number and location of affected lymph nodes, the type of lymphoma, and whether the disease has spread to the bone marrow or organs outside the lymphatic system. Pinpointing the exact type requires that you be tested carefully before a diagnosis is made.

What You Need to Know About Hodgkin's Disease and Non-Hodgkin's Lymphoma

- Lymphoma is a general term for cancers that develop in the lymph system. They account for about three percent of all cases of cancer in this country.

- The cure rate for early stage Hodgkin's disease is nearly 90 percent in some treatment centers.

- Many special tests are needed to diagnose and stage lymphoma.

- Because treatment decisions for lymphomas are very complex, it is especially important that treatments be carried out at institutions that have skilled pathologists, modern radiation equipment, and a team of physicians who are expert in treating the disease.

- Treatments usually include radiation and chemotherapy. Bone marrow or peripheral stem cell transplants are sometimes used in treating late-stage lymphomas. See Chapter 11, New Advances and Investigational Treatments.

What is the lymph system?
The lymph system is made up of a network of thin tubes that branch, like blood vessels, into the tissues throughout the body. The tubes carry lymph, a colorless, watery fluid that contains infection-fighting white blood cells, called lymphocytes, to all parts of the body. Situated along this network of vessels are groups of small glands, called lymph nodes. Other parts of the lymphatic system include the spleen, thymus, and bone marrow.

What is the role of the spleen?
The spleen, located on your left side near the stomach, is an organ that produces lymphocytes, filters the blood, stores blood cells, and destroys those that are aging. It is the only organ capable of mounting an immune response to antigens that are borne by the blood. Once the spleen is removed it does not grow back. However, its normal functions are taken over by other body tissues and its absence does not interfere with normal living.

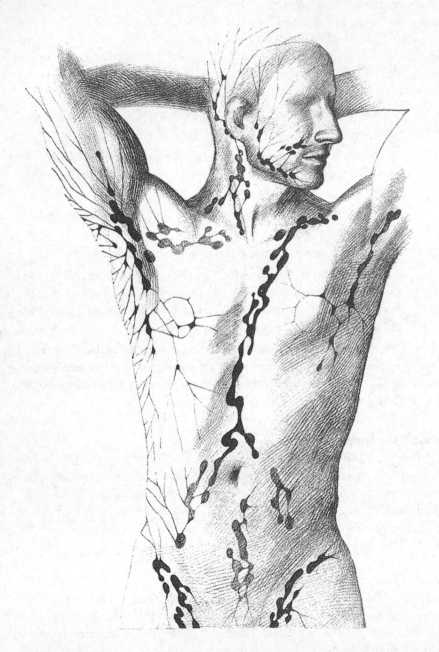

Lymph system

What is the thymus?
The thymus is an organ in which lymphocytes mature and multiply. It lies behind your breastbone.

What does the bone marrow do?
The bone marrow is soft, spongy tissue in the center of your large bones that produces white blood cells, red blood cells, and platelets.

Where are the lymph nodes found?
Clusters of lymph nodes are found throughout your body—behind the ears, in the groin, behind the knees, in the front of the elbow, under the armpit, at the angle of the jaw, deep inside the abdominal cavity, at the junction of the right and left bronchi and in many other areas. They trap and help destroy foreign particles and disease-causing agents. As the lymph passes through the nodes, they filter out foreign substances and pick up more lymphocytes. Lymph nodes are part of your body's immune system.

What is the role of the immune system?
The immune system is a complex network of specialized organs and cells that defends your body against infection. The organs of the immune system are often referred to as "lymphatic" organs because they are concerned with the growth, development and deployment of lymphocytes, the white blood cells that are the key workers of your immune system. Lymphatic organs include the bone marrow, thymus, spleen and lymph nodes, as well as the tonsils, appendix and clumps of lymphatic tissue in the small intestine known as Peyer's patches. Some nonlymphatic organs, like the skin, liver and lungs, also contain circulating lymphocytes and play a major role in immunity.

How does Hodgkin's disease differ from non-Hodgkin's lymphoma?
Hodgkin's disease, first identified by Thomas Hodgkin in 1832, has unique microscopic features that distinguish it from other lymphomas. Often, it is recognized by the presence of unique cells, called the Reed-Sternberg cells, in lymph tissue that has been removed by surgery for biopsy. Also Hodgkin's disease tends to follow a more predictable pattern of spread, which is generally more limited than that of the non-Hodgkin's lymphomas. By contrast, some non-Hodgkin's lymphomas (extra nodal) can begin in organs like the liver and bones rather than in the lymph nodes.

Has Agent Orange been associated with Hodgkin's disease or non-Hodgkin's lymphoma?
Agent Orange is a mixture of herbicides used during the Vietnam War mainly to defoliate forest trees. Both Hodgkin's disease and non-Hodgkin's lymphoma

have been associated with Agent Orange and herbicides used during the Vietnam War. If you are a Vietnam veteran and have been diagnosed with Hodgkin's disease or non-Hodgkin's lymphoma, you should qualify for VA disability compensation and the special access to medical care that the VA has offered to Vietnam veterans for health problems from Agent Orange exposure. You do not need to prove that your illness is related to your military service. It is presumed to be service-connected. For more information, see Chapter 4, What Is Cancer?

What are the symptoms of lymphoma?
The most common symptom is a painless swelling in the neck, underarm or groin, caused by enlarged lymph glands. The affected lymph node is usually painless, firm, rubbery in consistency, and freely movable.

If I have an enlarged lymph gland should I see a doctor immediately?
Lymph glands may be enlarged as a result of infections or other illnesses such as mononucleosis or rheumatoid arthritis—but if you have a lymph gland in the neck, armpit, or groin that remains enlarged for three weeks or longer, you should check with your doctor. If you have had a recent infection or another problem that could cause an enlarged lymph gland, the doctor may decide to delay doing the biopsy for a few days or a few weeks, while watching to see if it clears up. When lymph node swelling lasts more than six weeks and does not respond to antibiotics, it is suggestive of lymphoma. The only sure way to determine whether or not you have lymphoma is for the doctor to examine lymph tissue that has been surgically removed by biopsy.

Why is staging so important?
Because the symptoms, rate, pattern of spread, and the treatment of lymphomas vary greatly, it is important that the disease be accurately diagnosed by an experienced pathologist (or hematopathologist) who can recognize subtle cellular distinctions among the many lymphatic cancers. The nature and extent of your first treatment influences and can severely limit future treatments. Therefore, it is important for the doctor to stage your condition correctly before beginning treatment. The staging procedure may take several weeks.

Questions to Ask Your Doctor If You Have Hodgkin's Disease or Non-Hodgkin's Lymphoma

- **Is the disease confined to one area or more than one area?**
- **What are my treatment choices?**
- **Can you explain the cell type and how my disease has been staged?**

- **Will I become sterile as a result of the treatment? Is there anything I can do to avoid sterility? Can I bank my sperm? Can my fertility be preserved?**

- **If I am pregnant, must my pregnancy be terminated? Will I be able to have more children? Will my children's DNA be affected?**

- **Will I be able to continue to work? Will I be able to continue to exercise?**

- **Will I have long-term side effects as a result of the treatment?**

- **How long will the treatment last?**

- **What new treatments are being studied?**

- **Would a clinical trial be appropriate for me?**

Can sterility occur in a male as the result of treatment for lymphoma?

Yes, and this issue should be discussed with your doctor at the outset, because some of the treatments are known to cause sterility. There may be changes in sperm due to drugs and radiation therapy and sperm-banking may be needed.

Can treatment for lymphoma affect a woman's menstrual cycles and her fertility?

Radiation therapy in the abdomen or pelvic area can result in loss of ovarian function. Women may wish to have an oophoropexy (an operation which moves the ovaries to a protected spot behind the uterus) before beginning radiation therapy. This helps preserve ovarian function by shielding the ovaries from exposure to radiation during treatment. At some research centers, ovarian tissue is being frozen for future egg development, but the technology is at a basic stage.

Can lymphoma occur during pregnancy?

It is very rare, but both Hodgkin's and non-Hodgkin's lymphoma can occur during pregnancy. If the lymphoma is in the neck or underarm area only, it can usually be treated with radiation therapy, with the fetus shielded. If the disease is more extensive and the pregnancy is in its first four and a half months, a therapeutic abortion may be suggested. During the last half of pregnancy, treatment will depend on the stage of the pregnancy and the aggressiveness of the disease. Sometimes treatment is delayed.

Can I have a baby after I've been treated for lymphoma?

The doctor will usually advise that you wait for a period of time after remission before you become pregnant. Lymphoma itself does not necessarily have an adverse effect on fertility, the course of pregnancy, labor, or the baby. The treatment and its side effects, however, must be taken into consideration in making a judgment. If you have lymphoma, you should consult with your doctor about family planning. However, many women have become pregnant and delivered normal children after they have had intensive treatment for lymphoma. Furthermore, studies show that when compared to the general population, treatment for lymphoma does not appear to cause birth defects or medical diseases or cause damage to a future baby's chromosomes.

Are there other long-term side effects as a result of the treatment?
It depends upon the treatment being given. Some patients find they have relatively minor long-term complications. For others, the side effects may be severe. Organs, such as the lungs, heart, or kidneys may be affected. You may be at higher risk for leukemia in the future. You need to discuss the risks and management of these risks with your health care team.

What is a mini-transplant?
A mini-transplant, also known as a nonmyeloablative stem-cell transplant, is being used for older persons and others with leukemia, myeloma, and lymphoma who are not able to withstand the regular bone transplant. This investigational treatment uses lower level radiation—about six times less than a regular transplant. It means that the person's own bone marrow cells are not totally destroyed. No chemotherapy is used. Stem cells, from a donor are transplanted to strengthen the immune system to be able to fight the cancer.

What are the side effects of the mini-transplant?
The side effects, such as nausea, vomiting, hair loss, and fatigue are much fewer than with the regular transplant. The treatment is usually done as an outpatient treatment, so there is no hospital stay as with the traditional transplant.

HODGKIN'S DISEASE

The most common type of lymphoma is called Hodgkin's disease. Before 1970, most people with Hodgkin's disease often died within two years of diagnosis. Today, Hodgkin's disease is usually curable, particularly if it is discovered early. More than 75 percent of all newly diagnosed patients with Hodgkin's disease are curable with modern radiation therapy, chemotherapy, or a combination of the two treatments. Both adults and children are diagnosed with Hodgkin's disease. Treatment of Hodgkin's disease in children, is discussed in Chapter 24, When a Child Has Cancer.

WHO GETS HODGKIN'S DISEASE?

▪ Younger people, with the peak age between 15 and 34.

▪ People over the age of 54.

▪ More common in males than in females.

▪ Family history of Hodgkin's disease increases risk for other brothers and sisters.

▪ Those who have been exposed to Agent Orange.

What is Hodgkin's disease?

Hodgkin's disease is a type of lymphoma. In Hodgkin's disease, cells in the lymphatic system grow abnormally and the disease can spread to other organs. As the disease progresses, the body is less able to fight infection. Hodgkin's disease is rare. It accounts for less than one percent of all cases of cancer in this country.

What causes Hodgkin's disease?

The causes of Hodgkin's disease are not fully understood. There are many theories that have been explored, such as viruses, environment, and genetics. However, what causes the disease or what is required to prevent it are not known. People who have had mono—infectious mononucleosis—are slightly more susceptible than those who have not had mono. The Epstein-Barr virus has been suspected, but its role is unclear. People with AIDS or who take immune suppressing drugs have a slightly increased chance of getting Hodgkin's. It may have a hereditary factor, as some families often have a number of members with Hodgkin's. Hodgkin's disease usually starts in one lymph gland and spreads in an orderly pattern to nearby chains of lymph nodes. It can start anywhere in the body and spreads through the lymph system.

Are there different kinds of Hodgkin's disease?

Hodgkin's disease is divided into two classifications: Nodular lymphocyte-predominant Hodgkin's lymphoma that accounts for about three to eight percent of the Hodgkin's lymphomas. It is often localized and progresses slowly. The other classification which accounts for most cases of Hodgkin's is known as classical Hodgkin's lymphoma and it is divided into four different types:

- nodular sclerosis Hodgkin's (grades 1 and 2)
- lymphocyte rich classical Hodgkin's
- mixed cellularity Hodgkin's
- lymphocyte depletion Hodgkin's

The nodular sclerosis type is most common in women, adolescents, and young adults. The mixed cellularity type is less common, occurring in 20 to 40 percent of cases and is seen more often in males. Lymphocyte depletion Hodgkin's is quite rare, appearing in only three percent of cases, usually in older males or those with HIV.

What kinds of doctors and hospitals are best for treating Hodgkin's disease?

It is important to be in the hands of a team who has experience in treating this disease. A multidisciplinary team of cancer specialists, including radiation oncologists, surgeons, pathologists, and medical oncologists, should be consulted so that a proper treatment plan can be made. The high cure rates for this cancer are due to excellent results achieved with modern radiation therapy and effective combination chemotherapy. Be sure you are treated at a major institution that has modern equipment for giving radiation therapy and uses treatment planning simulators.

SYMPTOMS OF HODGKIN'S DISEASE

- Painless swelling in the neck, armpit, or groin.
- Fevers, night sweats, fatigue, and weight loss.
- Itching and reddened patches on the skin.

Are fever, weight loss, and night sweats often symptoms of Hodgkin's disease?

Fever, weight loss, and night sweats are symptoms often seen in Hodgkin's disease. A pattern of high fever alternating with normal or subnormal body temperature may also be seen.

Is itching a common symptom for those with Hodgkin's disease?

Sometimes itchy skin—or pruritus, as it is sometimes referred to by the medical profession—marks the early stages of Hodgkin's disease. The itchiness can be concentrated in one place, or all over the body. It usually disappears with treatment of the disease and some relief may be possible with antihistamines. It may return at a later time. Any recurrence should be reported to your doctor.

How is Hodgkin's disease diagnosed and staged?

Hodgkin's disease has special characteristics that distinguish it from the other lymphomas. It needs to be carefully staged because the extent of disease

TESTS THAT MAY BE DONE FOR HODGKIN'S DISEASE

- Complete history with special attention to unexplained fever, night sweats, or weight loss of more than ten percent in prior six months.

- Physical examination with particular attention to lymph nodes, liver, spleen and bone tenderness.

- Chest x-ray.

- CT scan.

- MRI scan.

- Ultrasound.

- Blood and urine tests.

- Bone marrow biopsy.

- Lymphogram.

- Gallium scan.

- Biopsy of lymph node.

Depending on condition, these may also be needed:

- Liver, spleen and bone scans.

- Splenectomy.

- Liver biopsy.

- Kidney tests.

- Staging laparotomy (in selected patients only.)

strongly influences the choice of treatment. Many different kinds of tests are involved. If Hodgkin's disease is suspected, the doctor will ask about your medical history and will do a thorough physical exam. In addition, blood tests, tests of the liver and urine, x-rays and scans of the chest or abdomen and a lymphogram may be ordered. A Gallium scan may also be used. The doctor will perform a biopsy, removing tissue from an enlarged lymph node. It is important that the disease be accurately diagnosed by an experienced pathologist who can recognize subtle cellular distinctions among the various lymphatic cancers. The pathologist will look at the tissue under the microscope for abnormal cells, called Reed-Sternberg cells that are usually found with Hodgkin's disease.

What are Reed-Sternberg cells?

These are abnormal cells that help confirm a diagnosis of Hodgkin's disease, but in general they are difficult to detect. They are named for the two scientists who first identified them. Finding the Reed-Sternberg cells alone is not enough to diagnose Hodgkin's disease, because they have been found in other diseases.

Why is the diaphragm important in diagnosis?

The diaphragm, a thin muscle below your lungs and heart that separates the chest cavity from the abdominal cavity, is important for determining treatment. You will hear the doctor talking about your disease being above or below the diaphragm or on one side or both sides of it. If you have it on one side of the diaphragm, either below or above it, it will be treated differently than if it is found on both sides.

What is a lymphogram?

A lymphogram or a lymphangiogram is an x-ray of the abdomen, pelvis, or chest. It shows the size of the lymph nodes and detects abdominal lymph node involvement which may not be seen through other tests. In many institutions today, CT scans or MRIs are used instead of, or in addition to, the lymphogram.

How is a lymphogram done?

Small incisions are made in the skin of the feet. After the local anesthetic has been given, an oil-based dye is injected into the lymph system. The lymph system carries the dye up the legs and into the abdominal lymph nodes. When the x-rays are taken, the dye outlines the lymphatic system. It shows the size of the various lymph nodes, their shape and even their internal structure. This allows the doctor to identify abnormal nodes. The patterns of lymph flow that show up on the x-rays are also important, because lymph does not pass easily through the nodes that are filled with cancerous cells, so abnormal patterns of lymph flow develop. Thus, the doctor is able to identify involved nodes and to choose several lymph nodes to remove and examine. Because the dye remains in the lymph vessels for a long period of time after a lymphogram, x-rays can be taken during and after treatment to monitor the effects of treatment on the cancer. Following the test, the skin may look blue or green and urine may also be colored blue or green. This color should disappear in 48 hours.

How long does it take to do a lymphogram?

The lymphogram takes several hours the first day, with follow-up x-ray films on the second day. Further testing is usually done and the dye remains in the lymph nodes for a few months to more than a year.

What else do I need to know about having a lymphogram?

Be sure to tell the doctor or nurse if you feel any shortness of breath after the dye has been injected. Wear loose shoes to avoid irritating the area where the incisions are made. Do not put your feet in water until the stitches are out. Clean the area every day with alcohol. Report any signs of redness or swelling to the nurse or doctor. You may have some possible side effects. They include: a bluish color in your feet and your urine, allergic reaction to the dye, infection where the incision was made, and fever within 24 hours of the injection.

How will the biopsy be done?

Usually, the biopsy is done under local anesthesia in a doctor's office or in a one-day surgery center. After the operation, depending on its location, you will need to wear loose-fitting clothing over the surgical site. You will also need to wait until the stitches are removed before bathing the area.

What is a laparotomy?

A laparotomy is an operation to explore the entire abdomen. It allows the doctor to determine the extent of disease and if it has spread to the abdomen.

Is a laparotomy routinely used to diagnose Hodgkin's disease?

No. Several years ago, laparotomy was a routine procedure for diagnosing Hodgkin's disease. It is usually restricted to patients in whom radiation alone will be used and is done only if the information gained will actually reduce the treatment. It is not necessary for patients who require combination chemotherapy.

What is the sedimentation rate?

This laboratory test determines the speed at which erythrocytes settle. An anticoagulant is added to the blood and placed in a long narrow tube. The distance the red cells fall in one hour becomes the sedimentation rate, sometimes referred to as the ESR. In Hodgkin's disease, a sedimentation rate of less than 50 is considered favorable.

What are the stages of Hodgkin's disease?

After the initial tests have been completed, the extent of disease is staged by a widely used system called the Ann Arbor Staging Classification of Hodgkin's disease. It divides Hodgkin's disease into four stages:

Stage I: Cancer is found in only one lymph node area or in only one area or organ outside of the lymph nodes. (If you have Stage I disease and none of the other symptoms, you would be listed as having Stage IA. If you had one or more of the B symptoms, you would be listed as having Stage IB.)

Stage II: Cancer is found in two or more lymph node areas on the same side of the diaphragm, or cancer is found in only one area or organ outside of the lymph nodes and in the lymph nodes around it. Other lymph node areas on the same side of the diaphragm may also be found to be cancerous.

Stage III: Cancer is found in lymph node areas on both sides of the diaphragm. The cancer may also have spread to an area or organ near the lymph node areas and/or to the spleen.

Stage IV: Cancer has spread in more than one spot to an organ or organs outside the lymph system. Cancer may or may not be found in the lymph nodes near these organs, or cancer has spread to only one organ outside the lymph system, but lymph nodes far away from that organ are involved.

Recurrent: Cancer has come back after it has been treated. It may come back in the area where it first started or in another part of the body.

What do the letters after the stage mean?

Stages of Hodgkin's disease are indicated by A, B, or E categories. If there are no symptoms, an "A" is used. B symptoms include the following: loss of more than 10 percent of weight in the previous six months, fever without any known cause other than Hodgkin's disease, or night sweats that leave the body soaked. (There is some disagreement about the importance of night sweats, but if they are recurrent and drenching, they may be considered in designating a stage "B" category.) "E" means that disease has been found in or extends to tissues beyond, but near, the major lymphatic clusters.

How and where does Hodgkin's disease spread?

Hodgkin's disease begins in a lymph node, often in the neck and spreads in a predictable pattern from the original site to lymph nodes in other areas. It usually spreads first to nearby lymph nodes and then to the nearby organ. In advanced Hodgkin's disease, the lungs, spleen, liver and bone marrow may also be affected.

How is Hodgkin's disease treated?

The treatment depends upon the person's medical history, age, type, and stage of disease. The usual treatment for most patients with early Hodgkin's disease is a combination chemotherapy, and high-energy radiation. New dose-intensive, time-condensed chemotherapy regimens, as well as chemotherapy with bone marrow transplants and mini-transplants are being studied in clinical trials for patients with advanced disease. Please see Chapter 11, New Advances and Investigational Treatments, for information on these transplants.

STAGES OF HODGKIN'S DISEASE

STAGE	DESCRIPTION
Stage I	Cancer is found in only one lymph node area (I) or in only one area or organ outside of the lymph nodes (IE).
Stage II	Cancer is found in two or more lymph node regions on the same side of the diaphragm (II); or Cancer is found in only one area or organ outside of the lymph nodes and in the lymph nodes around it. Other lymph node areas on the same side of the diaphragm may also have cancer (IIE).
Stage III	Cancer is found in the lymph node regions on both sides of the diaphragm (III). The cancer may also have spread to an area or organ near the lymph node areas (IIIE), or to the spleen (IIIS) or both (IIIE + S). Stage III (1) indicates the cancer is limited to the upper abdomen. Stage III (2) indicates involvement of pelvic and/or para-aortic nodes. Zero to four nodules on the spleen are classified as minimal disease in the spleen. Five or more nodules constitute extensive disease in the spleen.
Stage IV	Cancer has spread in more than one spot to an organ or organs outside the lymph system. Cancer cells may or may not be found in the lymph nodes near these organs; or Cancer has spread to only one organ outside the lymph system, but lymph nodes far away from that organ are involved.
Recurrent	Cancer has come back after it has been treated. It may come back in the area where it first started or in another part of the body.

Is it wise to be vaccinated against the flu or pneumonia before treatments begin?

It is recommended that vaccinations for flu, pneumonia and meningitis be given at least a week or two before treatments begin.

How successful are the treatments for Hodgkin's disease?

The success of the treatment for Hodgkin's disease is one of the outstanding stories of modern oncology. Before 1970, few patients with advanced Hodgkin's disease recovered from their illness. Most died within two years. Today the outlook is much brighter. More than half of all patients with **advanced** Hodgkin's disease are disease-free after follow-up of more than ten years. For early stage Hodgkin's patients, the news is even better. The cure rate has risen to nearly 90 percent in major cancer centers. This success has been due mainly to the use of new combinations of chemotherapy and modern radiation treatment techniques that allow large doses of radiation to be given, while shielding normal tissues to prevent unnecessary damage.

How is radiation treatment planned?

A technique called a treatment planning simulator is used to plan your radiation treatment and is essential in treating Hodgkin's disease. The simulator takes detailed x-rays of the position you will be in when you get your treatment so that the radiation fields can be designed to conform to your body. Individually shaped protective blocks are made to shield your normal tissues.

What is the mantle field?

This is a term used by the radiation oncologists to describe the part of the upper area of the body to be treated by radiation. It has the shape of an arrow, with the point starting at the neck and the base extending to the diaphragm. It encompasses the lymph nodes in the upper part of the body. The heart and lungs are protected during treatment by lead shields, to reduce the risk of complications to these organs.

What is the inverted Y?

This term is used to describe the part of the lower area of the body to be treated by radiation. Shaped like an upsidedown Y, it extends from the diaphragm to the lower border of the pelvis and includes the lymph nodes in the lower part of the body.

What kind of chemotherapy treatments are used to treat Hodgkin's disease?

The standard treatment is a drug combination, ABVD (doxorubicin, bleomycin, vinblanstine, and DTIC). Sometimes, MOPP (mechlorethamine, Oncovin, procarbazine, and prednisone) and ABVD are given as alternating treatments. In addition, there are other combinations that have proved to be effective and are now also considered standard options when chemotherapy is needed.

How long will it take after all these treatments for my energy level to return?

It depends on your age, stage of disease, and intensity of the treatment. It takes longer for older patients and patients with advanced disease who received combined treatments. The return to normal energy levels may take up to a year or more.

TREATMENTS FOR HODGKIN'S DISEASE

STAGE	TREATMENT
Stage IA	*If your cancer is above the diaphragm and does not involve a large part of your chest, your treatment may be one of the following*:
	Combination chemotherapy (ABVD) and radiation therapy **or**
	Radiation to upper part of the body (mantle field) and to the lymph nodes in the upper abdomen; **or**
	Radiation to mantle field and lymph nodes in upper area; **or** radiation to mantle field only after surgery to determine stage of tumor; **or**
	Clinical trial of combination chemotherapy alone.
	If your cancer is above the diaphragm but involves a large part of your chest, your treatment may be one of the following:
	Radiation to the upper body (mantle field) plus combination chemotherapy **or**
	Radiation therapy to mantle field and to the lymph nodes in the upper abdomen.
	If your cancer is below the diaphragm, your treatment may be one of the following:
	Radiation to the lymph nodes in the upper abdomen and pelvis. The spleen or the groin may also be treated if needed **or**
	Combination chemotherapy with radiation therapy **or**
	Clinical trials of chemotherapy alone.
Stage IB	Combination chemotherapy with radiation therapy **or**
	Clinical trials of chemotherapy alone.
Stage IIA	*If your cancer is above the diaphragm and does not involve a large part of your chest, your treatment may be one of the following*:
	Combination chemotherapy and radiation therapy **or**
	Radiation to the upper body (mantle field) and to the lymph nodes in the upper abdomen **or**
	Radiation to mantle field only after surgery to determine stage of tumor **or**
	A clinical trial of combination chemotherapy.
	If your cancer is above the diaphragm, but involves a large part of your chest, your treatment may be one of the following:
	Radiation to upper body (mantle field) plus chemotherapy

(continued)

TREATMENTS FOR HODGKIN'S DISEASE *(continued)*

STAGE	TREATMENT
Stage IIB	Combination chemotherapy with or without radiation **or**
	Clinical trials of chemotherapy alone.
Stage IIIA	*If your cancer does not involve a large part of your chest, your treatment may be one of the following:*
	Combination chemotherapy alone **or**
	Combination chemotherapy plus radiation **or**
	Clinical trial of chemotherapy.
	If the cancer involves a large part of the chest, treatment may be:
	Combination chemotherapy with radiation therapy.
Stage IIIB	Combination chemotherapy with radiation therapy **or**
	A clinical trial of chemotherapy.
Stage IV	Combination chemotherapy **or**
	Combination chemotherapy and radiation **or**
	Clinical trials of chemotherapy with bone marrow transplantation.
Recurrent disease	Treatment depends on where disease has returned and treatment received before.
	If previous treatment was radiation therapy without chemotherapy, treatment may be chemotherapy.
	If treatment was chemotherapy without radiation therapy and cancer comes back only in lymph nodes, treatment may be radiation therapy to the lymph nodes, with or without more chemotherapy. If disease comes back in more than one area, treatment may be more chemotherapy or a clinical trial of high doses of chemotherapy with bone marrow or peripheral stem cell transplantation.

Will there be sexual side effects?

Impotence and inadequate sperm counts have been reported in men even before treatment begins. Radiation to the pelvic area and some of the chemotherapy drugs can cause sexual problems for both men and women, including infertility, low sexual desire, erection problems, weaker orgasms, vaginal dryness, painful intercourse, and reduced vaginal size. There is more information on side effects in Chapter 9, Radiation Treatments, and Chapter 10, Chemotherapy. Sexuality is discussed in Chapter 27, Living with Cancer.

Is there any long-term danger to this intensive radiotherapy and chemotherapy?

In spite of the effectiveness of the treatments, there is the possibility of long-term effects. Several studies have shown an association between certain therapies and the development of leukemia many years later. The risk of leukemia is about three percent at ten years according to most studies. It seems to be highest in patients over 40 who have been treated with both intensive radiotherapy and intensive chemotherapy. Recent research at the National Cancer Institute indicates that the risk of leukemia seems to decline after ten years. In the past, women treated for Hodgkin's disease with radiation before the age of 30 were at a markedly increased risk for breast cancer, with the risk increasing dramatically more than 25 years after therapy. The newer treatments and drug combinations will hopefully show a decrease in these risks. Infertility has been seen in those who have had MOPP chemotherapy regimens. ABVD treatment does not seem to have an effect on testicular and ovarian function. ABVD appears to be the treatment with the least overall toxic side effects.

What treatment is available for a patient who relapses after the first set of treatments?

It depends on the first treatment and also on the stage of the disease. If the treatment was radiation, chemotherapy may be administered. If chemotherapy had been given, another combination of drugs may be used. A bone marrow or peripheral stem cell transplant may be considered. There is more information on bone marrow transplants in Chapter 11, New Advances and Investigational Treatments.

Do people who have AIDS get Hodgkin's disease?

Some people with AIDS also may get Hodgkin's disease. This may be explained by the fact that many AIDS patients are young or because AIDS patients have a weakened immune system. AIDS patients usually have Stage III or IV Hodgkin's disease when they are diagnosed. The disease may be found in the skin or bone marrow, which is not usual in other patients.

Is the treatment different for persons with AIDS?

The treatment is similar, but it depends on the health of the patient. Most patients with AIDS do not tolerate the chemotherapy drugs as well as other patients. They get more infections during treatment. While their remission rates are similar to other patients, because of their other complications, they live a shorter time than is usually expected for persons with the same stage of disease.

How often should I see a doctor for checkups after being treated for Hodgkin's disease?

Careful follow-up will be needed, and may vary for different types and stages of Hodgkin's disease. Generally, you will have regular visits with your doctor every month or two for the first year; then every three to six months for the next four years, and every year after that. Chest x-rays and blood tests will probably be done at every visit. At the end of the first year, your doctor may order CT scans of the chest and abdomen. The critical time is the first five years. If you are disease-free after five years, you are probably cured.

Are there any symptoms I should report to the doctor?

Yes. You should report any unusual fever, itching, night sweats, lumps, or breathing problems.

NON-HODGKIN'S LYMPHOMA

The term non-Hodgkin's lymphoma encompasses a host of different lymphomas. They have been lumped together in the past because they all affect the lymph system. Most of them start within a lymph node, but a significant number start in places such as the jaw or brain. Modern technology now makes it possible to differentiate between different subtypes. Some lymphomas seem to be more like leukemias than lymphomas and the medical profession is constantly reclassifying the various subtypes. That's why it is important that you remember, in comparing yourself with others who seem to have the same diagnosis, that there are many subtle differences that may explain the difference in treatment. Some lymphomas spread more quickly than others, and are more difficult to treat. However, major advances have been made in treating non-Hodgkin's, though the annual number of new cases of non-Hodgkin's lymphoma has nearly doubled since the 1970s.

What is non-Hodgkin's lymphoma?

Non-Hodgkin's lymphoma is a cancer that develops in the lymph system—but can spread to organs other than lymph nodes—such as the liver or the bones. It is seven or eight times more common than Hodgkin's disease. There are at least ten types of non-Hodgkin's lymphomas. Often they are grouped by how fast they grow—low grade (slow growing), intermediate grade, and high grade (rapidly growing). Or they may be grouped by immunology-oriented classifications. It's important that you learn from your doctor exactly which type you are dealing with and what the various names are for the type you have.

How is non-Hodgkin's lymphoma different from Hodgkin's disease or leukemia?

Epstein-Barr virus is seldom found in the more common non-Hodgkin's lymphomas. Where most leukemias release large numbers of easily detectable cancerous cells into the blood stream, non-Hodgkin's lymphomas do not.

Who is most likely to have non-Hodgkin's lymphoma?

More males than females get non-Hodgkin's lymphoma. It can strike people as young as age 40, although those over age 65 are at highest risk. Childhood non-Hodgkin lymphomas, which are quite rare, may resemble lymphoblastic leukemia, and are often successfully treated with aggressive chemotherapy. Those with deficiencies in their immune system, whether inherited (Wiskott-Aldrich syndrome and Bloom's syndrome), a result of autoimmune disease (rheumatoid arthritis, systemic lupus erythematosus) or acquired (organ transplant patients, AIDS patients) and those exposed to Agent Orange are at increased risk for developing the disease. For reasons not understood, the incidence of lymphoma is increasing yearly, especially in people with autoimmune deficiencies, such as AIDS. Interestingly, people who have an allergy to plants, those who experience multiple bee and wasp stings, and those who have had five or more vaccinations, are less likely to develop the disease.

What causes non-Hodgkin's lymphoma?

The cause of non-Hodgkin's lymphoma remains unknown. It is thought that certain viruses, deficiencies in the immune system and chromosome abnormalities play a part. Some people who have had long-standing Sjögren's syndrome develop diffuse aggressive lymphomas or immunoblastic lymphomas. It is believed that there may be an association between the two diseases.

SYMPTOMS OF NON-HODGKIN'S LYMPHOMAS

- Painless swelling in the neck, armpit, or groin.
- Fevers, night sweats, fatigue, and weight loss.
- Itching and reddened patches on the skin.
- Nausea and vomiting or abdominal pain.

What kind of doctor is best for treating non-Hodgkin's disease?

The treatment planning for non-Hodgkin's disease is complex. Therefore, it is extremely important that you are in the hands of doctors who have experience in treating lymphoma. The best solution is to find a well-trained multidisciplinary team of cancer specialists, including radiation oncologists, surgeons, pathologists, and medical oncologists. Since the treatment is influenced by the cell type, it is important that the biopsy results be carefully reviewed by a pathologist who is experienced in diagnosing lymphoma. Be sure that the institution where you are being treated has modern radiation equipment and treatment planning simulators, as well as medical oncologists who are experts in chemotherapy.

Are there any new treatments for non-Hodgkin's lymphoma?

After years of research, a monoclonal antibody called Rituxan was approved by the FDA for use in patients with non-Hodgkin's lymphoma. Bexxar is another drug that combines monoclonal antibodies with radioactive iodine, enabling the iodine to kill cancer cells at close range. On the horizon are two vaccine treatments for the indolent form of non-Hodgkin's lymphoma. The outlook for patients with many types of non-Hodgkin's lymphoma is very promising.

How is non-Hodgkin's disease diagnosed and staged?

Non-Hodgkin's disease needs to be carefully staged because the type of tumor and the extent of disease strongly influence the choice of treatment. Many different kinds of tests are involved. If non-Hodgkin's disease is suspected, the doctor will ask about your medical history and will do a thorough physical exam. The doctor will perform a biopsy of an enlarged lymph node, removing tissue that will be examined under the microscope. In addition, blood tests, tests of the liver and urine, x-ray of the chest, CT scan of the abdomen and biopsy of the bone marrow, liver and other accessible sites will be done. A gallium scan may also be used.

How will the lymph node biopsy be done?

Usually, the lymph node biopsy is done under local anesthesia in a doctor's office or in a one-day surgery center.

What is a lymphogram?

A lymphogram, or a lymphangiogram as it is sometimes called, is a test done to look for evidence of lymphoma in the abdominal lymph nodes, which usually cannot be felt.

When is a lymphogram used in non-Hodgkin's lymphoma?

It is rarely used, but may be necessary in some patients to verify early-stage disease in the lower abdomen. It is not used in patients whose disease is more advanced. (You will find details on how a lymphogram is done in the section on Hodgkin's disease earlier in this chapter.)

Is a laparotomy commonly used to stage non-Hodgkin's disease?
No. A laparotomy, an operation to explore the entire abdomen to determine the extent of disease, is not routinely used in non-Hodgkin's lymphoma because most non-Hodgkin's lymphoma patients have the disease below the diaphragm and do not require the operation for staging. Laparotomy, if used, is reserved for the few patients with early stage disease, in whom evidence of the disease in the abdomen would change the treatment from radiation therapy to chemotherapy.

How are the different types of non-Hodgkin's lymphoma classified?
Around the world, there are at least six different systems to classify the many different types of non-Hodgkin's lymphomas. This fact alone points to the difficulty that the medical profession has in categorizing the various types of lymphoma. In fact, some professionals feel that lymphoma and leukemia result from the same malignant cell. Some of the systems place major emphasis on structure of the cell that becomes cancerous; others on the arrangement of the cells when examined under the microscope. In 1982, an international panel of expert pathologists developed a classification system, called the International Working Formulation, to help standardize terms and apply new knowledge gained from the science of immunology. In the Working Formulation, lymphomas are classified depending upon the type of cell found in the cancer and on the arrangement of the cells. The types fall into three basic groups: low grade, intermediate grade, and high grade. A newer system called the REAL classification system was introduced in 1994. It was further refined in 1997 and called the WHO classification. This system divides B-cell neoplasms into two major categories with a long list of subcategories and T-cell and NK-cell types into two major categories with a long list of subcategories. The PDQ has modified the REAL classification into two main categories, indolent and aggressive.

What types are low grade lymphomas?
The low grade lymphomas are small lymphocytic, follicular small cleaved cell, and follicular mixed small-cleaved and large cell.

What types are intermediate grade lymphomas?
The intermediate grade lymphomas are follicular large cell, diffuse small cleaved cell, diffuse mixed cell, and diffuse large cell.

What types are classified as high grade lymphomas?
The high grade lymphomas are immunoblastic large cell, lymphoblastic convoluted or nonconvoluted cell, small cleaved cell (Burkitt's or non-Burkitt's) and HTLV-1.

TESTS FOR NON-HODGKIN'S LYMPHOMA

- Complete history with special attention to unexplained fever, night sweats or weight loss of more than ten percent in prior six months.

- Physical examination with particular attention to lymph nodes, liver, spleen, and bone tenderness.

- Fine needle aspiration.

- Biopsy of lymph node.

- Spinal tap.

- Bone marrow tests.

- Chest x-rays.

- CT scan.

- MRI scan.

- Ultrasound tests.

- Blood and urine tests.

- Liver and kidney function tests.

- Gallium scan (in selected patients.)

- Lymphogram (in patients, with abdominal CT scans that are negative.)

- PET scan.

Who is at highest risk for intermediate and high grade lymphoma?

Intermediate and high grade lymphomas are often seen in patients with AIDS, who require special treatment.

Are low grade lymphomas easier to treat than high grade lymphomas?

Not necessarily. Aggressive non-Hodgkin's lymphomas can sometimes be more successfully treated than low grade or indolent tumors.

What is the Rappaport system?

You may hear references to the Rappaport system, an older system of classification that is now less commonly used. In this system, a non-Hodgkin's lymphoma is described as either nodular or diffuse, based on the growth pattern of the cancer cells as seen through the microscope. The disease is further classified by cell type. If the cancer cells are small and resemble lymphocytes, it is called lymphocyte lymphoma. If the cancer cells are large and resemble macrophages or histiocytes, it is called histiocytic lymphoma. If the cells have both features, it is called mixed lymphoma. The Rappaport system also describes lymphoma cells as either poorly differentiated or well differentiated. Poorly differentiated cancer cells have poorly defined borders and are irregular in structure and size. Cancer cells that are more normal when looked at under the microscope are referred to as well differentiated.

What is meant by an indolent lymphoma?
Indolent lymphomas spread slowly and often take years to develop into aggressive disease. Most nodular lymphomas are called indolent or favorable histiocytic lymphomas. These include: follicular small cleaved cell lymphoma, follicular mixed cell lymphoma, follicular large cell lymphoma, adult diffuse small cleaved cell lymphoma, and small lymphocytic lymphoma. Also included in this group are a number of rarer types, including mycosis fungoides and Sezary syndrome.

What are aggressive lymphomas?
Most of the diffuse types, which tend to progress rapidly, are called aggressive, or unfavorable, histology lymphomas. These include: adult diffuse mixed cell lymphoma, adult diffuse large cell lymphoma, adult immunoblastic large cell lymphoma, adult lymphoblastic lymphoma, adult small noncleaved cell lymphoma, and at least 14 other, rarer subtypes. Without treatment, these rapidly growing lymphomas can progress very quickly. However, these lymphomas respond favorably to chemotherapy treatment.

What is the most common type of non-Hodgkin's lymphoma?
The most common type is diffuse large B-cell lymphoma that accounts for 31 percent of all newly diagnosed cases.

What is primary CNS lymphoma?
CNS is shorthand for central nervous system. Primary CNS lymphomas are tumors of the lymph system that begin in the brain. You also can have a lymphoma that begins in another part of the body and spreads to the brain. The primary CNS lymphomas that are not AIDS related are usually B-cell lymphomas that begin in the central nervous system. They occur at random in the general population and in patients with deficiencies in their immune systems.

Are there any other types of lymphomas?
There are certain types of non-Hodgkin's lymphomas that have unique features that distinguish them. They include Burkitt's lymphoma (a childhood B-cell lymphoma generally found in tropical Africa), lymphoblastic lymphoma (a childhood lymphoma most often of T-cell origin), and cutaneous T-cell lymphoma (originally called mycosis fungoides).

TYPES OF NON-HODGKIN'S LYMPHOMA AND HOW THEY ARE REFERRED TO UNDER TWO SYSTEMS

WORKING FORMULATION	PDQ MODIFICATION OF REAL CLASSIFICATION
Low Grade	**Indolent**
A. Small lymphocytic (SL)	Follicular lymphoma
B. Follicular, small cleaved cell (FCS)	Small lymphocytic lymphoma Lymphoplasmacytic lymphoma
C. Follicular, mixed cell, cleaved and large cell (FM)	Extranodulal marginal zone-Bell cell lymphoma
	Nodal marginal zone B-cell lymphoma Splenic marginal zone lymphoma
	Mycosis fungoides
	Primary cutaneous anaplastic large cell lymphoma
Intermediate Grade	**Aggressive**
D. Follicular, large cell (FL) E. Diffuse, small cleaved cell (DSC) F. Diffuse, mixed cell, small and large cell (DM) G. Diffuse, large cell, cleaved or noncleaved cell (DL)	Diffuse clear cell lymphoma (includes diffuse mixed cell, diffuse large cell, immunoblastic, T-cell rich large B-cell lymphoma) Burkitt's lymphoma Precursor B- or T-cell lymphoblastic lymphoma Primary CNS lymphoma Adult T-cell lymphoma
	Mantle cell lymphoma
	Polymorphic posttransplantation lymphoproliferative disorder
	AIDS-related lymphoma
	True histiocytic lymphoma
	Primary effusion lymphoma
	Aggressive NK-cell lymphoma

(continued)

TYPES OF NON-HODGKIN'S LYMPHOMA AND HOW THEY ARE REFERRED TO UNDER TWO SYSTEMS (continued)

WORKING FORMULATION	PDQ MODIFICATION OF REAL CLASSIFICATION
High grade	
H. Immunoblastic, large cell (IBL)	
I. Lymphoblastic, convoluted or nonconvoluted cell (LL)	
J. Small noncleaved cell, Burkitt's or non-Burkitt's (SNC)	

What are the stages of non-Hodgkin's disease?

After the initial tests have been completed, the extent of disease is staged by a widely used system called the Ann Arbor Staging Classification. It divides non-Hodgkin's disease into four stages:

Stage I: Cancer is found in only one lymph node area, or in only one area or organ outside of the lymph nodes.

Stage II: Cancer is found in two or more lymph node areas on the same side of the diaphragm, or cancer is found in only one area or organ outside of the lymph nodes and in the lymph nodes around it. Other lymph node areas on the same side of the diaphragm may also have cancer.

Stage III: Cancer is found in lymph node areas on both sides of the diaphragm. The cancer may also have spread to an area or organ near the lymph node areas and/or to the spleen.

Stage IV: Cancer has spread to more than one spot to an organ or organs outside of the lymph system. Cancer may or may not be found in the lymph nodes near these organs, or cancer has spread to only one organ outside of the lymph system, but lymph nodes far away from that organ are involved.

Recurrent: Cancer has come back after it has been treated. It may come back in the area where it first started, or in another part of the body.

What does an A, B or E added to the stage mean?

An "A" means there are no general symptoms. A "B" designates that the patient has any of the following symptoms: unexplained loss of more than

STAGES OF NON-HODGKIN'S DISEASE

STAGE	DESCRIPTION
Stage I	Involvement of only one lymph node region (I); **or**
	Localized involvement of a single extralymphatic organ or site (IE).
Stage II	Cancer is found in two or more lymph node regions on the same side of the diaphragm (II) **or**
	Cancer is found in only one associated extralymphatic organ or site and its regional lymph nodes with or without other lymph node regions on the same side of the diaphragm (IIE).
	Lymph node regions involved may be indicated by a number (II3).
Stage III	Cancer is found in the lymph node regions on both sides of the diaphragm (III). The cancer may also have spread to an area or organ near the lymph node areas (IIIE), or to the spleen (IIIS) or both (IIIE + S).
Stage IV	Cancer has spread to more than one organ or organs outside of the lymph system. Cancer cells may or may not be found in the lymph nodes near these organs **or**
	Cancer has spread to only one organ outside of the lymph system, but lymph nodes far away from that organ are involved.
Recurrent	Cancer has come back after it has been treated. It may come back in the area where it first started or in another part of the body.
Primary CNS lymphoma	Tumors of the lymph system that begin in the brain.

10 percent of body weight in the six months before diagnosis, unexplained fever, or drenching night sweats. Thus, your stage could be designated as IA or IB, depending upon the absence or presence of these symptoms. An "E" denotes that the disease has extended into nearby tissues.

What do the other letters added to the stage mean?
Other letters indicate where there is other involvement. "N" means that nodes are involved, "S" refers to spleen, "H" to liver, "P" to pleura, "L" to lung, "O" to bone, "M" to bone marrow and "D" to skin.

Are there any other factors used for staging non-Hodgkin's lymphoma?

Several other factors are taken into account by the doctor when staging non-Hodgkin's lymphoma. These include the grade of disease, its cell type, size of the tumor, sites of involvement, age of the patient, and LDH values.

How and where does non-Hodgkin's lymphoma spread?

In many cases, by the time non-Hodgkin's lymphoma is diagnosed, cancer cells often have already spread throughout the body, including abdominal lymph nodes, liver, bone marrow, and the gastrointestinal tract.

How is non-Hodgkin's lymphoma treated?

The treatment depends upon the person's medical history, age, type, grade, stage of disease. The treatment can include radiation of the lymph nodes, combination chemotherapy or drugs and radiation given together. Bone marrow and peripheral stem cell transplants are being studied in clinical trials for certain patients. See Chapter 11, New Advances and Investigational Treatments.

Are monoclonal antibodies being used to treat non-Hodgkin's Lymphoma?

Some monoclonal antibodies have been designed to attack lymphoma cells. (Monoclonal antibodies are made to link up with matching antigens on the surface of a particular cell.) When used alone, the treatment, unlike standard chemotherapy or radiation, does not cause cumulative toxic effects. The drug is genetically engineered to latch onto the surface of the malignant white blood cells that form in patients with non-Hodgkin's lymphoma. The body recognizes this antibody as a foreign invader and the immune system begins an attack that destroys only those cells to which the antibody is attached. One such product called Rituxan, or rituximab, is being used together with combination chemotherapy for the initial treatment of people with lymphoma. It is also used if the lymphoma reoccurs following chemotherapy.

How is primary CNS lymphoma treated?

Primary CNS lymphoma is treated either with chemotherapy or chemotherapy and radiation. Clinical trials with different kinds of drugs are under study. In patients over 60, radiation can cause dementia over time so use of radiation in older patients is usually reserved for use with recurrent CNS lymphoma.

What kinds of lymphoma are most common in persons infected with HIV?

People who test positively for HIV are four times more likely to develop non-Hodgkin's lymphoma than the general public. Most of them will have high grade B-cell lymphoma (small noncleaved Burkitt's and non-Burkitt's or immunoblastic), intermediate grade B-cell lymphoma (large cell), or central nervous system lymphoma. In over 50 percent of the patients, the lymphoma will be found after AIDS has been diagnosed. The lymphomas are found in all of the major risk groups, including homosexual men, intravenous drug users, and children of HIV-positive individuals.

Is the treatment for patients with AIDS-related lymphoma different?

Both the treatment and the response to the treatment are different. AIDS-related lymphoma is usually diagnosed with advanced disease that has spread outside of the lymph nodes and is less responsive to chemotherapy, thus the treatment is more aggressive.

What factors need to be considered when selecting treatment for AIDS-related lymphoma?

Several factors need to be considered, such as how severe the deficiency of the immune system is, what kind of infectious illnesses the person has had, whether the bone marrow and other organs are involved, and how healthy the patients are at the time of treatment.

TREATMENTS FOR AGGRESSIVE NON-HODGKIN'S DISEASE

STAGE	TREATMENT
Aggressive Stage I and Contiguous Stage II	Chemotherapy plus radiation therapy.
Aggressive, Noncontiguous Stage II, III and IV	Combination chemotherapy **or** Bone marrow transplantation or peripheral stem cell transplant (being evaluated). *Clinical trials*: evaluating new combination chemotherapy
Recurrent Aggressive Non-Hodgkin's	Bone marrow transplant **or** Bone marrow transplant plus radiation. *Clinical trials*: chemotherapy, bone marrow transplant or peripheral stem cell transplant and radiation, immunotherapy

TREATMENTS FOR INDOLENT NON-HODGKIN'S DISEASE

STAGE	TREATMENT
Indolent	Radiation to the area where cancer cells are found **or**
Stage I and contiguous	Radiation to area where cancer cells are found and extended to nearby lymph nodes **or**
Stage II	Radiation to part or all of the lymphatic system **or**
	Chemotherapy plus radiation therapy are being evaluated **or**
	Chemotherapy alone **or**
	Watchful waiting if radiation therapy is not possible.
Indolent, noncontiguous	If you do not have symptoms, treatment may be delayed until symptoms appear.
Stages II, III, IV	Chemotherapy with a single drug **or**
	Chemotherapy with single drug with or without steroids **or**
	Combination chemotherapy.
	Clinical trials: radioimmunotherapy with or without combination chemotherapy (NOTE: Anti CD20 monoclonal antibody (rituximab) sometimes used as first line therapy either alone or with combination chemotherapy); chemotherapy plus radiation therapy plus bone marrow transplant or peripheral stem cell transplant; chemotherapy with or without immunotherapy
Recurrent indolent (low grade)	Bone marrow transplant or Bone marrow transplant plus radiation therapy.
	Clinical trials: chemotherapy, bone marrow transplant or peripheral stem cell transplant and radiation; radioimmunotherapy

What other areas are usually involved in AIDS-related lymphoma?

The most common sites are the GI (gastrointestinal) tract, central nervous system, bone marrow, and liver. Some patients have involvement of the rectum, heart or the sac around it, lungs, bile ducts, mouth or soft tissues.

How often should I see a doctor for checkups after being treated for non-Hodgkin's lymphoma?

Careful follow-up will be needed and may vary for different types and stages of non-Hodgkin's disease. Generally, you will be checked every three months for the first year; every four months for the second to the fifth years, then yearly thereafter. You will probably have chest x-rays and blood tests at every visit. Every year, you may have ultrasound or CT scans of the abdomen and pelvis.

What symptoms should I be looking for to report to the doctor?

You should watch out for loss of appetite or loss of weight, fever, pain, lumps, difficulty in breathing, intestinal symptoms, problems with your balance, or a change in personality.

What is primary lymphoma of the stomach?

Malignant lymphoma sometimes is limited to the stomach. Sometimes these cancers, when they are small, disappear with antibiotic therapy. If the cancer involves the entire gastric wall and if it involves the lymph nodes in the surrounding area, it is usually treated with chemotherapy drugs and possibly, radiation. If there is upper gastrointestinal bleeding, surgery may be used before chemotherapy is given.

What is anaplastic large cell lymphoma?

Anaplastic large cell lymphoma is an aggressive lymphoma that is sometimes confused with Hodgkin's disease or melanoma. It can be successfully treated in 70 percent of cases with combination chemotherapy such as CHOP.

What is mantle cell lymphoma?

Mantle cell non-Hodgkin's lymphoma is a rare type of lymphoma that is difficult to diagnose. It involves lymph node groups and infiltrates the bone marrow. It may also involve the spleen, liver, gastrointestinal system, peripheral blood and Walyer's ring (tonsillar tissue). It is considered an intermediate grade lymphoma. Aggressive combination chemotherapy treatment can bring about complete remissions in many cases. Retuxin (Retuximab, Mabthera) is being used with success in many cases. Promising results have also been achieved using aggressive acute leukemia-like treatments with bone marrow transplants.

CUTANEOUS T-CELL LYMPHOMA
(MYCOSIS FUNGOIDES)

What is cutaneous T-cell lymphoma?

Cutaneous T-cell lymphoma is a rare chronic type of malignancy (also known as mycosis fungoides) that usually affects the skin and can be present for many years. In its early stages it may stay confined to one area for long periods of time. The disease progresses slowly and patients may live for many years with localized disease. Eventually the lymph nodes and internal organs may become involved. When large numbers of the tumor cells are found in the blood, the condition is called the Sezary syndrome. Cutaneous T-cell lymphoma is frequently difficult to diagnose in its initial stages, and several biopsies may be required before it is accurately diagnosed.

Is cutaneous T-cell lymphoma a fungus?

The disease was named mycosis fungoides several centuries ago when it was thought to be caused by a fungus. It has long been recognized as a disease primarily affecting the reticuloendothelial system—cells scattered throughout the body that destroy other cells, bacteria, and fragments of foreign materials, form antibodies, as well as regulate immune reaction and blood cells.

What kind of doctor should be treating cutaneous T-cell lymphoma?

It is a rare disease and needs to be treated in a major medical center. Treatments should be made by the joint decisions of dermatologist, medical oncologist, and radiation oncologist.

What are the symptoms of cutaneous T-cell lymphoma?

Reddish plaquelike tumors of scaly, thickened skin may develop. They may resemble eczema or psoriasis and may be found on the back, arms, stomach, face, scalp or other parts of the body. They may itch or spread and ulcerate. In the next stage, called the infiltration stage, lymph nodes may be enlarged and the skin becomes infiltrated with an overgrowth of reticuloendothelial cells of several kinds that allow a microscopic diagnosis to be made. In the third stage the tumors on the skin may become painful, itchy, uncomfortable and may

---

TREATMENT FOR CUTANEOUS T-CELL LYMPHOMA (MYCOSIS FUNGOIDES)

STAGE	TREATMENT
Stage I	
Appears only in patches of skin, no tumors, lymph nodes normal.	Phototherapy (PUVA) with or without biological therapy **or** Total skin electron beam (TSEB) radiation **or** Topical chemotherapy **or** Local electron beam or x-ray therapy to reduce size of tumor or relieve symptoms. *Clinical trials:* Phototherapy **or** Alpha interferon alone or in combination with topical therapy.

(continued)

TREATMENT FOR CUTANEOUS T-CELL LYMPHOMA (MYCOSIS FUNGOIDES) *(continued)*

STAGE	TREATMENT
Stage II	
Lymph nodes larger than normal but no tumors **or** Tumors on skin but lymph nodes normal or, if larger, do not contain cancer.	Phototherapy (PUVA) with or without biological therapy **or** Total skin electron beam radiation (TSEB) **or** Topical chemotherapy **or** Local electron beam or x-ray therapy **or** Alpha interferon alone or with topical therapy.
Stage III	
Nearly all skin affected but lymph nodes are free of cancer.	Phototherapy (PUVA) with or without biological therapy **or** Topical chemotherapy **or** Local electron beam or x-ray therapy **or** Systemic chemotherapy with or without therapy to skin **or** Chemotherapy for mycosis fungoides and Sezary syndrome **or** Extra coporeal photochemotherapy **or** Alpha interferon alone or in combination with topical therapy **or** Retinoids.
Stage IV	
Skin is involved and cancer cells are found in lymph nodes or cancer has spread to other organs.	Systemic chemotherapy **or** Topical chemotherapy **or** Total skin electron beam (TSEB) radiation **or** Phototherapy **or** Local electron beam or x-ray therapy **or** Chemotherapy for mycosis fungoides and Sezary syndrome **or** Monoclonal antibodies **or** Extra coporeal photochemotherapy **or** Retinoids.

TREATMENT FOR CUTANEOUS T-CELL LYMPHOMA (MYCOSIS FUNGOIDES) *(continued)*

STAGE	TREATMENT
Recurrent Cancer returns after being treated.	Depends upon many factors including previous treatment, may include: Local electron beam or x-ray therapy **or** TSEB radiation therapy **or** Phototherapy **or** Topical chemotherapy **or** Systemic chemotherapy **or** Extra coporeal photochemotherapy. *Clinical trials:* biological therapy **or** bone marrow transplant.

become infected. In the fourth stage, the lymph nodes, liver, or lung may be involved.

How is cutaneous T-cell lymphoma staged?
Staging depends on how the cancer has spread.

Stage I: The cancer only affects parts of the skin. There are red, dry, scaly patches, but no tumors. The lymph nodes are not enlarged.

Stage II: The skin has scaly patches but no tumors; lymph nodes are larger than normal, but do not contain cancer cells, or there are tumors on the skin but the lymph nodes do not contain cancer cells.

Stage III: Nearly all the skin is red, dry, and scaly. The lymph nodes are either normal or are larger than normal, but do not contain cancer cells.

Stage IV: Cancer cells are found in the lymph nodes, or the cancer has spread to other organs, such as the liver or lung.

Recurrent: The cancer returns after being treated.

MULTIPLE MYELOMA

Multiple myeloma begins in the plasma cells that are part of the immune system. In a healthy person, these blood cells produce antibodies to fight infection. Multiple myeloma weakens and damages bones, destroying the normal bone tissue and creating an environment for bone breakdown by osteoblasts. When plasma cells grow out of control, they can produce tumors that grow in multiple places in the bone marrow—giving the disease its name.

Is multiple myeloma the same as bone cancer?
No, it is not. Although multiple myeloma affects the bones, it begins in the cells of the immune system. Bone cancer, on the other hand, begins in the cells that form the hard, outer part of the bone. Multiple myeloma is treated differently than bone cancer.

What is a plasmacytoma?
If the myeloma cells are collected in only one bone and form a single tumor, it is called plasmacytoma. If plasma cell tumors are found in the soft tissues of the tonsils or tissues around the nose, it is referred to as an extramedullary plasmacytoma. If the myeloma cells collect in many bones and form many tumors, it is called multiple myeloma. Some people with plasmacytoma may develop multiple myeloma eventually.

How is plasmacytoma of the bone treated?
If you have a single tumor of the plasma cells that is found in the bone, with no M-protein found in the blood or urine, you will probably be treated with radiation therapy. However, sometimes surgery is used to remove a single plasmacytoma.

What is MGUS?
MGUS is an abbreviation for monoclonal gammopathy of undetermined significance. It is a precancerous condition with characteristics that are similar to multiple myeloma. Patients with this diagnosis have no symptoms of multiple myeloma and usually do not receive treatment. They are closely monitored for plasma cell and M-protein changes.

What is smoldering myeloma?
Smoldering myeloma is a slowly progressing or stable form of multiple myeloma. No symptoms are evident and no treatment is recommended unless the disease begins to progress.

What is macroglobulinemia?

This is a type of plasma cell abnormality in which lymphocytes that make an M-protein build up in the blood. This condition is sometimes referred to as Waldenstrom's macroglobulinemia. Lymph nodes and liver and spleen may be swollen. If there are no symptoms, treatment may not be needed. If symptoms develop, treatment may be chemotherapy, biologic therapy, or immunotherapy. New drugs and drug combinations are being tested. Stem cell support or transplant may be used in addition to chemotherapy.

Who usually gets multiple myeloma?

Multiple myeloma is most often seen in adults between the ages of 50 and 70. Only 2 percent of cases are found in people younger than age 40. More men than women have multiple myeloma and it is more common among blacks than whites.

Has Agent Orange been associated with multiple myeloma?

Agent Orange is a mixture of herbicides used during the Vietnam War mainly to defoliate forest trees. Multiple myeloma has been associated with Agent Orange and other herbicides used during the Vietnam War, but not as strongly as some other cancers. It is classified in the second category: limited/suggestive evidence of an association. However, if you are a Vietnam veteran and have been diagnosed with multiple myeloma, you should qualify for VA disability compensation and the special access to medical care that the VA has offered to Vietnam veterans for health problems from Agent Orange exposure. You do not need to prove that your illness is related to your military service. It is presumed to be service-connected. For more information, see Chapter 4, What Is Cancer?

What are the symptoms of multiple myeloma?

Symptoms of multiple myeloma depend on whether the disease is in an early or late stage. In the earliest stage, there may be no symptoms and the disease may be discovered through blood and urine tests. If there are symptoms, there may be anemia, or bone pain in the back or ribs. Broken bones may also occur. Other possible symptoms include: weakness, a tired feeling, weight loss, nausea, vomiting, constipation, night sweats, problems with urination, repeated infections, scrapes, cuts or bruises which cause serious bleeding, lowered resistance to infections such as pneumonia, and weakness or numbness in the legs.

How does the doctor diagnose multiple myeloma?

Multiple myeloma in the early stages may be found during routine blood and urine testing. If anemia is detected, and high levels of M-proteins are seen, an immunoelectrophoresis test is done to confirm the diagnosis. In more advanced cases, x-rays may show the patches of bone that have been destroyed, along with the number and size of tumors in the bones. Blood and urine tests are used to detect whether they contain high levels of antibody proteins (M-proteins) which suggest the presence of this disease. A bone marrow aspiration or a bone marrow biopsy is often done to check for myeloma cells. In the bone marrow aspiration, the doctor inserts a needle into the hipbone or breastbone to withdraw a sample of fluid and cells from the bone marrow. To do a bone marrow biopsy, the doctor uses a larger needle to remove a sample of solid tissue from the marrow (a more detailed description of these tests is in Chapter 6, How Cancers Are Diagnosed). Magnetic resonance imaging (MRI) and PET may be used to give close-up views of the bones.

What kind of doctor treats multiple myeloma?

Treatments for multiple myeloma are extremely complex and difficult. You need to be under the care of a doctor—preferably an oncologist or a hematologist—who has experience in treating multiple myeloma.

Are most myeloma patients anemic?

Since cancer cells may prevent the growth of new red blood cells and disease-fighting white blood cells, people with multiple myeloma may be anemic and susceptible to infections, such as pneumonia. They may also have too much calcium in their blood (hypercalcemia), causing loss of appetite, nausea, thirst, fatigue, muscle weakness, restlessness, and confusion. In addition, multiple myeloma patients may have serious problems with their kidneys because they are not filtering and cleaning the blood properly. Transfusions of red blood cells are sometimes given to reduce symptoms of anemia such as shortness of breath and fatigue.

How is multiple myeloma treated?

The treatment depends on the type and stage of disease, your medical history, and age. If you do not have any symptoms of the disease, even though you test positive for it, you will probably not be given any treatment. Rather, the doctor will monitor you carefully and watch for any changes. Your blood protein levels will be checked with immunoelectrophoresis. Chemotherapy is the main treatment for multiple myeloma. Among the drugs being used are melphalan and cyclophosphamide, in combination with prednisone. High-dose chemotherapy with melphalan has been successful, especially for younger patients in good health. Pamidronate is sometimes given monthly to reduce fractures and bone pain. If the spleen is swollen, it may be removed. Bone marrow transplantation may be used to replace the bone marrow with healthy bone marrow. Sometimes radiation therapy will also be used, especially to treat local symptoms in bones. Alpha interferon therapy, monoclonal

STAGES OF MULTIPLE MYELOMA

STAGE	DESCRIPTION
Stage I	Relatively few cancer cells have spread throughout the body. Number of red blood cells and amount of calcium in blood are normal. No tumors (plasmacytomas) found in bone. Amount of M-protein in blood or urine is very low. There may be no symptoms of disease.
Stage II	A moderate number of cancer cells have spread throughout the body.
Stage III	A relatively large number of cancer cells have spread throughout the body. One or more of the following may also be present: a decrease in the number of red blood cells, causing anemia; the amount of calcium in the blood is very high causing bone damage; more than three bone tumors are found; high levels of M-protein are found in the blood or urine.

antibodies, bone marrow transplantation, peripheral stem cell support, and treatment with colony-stimulating factors are being studied in clinical trials for certain patients.

Is thalidomide being used in treating myeloma?
Clinical trials are being done using oral thalidomide for advanced myeloma and for patients who have had high-dose chemotherapy that has failed.

What are zoledronic acid and pamidronate?
Zoledronic acid and pamidronate are bisphosphonates. They have been shown to reduce fractures, compression, hypercalcemia, and the need to give radiation to the bones. They help to maintain strong bones and reduce bone pain and the need for pain medicine, while keeping the disease in check. Both zoledronic acid (Zometa) and pamidronate (Aredia) have been approved by the Food and Drug Administration for use in patients with multiple myeloma. Zoledronic acid is the newer agent and appears to be more effective, takes less time to administer and has fewer side effects.

Are there any other new treatments for multiple myeloma?
According to the Multiple Myeloma Research Foundation, a number of new treatments are being tested. The drug Velcade (sometimes referred to as PS341 or MLN341) appears to block the myeloma cells' ability to resist traditional chemotherapy. The biotech company Celgene is working to produce a variety of thalidomide called Revimid that is safer and more potent. It appears to block the formation of new blood vessels and inhibits the pro-

TREATMENTS FOR MULTIPLE MYELOMA

STAGE	TREATMENT
Stage I	*If you have no symptoms:* Careful monitoring to see if disease progresses. *If you have symptoms:* Chemotherapy, with localized radiation therapy, if needed to treat bone tumors **or** Clinical trial of new treatment methods.
Stage II	Chemotherapy, with radiation therapy, if needed to treat bone tumors **or** Clinical trial of new treatment methods.
Stage III	Chemotherapy, with radiation therapy, if needed to treat bone tumors **or** Clinical trial of new treatment methods. Monthly intravenous pamidronate used to reduce fractures.
Isolated plasmacytoma of bone	External radiation therapy to tumor. If other symptoms appear, chemotherapy may be needed.
Extramedullary plasmacytoma	External radiation therapy to tumor **or** Surgery to remove tumor, usually followed by external radiation therapy. If other symptoms appear, chemotherapy may be needed.
Macroglobulinemia	*If you have no symptoms:* Careful monitoring to see if symptoms develop. *If you have symptoms:* Chemotherapy treatment **or** If blood becomes too thick, plasmapheresis to filter cells from blood. *Clinical trials:* new chemotherapy drugs and combinations of drugs.
Monoclonal gammopathy of undetermined significance	Close monitoring to see if symptoms of plasma cell neoplasm or lymphoma develop.
Refractory plasma cell neoplasm	Chemotherapy. *Clinical trials:* new drugs and combinations of drugs.

duction of growth factors as well as boosting the body's immune response. In addition, antiangiogenesis agents and proeasome inhibitors are being tested. Mini-transplants are also being studied (they are discussed earlier in this chapter, as are tandon transplants in which two transplants are being done instead of one).

Is exercise important to the myeloma patient?

Talk to your doctor and nurses about what kind of exercise is appropriate for you. Because exercise helps reduce calcium loss in the bones, it is important to be as active as possible. If movement is a problem, a cane or a walker can help provide a wider base of support and make it possible for you to get more exercise.

What kind of medical risks do myeloma patients face?

Because myeloma places such a burden on the body, many of the body systems are put under unusual stress. Hypercalcemia—excessive calcium in the blood—can lead to kidney failure or coma. Vertebral compression fractures can immobilize the body, causing paralysis of the body and the limbs. There is a susceptibility to serious infections, such as pneumonia and staph infections, because the immune system is seriously impaired.

What can be done to relieve bone pain?

If you have bone pain, make sure you discuss it with your health team so that pain medicine can be prescribed. Back and neck braces are also helpful. Some people have found that relaxation and imagery can help reduce their pain. Radiation therapy may be used to control severe bone pain and to stabilize areas that are likely to fracture. There is more information on controlling pain in Chapter 27, Living With Cancer.

What can be done to help prevent kidney problems?

Drinking plenty of fluids is important, since it helps the kidneys to get rid of excess calcium in the blood and prevents problems that occur when calcium collects in the kidneys. Dialysis may be used if kidneys are not working well. In dialysis, wastes are removed by machine and cleansed blood is returned into the body.

What can be done if the blood becomes very thick?

Plasmapheresis is helpful when an accumulation of myeloma proteins causes the blood to become very thick, interfering with circulation and causing stroke-like symptoms. Plasmapheresis removes excess blood from the veins and separates blood cells from blood plasma. Plasmapheresis helps relieve threatening symptoms but it does not kill the myeloma cells.

Can I do anything to prevent infections?

Since multiple myeloma weakens the immune system, you must do everything possible to protect yourself from infection. Don't get any inoculations of vaccines made with live materials. Drink plenty of liquids and eat a diet high in calories and protein. Try to stay away from people who have colds, coughs, or sore throats. Tell your doctor if you have signs of infection, such as a fever, sore throat, rash, tired feeling, or difficult or painful discharge of urine. Get enough sleep. Nap if you feel tired.

Web Pages to Check Out

www.cancer.gov: General up-to-date information and for clinical trials.

www.cancer.org: General up-to-date information and community resources.

www.leukemia-lymphoma.org: Patient information from Leukemia and Lymphoma Society.

www.lymphomainfo.net: Lymphoma Information Network.

www.ohsu.edu/cliniweb: Cliniweb International.

www.lymphoma.org/lymphoma.html: Lymphoma Research Foundation.

www.curehodgkins.com: On-line news magazine for Hodgkin's patients.

www.multiplemyeloma.org: Clinical trials and other information from the Multiple Myeloma Research Foundation.

www.Novartis.com: Information on Zometa.

Also see Chapter 2, Searching for Answers on the Web, for more information.

Other Resources

Non-Hodgkin's Lymphomas: Making Sense of Diagnosis, Treatment and Options, Lorraine Johnston (O'Reilly & Associates, 1999).

Twenty

GYNECOLOGICAL CANCERS

The female reproductive system remains a mystery to many women, even though we are reminded of its existence by monthly menstrual periods. Although most women know that a lump in the breast is not to be ignored, many remain uninformed about the danger of ignoring symptoms of problems in the reproductive tract. Since so many of the cancer problems that occur in this part of a woman's body are silent, regular checkups are a wise insurance policy. Though many women consider the pelvic examination a nuisance at best, and an embarrassing experience at worst, the examination takes on a whole different aspect when you stop to appreciate the incredible biological design of this part of the body. The better we understand how it all works, the better able we are to listen to our bodies and detect problems at a point when something can be done. Human papilloma virus (HPV) infections are found in the majority of cancers of the cervix, vulva, and vagina.

WHEREVER YOUR CANCER is located in your reproductive system, it is helpful to know as much as you can so you can ask the right questions and make the right decisions about your treatment.

What You Need to Know About Cancers of the
Female Reproductive Organs

- Many operations for these kinds of cancers affect your ability to have children. They also may affect your ability to have sexual relations.

- Since each part of the female reproductive system is unique, treatment varies depending upon the location of the tumor.

- Make sure you understand exactly what is going to be done to you, what organs will be affected and what side effects you can expect before you have any treatments.

- A Pap test can accurately detect cancer of the cervix. It is not a test for detecting cancer of the endometrium, fallopian tubes, or ovaries.

- Minimally invasive surgery, which makes several little incisions in your body, is being used for many gynecologic operations. This is also called laparoscopic or keyhole surgery.

Where do female reproductive system cancers occur?

The areas involved include:

- Cervix

- Endometrium (also called the uterus or womb)

- Ovaries and fallopian tubes

- Vagina

- Vulva

What is the doctor looking for when doing a pelvic exam?

The pelvic exam lets the doctor see the vagina and cervix. The doctor can also feel the uterus, vagina, ovaries, and fallopian tubes and can take a Pap smear. The doctor uses a speculum to widen the opening of the vagina to make it easier to see the upper part of the vagina and cervix. Once this portion of the examination is complete, the doctor usually examines the rectum. By inserting one finger into the rectum and one finger into the vagina, the physician is actually examining both areas at the same time, providing another opportunity to feel the uterus and ovaries. The doctor is looking for irritations, infections, and warts, as well as any abnormalities in shape and size.

Can the Pap test detect cancers in the female tract?

A Pap test can accurately detect cancer of the cervix, but it is not a test for detecting cancer of the endometrium, fallopian tubes, or ovaries. In cases

WHO IS AT RISK?

SITE	AGE	RISK AND PREVENTIVE FACTORS
Cervix	30–60	Human papilloma virus (HPV) infections in genitals; sexual intercourse before age 16; multiple sex partners; sex with partners who have had multiple partners; younger women whose mothers took DES; genital herpes virus; smoking; HIV infection; possibly oral contraceptives.
Endometrium (Lining of uterus or womb)	55–70	Heavy women; high calorie, high-fat diets; women with high blood pressure, diabetes, endometrial hyperplasia, or inherited form of colorectal cancer; women who use hormone replacement therapy or take tamoxifen; infertility due to ovulation failure; family history; few or no pregnancies; early menstruation; late menopause.
Ovarian	40–70	History of breast cancer or hereditary non-polyposis colorectal cancer; Ashkenazi Jewish descent; no pregnancies; family history of several members with ovarian cancer—mother, sister, daughter, grandmother, aunt, cousin; use of talc in genital area; use of postmenopausal estrogen.
Vagina	60–80 (12–30 if mother took DES)	Genital viruses; chronic irritation; women who have had hysterectomies. Mother took DES during pregnancy.
Vulva	Fifty percent with preinvasive are 20–40; older women (60 and over) at risk for invasive	Chronic vulvar disease; previous malignancy of lower genital tract; history of breast cancer; herpes papilloma virus; herpes simplex 2; exposure to coal tar derivatives.

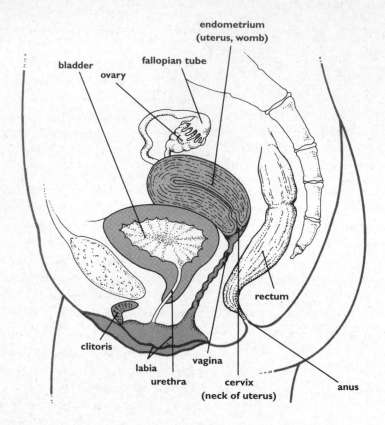

Female reproductive organs (ILLUSTRATION BY DOLORES BEGO)

where these types of cancer are discovered through a Pap smear, it is because the cancer cells have passed down into the cavity of the uterus and continued through the cervix and into the vaginal discharge.

What kinds of sexual side effects can result from treatment of cancers of the female reproductive organs?

Side effects vary, depending upon the location of the cancer, and the type of treatment. Some treatments have little or no effect on sexuality. Some women find that after a hysterectomy, for example, they are more relaxed and enjoy sex because they are no longer worried about becoming pregnant. Other women report vaginal problems that may be associated with surgery, radiation, or chemotherapy.

SYMPTOMS OF CANCERS OF THE FEMALE REPRODUCTIVE TRACT

SITE	SYMPTOMS
Cervix	Abnormal bleeding, may start and stop between regular periods, or may occur after intercourse, douching, orpelvic exam. Increased vaginal discharge. Often NO symptoms.
Endometrium (Lining of the uterus or womb)	Abnormal bleeding after menopause, pain during sexual intercourse; difficult or painful urination; pain in the pelvis. May begin as watery, blood-streaked discharge.
Ovarian	Swelling, bloating, discomfort in lower abdomen; loss of appetite, feeling full even after light meal; gas, indigestion, nausea, weight loss. Often no **early** symptoms.
Vagina	Vaginal bleeding, vaginal discharge, pelvic pain. Often NO symptoms.
Vulva	Intense itching; lesions sometimes seen, may be white, red, or darkly pigmented.

What can be done if the vagina becomes narrowed after treatment for gynecological cancer?

Treatments for cancers in the gynecological area sometimes result in a condition called vaginal stenosis that causes the narrowing of the muscles and tissues that form the walls of the vagina. Vaginal stenosis can result from the formation of scar tissue, making essential pelvic exams or sexual intercourse difficult. Information on using a dilator to help keep vaginal opening flexible can be found later in this chapter.

Is high-dose rate brachytherapy used in treating gynecologic cancers?

High-dose rate brachytherapy is sometimes used in treating gynecologic cancers, depending on the cancer and its stage. It may be used alone as an intracavitary or an interstitial implant to deliver a precisely targeted dose of radiation to tissues, or it may be used in combination with external beam radiation.

CANCER OF THE CERVIX

What You Need to Know About Cancer of the Cervix

- Many women's Pap tests show changes in the cells of their cervix. Most of these changes do **NOT** lead to cancer. Most clear up on their own without any treatment.

UNDERSTANDING THE MEANING OF GYNECOLOGICAL OPERATIONS

OPERATION	PROCEDURE	WHAT YOU SHOULD KNOW
Laparoscopy	Small incisions made in lower abdominal wall; laparascope and other surgical instruments inserted through the scope or through another small cut.	Sometimes used in diagnosis in ovarian, fallopian tubes, and uterus or to remove organs in abdomen or pelvis. General anesthesia used.
Leep loop electrosurgical excision procedure	Removal of tissue using electrical current passed through a thin wire loop which acts as knife.	Can be used for biopsy or for treatment. Local anesthesia to numb cervix. Treatment lasts only a few minutes.
Cone biopsy (Conization)	Cone-shaped removal of localized abnormal cervical tissue to evaluate extent of disease.	More extensive than simple biopsy. Usually performed under general anesthesia but sometimes done under local anesthesia in doctor's office. Increased risk of miscarriages, difficulties with labor, and possible infertility.
Subtotal or **Supracervical hysterectomy**	Uterus is removed, but cervix remains.	Will be unable to have children. Normal sexual relations.
Vaginal hysterectomy	Uterus removed through vagina.	Not advisable if uterus is enlarged or not fully movable. More difficult to perform than hysterectomy. Lose ability to become pregnant.
Total hysterectomy	Removal of cervix and uterus.	No longer fertile. Will not menstruate. Normal sexual relations.
Radical hysterectomy, also called Wertheim's operation	Removal of uterus, fallopian tubes, and ovaries as well as much of tissue surrounding uterus, regional lymph nodes and part of vagina.	Because of extent of operation, may have postoperative complications, which involve vital body systems, bladder, and bowel dysfunctions. If premenopausal, causes abrupt menopause and menopausal symptoms. No longer fertile. Sexual relations still possible.

UNDERSTANDING THE MEANING OF GYNECOLOGICAL OPERATIONS *(continued)*

OPERATION	PROCEDURE	WHAT YOU SHOULD KNOW
Myomectomy	Fibroid tumors removed from wall of uterus, but uterus left intact.	Recommended for younger women with fibroid tumors who wish to retain ability to become pregnant.
Oophorectomy or **Ovariectomy**	Removal of one or both ovaries.	Abrupt menopause if both ovaries removed. If only one removed, may continue to menstruate and can become pregnant. Normal sexual relations.
Salpingectomy or **Bilateral Salpingo oophorectomy**	Removal of fallopian tubes and ovaries.	Menstruation ceases. No longer fertile. Normal sexual relations.
Simple Vulvectomy	Removal of skin of major and minor lips of vulva and clitoris.	Sexual relations still possible.
Radical Vulvectomy	Removal of vaginal lips, clitoris, skin surrounding vulva and lymph glands.	Preoperative radiation often prescribed prior to operation. Sexual relations still possible.
Vaginectomy	Removal of vagina.	Vagina may be smaller or shorter after surgery. Plastic surgery may be necessary.
Pelvic Exenteration	Radical hysterectomy plus removal of rectum and bladder.	For very advanced cancer of cervix. Leaves patient with both bowel and urinary openings on abdomen. Very extreme operation.

- Human papilloma virus (HPV) infection is found in nearly all cases of cervical cancer. An HPV DNA test is now available for cervical screening.

- Research is underway to determine whether or not vaccines can be used against the viruses that cause HPV.

- The number of deaths from cancer of the cervix has **decreased more than 70 percent** during the last 40 years, mainly due to the Pap test and regular checkups.

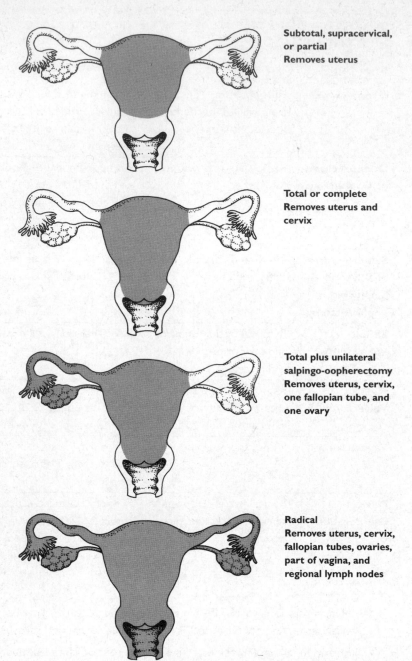

Subtotal, supracervical, or partial
Removes uterus

Total or complete
Removes uterus and cervix

Total plus unilateral salpingo-oopherectomy
Removes uterus, cervix, one fallopian tube, and one ovary

Radical
Removes uterus, cervix, fallopian tubes, ovaries, part of vagina, and regional lymph nodes

Types of hysterectomies (ILLUSTRATIONS BY DOLORES BEGO)

- In its early stages, cancer of the cervix is a highly curable disease—almost 100 percent curable, in fact.

- The accuracy of your Pap test depends on the quality of the laboratory interpreting the slide your doctor sends. You can ask for a reading from another lab or for a second pathology report before action is taken. The new, more accurate liquid Pap test and computerized readings are increasing the accuracy of the test.

- To help insure a more accurate reading it is wise to arrange your appointment between days 15 and 20 of your menstrual cycle. The first day of your period counts as day one.

- Do not douche for at least three days before your Pap test. If you do, there won't be enough loose cells in your vaginal fluid for an accurate test.

- Don't use birth control foam or jelly for five days before the test.

Where is the cervix located?
The cervix connects the uterus (or womb, where a baby develops) with the vagina (birth canal).

Is the cervix part of the uterus?
The cervix is the lower part or neck of the uterus. It protrudes into the vagina and is the segment of the uterus that can be seen by the doctor during a pelvic examination. Cancer of the cervix, or neck of the uterus, and cancer of the endometrium, or body of the uterus, present two very different sorts of problems. It is important for you to find out exactly where your particular cancer is. NOTE: References to endometrium and uterus are used interchangeably in common usage even though endometrium is a more accurate description.

How is the Pap test done?
The Pap smear is a simple, nearly painless test that can be done in a doctor's office, a clinic, or a hospital. Its purpose is to detect abnormal cells in and around the cervix. While a woman lies on an examining table, the doctor inserts a speculum into her vagina to widen the opening. Living cells are collected in and around the cervix, usually with a small cervical brush or a wooden scraper. The specimen is put on a glass slide and sent to a medical laboratory for evaluation. The test is usually done by a gynecologist or other specially trained healthcare professionals, such as physician assistants, nurse midwives, and nurse practitioners. The interpretation of the slide by the laboratory is an important factor in the diagnosis. The percentage of misinterpretations has been shown to be quite high, so it is important to have the test verified before any treatment is undertaken.

WHO IS MOST LIKELY TO GET CERVICAL CANCER?

- Women who have human papilloma virus (HPV) infections in the genitals.
- Women who began having sexual intercourse before 16 years of age.
- Women who have had many sexual partners.
- Women who have sex with partners who have had many sexual partners.
- Women who smoke cigarettes.
- Women over 60 years of age.
- African-Americans, Native Americans and Hispanics.
- Women who have been infected with HIV.

What is a liquid-based Pap test?

This is a new, more accurate type of lab test (it is also known by the brand names such as ThinPrep or AutoCyte). The doctor collects the cells in the same manner as for a regular Pap test. The cells are rinsed or put on liquid fixative and are placed on slides by special machines. The liquid Pap test is more sensitive to finding high and low grade cervical lesions than the regular Pap test, but it is also more expensive.

What do the results of the Pap test mean?

There are usually four terms that are used to describe Pap test results. They are part of a standard set of terms called the Bethesda System, which was first introduced in 1988, revised in 1991, and recently updated. What you will hear are four abbreviations: ASC-US, ASC-H, AGC, and AIS. The first three represent changes in cells, but they are not definite enough for a doctor to know what these changes mean. Fifty percent of the time the changes are caused by minor infection, tissues that are swollen, changes in your menstrual cycle or changes that are part of growing older. The other 50 percent are a sign of human papilloma virus. AIS denotes precancerous cells. If your doctor tells you that you have any of these results, you will need to get more tests or treatment.

Are the terms to describe the results of Pap tests new?

Over the past ten years, this set of terms, called the Bethesda System, has evolved through several changes. A series of studies has identified groups of women who have early cervical cell changes, some of which put the women at higher risk for cervical cancer.

WHAT THE RESULTS OF YOUR PAP TEST MEAN

TERM	WHAT IT MEANS	FOLLOW-UP NEEDED
Negative for intraepithelial lesion or malignancy	There are no atypical cervical changes. There may be some changes in the cells but they are benign.	None
ASC-US Atypical squamous cells of undetermined significance	There are some squamous cells that don't look normal but no one knows exactly what these changes will mean.	Repeat Pap test. Colposcopy with biopsy. Endocervical curettage. May be tested for HPV.
ASC-H Atypical squamous cells—cannot exclude HSIL	Some of the squamous cells do not look normal; it may be a high grade lesion or it may be something imitating a high grade lesion.	Colposcopy with biopsy and/or endocervical curettage.
LSIL Low grade squamous intraepithelial lesion (CIN-1)	Precancerous cells have been found in the lining of the cervix. May go away without treatment.	Repeat Pap test. Colposcopy with biopsy and/or endocervical curettage.
HSIL High grade squamous intraepithelial lesion (CIN 2-3)	Precancerous cells found in lining of cervix. Less likely than LSIL to go away without treatment. More likely to develop into cancer.	Colposcopy with biopsy and/or endocervical curettage.
AGC Atypical glandular cells	Cells in the upper part of the opening in the cervix have changed.	Colposcopy with biopsy and/or endocervical curettage.
AIS Endo-cervical adenocarcinoma *in situ*	There are cells in the tissues that are precancerous.	Colposcopy and biopsy and/or endocervical curettage.
Squamous Cell Carcinoma	Indicates likelihood of squamous cell cancer.	Further testing to insure diagnosis.

What does ASC-US mean?

ASC-US stands for atypical squamous cells of undetermined significance. It means that there are some squamous cells that don't look normal. No one knows exactly what these changes will mean and whether or not they will go away without treatment. You may need to have another Pap test, a colposcopy, and biopsy. The doctor also may test for HPV.

What does ASC-H mean?

ASC-H stands for atypical squamous cells. The H means that the test cannot exclude HSIL. That tells the doctor that some of the squamous cells do not look normal, that a high grade lesion (HSIL) is suspected but the cells have not changed enough to be sure. This diagnosis means that you will probably need to have a colposcopy and biopsy.

What is AGC?

AGC stands for atypical glandular cells. It means that the cells in the upper part of the opening of your cervix have changed. The doctors are not sure what these changes mean. You will probably need to have a colposcopy and biopsy and/or endocervical curettage.

What is meant by "positive" and "negative" Pap test results?

If the lab finds changes, the Pap test results are called "positive." If no changes are found, the result is called "negative."

What is human papilloma virus?

Human papilloma virus, often referred to by its initials HPV, includes some 100 similar viruses that tend to cause warts, including the fairly common warts that grow on hands and feet. About 30 of the wart strains affect the cervix, with about 12 of them known to cause cancer of the cervix.

How do women get HPV infection of the cervix?

Almost all of the HPV of the cervix is passed through sexual interaction. It's easy to get by having sex with someone who carries the virus, since it can be spread through skin contact with any part of an infected person's genital area. Frequent sex with many partners, sex at an early age, or having partners who have had many sexual partners increase the odds of getting cancer of the cervix. A girl who begins having sex before age 18 is more likely to get HPV because her cervix is much less mature.

Who gets HPV infection?

HPV infection is found mostly among teenage girls and young women. It is estimated that between 10 and 20 million women in the United States have

HPV of the cervix. Studies consistently find many fewer infections in older women. It is not yet known whether or not condoms help prevent HPV and cancer of the cervix.

Are vaccines being used to prevent cervical cancer?

There are several studies presently underway that are testing vaccines to prevent cancer of the cervix. There are some early results of one study. The vaccine would be given to women before they became sexually active to make them immune to HPV-16, the papillomavirus that causes half of all cervical cancers. This vaccine, given in three injections over a period of six months, would prevent a woman from developing infections or precancerous lesions associated with HPV-16. Further studies are needed to determine whether or not this vaccine is safe and effective.

When should a woman get her first Pap test?

According to the American Cancer Society, you should begin having Pap tests about three years after you have begun having vaginal intercourse, but no later than 21 years of age. You should be screened every year if you are having a regular Pap test or every two years if you are having the liquid-based test. After you have reached the age of 30, if you have had three normal test results in a row, you can get screened every two to three years. However, if you have risk factors such as DES exposure before birth, HIV infection, or if your immune system is weak because of an organ transplant, chemotherapy, or chronic steroid use, you should continue to have yearly exams. There is more information on DES later in this chapter.

Should an older woman continue to have Pap tests?

American Cancer Society recommends that women 70 years of age or older, who have had three or more normal Pap tests in a row and have had no abnormal Pap test results in the last ten years, may decide to stop having this screening. If you have a history of cervical cancer, DES exposure before birth, HIV infections, or if your immune system is weak because of an organ transplant, chemotherapy, or chronic steroid use, you should continue to have the screening.

Is it necessary to have a Pap test after a woman has had a hysterectomy?

If you had a total hysterectomy, with both your uterus and cervix removed, you may choose to stop having cervical cancer screening, unless you had a hysterectomy as a treatment for precancer or for cancer of the cervix. If your cervix was not removed as part of the hysterectomy, you need to continue to have a Pap test according to the regular guidelines.

Is there anything I should do to make sure my Pap test results are accurate?

A recent study by the AHCPR (Agency for Health Care Policy and Research) found that anywhere from 10 to 30 percent of Pap test results that were called "normal" were not. In addition, some results that are reported as positive for cancer turn out to be normal. This is very troubling because errors of this type can lead to a wrong or a delayed diagnosis. Here are some steps you can take:

- Ask your doctor what labs your test is being sent to and why. Is the lab chosen because the doctor has business ties to it? Is it the health plan that is requiring where the tests will be read?

- Check to see if the lab is accredited by the College of American Pathologists (1–800–323–4040) or by the Joint Commission on Accreditation of Healthcare Organizations (www.jacho.org).

New screening techniques are being tested to see if they can help improve the accuracy of the Pap test.

If I have HPV will I get cancer?

HPV is the main cause of cervical cancer, but having an HPV infection does not necessarily lead to cervical cancer. As a matter of fact, most of the time, women with HPV do not end up with cervical cancer.

What is LSIL?

LSIL is the abbreviation for low grade squamous intraepithelial lesion. You might also hear it called mild dysplasia or CIN-1 (cervical intraepithelial neoplasia-1). More than half of the women who have HPV will get LSIL sometime within four years after getting the virus. In LSIL, an area of cells on the surface of the cervix do not look normal but they behave much like healthy cells—growing for a time and then dying. About 80 percent of the time, these cells disappear on their own in a few months with healthy cells replacing them. Sometimes, a low grade lesion will turn into a high grade one (HSIL).

What is HSIL?

HSIL is high grade squamous intraepithelial lesion. It may also be referred to as CIN 2–3. That means that the HPV infection has not gone away on its own and that there are more abnormal cell changes. HSIL needs to be treated so that it does not turn into cancer.

Does everybody who has HSIL get cervical cancer?

No. Only a small percentage of women who have abnormal cell changes with high-risk types of HPV will develop cancer, if the abnormal cells are not removed. Studies also show that other factors, such as smoking, HIV infection, and having many children, may increase the risk of cancer in women with HPV infections.

How long does it take HSIL to turn into cancer?

The average time it takes for HSIL (CIN3) to turn into cancer is estimated to be 10 to 15 years, which means that follow-up is essential for anyone with this problem. A small group of these progressive cancers, however, are more rapidly growing and could become cancer within three years. These usually occur in younger women.

Can a Pap test tell whether a woman has LSIL or HSIL?

A Pap test cannot tell for certain whether a woman has low grade or high grade squamous intraepithelial lesion. It can tell that there are abnormal lesions that indicate that the disease may be present. However, additional testing is needed to make a final diagnosis.

Is human papilloma virus (HPV) DNA typing done if there are abnormal cells in the cervix?

Studies are still ongoing to determine whether or not HPV DNA typing would be helpful in deciding who is at high risk and may need more aggressive evaluation and follow-up. At the present time, studies suggest that HPV testing would be useful as follow-up for women with an ASC-US Pap test result.

What kind of cancer are most cancers of the cervix?

Most cancers of the cervix are squamous cell cancers. Some are adenocarcinomas. Among other cell types are adenosquamous, endocervical, clear cell, endometroid, small cell cervical sarcoma, and malignant lymphoma of the cervix.

What are the symptoms that alert me to cervical cancer?

There are usually no visible symptoms or signs in the early stages of cervical cancer. As the cancer grows, there may be unusual bleeding or discharge. You may have longer menstrual periods, a heavier flow, bleeding between periods or after intercourse, or bleeding after menopause. The bleeding is usually bright red and unpredictable as to when it appears, its amount, or its duration. Although these symptoms may not be cancer they should be checked by the doctor. Cancer of the cervix is usually found through a Pap smear. It is almost 100 percent curable in its earliest stages. Thanks to the Pap smear, more than two-thirds of cervical cancers are now detected in the early, *in situ* stage.

At what age do women usually get cervical cancer?

The age varies, with the peak for cancer *in situ* being between 25 and 35, and for invasive cancer between 45 and 50. However, cervical cancer may occur at any age. About 25 percent are seen in women under the age of 35.

Why must a biopsy be done if the Pap smear already indicates there are cancerous cells?

The Pap smear is only a screening tool. Although it is very accurate as a screening device, a biopsy must be done to give a definite diagnosis of cancer so that treatment can be properly staged.

What is a colposcopy?

A colposcopy is a procedure used to evaluate abnormal tissue in the vagina and cervix. The colposcope itself is basically a microscope on a stand. It gives a lighted, magnified view showing greater detail than can be seen with the naked eye. Your cervix will be painted with a solution of acetic acid that removes excess mucus and helps highlight abnormal tissues. You will lie on your back on an examining table with your knees bent and feet resting in stirrups. The doctor gently inserts a speculum into your vagina. The colposcope is passed through the speculum and focused on the cervix. The doctor will note abnormal areas. If a biopsy is performed, a special scissors-like instrument is inserted and used to take tiny specimens from the cervix.

Is the colposcopy painful?

If tissue is removed for a biopsy, you may have some minor discomfort, as well as some cramping and bleeding. The procedure takes 10 or 15 minutes and is usually done in a doctor's office. You may have a brown vaginal discharge for a few days as well as slight bleeding and possibly an unpleasant smelling vaginal discharge. You should not use tampons, douche, lift heavy objects or have sexual intercourse for several days while your cervix heals.

How is endocervical curettage done?

The doctor will use a small instrument, called a curette, to scrape cells from inside the opening in the center of your cervix. It will only take a few seconds to do this test. You might feel some mild pain and cramps.

What will happen after the biopsy?

After the biopsy, the doctor will decide on what treatment will be needed. If your tissue looks normal or you have slight changes in your cells, you will probably have your Pap test repeated every four to six months until you have three normal Pap tests in a row. Or the doctor may order HPV testing or a colposcopy. If the results are unclear, more invasive testing, usually a cone biopsy may be necessary. If high grade changes or if cancer cells have been found, you will need to have further treatment.

What is a cone biopsy?

A cone biopsy, also called conization, removes a cone-shaped piece of tissue from the cervix. Doctors may use a laser, LEEP or harmonic scalpel for this operation. (Cold knife surgery for this procedure has been replaced by these newer methods.) Conization may be done in a hospital with general anesthesia or in a doctor's office with local anesthesia. The doctor removes a cone-shaped portion of tissue from the center of the cervix. The widest part of the cone is taken from the opening of the cervix, while the middle and tip of the cone are taken from the cervical canal leading to the uterus. The edges of the cervix are sutured or may be sealed with electric current. Conization takes out a part of your cervix and can result in scarring. Cone biopsy may lead to increased risk of miscarriages and possible infertility because the cervix may be weakened by the surgery. Scar tissue from the biopsy may also interfere with labor and reduce the chances for vaginal childbirth. The procedure takes about 30 minutes to perform.

When is conization or laser used for early stage cervical cancer?

If your cervical canal is involved and you wish to preserve the uterus and avoid radiation therapy and/or more extensive surgery, conization may be used. If you are past childbearing age, you may be treated by total abdominal or vaginal hysterectomy.

What is the loop electrosurgical excision procedure (LEEP)?

This is a surgical procedure for treating abnormal, precancerous tissue in the cervix. It uses an electrified wire loop through which high frequency current passes. This technique is also referred to as LOOP diathermy, or LLETZ, large loop excision of the transformation zone. Your cervix is numbed, the loop is inserted into the vagina and the precancerous cells are removed, producing a button-size sample of tissue. Your wound is packed with a medicinal paste that hastens healing and the tissue is sent to a pathologist for further analysis. After two or three months, your cervix is completely healed. This technique is less costly, can be done in a doctor's office, has a

FOLLOW-UP AFTER BIOPSY OR CURETTAGE

RESULT	FOLLOW-UP
Tissue looks normal	Repeat Pap tests every four to six months until three normal Pap tests in a row. HPV test or repeat colposcopy may be ordered.
Tissue shows mild changes	HPV test or colposcopy may be ordered. Or repeat Pap tests every four to six months until three normal Pap tests in a row.
Uncertain results	Additional testing including conization.
High-grade changes	LEEP, cryotherapy, laser therapy, or conization.
Invasive cancer cells	Tests to determine stage of cancer followed by treatment.

shorter recovery time and, when done by a well-trained physician, fewer complications.

How is cryosurgery done?

Cryosurgery or cryocautery uses liquid nitrogen or carbon dioxide to destroy tissue by freezing. The substance is placed in a hollow metal probe that is inserted into the tumor or applied to its surface. The doctor freezes enough tissue to destroy the cells that are not normal. Cryosurgery can be done in a doctor's office. You will not need anesthetic. You may have some cramping and pain as well as a watery brown discharge for several weeks. You should not use tampons or have sex for several weeks following cryotherapy. Cryosurgery may lead to scarring. In rare cases, this will mean you might have problems getting pregnant. Be sure you discuss this issue with your doctor before you decide to have this treatment.

Is laser surgery used in treating CIN?

Yes. The laser is mounted on the colposcope and the laser beam is directed at the affected area. The laser allows for great accuracy in removal of the diseased tissue, sparing disease-free tissue. There may be some discomfort but there is little vaginal discharge and healing occurs in about two weeks. There may be thermal damage to tissue, which may make future detection of invasive cancer difficult.

What is an harmonic scalpel?

An harmonic scalpel uses ultrasound vibrations to cut tissues and seal blood vessels. The scalpel vibrates at more than 55,000 times per second. It is being used in various operations, including conization and hysterectomy.

Questions to Ask Your Doctor Before Being Treated for Cervical Cancer

- **Has my Pap test been rechecked to make absolutely certain that I do have a cancerous condition?**
- **What kind of cancer is it and where is it located?**
- **Has there been any spread?**
- **What kind of treatment are you planning?**
- **Is this treatment necessary or is it elective?**
- **Is there an alternative way of treating this condition?**
- **Will this treatment mean I can't have a baby?**
- **Will this treatment affect my sexual functioning?**
- **Will it affect my urinary function or control?**
- **If radiation therapy is being used, what complications will these treatments cause in my case?**
- **Are there clinical trials for my stage of cervical cancer?**

What treatment is recommended for Stage 0 cancer of the cervix?

It is very important that the stage and extent of the disease be properly determined. If the cancer is Stage 0, it may be treated with conization, laser surgery, or cryosurgery. Hysterectomy, to take out the area where the cancer is found, the cervix, and the uterus may be the recommended treatment if you cannot have or no longer wish to have children. The cure rate for Stage 0 cancer of the cervix, when properly treated, can be 100 percent.

What treatments are recommended for Stage I-A cervical cancer?

It depends on how deeply the cancer has been found in the tissues of the cervix. You may have conization or a hysterectomy to remove the cancerous area, cervix, and uterus; ovaries may also be removed. If the cancer is deeper in the tissues, a hysterectomy may be done to remove cancerous area, cervix and uterus, part of the vagina, along with lymph nodes in the pelvic area. Internal radiation therapy also may be a treatment choice for cancers that are not too deep.

What are the preferred treatments for Stage I-B cervical cancer?

Radiation therapy (internal or external) or radical hysterectomy (removing the uterus, cervix, ovaries, part of the vagina and lymph nodes in the pelvic area). This may be followed by radiation therapy plus chemotherapy. Or radiation plus chemotherapy may be the treatment. The size of the tumor will be an important factor in deciding what treatment is appropriate for you.

TREATMENT CHOICES FOR CANCER OF THE CERVIX

STAGE	TREATMENT
Stage 0 Cancer *in situ*, very early stage found only in first layer of cells of lining of cervix.	*It is mandatory to know the extent of the disease. If Stage 0, one of following treatments:* Conization **or** Laser surgery **or** LEEP **or** Cryosurgery **or** Hysterectomy to remove cancerous area, cervix, and uterus (for women who cannot have, or no longer want, children) **or** *Clinical trials.* Properly treated, cure rate can be 100 percent.
Stage I-A Cancer is found throughout cervix, with small amount of cancer found deeper in tissues of cervix.	Hysterectomy to remove cancerous area, cervix and uterus; ovaries may be removed **or** Conization **or** Hysterectomy to remove cancerous area, cervix, uterus, and part of vagina, along with lymph nodes in pelvic area (if cancer is deeper in the tissues) **or** Internal radiation therapy **or** *Clinical trials.*
Stage I-B Larger amount of cancer in tissues of cervix.	Internal and external radiation combined **or** Radical hysterectomy to remove uterus, cervix, ovaries, part of vagina, and lymph nodes in pelvic area **or** same as above followed by radiation therapy plus chemotherapy **or** Radiation therapy plus chemotherapy **or** *Clinical trials.*
Stage II-A Cancer has spread beyond cervix to upper two-thirds of vagina but still inside pelvic area.	Combined internal and external radiation **or** Radical hysterectomy with lymph node dissection **or** Radical hysterectomy with lymph node dissection followed by radiation therapy plus chemotherapy **or** Radiation therapy plus chemotherapy. *Clinical trials:* Radical hysterectomy, lymph node dissection followed by radiation.
Stage II-B Cancer has spread to tissue around cervix.	Combined internal and external radiation plus chemotherapy **or** Radical hysterectomy plus lymph node dissection **or**

TREATMENT CHOICES FOR CANCER OF THE CERVIX *(continued)*

STAGE	TREATMENT
Stage II-B *(continued)*	Radical hysterectomy and lymph node dissection, plus radiation, plus chemotherapy **or** Radiation therapy plus chemotherapy. *Clinical trials.*
Stage III Spread throughout pelvic area, or to lower part of vagina, and/or block ureters.	Combined internal and external radiation plus chemotherapy. *Clinical trials.*
Stage IV-A Cancer spread to organs close to cervix such as bladder or rectum.	Combined internal and external radiation plus chemotherapy. *Clinical trials.*
Stage IV-B Cancer spread to faraway organs such as lungs.	Radiation therapy to relieve symptoms such as pain **or** systemic chemotherapy *Clinical trials*: new, or new combinations of, chemotherapy drugs.
Recurrent Disease has come back in cervix or another place.	Depends on where recurrence occurs. *In pelvis:* Radiation therapy and chemotherapy **or** Chemotherapy to relieve symptoms. *Clinical trials.*

Is treatment different for those with Stage II-A cervical cancer?

Radiation therapy (internal combined with external) or radical hysterectomy (removing the uterus, cervix, ovaries, part of the vagina and lymph nodes in the pelvic area) followed by radiation therapy plus chemotherapy may be used. Or radiation plus chemotherapy may be the treatment. The size of the tumor and the medical expertise available in your community are the most important factors.

What are the standard treatments recommended for Stages II-B, III, and IV-A cervical cancer?

The treatment of choice is external beam radiation with the addition of radiation implants plus chemotherapy (cisplatin or cisplatin/fluorouracil).

What treatments are used for Stage IV-B cervical cancers?

Usually radiation therapy is used to relieve the symptoms of cervical cancer. A number of chemotherapy drugs, alone or in combination, are being tested in clinical trials.

Are there urinary or sexual side effects to treatment for cervical cancer?

Some treatments, such as radiation, can shorten the vagina, and some cancers of the cervix may extend into the vagina. Some of the treatments also produce sexual side effects. For information on sexual and urinary side effects, see information later in this chapter entitled "Sexual and Urinary Problems Following Gynecological Treatment" as well as in Chapter 9, Radiation Treatment, Chapter 10, Chemotherapy, and Chapter 27, Living with Cancer.

What treatment is used if cervical cancer recurs?

If the cancer recurs in the pelvis, surgery may be done to remove the area where the cancer has spread, as well as surgical removal of the cervix, uterus, and vagina (called an exenteration). Or further radiation therapy and chemotherapy may be used. If the cancer has recurred outside the pelvis, combination chemotherapy may be used and there are clinical trials available that are testing new drugs or combinations of drugs.

What are the consequences of a total pelvic exenteration?

This surgery, which includes the removal of the lower colon, rectum, or bladder as well as the cervix, uterus, and vagina, is the most radical kind of pelvic surgery. Two ostomies are usually created, one for urine and one for rectal waste. In addition, the vagina is usually reconstructed. The clitoris and outer genitals are usually not removed, so that many women find they can still have sexual desire, pleasure, and orgasm.

What kind of checkups should be scheduled following treatment for cancer of the cervix?

The first year, you will probably see the doctor every three months and your Pap smear will be repeated at six, nine and 12 months. Chest x-rays and CT scans will be done at the end of the first year. The second to fifth year, checkups will probably be scheduled each six months, and after that yearly checkups should suffice. Be sure to tell your doctor if you have vaginal discharge or bleeding, bone pain, weight or appetite loss, bowel or bladder problems, or swelling of the legs. Life-long follow-up on a regular basis is important.

CANCERS OF THE UTERUS

What You Need to Know About Cancers of the Uterus

- There are many tumors in the uterus that are not cancer.

- There are two kinds of cancer of the uterus: endometrial, a disease in which cancer cells start growing in the lining of the uterus, and uterine sarcoma, in which the cells of the muscles or other supporting tissues of the uterus are involved.

- Most cancers of the uterus are endometrial. Uterine sarcoma is a rare cancer.

- Most endometrial cancer occurs in women who are between 50 and 59 and are postmenopausal.

- Taking tamoxifen for breast cancer, or taking estrogen alone (without progesterone), can put you at higher risk for developing endometrial cancer.

- Most uterine sarcomas occur in women over 50 who received high doses of external radiation therapy in the area of the pelvis. This radiation was given to women some five to 25 years earlier to stop noncancerous bleeding of the uterus.

Uterine Endometrial Cancer

What is the endometrium?

The endometrium is the lining of the uterus, or womb, where a baby grows. The body, or corpus, of the uterus is a muscular, hollow, pear-shaped organ, which is lined with epithelial cells. Cancer in this area is referred to as uterus or uterine cancer, or endometrial cancer. The wall of the uterus has two layers of tissue. The inner layer, or lining, is the endometrium. The outer layer of muscle tissue is the myometrium. When a woman is menstruating, the endometrial tissue grows and thickens in preparation for receiving a fertilized egg. Menstruation occurs when this tissue is not used and passes out through the vagina.

Do fibroid tumors become cancerous?

Fibroid tumors (sometimes called leiomyomas) are noncancerous tumors in the uterus, usually found in women in their 40s. When a woman stops having menstrual periods, fibroids may become smaller and sometimes disappear. Often fibroids do not cause symptoms and do not need to be treated, although they should be checked often. Symptoms of fibroids depend on the size and location of the tumors and may include irregular bleeding, vaginal discharge, and frequent urination. When fibroids press against nearby organs and cause pain, surgery or other treatment may be needed. It is estimated that about 20 percent of women over 30 have fibroid tumors.

What is endometrial hyperplasia?

Endometrial hyperplasia (also called atypical hyperplasia) is an abnormal increase in the number of endometrial cells and of stromal cells—cells that support endometrial tissue. Many scientists regard it as a precancerous condition. Severe hyperplasia is often called *in situ* cancer of the endometrium. Symptoms may include heavy bleeding during menstruation, erratic bleeding between periods, or abnormal or heavy bleeding during menopause. Though every case of hyperplasia does not develop into cancer, uterine cancer goes through a hyperplastic stage before becoming cancerous. Therefore, hyperplasia is a warning that cancer may develop. Endometrial hyperplasia may be mild, moderate, or severe. Endometrial hyperplasia can occur in menopausal and postmenopausal women as well as in young women who have irregular menstrual cycles. It is most common after age 40.

What is the treatment for endometrial hyperplasia?

Treatment depends upon age and how advanced the hyperplasia is at the time it is diagnosed. For younger women who wish to remain fertile, endometrial hyperplasia may be treated with dilation and curettage (D&C). For women with severe hyperplasia and those for whom fertility is no longer a concern, hysterectomy may be recommended. If surgery is not possible because of other medical problems, progesterone is usually prescribed.

What is endometriosis?

Endometriosis is a condition in which the kind of tissue which normally lines the uterus is found in abnormal places, such as on the outside of the uterus, the surface of the ovaries, in tissues between the vagina and rectum, in tissue in the lower abdomen. It is not a cancerous condition, but it does cause painful menstrual periods, abnormal bleeding, general discomfort, and sometimes the loss of fertility. It is most common in women in their 30s and 40s. Endometriosis may be treated with hormones or surgery.

What are the symptoms of endometrial cancer?

Abnormal bleeding after menopause is the most common symptom. The bleeding may begin as a watery, blood-streaked discharge. Later, the discharge may contain more blood. If there is reappearance of bleeding around the time of menopause, it is important to be checked as soon as possible by the doctor. Cancer of the endometrium usually occurs in women of this age group, so any abnormal bleeding should be checked and diagnosed.

What causes endometrial cancer?

The causes of endometrial cancer are not well understood, but there are a number of factors that seem to increase the risk of developing it. One factor

WHO IS MOST LIKELY TO GET ENDOMETRIAL CANCER?

- Women who are obese.
- Women who have high blood pressure or diabetes.
- Women who have endometrial hyperplasia.
- Women over 50 years of age.
- Women who use hormone replacement therapy.
- Women who take the drug tamoxifen.
- Women who have had an inherited form of colorectal cancer.
- Women who have no children.
- Women who begin menstruation at a very young age.
- Women who enter menopause late in life (after 52 years old.)
- Women with a family history of cancer of the uterus.

that appears to be related is hormone production. It is known that fatty tissue converts certain hormones into estrone, a form of estrogen. Scientists believe that an elevated estrogen level may be the reason why obese women are twice as likely to develop endometrial cancer as are women of normal weight. Many studies suggest that the development of endometrial hyperplasia, which often precedes endometrial cancer, is related to hormones.

Who is at risk for endometrial cancer?

Being obese—50 pounds overweight or more—makes you nine times more likely to develop this cancer than women of average weight. Taking tamoxifen for breast cancer or taking estrogen alone (without progesterone) puts you at a higher risk. Diabetes and high blood pressure may also be risk factors. If you have had an inherited form of colorectal cancer (hereditary nonpolyposis), have a family history of cancer of the uterus, have no children, began menstruation at a very young age, or entered menopause late in life (after 52), you also are at a higher risk for the disease.

What are the major cell types of cancer that develop in the endometrium?

Three-quarters are several varieties of endometroid adenocarcinomas— ciliated adenocarcinoma, secretory adenocarcinoma, papillare or villoglandular, adenocarcinoma with squamous differentiation, adenoacanthoma, or adenosquamous. Other types include mixed, (accounts for 10 percent); uterine papillary serous (accounts for less than 10 percent); clear cell carcinoma (is responsible for 4 percent) and mucinous, squamous, and undifferentiated (each account for 1 percent or less).

How is endometrial cancer diagnosed?

The diagnosis usually begins with a review of symptoms and medical history. The physician will perform a pelvic exam—checking the uterus, vagina, ovaries, fallopian tubes, bladder, and rectum. Routine laboratory tests, including blood tests and urinalysis, also are done. A Pap test may also be done, although it is not a specific test for uterine cancer because it only detects those cancer cells from the endometrium that have passed through the cervix into the vaginal discharge. The only way to get a definitive diagnosis is by doing a uterine biopsy that takes a sample of the cells from the uterine wall. This is usually done with aspiration curettage or with a D&C (dilation and curettage).

How are uterine biopsies done?

Uterine biopsies (also called endometrial biopsies) can be done in one of two ways. Aspiration curettage is usually done in the doctor's office with an endometrial aspirator that consists of a disposable tube connected to a suction device. The tube is inserted through the cervix into the uterus and tissue samples are taken from the uterine lining. The tissue samples are studied to see if there are abnormal cell changes. Suction biopsy may be performed using local anesthesia, but anesthesia is not usually required. The other procedure is a D&C (dilation and curettage). This is a minor surgical procedure in which the uterus is scraped with an instrument known as a curette to obtain a sample of tissue. The procedure is also sometimes used to remove the cancerous cells in cases of hyperplasia, as well as to stop heavy bleeding or remove tissue after miscarriage or abortion. It is usually done on an outpatient basis by a gynecologist, either in the hospital or in a surgery clinic. Local or general anesthesia may be used.

What is transvaginal ultrasound?

The doctor inserts an instrument into the vagina, that produces sound waves. The pattern of the sound waves produces an image of the uterus on the computer screen. If the endometrium looks too thick, the doctor will do a biopsy. Sometimes, a color Doppler is added which lets the doctors see the blood flowing in the tissue.

What is the next step if a biopsy confirms endometrial cancer?

Additional tests are needed to determine the extent of the disease. X-ray exams, such as intravenous pyelography (IVP), CT scans, ultrasound, MRI, sigmoidoscopy, or colonoscopy may be done before surgery. A test measuring the CA-125 tumor marker may also be done.

TESTS THAT MAY BE USED TO DIAGNOSE
ENDOMETRIAL CANCER

- Health history and physical examination
- Pap test
- Aspiration curettage
- Dilation and curettage (D&C)
- Intravenous pyelography (IVP)
- Transvaginal ultrasound
- CT scans
- MRI
- Bone scans
- CA-125 test

Questions to Ask Your Doctor About Endometrial Cancer Treatment

- **How extensive do you think the surgery will be?**
- **What grade and stage is it?**
- **Will you show me exactly what the operation entails and what will be removed?**
- **Where will the scar be? Will the scar be vertical or horizontal? How long will it be?**
- **Will this operation change my bowel functions, urinary control, or sexual life in any way?**
- **Is there an alternative way of treating this condition?**
- **Has it spread? Is it in the lymph nodes?**
- **Have the progesterone and estrogen receptor levels been checked?**
- **What are the risks and side effects I should expect?**
- **How long will it be before I can return to normal activities?**

What kind of surgery is done for endometrial (uterine) cancer?

A hysterectomy, the surgical removal of the uterus, is the most common treatment for endometrial cancer. Usually, if the cancer has not spread beyond the endometrium, the uterus as well as the fallopian tubes and ovaries will be removed. Radiation therapy, internal and external radiation, and hormone therapy are also used for later stages of endometrial cancer.

Is it important to have progesterone and estrogen receptors checked?
It has been found that progesterone receptor levels are an important part of the evaluation process for treatment of those with Stage I, and Stage II endometrial cancer. Progesterone levels greater than 100 were found to be a good sign that the cancer probably would be contained.

Does it make a difference whether the cancer cells are well or poorly differentiated?
Besides being staged, endometrial cancers are also grouped according to their degree of differentiation. Grade 1 means the cells are well differentiated. They resemble normal cells. Grade 2 means they are moderately well differentiated. Grades 3 and 4 refer to poorly differentiated cells. Poorly differentiated cells are abnormally shaped and bear little resemblance to normal cells. These cells often spread more rapidly than those that are well differentiated. For example, treatment for Stage I cancer depends on the location of the tumor, and whether the cells are well or poorly differentiated. When only part of the myometrium (muscle layer) is affected and cells are reasonably well differentiated, and when the tumor is not invasive, hysterectomy and removal of the ovaries and fallopian tubes is recommended. In addition, a few lymph nodes in the adjacent areas are removed to determine whether cancer has spread. If no cancerous cells are found in the nodes, no further treatment is necessary. However, in all other cases and cell types, a more drastic node dissection is done and radiation therapy will follow the surgery.

Will I have urinary or sexual side effects after my treatment for endometrial cancer?
There can be both urinary and sexual side effects, depending upon the extent of the disease and the type of treatment. If you have a hysterectomy, you will no longer have menstrual periods. When ovaries are removed, menopause occurs at once. Some treatments, such as radiation, can give you dryness, itching, tightening, and burning in the vagina. For information on sexual and urinary side effects, see information later in this chapter entitled "Sexual and Urinary Problems Following Gynecological Treatment," as well as discussion of sexual side effects in Chapter 9, Radiation Treatment, Chapter 10, Chemotherapy, and Chapter 27, Living with Cancer.

What kind of follow-up exams will be needed after being treated for endometrial cancer?
The doctor will probably schedule follow-up visits every three months for the first year, every six months for the second to fifth year and yearly thereafter. Examination will probably include pelvic exam, stool, blood, and urine

TREATMENT CHOICES FOR ENDOMETRIAL CANCER

STAGE	TREATMENT
Stage IA Cancer limited to the endometrium. **Stage IB** Cancer found in less than one-half the myometrium. **Stage IC** Cancer found in more than one-half of the myometrium.	Total hysterectomy, plus removal of ovaries, fallopian tubes & lymph nodes **or** Same as above with or without removal of lymph nodes, followed by internal or external radiation therapy to pelvis and internal radiation to vagina **or** For patients who cannot have surgery, radiation therapy alone. *Clinical trials*: radiation and/or chemotherapy following surgery.
Stage IIA Cancer cells have spread to cervix, with glandular involvement only.	Total hysterectomy, plus removal of ovaries, fallopian tubes & lymph nodes **or** Same as above, with or without removal of lymph nodes, followed by internal or external radiation therapy to pelvis and internal radiation to vagina **or** For patients who cannot have surgery, radiation therapy alone. *Clinical trials*: radiation and/or chemotherapy following surgery.
Stage IIB Cancer cells have spread to the cervix, in both glandular and connective tissue.	Total hysterectomy plus removal of ovaries and fallopian tubes; with removal of lymph nodes, followed by radiation therapy; **or** Internal and external radiation followed by total hysterectomy plus ovaries and fallopian tubes with removal of lymph nodes **or** Radical hysterectomy plus ovaries, fallopian tubes, and removal of part of vagina with or without removal of lymph nodes. *Clinical trials*.
Stage IIIA Cancer has spread outside uterus to lining or abdominal wall. **Stage IIIB** Cancer spread to vagina.	Radical hysterectomy, plus removal of ovaries, fallopian tubes, ovaries and part of vagina; lymph node dissection followed by internal and external radiation **or** If patient cannot have surgery, radiation therapy alone **or** If patient cannot have surgery or radiation, hormone therapy. *Clinical trials*.

(continued)

TREATMENT CHOICES FOR ENDOMETRIAL CANCER (continued)

STAGE	TREATMENT
Stage IIIC Cancer found in pelvic and/or nearby lymph nodes.	Same as Stages IIIA and IIIB.
Stage IVA Cancer spread to bladder or linings of bowels. **Stage IVB** Cancer spread to distant areas and lymph nodes.	Internal and external radiation **or** Hormone therapy. *Clinical trials*: chemotherapy using either one or a combination of drugs.
Recurrent Cancer returns after being treated.	Radiation if occurs in vagina when no radiation previously used **or** Radiation to relieve pain, nausea, and abnormal bowel functions **or** Hormone therapy using progestins or tamoxifen. *Clinical trials*: Chemotherapy.

tests, and a Pap test. Tumor markers, like CA-125, which can detect a protein shed by cancerous tissue, will usually be done at each visit. Chest x-rays are done yearly. Tell your doctor if you have any vaginal bleeding, pelvic pain, change in the size of your stomach, or swelling of the legs. The most crucial follow-up time is the first three years, but lifetime follow-up is important.

Is it safe for me to take estrogen replacement therapy after I've had endometrial cancer?

One of estrogen's primary roles is to promote the growth of cells in the breast and uterus. Thus, there is some concern whether or not the use of postmenopausal estrogen after cancer will promote further tumor growth. There has been only a small amount of research to look at the risk to women who have had cancer of the uterus in taking estrogen replacement therapy. Thus, at the present time, it is not certain whether or not it is safe for women who have had early stage cancer of the uterus to take it. The Estrogen Replacement Therapy Study, sponsored by the National Cancer Institute and now underway, is designed to answer this question.

Uterine Sarcoma

What is uterine sarcoma?
Sarcoma of the uterus is a rare kind of cancer in women in which cancer cells start growing in the muscles (myometrium), called leiomyosarcoma, or from the epithelium, called mesodermal and stromal sarcomas.

TREATMENT CHOICES FOR UTERINE SARCOMA

STAGE	TREATMENT
Stage I Cancer found only in the main part of uterus, not in the cervix.	Surgery to remove uterus, fallopian tubes, ovaries, and some of lymph nodes in pelvis and abdomen **or** Surgery as above followed by radiation therapy to pelvis **or** Surgery followed by chemotherapy **or** Surgery followed by radiation therapy. *Clinical trials.*
Stage II Cancer has spread to cervix.	Surgery to remove uterus, fallopian tubes, ovaries and some of lymph nodes in pelvis and abdomen **or** Surgery as above followed by radiation therapy to pelvis **or** Surgery followed by chemotherapy **or** Surgery followed by radiation therapy. *Clinical trials.*
Stage III Cancer has spread outside uterus but not outside pelvis.	Surgery to remove uterus, fallopian tubes, ovaries, and some of lymph nodes in pelvis and abdomen, plus as much as possible of cancer that has spread to nearby tissues **or** Surgery as above followed by radiation therapy to pelvis **or** Surgery followed by chemotherapy. *Clinical trials.*
Stage IV Cancer spread beyond pelvis, to other parts of body or into lining of bladder or rectum.	*Clinical trials:* chemotherapy.
Recurrent Cancer has come back after treatment.	*Clinical trials:* chemotherapy or hormone therapy **or** Radiation therapy to relieve symptoms.

Who is at risk for uterine sarcoma?
If you have received high doses of external radiation therapy in the area of your pelvis, you are at a higher risk in developing sarcoma of the uterus. Radiation was sometimes given to women five to 25 years ago to stop non-cancerous bleeding of the uterus. Most women who have this kind of cancer have already had menopause.

What are the symptoms of uterine sarcoma?
The major symptom is between-period bleeding or bleeding after menopause.

How is uterine sarcoma diagnosed?
If you have abnormal bleeding, the doctor will do an internal examination, feeling for lumps or changes in the shape of your organs. A Pap test will be done. However, because sarcoma of the uterus begins inside the uterus, it will not usually show up on a Pap test. A dilation and curettage (D&C) will be done, removing pieces of the lining of the uterus, to be looked at under a microscope. If uterine sarcoma is found, additional tests will be done to determine whether it has spread to other parts of the body.

How is uterine sarcoma treated?
Treatment will depend on the stage of the cancer. Surgery—taking out the uterus, fallopian tubes, ovaries, and some lymph nodes in the pelvis and around the aorta—is the most common treatment for uterine sarcoma. Radiation, with or without surgery, may be used. Chemotherapy or hormones may also be part of the treatment for this cancer.

OVARIAN CANCER

What You Need to Know About Cancers of the Ovary

- There are several different cell types of cancer of the ovary that require different treatments.

- Ovarian epithelial cancer is the most common, and half of the cases occur in women over 65.

- Ovarian low malignant potential tumor is a precancerous condition that can be treated successfully.

- Germ cell ovarian tumors form in the egg cells of the ovary.

- Women who have a family history of ovarian cancer have an increased risk of developing ovarian cancer.

- If cancer of the ovary is suspected, it would be wise to be under the care of a gynecological oncologist.

Where are the ovaries located?

The ovaries are located in the pelvis, one on each side of the uterus. Each of these female reproductive organs is the size and shape of an almond. During each monthly menstrual cycle, one ovary releases an egg that travels from the ovary through the fallopian tubes to the uterus. The ovaries are the body's main source of female hormones—estrogen and progesterone—which regulate the menstrual cycle and pregnancy. These hormones control the development of female body characteristics, such as the breasts, body shape, and body hair.

What are the symptoms of ovarian cancer?

Most women who have cancer of the ovary do have symptoms and often delay diagnosis because the symptoms are similar to those of other illnesses. Several studies of ovarian cancer patients show that most of the symptoms relate to abdominal bloating or gastrointestinal disturbances. Symptoms include:

- Abdominal swelling or bloating.
- Discomfort in the lower part of abdomen.
- Feeling full after a light meal.
- Nausea or vomiting.
- Not feeling hungry.
- Gas or indigestion.
- Unexplained weight loss.
- Diarrhea, constipation, or frequent urination.
- Shortness of breath.
- Bleeding with intercourse, or bleeding that is not part of regular menstruation pattern.
- Pain in the back, abdomen, or pelvis during or after intercourse.

Who is most likely to develop ovarian cancer?

Most cases of ovarian cancer are found in women over the age of 50. But the disease is also sometimes found in younger women. Ovarian cancer is relatively rare, affecting about one in 55 women. Risk rises with age, with most cases occurring after menopause. Risk doubles for older women who have never had children or who have previously had breast or endometrial cancer. The highest risk appears to be in women with two or more first-degree relatives—mother, daughter, or sister—with the same problem. A family or personal history of

WHO IS MOST LIKELY TO GET OVARIAN CANCER?

- Women whose mother, daughter, or sister has had ovarian cancer.
- Women whose other relatives—grandmother, aunt, cousin—have had ovarian cancer.
- Family history of breast cancer or hereditary nonpolyposis colorectal cancer.
- Ashkenazi Jewish descent with family or personal history of ovarian or breast cancer.
- Women over 50, with those over 60 at highest risk.
- Women who have never had children.
- Women who have had breast or colon cancer.
- Women who have used talcum powder in the genital area.
- Women who have taken postmenopausal estrogen.

breast or colon cancer is also a risk, as is hormone replacement therapy. Use of talcum powder in your genital area for many years may also put you at higher risk.

Does estrogen cause cancer of the ovary?
There are recent studies that show that estrogen use is associated with a higher risk of cancer of the ovary. In a recent large study women who used estrogen alone for 10 to 19 years were twice as likely to develop ovarian cancer as were women who did not take estrogen. And those women, who took it for 20 years or more, had an increased risk three times that of those who had not taken it.

Do women who have taken fertility drugs have a higher risk for ovarian cancer?
There has been debate around this issue, and the findings are not consistent. A recent analysis of a series of studies indicates that infertility itself is associated with ovarian cancer. It may be that an early undetectable cancer is causing the infertility rather than the drugs used to treat infertility.

Should women with a family history of ovarian cancer take special precautions?
About 10 percent of ovarian cancers are found in women with a family history. It may be that they are carrying mutations in genes for BRCA1, BRCA2, HBOC (hereditary breast/ovarian cancer) or HNPCC (hereditary nonpolyposis

colorectal cancer syndrome). Several organizations have offered guidelines for screening. Most agree that an annual pelvic examination and transvaginal ultrasound and annual or semiannual CA-125 tests are essential.

For women with a family history of ovarian cancer, can removal of one or both ovaries be used for preventive purposes?

Removal of one or both ovaries as a precaution is a viable option. Women with a family history of ovarian cancer would be wise to undergo cancer risk counseling as an essential first step. For more information, see Chapter 4, What Is Cancer?

Is cancer of the ovary curable?

Eighty-five to 90 percent of cancers that have not spread beyond the ovary are curable. The real problem is that they are difficult to detect at an early stage, since often there are no symptoms in the early stages and even when symptoms appear, they may be ignored because they are so vague. Often when cancer of the ovary is found, it has spread to other organs.

What kind of doctor should I see if cancer of the ovary is suspected?

You should be in the care of a doctor who is well versed in diagnosing and treating ovarian cancer. A gynecological oncologist would be the preferred specialist since surgery is the foundation of the diagnosis and treatment of ovarian cancer. Depending on the stage of disease, a team of doctors may be needed including a gynecologic oncologist, a medical oncologist, and/or a radiation oncologist.

What kinds of tests are used to detect ovarian cancer?

The first step is usually a pelvic exam, with a Pap smear being done at the same time. The Pap smear, however, is a test for cancer of the cervix and should not be depended upon to find or to accurately diagnose ovarian cancer. An ultrasound may be done of the ovaries to help differentiate between healthy tissues, fluid-filled cysts, and tumors. CT scans may be ordered as well as a lower GI series and an intravenous pyelogram (IVP). This is a series of x-rays of the kidneys, ureter, and bladder to help determine if the cancer has spread. A blood test to measure a substance that is produced by ovarian cancer cells, called CA-125, may be ordered. If these tests raise the suspicion that cancer may be the problem, the only sure way is to have a biopsy to examine a sample of the ovarian tissue under the microscope. This requires surgery.

How is the ultrasound done?

The doctor inserts an instrument, which produces sound waves, into the vagina. The pattern of the sound waves produces a sonogram (a picture of the ovaries) on the computer screen, allowing the doctors to find signs of ovarian cancer. Sometimes, a color Doppler is added which lets the doctor see the way the blood flows in the tissue.

What is the CA-125 assay test?

This is a blood test to measure a protein found on the surface of ovarian cancer cells and in some normal tissue. This cancer antigen test has proved useful for monitoring the success of ovarian cancer treatment, indicating whether a tumor has shrunk or if it has recurred. This test works less well at detection, missing about half of all early tumors. Endometriosis and fibroids, both benign uterine tumors, can also elevate CA-125 levels, as can menstruation, pregnancy, pelvic inflammatory disease, hepatitis, and endometriosis.

How will the CA-125 test be done?

You will have blood taken from a vein in your arm. The doctor will do a baseline test and will compare your future tests to it. Usually the test is reported in numbers, which may vary depending on the test that is being used and the laboratory reading it. If your levels are falling during treatment, this normally confirms that the treatment is working.

What kind of surgery will be required for the biopsy?

If the doctor suspects cancer, a laparotomy may be done. This is an operation that requires a surgical incision in the wall of the abdomen. The entire ovary will be removed because, if the problem is cancer, cutting through the outer layer of the ovary to get a sample of tissue may cause spread. If the pathology report shows that the ovary is cancerous, further surgery is usually necessary. The second ovary, uterus, and fallopian tubes are usually removed. In addition, the surgeon will also take samples of nearby lymph nodes, and check the diaphragm and fluid from the abdomen to determine whether or not the cancer has spread.

What kinds of cancers develop in the ovaries?

Epithelial ovarian cancer occurs in the lining of the ovary, and accounts for 90 percent of all ovarian cancers. Of these epithelial ovarian cancers, about 15 percent are called tumors of low malignant potential, and are treated differently than the more common and more invasive ovarian cancers of the epithelium. Other ovarian cancers include germ cell cancer and stromal tumors (sex cord tumor), which are quite rare. Germ cell tumors affect the egg-making cells in the ovary and most often affect young women. Stromal tumors include granulosa cell tumors and Sertoli-Lydig tumors.

What is meant by tumors of low malignant potential?

When the pathologist looks at the tissue from this tumor under the microscope, the cells of the tumors of low malignant potential, sometimes called borderline tumors, do not clearly look like cancer.

What is meant by the grade of an ovarian tumor?

Epithelial ovarian cancers, besides being given a stage number, are also given a grade number. The grades are 1, 2 and 3. If your tumor is grade 1, the cells look more like normal cells. Grade 3 cells look less like normal cells.

Questions to Ask Your Doctor Before You Have Surgery and Other Treatments for Cancer of the Ovary

- What kind of ovarian cancer do I have?

- What stage and grade is it?

- What kind of operation will I have?

- Exactly what parts of my reproductive tract will you be taking out?

- How long will I have to be in the hospital? Recuperating at home? When will I be able to get back to my normal routine?

- Will I have pain after the operation? For how long? How will it be treated?

- Will I still be able to have sex after the operation?

- Will I need chemotherapy or radiation treatment after the operation? When will it start? For how long? Will I be able to continue my normal activities?

- Will you be planning to do second-look surgery?

How is ovarian cancer treated?

Surgery is the most common treatment. The type of surgery depends upon the extent of the cancer. A *total abdominal hysterectomy and bilateral salpingo-oophorectomy* means that the ovaries, fallopian tubes, and uterus are removed. If the area that stretches from the stomach to the nearby organs in the abdomen is affected, this operation is called an *omentectomy*. If only one ovary is removed along with the fallopian tube on the same side of the body, the operation is called a *unilateral salpingo-oophorectomy*. *Tumor debulking* means taking out as much of the cancer as possible. *Laparotomy* refers to any surgical procedure in which the abdominal cavity is opened either to examine it (*exploratory surgery*) or to perform surgery. Radiation is also used in treating ovarian cancer. It may be external radiation, from a machine or it may be put directly into the sac that lines the abdomen in a liquid that is radioactive, called *intraperitoneal radiation.* Chemotherapy is also used. It may be taken by pill, put into the bloodstream intravenously or given directly to the affected area.

Will I still have menstrual periods after the operation?

It depends on whether both ovaries are taken out, your age, and your general condition. If both ovaries are removed, you will begin to have symptoms of menopause soon after the operation, no matter what age you are.

Will I need to take hormone replacement therapy after my hysterectomy?

This is a subject of much debate in the medical community. Data from the Women's Health Trial give concern that use of postmenopausal estrogen after cancer may promote further tumor growth. This trial has shown that postmenopausal women, who had not had cancer and who had taken estrogen for 10 to 20 years, had an increased risk of ovarian cancer. You need to talk with your doctor. Usually if prescribed, it is for women with very early stage disease, or for young women.

What happens to my sexual desire after the ovaries are removed?

Many women have a very low interest in sex during treatment due to all the stresses and the side effects of the treatment itself. On the other hand, because the ovaries are not the only production sites for estrogens—the adrenal glands also produce androgens that govern sexual desire—there should be no change in your desire in the long term. A decrease in vaginal lubrication may make it necessary for you to use extra lubrication during intercourse.

Will I have urinary or sexual side effects after my treatment for ovarian cancer?

There can be both urinary and sexual side effects, depending upon the extent of the disease and the type of treatment. Some treatments, such as radiation, can cause dryness, itching, tightening, and burning in the vagina. For information on sexual and urinary side effects, see information later in this chapter entitled "Sexual and Urinary Problems Following Gynecological Treatment," as well as information on sexual side effects in Chapter 9, Radiation Treatment, Chapter 10, Chemotherapy, and Chapter 27, Living with Cancer.

What is second-look surgery?

Following chemotherapy, an operation called a second-look laparotomy is sometimes done. During the second-look operation, the doctor will take samples of lymph nodes and other tissues in the abdomen to see if the treatment has been successful. This helps to determine whether therapy can be stopped or whether a change in therapy is indicated. This operation is usually performed through a vertical incision in the abdomen. If cancer is still present, radiation or chemotherapy may be considered.

Are any other treatments being studied in clinical trials?

Biological therapy, stimulating your own immune system to fight cancer, as well as high-dose chemotherapy with bone marrow transplantation or peripheral blood stem cells transplantation are being studied in clinical trials.

What kind of follow-up is recommended for women who have had ovarian cancer?

Your doctor will probably ask you to come back every three months for the first year, and every six months thereafter. You will have blood, urine, and Pap tests every six months, tests for tumor marker CA-125 every six months, and chest x-rays or CT scans every year. You should tell the doctor if you notice changes in the size of your stomach, pain in your pelvic area, bleeding in the vagina, swelling of the legs, or signs of masculinization.

What is an ovarian low malignant potential tumor?

This is an ovarian epithelial tumor but it is considered precancerous—which means that it may or is likely to become cancer. It forms in the tissue covering the ovary and seldom spreads beyond the ovary. About 15 percent of all epithelial cancers fall into this category. Because these tumors are not as malignant as the other epithelial cancers, they are treated differently. In most cases, ovarian low malignant potential tumor can be treated successfully.

How are Stage I and II ovarian low malignant potential tumors treated?

Surgery is the usual treatment and the type depends on whether or not the woman plans to have children. In stages I and II, for those women who do not plan to have children, the treatment may be a hysterectomy and bilateral salpingo-oopherectomy. For women who plan to have children, a unilateral salpingo-oophorectomy or a partial oophorectomy is the usual treatment. If a woman does not plan to have more children, most physicians favor removal of the remaining ovarian tissue as it may be at risk of recurrence.

What is the treatment for Stage III or recurrent ovarian low malignant potential tumor?

For Stage III tumors, a hysterectomy, bilateral salpingo-oophorectomy, and omentectomy (taking out part of the lining of the abdominal cavity) is the

TREATMENT CHOICES FOR OVARIAN EPITHELIAL CANCERS

STAGE	TREATMENT
Stage IA Cancer is in one ovary. **Stage IB** Cancer is in both ovaries.	Total abdominal hysterectomy, bilateral salpingo-oophorectomy with omentectomy with lymph node sampling **or** *For those who hope to remain fertile and have Grade I cancer:* ovary and fallopian tube on affected side removed (unilateral salpingo-oophorectomy), lymph nodes in pelvis and abdomen biopsied. *Clinical trials.*
Stage IC Cancer is found in one or both ovaries and on surface of one or both ovaries; or cancer is in one or both ovaries and tumor has ruptured ovary wall; or cancer is found in one or both ovaries and fluid contains malignant cells.	Intraperitoneal radiation therapy **or** Internal or external radiation therapy **or** Chemotherapy. *Clinical trials.* For selected patients, careful observation without immediate treatment.
Stage IIA Cancer in one or both ovaries and/or spread to uterus and/or fallopian tubes. **Stage IIB** Cancer in one or both ovaries and spread to other tissue within pelvis. **Stage IIC** Tumor either stage IIA or IIB and/or surface of one or both ovaries or tumor has ruptured ovary wall or fluid contains malignant cells.	Total abdominal hysterectomy and bilateral salpingo-oophorectomy with omentectomy and tumor debulking. Lymph node sampling. Following operation either: systemic chemotherapy **or** Depending on amount of tumor that remains, external beam radiation to abdomen and pelvis **or** Intraperitoneal radiation may be used. *Clinical trials*: new drugs and combinations of drugs.

TREATMENT CHOICES FOR OVARIAN
EPITHELIAL CANCERS *(continued)*

STAGE	TREATMENT
Stage IIIA Cancer in one or both ovaries, spread to surface of abdominal wall and surface of liver. **Stage IIIB** Cancer in one or both ovaries, spread to abdominal wall and surface of liver, but not larger than 1 inch in diameter. **Stage IIIC** Cancer in one or both ovaries, spread to abdominal wall and surface of liver, larger than 1 inch in diameter, and/or spread to lymph nodes in abdomen.	Total abdominal hysterectomy as above. Depending on amount of tumor that remains, Combination chemotherapy. *Clinical trials*: New chemotherapy drugs or intraperitoneal chemotherapy. Second-look surgery may be done.
Stage IV Cancer in one or both ovaries and spread outside abdomen to other parts of the body. Cancer is found inside liver.	Combination chemotherapy with or without surgery to reduce size of tumor. *Clinical trials*: New drugs and/or combinations or biological therapy.
Recurrent Cancer recurs after treatment, either in remaining ovary or elsewhere.	Systemic chemotherapy **or** Surgery to relieve symptoms. *Clinical trials*: intraperitoneal chemotherapy or new chemotherapy drugs and combinations of drugs.

usual treatment. Your lymph nodes may also be looked at. If your cancer has come back after treatment, surgery is the usual treatment. It may be followed by chemotherapy.

What is the difference between ovarian epithelial cancers and ovarian germ cell cancers?

Germ cell cancers, of which there are a number of different types, appear to be more aggressive than epithelial cancers, and therefore different treatments are prescribed. The most common type of germ cell cancer is dysgerminoma. These rare tumors are seen most often in young women or adolescent girls and usually affect only one ovary. They are generally curable if found and treated early. The use of chemotherapy after initial surgery is very successful in treating germ cell cancers of the ovary. Dysgerminomas, when they are confined to the ovary, are less than 10 centimeters in size and have an intact, smooth capsule unattached to other organs have a high cure rate when treated with conservative surgery. One or more successful pregnancies following unilateral salpingo-oophorectomy have been reported by women who were treated.

What tests are used to diagnose germ cell tumors?

Several tests might be used including laparotomy lymphangiography, CT scan, and blood tests. The blood tests measure the levels of alpha-fetoprotein (AFP) and human chorionic gonadotropin (HCG) in the blood. These substances may signal ovarian germ cell tumor if they are found at higher levels.

Is chemotherapy successful in treating ovarian germ cell cancers?

Many patients who have ovarian germ cell cancers can benefit from chemotherapy either before or after surgery. The use of platinum-based combination chemotherapy has improved the treatment of many types of ovarian germ cell cancers such as endodermal sinus tumors, immature teratomas, embryonal carcinomas, choriocarcinomas, and mixed tumors containing one or more of these elements.

Do primary cancers grow in the fallopian tubes?

Cancer that starts in the fallopian tubes, which transport eggs from the ovary to the uterus, is the rarest cancer of the female genital tract and is often difficult to distinguish from ovarian cancer. Many times cancer of the fallopian tubes has spread from another site.

What are the symptoms of cancer of the fallopian tubes?

Symptoms can include excessive bleeding, bloody or watery vaginal discharge, or pains in the abdomen or pelvis. Diagnosis is usually only possible with exploratory surgery. Usually treatment is hysterectomy with removal of the ovaries and fallopian tubes with lymph node dissection. Radiation and chemotherapy may be given following surgery.

TREATMENT CHOICES FOR OVARIAN GERM CELL CANCERS

STAGE	TREATMENT
Stage IA Cancer in one ovary. **Stage IB** Cancer found in both ovaries. **Stage IC** Cancer found in one or both ovaries but has spread to outside surface of one or both **or** the outer covering of the tumor has broken open **or** cancer is found in fluid of abdomen.	**Dysgerminoma:** Surgery to remove affected ovary and fallopian tube on same side (unilateral salpingo-oophorectomy), with or without lymphangiography or CT scan **or** Surgery to remove affected ovary and fallopian tube on same side (unilateral salpingo-oophorectomy) followed by close monitoring or radiation therapy **or** Chemotherapy **Other cell types:** Surgery as above followed by chemotherapy **or** Surgery as above with no further treatment.
Stage IIA Cancer in one or both ovaries and/or spread to uterus, and/or fallopian tubes. **Stage IIB** Cancer found in one or both ovaries and has spread to tissues within the pelvis. **Stage IIC** Cancer found in one or both ovaries has spread to uterus.	**Dysgerminoma:** Surgery to remove uterus and both ovaries and fallopian tubes (total abdominal hysterectomy and bilateral salpingo-oophorectomy) followed by chemotherapy or radiation therapy **or** If cancer is only in ovary and fallopian tube on same side and you wish to remain fertile, unilateral salpingo-oophorectomy followed by chemotherapy. **Other cell types:** Total abdominal hysterectomy and bilateral salpingo-oophorectomy. If cancer cannot be totally removed, tumor debulking will be done followed by chemotherapy **or** If cancer is only in ovary and fallopian tube on one side and you want to remain fertile, unilateral salpingo-oophorectomy can be done followed by chemotherapy. *Clinical trials.*
Stage III Cancer in one or both ovaries, spread to lymph nodes or to other parts of abdomen or to surface of liver or intestines.	**Dysgerminoma:** Total abdominal hysterectomy and bilateral salpingo-oophorectomy and tumor debulking **or** Same as above, but if remaining cancer is large, systemic chemotherapy following surgery **or** If you wish to remain fertile, surgery to remove

(continued)

TREATMENT CHOICES FOR OVARIAN GERM CELL CANCERS (continued)

STAGE	TREATMENT
	only ovary and fallopian tube involved followed by chemotherapy.
	Other Cell Types: Total abdominal hysterectomy and bilateral salpingo-oophorectomy and tumor debulking, with chemotherapy before or after surgery.
	or
	If cancer found only in ovary and fallopian tube on same side and you want to remain fertile, unilateral salpingo-oophorectomy followed by chemotherapy.
	Clinical trials.
Stage IV Cancer in one or both ovaries and spread outside abdomen or inside liver.	**Dysgerminoma:** Total abdominal hysterectomy and bilateral salpingo-oophorectomy plus tumor debulking. Chemotherapy following surgery. If cancer remains, additional chemotherapy with different drugs **or** If cancer found only in ovary and fallopian tube on same side and you want to remain fertile, unilateral salpingo-oophorectomy followed by chemotherapy. *Clinical trials.* **Other cell types:** Total abdominal hysterectomy and bilateral salpingo-oophorectomy plus tumor debulking. Chemotherapy before or after surgery **or** If only in one ovary and fallopian tube on same side and you want to remain fertile, unilateral salpingo-oophorectomy followed by chemotherapy. *Clinical trials.*
Recurrent Cancer recurs after treatment, either in remaining ovary or elsewhere.	**Dysgerminoma:** Systemic chemotherapy with or without radiation. **Other Cell Types:** Surgery with or without systemic chemotherapy. *Clinical trials.*

CANCER OF THE VAGINA

What You Need to Know About Cancer of the Vagina

- Squamous cell vaginal cancer is usually found in women between 60 and 80.

- Adenocarcinoma is more often found in women between the ages of 12 and 30.

- Clear cell adenocarcinoma has been seen in young women whose mothers took DES.

- Surgery is the most common treatment for vaginal cancer. Laser may be used for the surgery. Radiation and chemotherapy may follow the surgery.

What is cancer of the vagina?

Cancer of the vagina is an uncommon, highly treatable, often curable cancer that grows in the passageway between the cervix and the vulva. This part of the body is often referred to as the birth canal. Squamous cell vaginal cancer is most often found in women between the ages of 60 and 80. An even rarer type of vaginal cancer is clear cell adenocarcinoma, found most often in young women between the ages of 17 and 21. This type of cancer is associated with DES (diethylstilbestrol). It is believed that daughters of women who took DES to prevent miscarriage between 1945 and 1971 are at a risk of developing clear cell adenocarcinoma. There is more information on DES later in this chapter.

What are the symptoms of cancer of the vagina?

Bleeding or discharge not related to menstrual periods, difficult or painful urination and pain during intercourse or in the pelvic area are symptoms of cancer of the vagina.

If I have had a hysterectomy, can I still get cancer of the vagina?

Yes, you can get cancer of the vagina, even if you have had a hysterectomy.

**Are squamous cell and adenocarcinoma of the vagina
treated in the same manner?**

Different treatments are recommended for Stage I squamous cell cancer of the vagina and Stage I adenocarcinoma of the vagina. You should be sure that you understand which type of cancer you have and what treatment is being recommended. All other stages of squamous cell and adenocarcinoma of the vagina are treated in a similar manner.

What kind of follow-up is needed for vaginal cancers?

Life-long follow-up is important for women with vaginal cancers. For the first year, follow-up should be every three months. Pap smears and tumor

TREATMENT CHOICES FOR CANCER OF THE VAGINA

STAGE	TREATMENT
Stage 0 or *in situ* Found inside vagina only, and is only in a few layers of cells.	Removal of cancer and tissue around it with or without skin grafting **or** Removal of all or part of vagina with skin grafting **or** Intravaginal chemotherapy with five percent fluorouracil cream **or** Laser surgery **or** Intracavitary radiation.
Stage I Not spread outside vagina.	**Squamous cell:** Depending on thickening of tumor, internal radiation therapy with or without external radiation **or** Removal of cancer and tissue around it with or without skin grafting with or without radiation **or** Removal of vagina, with or without removal of lymph nodes. **Adenocarcinoma:** Removal of vagina, uterus, ovaries, fallopian tubes, and lymph nodes with or without skin grafting and with or without radiation therapy **or** Internal radiation with or without external radiation **or** Removal of cancer, tissue around it and lymph nodes with or without internal radiation.
Stage II Spread to tissues outside vagina, but not to bones of pelvis.	Radiation, both internal and external **or** Surgery with or without radiation.
Stage III Spread to bones of pelvis and to other organs and lymph nodes.	Combination internal radiation and external radiation **or** Surgery may be combined with above.
Stage IV-A Spread to bladder or rectum.	Combination internal and external radiation **or** Surgery may be combined with above. *Clinical trials* should be considered.
Stage IV-B Spread to other parts of body, such as lungs.	Radiation. *Clinical trials* should be considered.

TREATMENT CHOICES FOR CANCER OF THE VAGINA *(continued)*

STAGE	TREATMENT
Recurrent Comes back in vagina or another place.	Difficult to treat. Removal of cervix, uterus, lower colon, rectum, or bladder depending on where cancer has spread. Chemotherapy and radiation may be used. *Clinical trials* should be considered.

markers should be checked at this time with chest x-rays, urine, and stool testing every three months for the first six months, and then at six month intervals until the fifth year. Thereafter, yearly checkups should be scheduled. Tell the doctor if you have vaginal discharge or bleeding, bone pain, weight or appetite loss, bowel or bladder problems, or swelling of the legs. Routine examinations are an important factor in detecting problems early and raising the cure rates for vaginal cancer.

Must special care be taken after having a radiation implant in the vagina?
The procedure for radiation implants is explained in Chapter 9, Radiation Treatment. However, there are a few additional points that you will need to know about if you are having vaginal radiation implant treatments. For two to three weeks following the implant, you should not use tampons, should not have intercourse and should not douche or take tub baths. After this period, it is necessary, in the interest of proper healing, for you to either use a dilator or to have intercourse in order to prevent the vaginal cavity from closing and/or forming adhesions. Since the implant often causes vaginal dryness, use of a water-soluble lubricant may make intercourse more comfortable. It is advised that you have intercourse twice a week or use a dilator to help the tissues begin to stretch. Some degree of discomfort and perhaps a little bleeding may be noticed.

How is a dilator used?
A dilator is used to keep the vaginal opening from closing. You can apply a water-soluble lubricant to the rounded end of the dilator, lie on your back in bed with your knees bent and slightly apart. Insert the rounded end of the dilator into the vagina gently and as deeply as you can without causing discomfort. Let it stay in place for 10 minutes. Withdraw and clean the dilator with hot, soapy water, rising it well. Do not be alarmed if slight bleeding or spotting occurs following dilator use. If you are unable to insert the dilator easily, check with your nurse or doctor.

Is it normal for intercourse to hurt following vaginal surgery?

Intercourse may cause you some pain following this surgery. The cause may be a combination of physical and psychological factors. You should first check with your doctor or nurse to determine if there are physical reasons why you feel pain. The use of medicine, including antispasmodics and analgesics, may be advised to help you relax before intercourse and prevent a tightening of your pelvic muscles, which can make intercourse uncomfortable. Touching and exploring the vaginal area with your fingers may help you gain confidence. Short-term behavioral sex therapy, with instruction in relaxation and desensitization techniques, or consultation with a sex therapist, may be helpful.

Is reconstruction done following vaginal cancer surgery?

If possible, plans for reconstruction should be made before original surgery, although reconstruction may be possible at a later date even if not pre-planned. Just as women who have undergone mastectomies may have breast reconstruction, women who have vaginal surgery (or colpectomies) may have plastic surgery to reconstruct the vagina. Women who have had this reconstruction say it is possible to regain former sensations and feelings. Partners report pleasurable, successful sexual relations following this surgery. Reconstruction is often done in stages, and may involve several separate surgeries done several weeks or months apart. Consultation with a reputable plastic surgeon who will do the reconstruction, as well as with the surgeon who performs the vaginectomy, is necessary.

CANCER OF THE VULVA

What You Need to Know About Cancer of the Vulva

- This cancer is rare and when it is detected early it is very curable.

- Three-quarters of the women who get cancer of the vulva are over 50.

- Almost all cancer of the vulva develops slowly over the years from carcinoma *in situ* (or Stage 0 cancer), found in women from 30–35 years old.

- Surgery, with or without radiation therapy, is the usual treatment for this cancer. Chemotherapy may also be used.

- Be sure that you are treated at a major medical center by a gynecological oncologist who understands this disease.

What is cancer of the vulva?

The vulva is the outer part of the vagina and looks much like a pair of lips. It is made up of several structures including the clitoris, labia, hymen, vaginal opening, and bladder opening (urethra). Cancer in this area is rare, most often occurs in women over 50, although it can sometimes occur in women under the age of 40. Most of these cancers are found on the labia and are of the squamous cell type.

What causes cancer of the vulva?

It is thought that human papilloma virus (HPV) is responsible for about half of cancers of the vulva. Cigarette smoking and HIV infection also put a woman at higher risk of getting this cancer.

What are the symptoms of cancer of the vulva?

Itching, burning, bleeding, pain, and a lump or growth on the vulva are symptoms of this cancer. The doctor will usually do a punch biopsy to determine whether or not there is cancer in the area. Several other tests, such as cystoscopy, proctoscopy, and intravenous urography, may also be done to determine the stage of disease.

What is the usual treatment for cancer of the vulva?

Surgery is the most common treatment for vulvar cancer. Radiation therapy may precede or follow surgery for women with Stages III and IV vulvar cancer. For some patients, chemotherapy may also be used. Vulvar cancer is highly curable when diagnosed in an early stage, before the nodes become involved.

Questions to Ask Your Doctor Before Being Treated for Cancer of the Vulva

- How extensive will the surgery be?
- What exactly will be removed?
- Will the clitoris be removed?
- Where will the scars be located?
- Will this procedure change my normal urination, voiding and sexual patterns?
- How long will I be in the hospital?
- How long will recovery take?
- How long will the surgery take?
- How long before stitches are removed?
- Following surgery, what kinds of complications should I report to the doctor and what doctor will I report to?
- Should I expect swelling in my legs, groin, and feet due to the lymph node dissection?

- How long will it be before swelling from lymph node dissection ceases?
- Will my sexual responses be changed by the surgery?
- How long before I can resume sexual intercourse?
- How long before I can use tampons?
- Is it wise for me to use a vaginal douche?
- How long before I can resume normal activities?

TREATMENT CHOICES FOR CANCER OF THE VULVA

STAGE	TREATMENT
Stage 0 or *in situ*; very early stage. Found only in vulva on surface of skin.	Wide localized surgery and/or Laser surgery **or** Combination of both **or** Skinning vulvectomy with or without grafting. (NOTE: If simple vulvectomy is suggested, you should know that more limited surgical procedures produce equivalent results and are less drastic. Topical fluorocuracil is **not** a reliable first choice of treatment.)
Stage I Found only in vulva and/or in perineum (space between opening of rectum and vagina). Two centimeters (one inch) or less in size.	Wide localized surgery **or** Radical local surgery with removal of all nearby lymph nodes in groin and upper part of thigh on same side **or** Radical vulvectomy and lymph node removal in groin and on one or both sides **or** If unable to tolerate surgery, radiation therapy.
Stage II Found in vulva and in perineum (space between opening of rectum and vagina). Larger than two centimeters (one inch) in size.	Radical vulvectomy, removal of lymph nodes in groin on both sides plus radiation therapy if cancer found in lymph nodes **or** If unable to tolerate surgery, radiation alone.
Stage III Found in vulva and/or perineum (space between rectum and vagina) and has spread to lower part of urethra, vagina, anus and/or has spread to nearby lymph nodes.	Radical vulvectomy, removal of lymph nodes in groin and upper thigh on both sides of body. Radiation given to pelvis and groin if cancer found in lymph nodes or only to vulva if tumor is large but has not spread **or** Radiation and chemotherapy followed by radi-

TREATMENT CHOICES FOR CANCER OF THE VULVA *(continued)*

STAGE	TREATMENT
Stage III (continued)	cal vulvectomy and removal of lymph nodes on both sides of body **or** Radiation with or without chemotherapy (selected patients).
Stage IV Spread beyond urethra, vagina and anus into lining of bladder and bowel or pelvic bone, or spread to lymph nodes in pelvis or other parts of body.	Radical vulvectomy and removal of lower colon, rectum or bladder, depending on spread of cancer, along with removal of uterus, cervix and vagina (pelvic exenteration) **or** Radical vulvectomy followed by radiation **or** Radiation therapy followed by radical vulvectomy **or** Radiation therapy (selected patients) with or without chemotherapy and possibly surgery. *Clinical trials.*
Recurrent Cancer returns after treatment.	Wide local excision with or without radiation therapy or Radical vulvectomy plus pelvic exenteration **or** Radiation plus chemotherapy with or without surgery **or** Radiation of new cancer or to reduce symptoms. *Clinical trials.*

What are the surgical procedures used for cancer of the vulva?

The technical terms for the various operations include:

- Wide local excision which removes the cancer and some of the normal tissue around it.

- Radical local excision which takes out the cancer, and a larger portion of normal tissue. Lymph nodes may also be removed.

- Skinning vulvectomy which removes only the skin of the vulva that contains the cancer; Partial vulvectomy, which takes out less than the entire vulva; Simple vulvectomy which takes out the entire vulva, but no lymph nodes; and Radical vulvectomy which removes the entire vulva and the lymph nodes around it.

- If the cancer has spread outside the vulva and the other female organs, the doctor may perform a pelvic exenteration—the surgical removal of the lower colon, rectum, or bladder as well as the cervix, uterus, and vagina.

- Following surgery, reconstruction with plastic surgery and skin grafts may be done to create an artificial vulva or vagina.

What are the possible complications of a radical vulvectomy?

Following the operation, because of the removal of a large number of lymph nodes, fluid collects under the skin and may be a problem until other lymph channels have become established. For this reason, deep-breathing, coughing, and leg exercises are started immediately after surgery. Frequent irrigations with sterile saline solution, heat lamp treatments, and sitz baths are also used to promote healing.

Is sexual intercourse possible after vulvectomy?

Intercourse is still possible though you may have to change position or technique. Removal of the vulva may cause the remaining vaginal tissues to tighten, making intercourse and physical examination more difficult. Intercourse and/or stretching of the vagina right after the operation are important to make sure that the tissues will remain supple and elastic.

Is laser beam therapy used for cancer of the vulva?

Laser beam therapy may be used either alone or with wide local excision for Stage 0 vulvar cancer.

Sexual and Urinary Problems Following Gynecological Treatments

What sexual changes can I expect after treatment for gynecological cancer?

First and foremost, you should have a frank discussion with your doctor before the surgery, if possible, so that you know what to expect and so that you can mentally start dealing with the issues. When you first have sexual intercourse after having had treatment, you will probably worry about pain and think that your sexual life will never be the same as it was before. Don't be surprised if your first attempt is disappointing. You will probably have to make adjustments. Talk with your doctor or nurse about sex and discuss what the doctor tells you with your partner. Good communication is essential at this time. Tell your partner if you feel pain. Remember that no matter what kind of cancer treatment you have had, the ability to feel pleasure from being touched almost always remains. Even if some aspects of sexuality have changed, pleasure is still possible.

What are the most common symptoms that interfere with sexual functioning following gynecological treatment?
Lack of desire and pain are two of the most commonly heard problems. Lack of desire immediately after treatment may be caused by worry, depression, and pain. Pain during intercourse can be caused by changes in the body as the result of treatment. Pain can occur after surgery, radiation, chemotherapy or other treatment that affects the hormonal balance. The pain can set off a series of further problems. Sometimes just one incidence of painful intercourse can cause the muscles around the opening of the vagina to tense up and make intercourse impossible and unpleasant.

How can I learn to relax my vaginal muscles?
There is a set of exercises called Kegels, which can help to teach you to relax, and thus lessen pain during intercourse.

- The muscles around the entrance to the vagina are the same ones that stop the flow of urine. When you urinate, try stopping the flow of urine for a few seconds. Be aware of the muscles you use to make this happen. Relax your muscles and let the urine flow again.

- Practice using those muscles when you are not urinating. First, tighten the muscles in the genital area. To check whether you are tightening the right muscles, try slipping one finger about two inches into your vagina. When you tense your vaginal muscles, you will feel a slight twitch of the vaginal walls around your finger.

- Once you know the muscles that need relaxing you can do the exercise anywhere—while reading, sitting in the car or watching television. Just tighten your vaginal muscles, count to three and relax. Do this ten times in a row, several times a day.

- During intercourse, make sure you are well lubricated. Use the same technique to tense and relax your vaginal muscles. The action will help you focus on your excitement and will add to your partner's pleasure.

- If you begin to feel tightness or pain, stay still for a moment while you gently squeeze your vaginal muscles. Notice the looseness when you relax your muscles.

- If you still have pain, you may need the help of your gynecologist or a sex therapist. Some doctors recommend using a series of vaginal dilators in different sizes to stretch the vagina.

How is a vaginal dilator used?
A vaginal dilator can be helpful in stretching the vagina. Dilators are cylindrical- or tube-shaped—and usually made of plastic. They come in various sizes.

Your doctor will prescribe the correct size for you. Usually you will start with one about the size of a finger, and then the size is increased until the vagina has stretched enough to allow penetration without pain. To use the dilator, lubricate it well with a water-based gel. Lie down in bed or put your foot up on the toilet and gently and slowly insert the dilator into the vagina. If you feel tight, tense and relax your muscles, then put the dilator farther into the vagina. You may need to squeeze and relax a few times before the dilator is fully inserted. Sometimes it is helpful to bear down as if having a bowel movement. When the dilator is in as far as possible, leave it in your vagina for about 10 minutes. NOTE: When the vagina has been rebuilt with skin grafts, a special dilator may be prescribed to be worn twenty-four hours a day for a period of time.

What is the effect of premature menopause on sexual intercourse?

Premature menopause, as caused by the removal of the ovaries, triggers severe and abrupt changes in the body. Besides causing hot flashes, the loss of estrogen causes the vagina to become tight and dry. Understanding the consequences of this type of treatment and compensating for it with the use of extra lubrication can help to make intercourse more comfortable. There are many water-based gel vaginal lubricants available. You may find that an over-the-counter vaginal moisturizer used three times weekly, keeps the vagina moist at all times, helps normalize the pH balance, and helps prevent yeast infections.

How does a radical vulvectomy affect sexual functioning?

When the whole vulva, including the inner and outer lips and the clitoris, and sometimes lymph nodes in the area are surgically removed, there may be a problem with reaching orgasm. The outer genitals, especially the clitoris, are the centers of sexual sensitivity. Additionally, there may be a feeling of numbness in the genital area, which may return over the period of a few months. When scarring is severe, the surgeon may do reconstructive surgery with skin grafts to correct the problem of a narrowed vaginal entrance.

How is the vagina reconstructed?

Several methods are used. Skin grafts are the most common method. Following such a reconstruction, a special vaginal mold is designed to be worn internally. At first it is worn twenty-four hours a day. Gradually, it is worn for part of the day. In about three months, regular sexual intercourse or the use of a plastic tube (dilator) to stretch out the vagina for a short time daily is enough to keep the vagina open. Without dilation, the vagina will shrink and close. If the entire vagina needs to be rebuilt, flaps of muscle and skin from both inner thighs may be used. The surgeon forms the flaps from each side into a closed tube that is lined by the skin surface, and then are sewn into the area where the vagina was removed. When the new vagina heals, it is similar in size and shape to the one that was surgically removed. Learning to live with a redesigned vagina means that you will need to make adjustments in your sexual patterns. You may need to try different intercourse positions to bring pleasure, since the muscles ringing the vaginal entrance no longer can be contracted at will, and nerve sensations are connected to the original nerve supplies at the inner thigh. Women who have had the surgery say that changes in sensations due to the surgery can be sexually interesting and stimulating.

What is the result of lymph node removal in the genital area?

When lymph nodes in the groin are removed or you have had radiation treatment to the lymph nodes, swelling can occur in the genital area and in the legs. The problems, referred to as lymphedema, can be similar to those described in Chapter 13, Breast Cancer, except that they occur in another part of the body. There are things you can do to help prevent lymphedema: wear loose clothes, avoid tight bands around your groin, knees or ankle, use support hose when you stand for a long time, don't sit with knees and hips bent for long periods of time and exercise so that you have muscle tone in this area. For more information about this side effect, get in touch with the Lymphedema Network. See Chapter 28, Where to Get Help.

Should I be concerned about infections?

Infections are potential problems, especially if you have lymphedema. Check for redness across the lower abdomen, groin, thigh, or vulva. Tell your doctor if you have fever or pain. Infections need to be treated promptly with antibiotics. There are a few precautions you can take: be careful about scraping or cutting your legs, ankles, and feet, don't go barefoot, make sure your shoes fit well, shave your legs with an electric razor, and don't cut your toenails too short.

Pregnancy and Gynecological Cancers

What happens if you get cancer in the reproductive area when you are pregnant?

The discovery of cancer during pregnancy is a highly traumatic event that needs to be carefully evaluated before any decisions are made. Pregnancy complicated by a diagnosis of cancer in the reproductive organs is very rare, but when it happens, it creates an incredible range of multiple problems, both physical and emotional. In general, most cancers do not, in and of themselves, impact on the outcome of the pregnancy although the pregnancy is certainly complicated by the diagnosis of cancer. Unless continued pregnancy will compromise treatment and thus prognosis, therapeutic abortion has not been shown to be of benefit in altering the progression of the cancer. The risk of abortion and fetal malformation from radiation and chemotherapy are highest during the first trimester and vary with treatments used. During the second and third trimesters, the evidence of increased risk appears to be minimal. Most doctors feel that if cure is a reasonable goal, treatment should not be compromised by modification or delay. However, if treatment for cure or significant relief is not possible, the goal must then shift to the protection of the fetus from damage. There is information concerning breast cancer and pregnancy in Chapter 11, Breast Cancer.

What happens when cancer of the cervix is found during pregnancy?

Most of the cancers of the cervix found during pregnancy are Stage 0 or *in situ* cancers. Invasive cancer of the cervix is seen in only two to five percent of all cases. Symptoms are similar to those found in non-pregnant women. Very often, with stage 0 or *in situ* cancers, pregnancy is allowed to continue and treatment delayed until after delivery, unless the disease appears to be spreading. If invasion is found during the first two trimesters, surgery or radiation therapy without therapeutic abortion is usually the treatment. During the third trimester, the baby, when viable, may be delivered by cesarean section, with appropriate treatment undertaken after the delivery. There is an unresolved controversy over the safety of vaginal delivery versus cesarean delivery. Some doctors recommend cesarean delivery because they feel that vaginal delivery may disseminate the cancer or cause hemorrhage or infection. One study reported recurrence in an episiotomy after vaginal delivery. Other doctors suggest that vaginal delivery actually may be beneficial and should be planned if possible. Careful follow-up is essential.

What is done when ovarian masses appear during pregnancy?

Though ovarian masses are common during pregnancy, only about two to five percent become malignant. There are a variety of approaches to treatment. Some doctors feel that a mass that is larger than five centimeters that continues into the second trimester should be explored. Others feel that a mass over six centimeters should be evaluated immediately. Yet others feel that a single, encapsulated, movable mass under 10 centimeters can wait until the second trimester for evaluation. However, if the mass is found to be cancerous, treatment can continue just as it would in someone who is not pregnant. Early stage disease may be managed by removal of the affected ovary and biopsy of the other ovary. The pregnancy may be allowed to continue. If the patient is near delivery, a cesarean section, followed by the appropriate therapy is usually the choice. For other stages and scenarios, standard treatment can be followed. As in the treatment of all cancers, the wishes of the patient will be considered. It is not uncommon for a pregnant woman with advanced disease to delay treatment until the fetus is viable. In every case, treatment should be started at the earliest possible time.

What are gestational trophoblastic tumors?

A group of rare cancers known as gestational trophoblastic tumors grow in the uterus in tissues that are formed after a woman conceives. In the last 30 years this type of cancer has gone from one of the most fatal gynecological cancers to one of the most potentially curable. Hydatidiform moles and choriocarcinoma are the two most common of these cancers. They can be diagnosed by a sonogram. Hydatidiform mole, sometimes called molar pregnancy, occurs when the sperm and egg cells join but do not succeed in forming a fetus. The tissue that grows in the uterus resembles grape-like cysts and does not spread outside the uterus. Choriocarcinoma may develop from a hydatidiform mole or from tissue that remains in the uterus following an abortion or delivery of a baby. It can spread outside the uterus to other parts of the body. A third, very rare type of gestational trophoblastic tumor, which starts where the placenta was attached in the uterus, is known as placental-site trophoblastic tumor. Before chemotherapy, many of these cancers were considered fatal. Choriocarcinoma was the first malignancy that proved to be curable by chemotherapy after it had metastasized. Today, the cure rate is 97 to 100 percent for those that have not metastasized, and 75 percent for those that are listed as poor prognosis metastatic. The major factor is early diagnosis, proper treatment and careful follow-up. It is important to be treated by someone who understands this disease and treatments.

How is choriocarcinoma classified?

Choriocarcinoma is divided into three groups of gestational trophoblastic tumors: nonmetastatic, good prognosis metastatatic, and poor prognosis metastatic. The cancer is classified as good prognosis metastic if all of these are true: last pregnancy less than four months ago, level of HCG is low, cancer has not spread to liver or brain, you have not received chemotherapy previously. If you have poor prognosis metastatic gestational trophoblastic tumor, you need to be treated quickly by a gynecological cancer specialist or at one of the Regional Trophoblastic Disease Centers.

What is beta-HCG?

Beta-HCG measures serum beta human chorionic gonadotropin, which is produced normally during pregnancy. In patients with gestational

TREATMENT CHOICES FOR HYDATIDIFORM MOLE AND GESTATIONAL TROPHOBLASTIC TUMORS

TYPE	WHAT IT MEANS	TREATMENT
Hydatidiform mole **Invasive mole** (chorioadenoma destruens)	Confined to inside of uterus, does not spread outside uterus. Found in muscle of uterus.	D & C, suction evacuation, preservation of childbearing ability **or** Hysterectomy, ovaries not removed. Close monitoring. If levels of beta-HCG rise, tissue diagnosis shows choriocarcinoma, or post evacuation hemorrhage not caused by retained tissues occurs, chemotherapy is given.
Placental-site	Found where placenta was attached and in muscle of uterus, very rare.	Hysterectomy. (These tumors are relatively resistant to chemotherapy.)
Nonmetastatic gestational trophoblastic tumor (This is the most common type, considered 100 percent curable)	Found inside uterus from tissue remaining following hydatidiform mole or following abortion or delivery. Has not spread outside uterus.	Chemotherapy **or** Occasionally hysterectomy if fertility is no longer desired.
Good prognosis metastatic gestational trophoblastic tumor	As above, but spread outside uterus. Last pregnancy less than 4 months ago, beta HCG level is low, has not spread to liver or brain, and has never had chemotherapy.	Chemotherapy **or** Hysterectomy followed by chemotherapy **or** Chemotherapy followed by hysterectomy if cancer remains following chemotherapy.
Poor prognosis metastatic gestational trophoblastic tumor.	As above, with spread to other parts of the body and if any of the following: pregnancy more than four months ago, beta HCG level high, cancer spread to	Chemotherapy. Radiation to places where cancer has spread. Surgery may be necessary. Quick treatment needed at hospital with trophoblastic center. *(continued)*

TREATMENT CHOICES FOR HYDATIDIFORM MOLE AND GESTATIONAL TROPHOBLASTIC TUMORS (continued)

TYPE	WHAT IT MEANS	TREATMENT
	liver or brain, have had chemotherapy which did not eradicate cancer or tumor began after normal pregnancy.	
Recurrent	Cancer returns after treatment, either in uterus or other part of body.	Chemotherapy with or without radiation. For selected patients, surgery

trophoblastic tumors, beta-HCG is abnormally elevated in the blood and urine. The doctor measures the beta-HCG titer level that serves as a sensitive marker to indicate the presence or absence of activity of the cancer before, during, and after treatment.

What kind of follow-up is suggested for gestational trophoblastic tumors?
Careful follow-up is essential—an exam every three months for the first year, then every six months. Beta HCG testing should be done weekly until it has fallen to normal levels, then every two weeks for three months, then monthly for three months, every two months for six months and then every six months. Contraception should be used for at least the first year.

DES-RELATED CANCERS

What is DES and what is its connection to cancer of the cervix and vagina?
DES is a synthetic form of estrogen, also known as diethylstilbestrol. It was prescribed from the early 1940s until 1971 to help women with certain complications of pregnancy. It has been found that when given during the first five months of pregnancy, DES interfered with the development of the reproductive system in a fetus. A link has been found between DES exposure before birth and an increased risk of developing abnormal cells in the tissue of the cervix and vagina. These abnormal cells, sometimes called dysplasia,

cervical intraepithelial neoplasia (CIN) and squamous intraepithelial lesions (SIL) resemble cancer cells in appearance. However, they do not invade nearby healthy tissue the way cancer cells do. They usually occur between the ages of 25 and 35 in women whose mothers took DES. Although they are not cancer, they might develop into cancer if not treated. DES-exposed daughters may also have structural changes in the vagina, uterus, or cervix. Most of these changes do not cause medical problems but some women may have irregular menstruation and an increased risk of miscarriage, premature delivery, and infertility. There is some evidence that DES-exposed sons may have testicular abnormalities, such as undescended testicles or abnormally small testicles although the risk of testicular or prostate cancer or infertility has not shown an increase. New research looking at grandchildren of the DES-exposed women does not show any evidence that the grandchildren have been affected.

Are the women who took the DES at higher risk for cancer?
Women who used DES may have a slightly increased risk for breast cancer. If you used DES, it would be useful to know when you started taking it, what amount you were taking and how you were taking it. You need to make sure your doctor knows this and that you have yearly medical checkups with breast and pelvic exams and a Pap test. You also need to inform your children so that this information can be listed on their records.

Where can DES-exposed people get additional information?
DES Action is a consumer group organized by individuals who were exposed to DES. DES Cancer Network is a national organization for DES-exposed women and their families. The Registry for Research on Hormonal Transplacental Carcinogenesis is a worldwide registry for individuals who developed clear cell adenocarcinoma as a result of exposure to DES. See Chapter 28, Where to Get Help, for address information.

Web Pages to Check Out

www.cancer.gov: For general up-to-date information, and for clinical trials.
www.cancer.org: For general up-to-date information and community resources.
www.wcn.org: Women's Cancer Network, information on women's cancer.
www.jcaho.org: Joint Commission on Accreditation of Healthcare Organizations to see if lab is accredited.
www.personal.u-net.com/~njh/cgest.html: Gestational Trophoblastic Tumors.
www.desaction.org: DES Action USA.
www.descancer.org: DES Cancer Networks.

www.obgyn.bsd.uchicago.edu/registry.html: The Registry for Research on Hormonal Transplacental Carcinogenesis.

Web Sites for Ovarian cancer:

www.ovariancancer.org: Ovarian Cancer National Alliance.
www.ovarian.org: National Ovarian Cancer coalition.
www.ovariancancer.com: Gilda Radner Familial Ovarian Cancer Registry.

Also see Chapter 2, Searching for Answers on the Web, for more information.

Twenty-one

BONE AND SOFT-TISSUE SARCOMAS

Bone and soft-tissue sarcomas are cancers of the structural and connective tissues of the body. Bone cancers are extremely rare—only about 2,500 new cases are diagnosed each year. Soft-tissue cancers are also quite unusual, with about 8,300 new cases each year. Molecular genetics are being studied in both bone and soft-tissue sarcomas and perhaps in the future, genetic therapy will help to alleviate some of them.

FOR THOSE WHO are dealing with a diagnosis of sarcoma, it is reassuring to know that recent findings about bone and soft-tissue sarcomas and a multidisciplinary approach to treatment have improved the results of bone and soft-tissue tumor treatment in recent years. This chapter will deal with bone and soft-tissue cancers in adults. Osteosarcoma, Ewing's sarcoma, and rhabdomyosarcoma affect children; they are discussed in Chapter 24, When a Child Has Cancer. Multiple myeloma, a cancer of the white blood cells that affects bones is included in Chapter 19, Hodgkin's Disease, Non-Hodgkin's Lymphoma, and Multiple Myeloma. Cancer that has spread to the bone from another part of the body is covered in Chapter 26, When Cancers Recur or Metastasize.

WHAT YOU NEED TO KNOW ABOUT
BONE AND SOFT-TISSUE SARCOMAS

- Cancers that begin in the bone are quite rare. (Cancers that spread to the bone are more common. This chapter deals only with cancers that **start in the bone.**)

- Because these cancers are very rare, it is important to go to a major medical or research center where there are specialists who specialize in diagnosing and treating them.

- Most tumors in the bone are found to be benign. A very small percentage are cancerous.

- Cancer can occur in any of the 206 bones in the body—but it occurs most often in the arms and legs. Most bone cancers are sarcomas.

- Children and young people are more likely than adults to have primary bone cancers.

- Surgery is the most common treatment for most bone cancers (except for Ewing's sarcoma). Soft-tissue sarcomas are also most commonly treated with surgery. For both bone and soft-tissue sarcomas, radiation therapy, and chemotherapy may be used before or after surgery.

- Until recently, amputation was considered the best treatment for bone cancers in the arm or leg. Today, limb-sparing surgery is possible in many cases with the use of preoperative or postoperative chemotherapy. Even high-grade soft-tissue sarcomas in the arms and legs can often be treated while preserving the limb.

- **Inappropriately performed biopsy must be avoided** since it can ruin chances of having limb-sparing surgery.

- Sarcomas are cancers that begin in the connective tissues. They are divided into two groups: those that begin in the bone, and those that begin in the muscles, fat, and other connective or supportive tissues of the body (soft-tissue sarcomas).

- Soft-tissue sarcomas can grow anywhere in the body. The largest percentage develop at, or above, the knee or in the trunk. Fifteen percent develop in arms and hands, ten percent in the head and neck, and about ten percent in the back wall of the abdominal cavity. Some of these are so well hidden by overlying normal tissue that they may become quite large before being noticed.

- When bone sarcomas spread, they do so through the bloodstream, since bones do not have a lymph system.

Are bone and soft-tissue sarcomas difficult to diagnose?

Because they are seen infrequently, sarcomas may be misdiagnosed, confused with other benign disease, or overlooked. CT scans, MRI, and ultrasounds will show changes in bone or cartilage. They also can show abnormal changes in softer tissues. A bone scan can detect sarcomas of the bone. Arteriograms or angiograms depict blood vessels showing whether they are pushed aside or whether the tumor has an abnormal blood supply. Chemical changes in the blood are often found in sarcomas of bone. Chest x-rays are important in evaluating sarcomas because these cancers have a tendency to spread to the lungs. The biopsy is the final diagnostic procedure. It is usually done as an open biopsy rather than as a needle biopsy to get an adequate piece of tumor so that treatment can be properly staged. **If the sarcoma affects a bone in the arm or leg, the biopsy should be done by the surgeon who will be doing the limb-sparing surgery. A biopsy that is inappropriately done can make it impossible to achieve limb-sparing surgery.**

Is there a blood test that can detect cancer of the bone?

A blood test to determine the level of alkaline phosphatase, an enzyme produced by cells that form new bone tissue, is often used in detecting bone tumors. However, this enzyme is also found in large amounts found in the blood for other reasons, for instance when children or adolescents are growing, when a bone is mending, or when a disease causes the production of an abnormal amount of bone tissue. Therefore, this blood test can be used only as an indicator, not as a definite diagnostic test.

What kind of doctor should be treating bone or soft-tissue sarcomas?

Since these two types of cancers are extremely rare, specialists experienced in treating these types of cancer are most likely to be found at large cancer treatment and research centers. Since the selection of treatment is determined by the information gleaned from a biopsy, careful study of the biopsy tissue by a pathologist experienced in these types of cancers is important. Complete staging and planning treatment by a multidisciplinary team of cancer specialists—pathologists, surgeons, radiation oncologists, and medical oncologists—who can review all of the information gathered in the diagnostic and staging procedures, will assure that the very latest and best treatment is given. In addition, there are musculoskeletal oncologists who specialize in limb reconstruction after bone cancer.

Why is the biopsy so important in staging bone and soft-tissue sarcomas?

Treatment will be based on the type of cells found in the biopsy tissue. Having the advice of an orthopedic surgical oncologist **before** biopsy is important since the biopsy may have an impact on how subsequent surgery is performed.

What causes bone and soft-tissue sarcomas?

Relatively little is known regarding the cause of these cancers. It does appear that prior cancer therapy in the form of high-dose radiation and some chemotherapy drugs (the alkylating agents) may be linked to the development of primary bone cancer. People with inherited diseases such as Li-Fraumeni syndrome or von Recklinghausen's disease are at increased risk for soft-tissue sarcoma. Doctors stress that sarcomas are definitely not related to common injuries. Some studies suggest that workers who have been exposed to phenoxy herbicide, vinyl chloride, dioxin, arsenic, or thorotrast may have an increased risk for developing soft-tissue sarcomas. Researchers believe that a retrovirus may play an indirect role in Kaposi's sarcoma often found in people with AIDS.

Has Agent Orange been associated with soft-tissue sarcoma?

Agent Orange, a mixture of herbicides used during the Vietnam War mainly to defoliate forest trees, and other herbicides used during the Vietnam War have been associated with soft-tissue sarcoma (other than osteosarcoma, chondrosarcoma, Kaposi's sarcoma, or mesothelioma). If you are a Vietnam veteran and have been diagnosed with soft-tissue sarcoma, you should qualify for VA disability compensation and the special access to medical care that the VA has offered to Vietnam veterans for health problems from Agent Orange exposure. You do not need to prove that your illness is related to your military service. It is presumed to be service-connected. For more information, see Chapter 4, What Is Cancer?

Questions to Ask Your Doctor Before Treatment for Bone or Soft-Tissue Sarcomas

- **Where can I get the best possible treatment? Can you help me find the best doctor in the area to consult about my cancer?**
- **How many patients with my kind of cancer have you treated?**
- **Is it possible for me to have radiation before surgery to shrink the tumor?**
- **Is it possible for me to have limb-sparing surgery?**
- **What are the steps involved in treating me without removing my limb?**
- **How many operations are involved and how long will it take?**

- Will I still be able to use my limb after surgery?

- Is it likely that I will limp after surgery?

- How long will it take the wound to heal?

- What kind of therapy will I need?

- Will I need radiation or chemotherapy before or after the surgery?

- How soon after surgery will I be able to get up and move about?

- Can you arrange for me to talk with someone who has had this operation?

If an amputation is planned:

- If I have to have an amputation, how much of the limb will be removed?

- What kind of reconstruction will be done after the surgery?

- Can I be referred to a musculoskeletal oncologist before surgery so I can see what the different options are and how they work?

- Will I get my artificial limb before I leave the hospital?

BONE CANCERS

What is bone cancer?

Bone cancer occurs when the cells in the bone begin to grow in a disorderly or uncontrolled way. Tumors in bones may be benign or cancerous. Benign tumors are more common than cancerous ones. Both grow in the same way, compressing adjacent healthy bone tissue, sometimes absorbing the healthy tissue and replacing it with abnormal tissue. A benign tumor is limited to the bone in which it develops. Bone cancers destroy the outer layer of the bone and can invade surrounding soft tissues and other bones. Sometimes cells from bone cancers, like all other types of cancer, break away from the primary tumor and spread.

How are bone cancers staged?

Information collected from the physical examination, laboratory tests, including determining the level of alkaline phosphatase will be done. X-rays, bone or CT scans, MRIs, and radio nuclear scans may be used to show the location, size, and shape of the tumor. Finally a biopsy will be needed to determine whether or not the tissue is cancer. For some bone cancers, the pathologist's determination of the grade of the cancer cells is needed to help predict the aggressiveness of a tumor based on the appearance of the cells. Bone cancers have two grades. Low-grade tumors are likely to spread outward

SYMPTOMS OF CANCER OF THE BONE

- Pain
- Swelling or mass
- Stiffness, swelling, or tenderness in the affected area
- Loss of bladder or bowel function (if cancer is in pelvic bones or base of spine)
- Bone fracture
- Tiredness
- Fever
- Weight loss
- Anemia

from the original tumor but are not likely to metastasize. High-grade tumors grow rapidly, spread to surrounding tissues and metastasize to other parts of the body. Stage I disease includes low-grade tumors without metastases; Stage II, high-grade tumors without metastases; Stage III, any grade tumors with metastases. In general, the type of bone cancer is not as important in selecting treatment as its location, size, and extent of spread.

What is osteosarcoma?

Osteosarcoma (sometimes called osteogenic cancer), the most common type of bone cancer, originates in the newly forming tissue of the bone and develops in the long bones of the arms, legs, and pelvis. It contains immature bone cells that destroy and replace normal tissue, weakening the bone.

Has treatment and outlook for those with osteosarcoma changed in the last twenty years?

Twenty years ago, only about 20 percent of patients with osteosarcoma lived five years or more after diagnosis. The only effective treatment was amputation and there was no known way to control metastasis. With the advent of adjuvant chemotherapy for this disease, five-year survival rates for osteogenic bone cancer patients who have no signs of metastasis at diagnosis are now up to 60 to 80 percent. Osteosarcoma is discussed in more detail in Chapter 24, When a Child Has Cancer.

What is chondrosarcoma?

Chondrosarcomas are sarcomas that grow in the cartilage. They can often cause swollen joints or restrict motion. They are found in the pelvic bone, arms, legs, scapula, and ribs and less frequently in the bones of the hand, foot, nose, and base of the skull. They can remain rather slow growing, but when they become aggressive, can metastasize to the lungs and heart.

What is fibrosarcoma?

This is a very rare form of bone cancer, which usually develops from soft tissues such as ligaments, tendons, fat and muscle. Fibrosarcomas may occur at any age but are most often seen in middle-aged and elderly adults. Bones most often affected include those of the legs, arms, and jaw. Adults who have Paget's disease are more likely to get fibrosarcoma. Fibrosarcomas may also develop in persons who have had radiation or at the site of a past bone fracture.

What is the usual primary treatment for most bone cancers?

The primary treatment is usually surgery. The most important consideration in planning surgery is to be certain that the primary tumor and all surrounding tissue where it may have begun to spread are removed. Whenever possible, a margin of healthy tissue also is removed to further reduce the chance that tumor cells remain. For the cancers that occur in the arm and leg, amputation was once considered the best treatment. However, preoperative and postoperative chemotherapy now makes it possible to perform limb-sparing surgery in many cases. This allows parts of the bone to be taken out and replaced with bone grafts or rods so that the arm or leg can still be used. Some bone cancers are also treated with radiation therapy or chemotherapy, either alone or before or after surgery. (Treatment for Ewing's sarcoma, which has different treatment options, is discussed in Chapter 24, When a Child Has Cancer.)

What steps are necessary in limb-sparing operations?

A limb-sparing operation requires three steps. First the tumor must be removed, along with a margin of healthy tissue. The removed segment is replaced with a bone graft or a metal prosthetic bone. The final step is the replacement of the removed margin tissue, usually muscle, with healthy tissue taken from another part of the body.

What circumstances might require amputation of a leg or arm?

In the past, many patients with bone cancers needed amputation. However, the use of radiation, both before and after surgery has meant that many patients can have their limbs spared. Although every effort is made to avoid amputation and to preserve as much normal function as possible, there are some cases where it becomes necessary to amputate. For example, if it is impossible to remove an adequate amount of healthy tissue to assure that the tumor is totally removed, or if the nerves and blood vessels are involved by the tumor, amputa-

MAJOR TYPES OF BONE CANCER

TYPE	DESCRIPTION
Osteosarcoma or osteogenic sarcoma (Also discussed in Chapter 24, When a Child Has Cancer)	Most common type, contains immature bone cells that destroy and replace normal tissue, weakening bone. Usually occurs in knee, upper leg, upper arm. Common ages: 10–25; about 10 percent in people over 60.
Chondrosarcoma	Made up of abnormal cartilage. Usually occurs in pelvis, upper leg, ribs, shoulder. Common ages: 50–75, although can also appear in people 20 and older.
Ewing's sarcoma (See Chapter 24, When a Child Has Cancer)	Begins in immature nerve tissue, usually in bone marrow. Occurs in pelvis, upper leg, ribs, arm. Common ages: 10–20.
Malignant giant cell tumor	There are benign and malignant forms of this cancer. Begins in connecting tissue of bone marrow. Weakens knee or vertebra, causes bone fractures. Occurs in 40–55 age group.
Fibrosarcoma of bone	Begins in connective tissue. Seen in leg, arm, jaw. Occurs mostly in middle-aged and elderly.
Chordoma	Cellular remnants of fetal spinal cord. Occurs at base of skull and bones of the spine. Nerve involvement makes treatment difficult. May recur, even long after treatment. Occurs in 55–65 age group.
Parosteal sarcoma	Involves midshaft of bone. Can often be cured by removing affected section of bone. Slow growing. Occurs in 10–25 age group.
Adamantinoma and a group of types previously known as reticulum cell sarcomas of the bone now referred to as **malignant fibrous histiocytoma, small round cell sarcomas, and diffuse large cell lymphoma of bone**	Rare. Usually occur in elderly and middle-aged adults.

tion may be necessary. Amputation also is recommended if a nonfunctional limb would result from the operation. Sometimes in children younger than ten years of age, amputation is recommended because of skeletal development problems, although new expandable prosthesis and rotationplasty are possible options that should be explored before any treatment is done. If amputation is required, it is essential you be treated at a multidisciplinary medical center, with experienced pathologists, radiologists, and other specialists.

What is rotationplasty?

This is a complex operation used to preserve as much movement of the arm or leg as possible. It may be suggested if the leg or arm need to be removed. If it is the leg, it is amputated mid-thigh, the lower leg and foot are rotated and attached to the thighbone where the ankle becomes the knee joint. If the cancer is in the upper arm, the tumor is taken out and the lower area reattached, so that the arm is shorter but is still useable.

Can reconstruction be accomplished when amputation occurs?

There are many new materials, new procedures, and new approaches to give the patient the best function possible. The doctor will explain the different kinds of reconstruction and decisions must be made depending on the patient's needs. There is an increasing use of metal and plastic materials as well as allografts—the use of freeze-dried or frozen bone—which is incorporated in the patient's own skeleton over time.

Is it wise before having surgery to meet with someone who has had the same operation?

It may be helpful and encouraging to talk with someone who has been through such a surgery. Your doctor or the social workers at the hospital may be able to put you in touch with someone. The American Cancer Society and the American Handicapped Association can be helpful. Rehabilitation requires patience, cooperation, coordination, and tremendous physical energy.

What is a skip metastasis?

A skip metastasis is a tumor nodule located in the same bone as the main tumor but not in continuity with the tumor. It is usually located in the joint adjacent to the main tumor, and is found mostly with high-grade sarcomas.

How are metastases to the lung treated in bone cancer?

If bone cancer does metastasize, more than 50 percent of the time it will occur in the lung. Surgery may be possible, depending on the size and number of metastatic tumors in the lung. Usually this surgery is preceded or followed by chemotherapy.

SYMPTOMS OF SOFT-TISSUE SARCOMAS

- Enlarging painless swelling or mass.
- Pain or soreness caused by tumor pressing against nearby nerves and muscles.

ADULT SOFT-TISSUE SARCOMA

What is adult soft-tissue sarcoma?

Sarcomas are cancers that are found in the soft tissues of the body—the muscles, connective tissues or tendons, the vessels that carry blood or lymph, joints, and fat. Because these soft tissues are present all over the body, the treatment can vary depending upon the location of the tumor. About half are found in the limbs, 40 percent in the trunk, and ten percent in the head and neck. Today, even high-grade sarcomas of the arm and leg can often be effectively treated while preserving the limb, with pre- or postoperative radiation playing an important role.

What are the different kinds of soft-tissue sarcomas?

The main types of soft-tissue sarcomas are malignant fibrous histiocytoma and liposarcoma. Soft-tissue sarcomas are also classified according to the cell of origin. They include alveolar soft-part sarcoma, angiosarcoma, dermatofibrosarcoma protuberans, epithelioid sarcoma, extraskeletal chondrosarcoma, extraskeletal osteosarcoma, fibrosarcoma, gastrointestinal stromal tumor, leiomyosarcoma, liposarcoma, malignant fibrous histiocytoma, malignant hemagiopericytoma, malignant mesenchymoma, malignant schwannoma, malignant peripheral nerve sheath tumor, peripheral neuroectodermal tumor, rhabdomyosarcoma, and synovial sarcoma.

What happens if a tumor is removed and then it is discovered to be a soft-tissue sarcoma?

It is not uncommon for this to happen. In this situation, surgery will need to be performed again to take a wider margin around the tumor. This is done to remove any microscopic tumor cells remaining, to lessen the likelihood of a local recurrence, and to forestall the possibility of spread.

How are soft-tissue sarcomas staged?

The size of a soft-tissue sarcoma is not as important as how the cancer cells look under the microscope. The more different the cancer cells look from

TREATMENT FOR ADULT SOFT-TISSUE SARCOMA

STAGE	TREATMENT
Stage IA: Cancer is low grade, small, superficial, and deep. **Stage IB:** Cancer is low grade, large, and superficial. **Stage IIA:** Cancer is low grade, large, and deep. CAUTION: Wide negative tissue margins of at least 2 centimeters necessary to prevent local recurrence.	*If in head, neck, abdomen, or trunk*: Surgery with or without radiation **or** Radiation before and after surgery **or** Fast neutron therapy. *If in other areas*: Surgery to remove cancer **or** Radiation therapy followed by surgery **or** Surgery followed by radiation **or** Radiation before and after surgery.
Stage IIB: Cancer is high grade, small, superficial, and deep. **Stage IIC:** Cancer is high grade, large, and superficial **Stage III:** Cancer is high grade, large, and deep. CAUTION: Wide negative tissue margins of at least several centimeters necessary to prevent local recurrence.	Surgery to remove cancer **or** Surgery followed by radiation **or** Radiation alone **or** Radiation before and after surgery **or** Chemotherapy followed by surgery followed by radiation therapy. *Clinical trials*: New forms of radiation **or** regional chemotherapy followed by surgery **or** surgery and adjuvant chemotherapy **or** chemotherapy.
Stage IVA: Cancer has spread to lymph nodes but not to other parts of body.	Surgery to remove cancer and lymph nodes (lymph node dissection) **or** Surgery as above followed by radiation **or** Radiation before and after surgery to remove cancer and lymph nodes (lymph node dissection). *Clinical trials*: Chemotherapy.
Stage IVB: Cancer has spread to other parts of body such as lungs.	*If in head, neck, abdomen, or trunk*: Surgery with radiation before or after **or** Surgery with radiation before or after and chemotherapy. *If in other areas*: Surgery to remove cancer with or without radiation after surgery **or**

TREATMENT FOR ADULT SOFT-TISSUE SARCOMA *(continued)*

STAGE	TREATMENT
Stage IVB: *(continued)*	Radiation before and after surgery **or** Radiation alone **or** Radiation with chemotherapy. *Clinical trials*: New chemotherapy drugs or biological therapy.
Stage IVB: Cancer has spread to other parts of body such as lungs.	*If in head, neck, abdomen, or trunk*: Surgery with radiation before or after **or** Surgery with radiation before or after and chemotherapy. *If in other areas*: Surgery to remove cancer with or without radiation after surgery **or** Radiation before and after surgery **or** Radiation alone **or** Radiation with chemotherapy. *Clinical trials*: New chemotherapy drugs or biological therapy.
Recurrent: Cancer has come back after being treated either in tissues where began or another part of body.	Depends on previous treatment. Surgery to remove cancer followed by radiation therapy. *Clinical trials*: chemotherapy and autologous bone marrow transplant

normal cells the higher the grade. The grade (G) of the tumor predicts the growth rate and its tendency to spread. Grades 1 and 2 are well differentiated and moderately well differentiated cancer cells. This means they look much like their normal counterparts. Grades 3 and 4 include poorly differentiated cells and undifferentiated cells (cells that look different from or very different from normal cells). Also involved in determining treatment is the size of the tumor, and whether or not it has spread to lymph nodes or other parts of the body. Since high-grade tumors are more likely to spread than low-grade ones, it is important for the physician to know this before making recommendations for treatment.

What tests are necessary to determine treatment?

X-rays and scans of the affected area must be done so that the exact location and dimensions of the tumor can be determined. Possible tests, in addition to laboratory studies and a thorough physical examination, may include:

- X-ray called a xerogram, or soft tissue radiograph
- CT scans to give three-dimensional map of tumor and surrounding tissues
- Arteriogram
- MRI
- Ultrasound
- Biopsy (should be done in conjunction with surgical oncologist for best possibility of sparing limb)
- Flow cytometry, electron microscopy, histochemistry, cytogenetics, tissue culture studies may be needed to identify the subgroups within the major categories.

It is very important, because these tumors are rare, because there are many types, and because the biopsy needs to be carefully done, that you go to a major medical or research center where there are specialists with expertise in diagnosing and treating these cancers and sophisticated equipment with which to do the tests. There can be disagreement even among expert pathologists as to the type of soft-tissue sarcoma.

What kind of follow-up is recommended for bone and soft-tissue cancer patients?

Because these tumors are unusual, follow-up must be customized. However, the first two years, repeat visits to the physician will probably be scheduled for every three months. The third year, every four months; the fourth and fifth year, every six months, and thereafter, every year.

Questions to Ask Your Doctor About Follow-up

- **Will you be doing my main follow-up?**
- **Will I also need to see any of my other doctors?**
- **How often will I need to see you?**
- **What tests will you be doing during my follow-up exam?**
- **What will you be looking for?**
- **What should I be watching for between my visits with you?**
- **What symptoms should I report? To whom?**

KAPOSI'S SARCOMA

What is Kaposi's sarcoma?

Kaposi's sarcoma is a cancer that is found in the tissues under the skin or mucous membranes. It causes red-brown or purple patches on the skin, often on the legs, without other symptoms. It spreads to other organs in the body, such as the lung, liver, or intestinal tract. Until the early 1980s, Kaposi's sarcoma was considered a very rare disease found mainly in older men, patients who had organ transplants, or African men. In people who do not have AIDS, the disease develops slowly.

How does Kaposi's sarcoma differ in AIDS patients?

In the 1980s, doctors began to see many cases of Kaposi's sarcoma in people with AIDS. In these cases, Kaposi's sarcoma may be found in the mouth, nose, lymph nodes, gastrointestinal tract, lung, liver, and spleen. Kaposi's sarcoma usually spreads more quickly in patients with AIDS. It may produce significant deterioration in the organ affected. About 20 percent of AIDS patients develop Kaposi's sarcoma.

What are the symptoms of Kaposi's sarcoma?

You will see raised spots on the skin, purplish or red-brown in color. In classic Kaposi's, spots are usually found on legs. In AIDS-related, they are often found in the mouth, on the face, and chest. Sometimes there will be swelling around the raised spots. Other symptoms include difficulty in eating, or coughing up blood.

How is Kaposi's sarcoma staged?

There is no true staging for Kaposi's sarcoma at this time. Patients are grouped according to the type of Kaposi's sarcoma:

- Classic Kaposi's sarcoma
- African Kaposi's sarcoma
- Immunosuppressive treatment-related Kaposi's sarcoma
- AIDS-related (epidemic) Kaposi's sarcoma
- Nonepidemic Kaposi's sarcoma

What is classic Kaposi's sarcoma?

This is considered a rare disease, usually found in older men (50–70) of Jewish, Italian, or Mediterranean heritage. This cancer is quite rare. The disease is usually limited to one or two patches, usually localized in one or both legs, often at the ankle or sole. It progresses slowly, sometimes over ten to 15 years.

TREATMENT FOR KAPOSI'S SARCOMA

Classic Progresses slowly, sometimes over ten to 15 years.	*Depends on extent of lesions:* Radiation therapy (low-voltage photon or electron beam) **or** Local surgery **or** Chemotherapy (systemic or intralesional) **or** Chemotherapy plus radiation therapy.
Immunosuppressive treatment-related May occur in people taking drugs to suppress immune system for liver or kidney transplant.	May be controlled if able to cease taking immunosuppressive drugs. If not or if does not work, Radiation therapy **or** Chemotherapy. *Clinical trials:* Chemotherapy.
AIDS-related epidemic Found in patients with AIDS. This type spreads more quickly than other kinds of Kaposi's sarcoma and often is found in many parts of body.	Surgery, using local removal, electrodesiccation and curettage or cryotherapy **or** Localized radiation therapy **or** Intralesional chemotherapy **or** Systemic chemotherapy **or** alpha interferon. *Clinical trials:* New chemotherapy drugs and combination **or** biological therapy.
Nonepidemic Found in homosexual men without HIV. May be on skin of arms and legs and on genitals.	Depends on location and extent of lesions.
Recurrent Kaposi's sarcoma comes back after being treated, either in same area or another part of body.	Depends on type, past treatment response and general health. May wish to take part in clinical trial.

The lower legs may swell and the blood may not be able to flow properly. After some time, it may spread to other organs and there is a possibility that another type of cancer may develop later on in life. Usually, the doctor will check the skin and lymph nodes of the patient at regular intervals.

What is African Kaposi's sarcoma?
Men who live in Africa near the equator are most at risk for this type of Kaposi's sarcoma. Although it is similar to the classic type, it develops at a

younger age and can be very aggressive. A type that strikes young children is even more aggressive.

What is immunosuppressive treatment-related Kaposi's sarcoma?
This type may occur in people who are taking drugs to suppress their immune system. Mostly it occurs in patients who have had kidney or liver transplants. In some cases, when patients are able to stop taking the immuno-suppressive drugs, the disease can be controlled. In some cases, the Kaposi's sarcoma regresses.

What is AIDS-related (epidemic) Kaposi's sarcoma?
This type is found in patients who have Acquired Immunodeficiency Syndrome (AIDS). AIDS, caused by a virus called HIV, weakens the immune system. In people with AIDS, the sarcoma usually spreads faster than other kinds of Kaposi's and is found in many parts of the body.

What is nonepidemic Kaposi's sarcoma?
Kaposi's sarcoma has been found in homosexual men who have no sign of HIV infection. It is usually found only on the skin of arms and legs although sometimes it is also found on the genitals.

Web Pages to Check Out

www.cancer.gov: For general up-to-date information, and for clinical trials.
www.cancer.org: For general up-to-date information and community resources.
www.sarcomaalliance.com: Patient advocacy, guidance, education, support.
www.sarcoma.net: Educational resources; on-line consultation service.
www.thebody.com: Kaposi's sarcoma, an AIDS and HIV resource.

Also see Chapter 2, Searching for Answers on the Web, for more information.

Twenty-two

CANCER OF
THE BRAIN AND
SPINAL CORD

The specter of brain cancer is one of the most terrifying of nightmares. We all instinctively fear any tampering with our brain because of its role as the center for controlling thought, emotion, and feeling. The incidence of tumors of the brain, spinal cord, and the rest of the central nervous system remains very low for the population as a whole, accounting for 1.5 percent of all cancers. With the aid of computer assisted diagnostic methods, such as magnetic resonance imaging (MRI) and stereotactic needle biopsy, new ways of doing surgery, and new chemotherapy drugs, doctors have changed the course of this disease. And the future is even brighter with new treatments and studies of gene therapy giving added hope to patients with cancers of the central nervous system.

NEW TECHNIQUES IN identifying tumors in the brain and spinal cord before the operation allow neurosurgeons to approach surgery with greater information, thereby making it possible to establish a firm diagnosis, relieve symptoms, and in the case of some tumors, provide cures. Fortunately most central nervous system tumors in adults develop in accessible parts of the brain—the frontal, parietal, occipital, and temporal lobes. New surgical techniques make it possible for extensive surgery to be done on these important parts of the brain with good results. In many instances, where surgery is not curative, other treatments, including radiation therapy and chemotherapy are being used. New developments in immunotherapy and gene therapy are being tested and promise to deliver even more effective treatment of brain tumors.

There is no doubt that cancers of the brain and spinal cord, which make up our central nervous system, represent a complex problem for the patient, family and the medical team. The biggest fear people have is that they will lose their minds or become "vegetables" as the result of an operation. The outlook for recovery today is not as bleak as might be believed. Progress is being made in many areas. The length of survival, as well as the quality of life, is improving for most people who have brain and spinal cord cancers. Unlike a generation ago, medical specialists now have a spectacular array of powerful scanning machines to see inside the brain, new, computerized diagnostic tools and new methods of tumor removal which help minimize damage to normal tissues. As with other types of cancer, many factors determine the outcome of brain and spinal cancer—the type and grade of tumor, the location of the tumor, and how it affects the tissues that surround it.

WHAT YOU SHOULD KNOW ABOUT
BRAIN AND SPINAL CORD TUMORS

- Together the brain and spinal cord form the central nervous system, which controls much of what we do—walking, talking, breathing, digesting food, seeing, hearing, touching, tasting, smelling, thinking, and remembering.

- There is a major difference between cancers **of** the brain (primary brain cancer) and cancers **in** the brain (metastatic brain cancer). Tumors **of** the brain originate there. Tumors **in** the brain come from other organs through the invasive process known as metastasis. The same is true for tumors of the spinal cord. This chapter will cover tumors **of** these two sites.

- The brain contains 10 million working cells. Research is now underway to determine how to work with the 19,000 genes that are in the brain, which will lead to new ways of diagnosing and treating brain cancer.

- Brain tissue does not regenerate, but the brain is a remarkably adaptable organ. One part of the brain can take over the functions of a disabled or missing part. Extensive surgery can be done on many accessible parts of the brain without causing severe neurological damage.

- Tumors of the central nervous system are diverse—there are 126 different types identified by the World Health Organization.

- Nearly half of all primary brain tumors can be cured by appropriate therapy, usually neurosurgery.

- There are new treatments using monoclonal antibodies, bio-engineered proteins that seek out malignant cells and kill them. Used with or without radioactive isotopes, the monoclonal antibodies react specifically with the cells associated with brain tumors.

- Chemotherapy is being given using wafers designed to deliver drugs directly to the area of the brain tumor, bypassing the blood brain barrier. The wafers, implanted into the space formed by the removal of the tumor at the time of the surgery, slowly release a higher dose of a drug to the tumor bed, with fewer side effects than chemotherapy given in the more traditional manner.

- Scientific advances, coupled with technological advances, are leading to better and better cure rates.

PRIMARY BRAIN CANCER

Who is most likely to get brain cancer?

Those most likely to have primary brain tumors include young children and young adults to age 20 and people over age 40, with peak ages between 50 and 60. Some brain tumors that are common in adults are almost never found in children and some childhood brain tumors are rarely found in adults. There seems to be an increase in the number of brain tumors in adults, particularly in the elderly. It is not known whether this is due to better detection, such as with MRI, or to the fact that most of these tumors occur in older ages, a population group that is increasing in this country. (There is more information about childhood brain tumors in Chapter 24, When a Child Has Cancer.)

What kind of doctor should be treating someone with brain cancer?

Initially, most people see their family doctors. This is where a diagnosis of brain tumor usually begins. A basic neurological examination usually follows the taking of a complete history of the symptoms. If the results of this examination lead your physician to suspect a brain tumor, you will probably be referred to a specialist in the brain tumor field, commonly a neurosurgeon. Diagnosis and treatment are best handled in a major cancer center, many of which have Brain Tumor Centers with multidisciplinary teams who have diverse expertise, the very latest equipment and doctors who are trained in the use of the new techniques. Experts in such specialties as neurology, neurosurgery, oncology, pathology, diagnostic radiology, imaging, and radiation therapy pool their cooperative efforts to provide the best-coordinated services.

What are the parts of the brain and what does each part do?

The brain is a soft grayish-white spongy mass of nerve and supportive tissue that is enclosed inside the protective bony helmet known as the skull. The bony casing that protects the brain from all outside matter is the reason why even the tiniest growth can cause serious trouble inside the skull. In the simplest of terms (hardly adequate to cover such a complex subject), the brain has three major parts: the cerebrum, the cerebellum, and the brain stem, all of which work together doing their specific tasks. The cerebrum, which is the largest part of the brain, fills most of the upper skull. Its functions include control of the muscles, speech, emotions, reading, thinking and learning. The cerebellum, under the cerebrum at the back of the brain, controls balance and complex actions like walking and talking. The brain stem connects the brain with the spinal cord. It controls hunger and thirst and most of the basic body functions such as body temperature, blood pressure, and breathing. The location of the brain tumor within the brain, is, of course, the most important determining factor in the outcome of any surgery or treatment.

How is the brain protected?

The brain is protected by the bony skull and three thin layers of tissue called meninges. Surrounding, cushioning, and protecting the brain and spinal cord like a moat, is a special liquid, produced by the brain, called cerebrospinal fluid. This fluid brings nourishment from the blood to the brain and takes away waste matter. The bony casing that protects the brain so well, however, complicates matters when new growths occur. There is very little or no space inside the brain for expansion. While other parts of the body can endure large cancerous growths, even a small growth inside the skull causes serious trouble.

Are there different types of brain cancer?

Brain cancers are divided into two types—those that start in the brain and those which metastasize to the brain from cancer in some other part of the body. There are estimated to be about 17,000 cases of primary brain cancers and cancers of the central nervous system and as many as 100,000 cases of cancer that have metastasized to the brain. This chapter deals with brain tumors that start in the brain, referred to as *primary brain tumors,* although much of the information will also be of interest to those with metastatic brain tumors. (Also see Chapter 26, When Cancers Recur or Metastasize.)

Do some symptoms relate directly to the part of the brain the tumor is in?

Sometimes the symptoms are produced by the tumor pushing into a particular area of the brain. Tumors located in the area controlling motion can produce

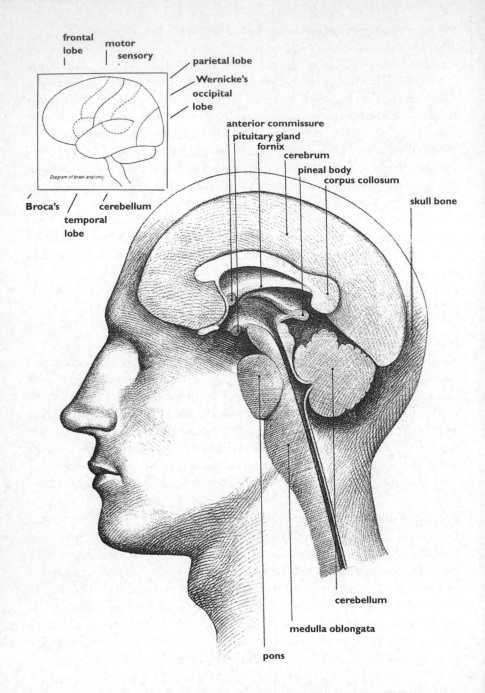

frontal lobe
motor
sensory
parietal lobe
Wernicke's
occipital lobe

anterior commissure
pituitary gland
fornix
cerebrum
pineal body
corpus collosum
skull bone

Broca's
temporal lobe
cerebellum

Diagram of brain anatomy.

cerebellum

medulla oblongata

pons

Brain

WHO IS MOST LIKELY TO GET PRIMARY BRAIN CANCER

- Adults 40 to 70 years old; children three to ten years old.
- Workers in oil refining, rubber manufacturing, drug manufacturing.
- Embalmers and chemists.
- People exposed to viruses.
- People who have a family history of brain tumors and nervous disorders.
- People who have had radiation to brain.

weakness in the arm, the leg, or both. A tumor located in the cerebellum, for instance, might produce loss of coordination, balance, or the ability to walk. However, since symptoms are usually difficult to pinpoint, may appear only occasionally, and are similar to those of other diseases, diagnosis may be delayed. For example, the key symptom in olfactory meningioma is loss of smell. Since loss of smell is considered a minor problem by many people, this symptom may be overlooked and not diagnosed until other symptoms become evident.

What is a benign brain tumor?
A benign brain tumor consists of benign cells and has distinct boundaries. Usually these tumors can be removed, and are not likely to recur. Surgery alone may cure this type of tumor. However, even benign tumors in the brain are dangerous because the skull cannot expand to make room for the extra growth. Although a benign tumor may not invade nearby tissue, it can press on sensitive areas of the brain. When an otherwise benign tumor is located in a vital area of the brain and interferes with vital functions, it may be treated as though it is malignant, even though it contains no cancer cells.

What is a malignant brain tumor?
A malignant brain tumor is life threatening. Malignant brain tumors are likely to grow rapidly, interfere with vital functions, and crowd or invade the tissue around them. If a malignant tumor remains compact and does not spread into healthy brain tissue, it is said to be encapsulated. A malignant brain tumor may spread to other locations in the brain or spinal cord, but seldom spreads outside the brain and spinal cord.

What are metastatic brain tumors?
Metastatic brain tumors are different from primary brain tumors because they are cancerous tumors that start somewhere else in the body and spread

SYMPTOMS OF BRAIN CANCER

- Headache, usually most severe after waking, and lessening as the day goes on.
- Seizures.
- Vomiting, usually after waking, with or without nausea.
- Weakness or loss of feeling in the arms or legs.
- Lethargy or mental sluggishness or drowsiness.
- Uncoordinated, clumsy movements when walking (ataxic gait).
- One-sided muscle weakness (hemiparesis).
- Difficulty in swallowing (dysphagia) or with speech (dysarthria).
- Ringing or buzzing in the ear (tintinitus).
- Dizziness (vertigo).
- Drowsiness.
- Loss of sense of smell (anosmia).
- Abnormal eye movements or changes in vision.
- Changes in personality or memory.
- Changes in speech.

to the brain. Because cancers can spread through the blood, it is not surprising that the brain is a frequent site of spread. The brain receives 20 percent of the blood flow of the heart, and the arteries within the brain have an "end-artery" pattern that can trap cancer cells, which then multiply and form a new cancer. Metastatic tumors are treated in a similar fashion to the primary cancer from which they spread. See Chapter 26, When Cancers Recur or Metastasize, for more information.

Why are brain tumors sometimes hard to diagnose?
Brain tumors may be difficult to diagnose because the bones of the skull hide brain tumors. The doctor cannot feel or see them during a routine examination. Scans are done to view the tumor, but only a sample biopsy of the tumor examined under a microscope can provide an exact diagnosis.

Why are brain tumors so dangerous?
Often, the damage done by brain tumors is due to their size. The skull cannot expand to make room for even a small mass growing within it. As a result, the tumor presses on and displaces normal brain tissue. This pressure may damage or destroy delicate brain tissue. Many of the symptoms of brain

tumors are caused by this pressure. Sometimes a tumor may block the fluid that flows around and through the brain. This can create increased pressure. Some brain tumors also cause swelling due to accumulation of fluid. The tumor may also grow into other areas of the brain. The mass effects of size, pressure, and swelling combine to make them destructive to the sensitive areas of the brain.

Why are some brain tumors inoperable?

Brain tumors sometimes occur in a part of the brain that cannot be reached by the neurosurgeon. In these cases, biopsy alone for diagnosis may be performed if the tumor cannot be taken out. Occasionally, biopsy may not be possible or advisable, even with the most advanced techniques. Treatment is then based on the assumed type of tumor.

Are gliomas the most common primary brain tumors?

About half of all primary brain tumors in adults are gliomas. These tumors begin in the glial tissue, which is the supportive tissue of the brain. They are divided into several types—astrocytoma, brain stem glioma, epedymoma, oligoendroglioma, mixed tumor, and medulloblastoma. There are many glial cells in the brain. They support and protect the nerve cells (neurons) that send and receive messages. These cells are responsible for a variety of tumors that are capable of behaving in either a benign or malignant fashion.

What are the characteristics of astrocytomas?

Astrocytomas may grow anywhere in the brain or spinal cord. They come from small, star-shaped cells called astrocytes. In adults, they are most often found in the cerebrum. In children, they occur in the brain stem, the cerebrum and the cerebellum. Noninfiltrating astrocytoma is a relatively slow-growing tumor that usually does not grow into the tissues around it. Well differentiated mild and moderately anaplastic astrocytoma is slow growing, but the tumor may start to grow into other tissues around it. A Grade III astrocytoma is sometimes called anaplastic astrocytoma and grows more rapidly. A Grade IV astrocytoma is usually called glioblastoma multiforme. It grows very rapidly.

What are brain stem gliomas?

These cancers occur in the lowest, stemlike part of the brain, where the brain is connected to the spinal cord. The brain stem controls many vital functions. Tumors in this area are usually not biopsied, generally cannot be removed and are treated by radiation therapy. Most brain stem gliomas are high-grade astrocytomas or glioblastomas.

CELL TYPES OF ADULT GLIOMAS

ASTROCYTOMA

Noninfiltrating

    Juvenile pilocytic

    Subependymal

Infiltrating

    Well differentiated mildly and moderately anaplastic astrocytoma

    Anaplastic astrocytoma

    Glioblastoma multiforme

BRAIN STEM GLIOMA
EPENDYMOMA

Myxopapillary and well differentiated ependymoma

Anaplastic ependymoma

Ependymoma blastoma

OLIGODENDROGLIOMA

Well differentiated oligodendroglioma

Anaplastic oligodendroglioma

MIXED TUMORS

Mixed astrocytoma-ependymoma

Mixed astrocytoma-oligodendroglioma

Mixed astrocytoma-ependymoma-oligodendroglioma

MEDULLOBLASTOMA

What are ependymomas?

Epenymomas usually develop in the lining of the ventricles, though they also occur in the spinal cord. They can develop at any age, but are most common in childhood and adolescence.

What are oligodendrogliomas?

These tumors arise in the cells that produce myelin, the fatty covering that protects nerves. They grow slowly and usually do not spread to surrounding brain tissue. They occur most often in people of middle age but have been seen in people of all ages.

What are mixed cell tumors?

These are brain tumor in which two or three type of brain cell types—astrocytoma, ependyoma, or oligodendroglioma—are involved.

What are medulloblastomas?

These tumors are usually found in the lower part of the brain. They arise from developing nerve cells that normally do not remain in the body after birth. Medulloblastomas are sometimes called primitive neuroectodermal tumors. Although they are sometimes found in adults, they are found more often in children and are more common in boys than in girls.

What are pineal parenchymal tumors?

These tumors occur in or around the pineal gland, a tiny organ near the center of the brain. The tumor may be slow growing (pineocytoma) or fast growing (pineoblastoma). They are sometimes called pineal region tumors. The pineal region is a very difficult one to operate on and these tumors often cannot be taken out.

What are germ cell tumors?

These tumors arise from primitive, developing sex cells known as germ cells. The most usual type of germ cell tumor in the brain is germinoma. Embryonal carcinoma, choriocarcinoma, and teratoma also fall into this category.

What are craniopharyngiomas?

Craniopharyngiomas start in the area of the pituitary gland near the hypothalamus. They are usually benign, but are sometimes considered malignant because they can press on, or damage, the hypothalamus and affect vital functions. They are most often found in children and adolescents.

What are meningiomas?

Meningiomas are common tumors, account for about 20 percent of adult primary brain tumors, and usually develop in women between the ages of 30 and 50. They are most often benign and the majority can be cured by surgery. They grow in the meninges and because they grow very slowly, the brain may be able to adjust to their presence. They grow in such a way that they usually indent the brain and cause symptoms by pressure or by producing a reaction in nearby brain tissue in the form of irritation or swelling. By the time they begin to cause symptoms, they are often quite large.

CELL TYPES OF ADULT NONGLINOMA TUMORS

PINEAL PARENCHYMAL

Pineocytoma

Pineoblastoma

Astrocytoma

GERM CELL TUMORS

Germinoma

Embryonal carcinoma

Choriocarcinoma

Teratoma

CRANIPHARYNGIOMA

MENINGIOMAS

Meningioma

Malignant meningioma

    Anapestic

    Hermagiopericytoma

    Papillary meningioma

Choriod plexus tumors

    Choroid plexus papilloma

    Anaplastic choroid plexus papilloma

Where are choroid plexus tumors found?

These are rare brain tumors that arise from the choroid plexus epithelial cells. Choroid plexus papilloma is not as serious as is anaplastic choroid plexus papilloma, which often spreads to the spinal cord.

What is Schwannoma?

These benign tumors begin in Schwann cells that produce the myelin that protects the hearing nerve (acoustic). The most common Schwannoma is acoustic neuroma (sometimes called vestibular schwannoma), which causes hearing loss as the earliest symptom. Schwannomas may also develop on other nerves—the trigeminal, facial, or vagal. Women get this type of cancer twice as often as men.

What does a neurologic exam consist of?

The doctor does several tests, including looking at your eye movement, the reflexes of your eyes, the reactions of your pupils, general reflexes in your body, hearing, movement, balance and coordination.

How are brain tumors diagnosed?

The diagnosis of brain tumors has been made more accurate and more precise by the enormous advances that have occurred in neuroimaging. Today, the most important test is an MRI (magnetic resonance imaging). Reactions to tumors, such as the swelling (edema) that forms as a result, can be assessed. The nature and extent of the blood flow of the tumor can be measured. CT scanning of the head is useful in the diagnosis of certain brain tumors and in instances where MRI is not available or feasible. PET scans may be used to determine the cell type and the growth pattern. As you can imagine, diagnosis of brain tumor requires the skills of highly qualified specialists.

How is the final diagnosis made?

The final diagnosis of brain cancer can only be made with a sample of the tumor tissue. A stereotactic biopsy or regular biopsy will be done to make a definite diagnosis. The neurosurgeon submits samples of the tumor tissue to a neuropathologist who can then establish an exact diagnosis.

How is a stereotactic biopsy done?

A small hole is made in the skull, and a thin needle is placed in the tumor, to obtain a biopsy. With the help of the MRI or CT scan, the neurosurgeon can find the exact location, touching as little normal brain tissue as possible. This is also referred to as stereotaxis.

When will a halo be used?

A special headframe that looks like a halo may be used to hold your head steady. It may be used for stereotactic biopsy or surgery or when gamma knife radiosurgery is being used.

How are brain tumors graded?

Some brain tumors are graded from low grade (Grade I) to high grade (Grade IV). The grade refers to the way the cells look under the microscope. Cells from higher grade tumors are more abnormal looking and generally grow faster than cells from lower grade tumors. Higher grade tumors are more malignant then lower grade tumors.

TESTS FOR BRAIN CANCER

Depending on results of physical and neurologic examinations, testing may include:

- MRI—the most important test.
- CT scan.
- PET scan (where available).
- X-ray of skull, using radioactive dye.
- Biopsy.
- Stereotactic biopsy.
- Spinal tap (lumbar puncture).

Questions to Ask Your Doctor Before Starting Treatment for Cancer of the Brain or Spinal Cord

- **Where is the tumor located?**
- **What kind of tumor is it?**
- **What is the plan for surgery?**
- **What kind of diagnostic tests will I still need? How painful or dangerous are they?**
- **Will you have to drill a hole in my skull?**
- **What are the expected benefits of treatment?**
- **Will there be side effects?**
- **What can be done about side effects?**
- **What are the risks?**
- **How long will I be in the hospital?**
- **Will I need special nursing care?**
- **How soon after the operation will we know how successful it was?**
- **Will there be any treatments following surgery? What kind and for how long?**
- **Where can I go for another opinion? Can I go to a specialized brain tumor center?**
- **Who is the most skilled doctor in dealing with this type of cancer?**
- **Where is the nearest hospital with a Brain Tumor Center?**
- **Are there any clinical trials being done for my kind of cancer?**
- **Will I need to change my normal activities? For how long?**

Will I be given any medicine to control my symptoms?
You may need to take drugs (steroids) to lessen the swelling in the brain, or medicine to prevent or to control seizures. If you have a buildup of fluid, you may need to have a shunt to drain it out. This would involve putting a long, thin tube into the brain and threading it under the skin to either the abdomen or the heart. The tube carries the fluid out of the brain down the tube and is then drained.

What kind of treatments are used for brain cancers?
The first step is usually surgery. Radiation, chemotherapy, and immunotherapy are all also being used to treat brain cancers.

What kind of surgery is used in treating brain cancers?
Surgery is one of the oldest techniques for treating brain cancers. Fortunately, new techniques have revolutionized brain surgery making it possible for the physician to perform the delicate job of tumor removal more accurately, with fewer surgical risks and better long-term results. Among the new techniques are stereotactic surgery, intraoperative brain mapping, and neuroendoscopy.

How is stereotactic surgery used in treating brain tumors?
Stereotactic surgery, also called stereotaxy or image-guided stereotactic surgery, uses computer-assisted techniques to allow the surgeon to remove tumors in some parts of the brain which are difficult to reach manually. MRI, in conjunction with special computer techniques, allows a tumor to be seen in three dimensions and to plan the surgery precisely in advance. The day before surgery, six plastic dots are attached to the skull and an MRI scan of the brain and the tumor is taken. In the operating room, the location of the dots is registered on a computer and matched. Navigation software allows special computer-assisted stereotactic instruments to be guided to the location of the tumor.

What is intraoperative brain mapping?
This technique, also called functional imaging or fMRI, uses high-speed MRI to map out areas of the brain that control vital functions such as vision, hearing, taste, touch, movement, speech, and language. The map allows the doctor to plan the surgery precisely to avoid disrupting sensitive areas and to remove more tumor while minimizing damage to critical brain tissue.

What is neuroendoscopy?
Some treatments are now being done using neuroendoscopy. The doctor works through a small opening in the skull, using a small telescope and video camera to look into the skull, brain, and spine. The advantages of this type of surgery

TYPES AND TREATMENTS FOR ADULT BRAIN CANCER

CELL TYPE	DESCRIPTION	TREATMENT
Astrocytoma, Adult Noninfiltrating	Starts in brain cells called astrocytes. Grows slowly and usually doesn't grow into surrounding tissues. Often curable.	Surgery to remove cancer **or** Surgery followed by external radiation therapy. If it recurs, reoperation and radiation, if not used before. *Clinical trials*: chemotherapy or biological therapy.
Astrocytoma, Adult Well Differentiated Mildly and Moderately Anaplastic	Starts in brain cells called astrocytes. Slow growing but grows more quickly than noninfiltrating astrocytoma. Can grow into surrounding tissues.	Surgery followed by external radiation **or** Surgery with or without radiation. *Clinical trials*: surgery followed by radiation and chemotherapy.
Astrocytoma, Adult Anaplastic	Starts in brain cells called astrocytes. Cells look very different from normal cells. Grows rapidly. Clinical trials should be considered.	Surgery followed by external radiation with or without chemotherapy. *Clinical trials*: internal radiation, **or** radiation given during surgery, **or** radiation given with drugs to make cancer cells more sensitive **or** radiation followed by chemotherapy or biological therapy **or** chemotherapy placed in body during surgery **or** hyperthermia.

Glioblastoma Multiforme, Adult. Also called Grade IV Astrocytoma	Grows very quickly. Cells look very different from normal cells. Clinical trials should be considered.	Surgery followed by external radiation with or without chemotherapy. *Clinical trials:* internal radiation **or** radiation given during surgery **or** radiation given with drugs to make cancer cells more sensitive **or** radiation followed by chemotherapy or biological therapy **or** hyperthermia **or** chemotherapy drugs placed in body during surgery.
Glioma, Adult Brain Stem	Located in bottom part of brain (brain stem) that connects to spinal cord.	External radiation. *Clinical trials:* chemotherapy or biological therapy.
Ependymoma, Adult Myxopapillary and Well Differentiated	Begins in the ependyma, cells that line passageways in brain where cerebrospinal fluid is made and stored. Cells look very much like normal cells. Grows slowly. Often curable.	Surgery to remove cancer **or** Surgery followed by external radiation. *Clinical trials:* chemotherapy or biological therapy. If it recurs, reoperation and radiation if not used before; otherwise, clinical trials of chemotherapy or biological therapy.
Ependymoma, Adult Malignant	Begins in the ependyma, cells that line passageways in brain where cerebrospinal fluid is made and stored.	Surgery to remove cancer followed by external radiation. *Clinical trials:* external radiation with chemotherapy **or** chemotherapy or biological therapy.

(continued)

TYPES AND TREATMENTS FOR ADULT BRAIN CANCER *(continued)*

CELL TYPE	DESCRIPTION	TREATMENT
Oligodendroglioma, Adult Well Differentiated	Begin in brain cells that provide support and nourishment for cells that transmit nerve impulses. Cells look very much like normal cells. Grows slowly.	Surgery to remove cancer with or without external radiation. *Clinical trials:* radiation plus chemotherapy
Oligodendroglioma, Adult Anaplastic	Begin in brain cells that provide support and nourishment for cells that transmit nerve impulses. Cells look very different from normal cells. Grows more quickly. Clinical trials should be considered.	Surgery to remove cancer followed by external radiation with or without chemotherapy. *Clinical trials:* internal radiation **or** radiation given during surgery **or** radiation given with drugs to make cancer cells more sensitive.
Mixed Glioma	Made up of two or three different cell types—astrocytoma, ependymoma and/or oligodendroglioma. The most malignant-appearing cells determine prognosis.	Surgery followed by external radiation with or without chemotherapy. *Clinical trials:* internal radiation **or** radiation given during surgery **or** radiation given with drugs to make cancer cells more sensitive **or** radiation followed by chemotherapy or biological therapy.
Medulloblastoma, Adult	Rapidly growing tumor. Has tendency to spread from brain to spine.	Surgery to remove cancer followed by external radiation. *Clinical trial:* surgery followed by radiation **or** chemotherapy.

Pineal Parencymal Tumor, Adult	Vary from slow-growing pinecytoma to more malignant and faster growing pineoblastoma. Astrocytomas also can grow in this area, as can some primary germ cell tumors: germinoma, embryonal carcinoma, choriocarcinoma and teratoma.	Surgery plus external radiation with or without chemotherapy. *Clinical trials:* internal radiation **or** radiation given during surgery **or** radiation given with drugs to make cancer cells more sensitive **or** hyperthermia **or** radiation followed by chemotherapy or biological therapy.
Central Nervous System Germ Cell Tumor, Adult	Includes germinoma, embryonal carcinoma, choriocarcinoma and teratoma.	Treatment depends on whether cancer can be removed, cell type, location of tumor, and other factors.
Craniopharyngioma, Adult	Arises from remains of structure found in developing embryo in area of the pituitary gland. Often curable. Presses on vital part of brain and spinal cord.	Surgery to remove cancer with or without radiation.
Meningioma, Adult	Arise from meninges surrounding brain and spinal cord. Usually curable with surgery if all tumor can be removed.	Surgery to remove tumor with or without radiation **or** Radiation if tumor cannot be removed.
Meningioma, Malignant, Adult Hemangiopericytoma Papillary Meningioma	More serious than meningioma.	Surgery followed by external radiation. *Clinical trials:* internal radiation **or** radiation given during surgery **or** radiation given with drugs to make cancer cells more sensitive **or** hyperthermia **or** external radiation followed by chemotherapy **or** biological therapy.

(continued)

TYPES AND TREATMENTS FOR ADULT BRAIN CANCER *(continued)*

CELL TYPE	DESCRIPTION	TREATMENT
Choroid Plexus Tumors	Arise from choroid plexus epithelial cells. Choroid plexus papilloma less serious than anaplastic choroid plexus papilloma, which is more likely to spread to spine.	Surgery followed by radiation.
Recurrent Adult Brain Tumor	Arises from meninges surrounding brain and spinal cord.	Surgery with or without chemotherapy **or** External radiation (if not used previously) with or without chemotherapy **or** Internal radiation **or** Chemotherapy. *Clinical trials:* chemotherapy drugs, may be placed in body during surgery.

include the fact that only a small incision is needed and the ability to perform microsurgery resulting in the least amount of damage to healthy tissues.

What is the aim of brain surgery?

The purpose of the surgery is to remove the entire tumor if possible, or as much tumor as possible. Even partial removal of the tumor provides relief of symptoms, and a smaller amount of tumor left after surgery makes it possible to treat it more easily with other forms of treatment. Surgery is also performed to establish an exact diagnosis, to determine the full extent of the tumor and to provide access for other treatments such as radiation implants or radiation. Usually an MRI will be done within a few days after surgery to discover whether there is any tumor remaining.

What is a craniotomy?

A craniotomy is an operation that exposes the brain so the surgeon can remove the diseased tissue. A craniotomy is usually performed under general anesthesia, although sometimes local anesthesia is used. The head is shaved in the area of the operation, and the scalp is cleaned with soap and water. An antiseptic is used and all but the portion to be operated on is covered with a sterile drape.

How is a craniotomy done?

Usually, the doctor makes an incision in the shape of a semicircle on the affected part of the scalp. The skin will be flapped down and holes drilled into the skull. The holes will be connected by sawing with a wire, air, or electric saw so that a block of bone (called a bone flap) can be removed from the skull. In effect, this creates a window into the skull through which the doctor will work. Directly underneath are the membranes that cover the brain. These will be cut so that the physician can see the brain.

Is the bone replaced after the operation?

After the operation, the doctor will return the bone flap to its location in the skull and stitch the skin back in place. Sometimes a metal or fabric mesh is used to close the opening. In some cases, replacing the bone is not necessary. Muscles in the back of the head, for example, are very strong and can protect the brain.

Can the doctor tell before the operation whether a brain tumor is malignant or benign?

The doctor may suspect what type of tumor is involved but the final diagnosis depends upon a careful study of biopsy samples taken from various parts of the tumor.

Do brain operations take a long time to perform?

The delicate surgery required to perform a brain operation requires the skills of highly trained surgeons. The location and complexity of the tumor, the procedure being used and the surgeons' dexterity all have a bearing on the length of time involved. Some operations are complete within an hour or two. Others may take three, four, or more hours.

Can biopsies be performed in most parts of the brain, even when surgery is not possible?

Computer-guided stereotactic methods now allow needle biopsies to be obtained safely in virtually any part of the brain.

Will I have intravenous feedings following brain surgery?

Sometimes feedings are through a tube in the stomach or vein. Often you can be fed by mouth.

Should I plan to have special nurses after brain surgery?

It depends upon the hospital where you have your surgery. Most large hospital centers use intensive care centers where patients are monitored constantly by nurses with clinical expertise in caring for patients who have had this kind of surgery. Otherwise, it is advisable to have special nurses.

What are the aftereffects of brain surgery?

Many people who have brain surgery are back to normal very soon after surgery. Usually the doctor will be able to give you some indication before the operation as to how long your recovery time will be, and whether or not you will have any defects after the operation—such as poor vision, hearing loss, difficulty in speaking, or problems with use of arms or legs. The operation itself usually does not cause the problems; the problems are usually caused by the location of the growth in the brain.

Are a number of samples of the brain tissues taken during the operation?

A number of samples, sometimes as many as a dozen or more, are taken from around the edges of tumors. These are sent from the operating suite to the surgical pathology laboratory where, within 15 minutes, the operating surgeon knows whether there are malignant cells. The remainder of the tumor tissue is processed for more extensive analysis.

What kinds of treatments besides surgery are used for brain cancer?

A variety of types of radiation therapy, chemotherapy and a number of investigational therapies are being used.

What kinds of radiation are used to treat brain cancer?
Radiation may be used to treat brain cancer that cannot be operated on or may be given after surgery to kill remaining cells. Different types of radiation are used for brain cancer including external beam, interstitial (brachytherapy) radiation, and stereotactic radiosurgery.

Is external beam radiation used for treating brain cancers?
Radiation is sometimes used, although the doses of radiation needed to kill a brain cancer can be dangerous to healthy tissues as well. Newer techniques such as three-dimensional treatment planning (conformal radiation) and stereotactic radiosurgery can help spare normal tissue surrounding the affected area.

How is external beam radiation given?
It is usually given five days a week for several weeks, depending on the type and size of tumor and age of the patient. Depending on need, it can be directed at the tumor and the areas close to it or to the entire brain.

How is interstitial radiation being used for brain cancer?
This type of radiation, which involves the computer directed placement of radioactive pellets into the tumor, is sometimes referred to as brachytherapy, tumor seeding, or radioactive pellets. The seeds may be implanted directly in the tumor or put into a catheter that will give precise doses to the tumor. The implant may be left in for a short time or permanently. Sometimes interstitial radiation is used as a boost following external beam radiation or in place of it.

How is stereotactic radiation or the gamma knife used to treat brain cancer?
This method (which may also referred to as sterotactic radiosurgery, fractionated stereotactic radiation, gamma knife, incisionless brain surgery, or conformal beam radiation, depending on the equipment and method that is being used), combines radiation with sophisticated computerized software to deliver a high dose of radiation to a small, precisely defined area. The high-energy rays are aimed from different angles, so that a high dose reaches the tumor without damaging other brain tissue. The instrument is very precise and delivers the radiation much closer to tumor boundaries. It spares the surrounding brain tissue from radiation. The painless, incisionless treatment takes about a day including preparation, although the treatment itself takes only about 20 minutes. An overnight stay in the hospital is not required. Smaller tumors, below an inch and a half or less in diameter, are the best candidates for this treatment. Additional information on this treatment can be found in Chapter 9, Radiation Treatment.

How are radiosensitizers used for brain cancer?

It is thought that cells exposed to certain drugs (radiosensitizers) are more responsive to radiation therapy. Radiosensitizers are usually given through an artery, followed by a course of conventional radiation. A number of different agents are under investigation.

What is hyperfractionation?

Hyperfractionation is a method of giving smaller daily doses of radiation more frequently—often twice a day—without a change in the overall treatment length.

Is chemotherapy used in treating brain cancers?

Chemotherapy may be used in addition to surgery and radiation. There are more than three dozen new drugs presently in clinical trials of all phases to treat brain tumors of all types, including metastases. Angiogenesis inhibitors, drugs that prevent the growth of new blood vessels, are also being studied in the treatment of brain tumors. (For more information about chemotherapy drugs, see Chapter 10, Chemotherapy.)

Is hyperthermia being used in brain cancer treatment?

Heat therapy (hyperthermia) is being investigated as a treatment. Several devices are used, including radiofrequency, microwaves, ultrasound, and electromagnetic equipment. This treatment is under investigation as an individual treatment as well as for use in combination with interstitial radiation.

Is gene therapy being used for brain tumors?

There are some 19,000 genes in the brain and the National Cancer Institute and the National Institute of Neurological Disorders and Stroke are working in this area. This should bring about not only new ways of diagnosing brain cancer but also new treatments for this difficult disease.

Questions to Ask Your Doctor About Follow-up

- **Will you be doing my main follow-up?**
- **Will I also need to see any of my other doctors?**
- **How often will I need to see you?**
- **What tests will you be doing during my follow-up exam?**
- **What will you be looking for?**
- **What should I be watching for between my visits with you?**
- **What symptoms should I report? To whom?**

What kind of medical follow-up will I have for my brain cancer?

You will usually have follow-up visits, including a complete checkup, at three month intervals for the first year; six month intervals for the second to fifth year, and yearly thereafter. During the first year, the doctor will check carefully for any physical changes, asking you questions about headaches, seizures, speech or mental changes, motor deficits and balance problems. Every six months you will have a complete physical, a chest x-ray, CBC, CT scan or MRI of the brain. If indicated, an EEG or skull x-ray will be done.

What causes brain cancer?

The cause of primary brain cancer is unknown. In most cases it appears that patients with a brain tumor have no clearly defined reason why they should be at risk. However, some studies have linked the risk for brain cancer to exposure to high doses of ionizing radiation—such as x-rays and gamma rays, which can cause chromosomal changes. Occupational exposure to organic solvents and some pesticides, and employment in electrical and electronic-related jobs, as well as oil refining, rubber manufacturing, and drug manufacturing have been studied. Other studies have shown that chemists and embalmers have a higher incidence of brain tumors. Genetic factors, including the familial Li-Fraumeni syndrome and neurofibromatosis have also been implicated. Studies in laboratory animals have found that certain chemicals and DNA viruses can cause brain tumors.

Do cellular phones cause brain cancer?

Four large studies have been completed that have looked at this question— one each in Sweden and Denmark and two in the United States comparing the cell phone use of people with brain cancer and people who do not have it. All studies have had the same results. Cell phone use was not associated with the increased risk of developing brain tumors. This was true whether all brain cancers were considered as a group or different types of brain cancers were looked at individually. Since cell phones are a relatively new technology, longer-term follow-up will need to be done. The phones in question are hand-held cellular phones, the kind that have a built-in antenna that is positioned close to the user's head during normal telephone conversations. You should be aware that the safety of so-called "cordless phones," which have a base unit connected to the telephone wiring in a house and which operate at far lower power levels and frequencies, have not been questioned.

SPINAL CORD TUMORS

What is the spinal cord?

The spinal cord begins at the end of the brain stem and runs down the center of the spine almost to its base. It connects the brain to most of the body's nerves, carrying both incoming and outgoing messages. The spinal cord is protected by the bones that make up the spinal column (vertebrae), is covered by three membranes (meninges) and has fluid to cushion it.

Does cancer occur in the spinal cord?
Primary cancer of the spinal cord is very rare. When it is found, it can be a tumor that starts in the spinal cord or a tumor of the brain that has extended down into the spinal cord. Much more often, however, cancers in the spinal cord have metastasized from another part of the body. See Chapter 26, When Cancers Recur or Metastasize.

Are most spinal cord tumors cancerous?
Tumors that grow within the spinal cord (referred to as primary spinal cord tumors) are more often cancerous than those that start outside the cord itself.

What are the symptoms of spinal cord tumors?
Pain is the most common first symptom of a spinal cord tumor. The kind of pain, as well as of any other symptom, depends on where the tumor is located. Usually the pain gets worse when you cough or strain. Spinal cord tumors may stop the flow of communication between the body and the brain in either one or both directions, similar to spinal cord injuries which occur as a result of accidents. Some symptoms can mimic other diseases such as sciatica, multiple sclerosis, or cervical disk disease. The difficulty in diagnosing spinal cord tumors is that the symptoms are similar to those of many other back problems.

How are spinal cord tumors diagnosed?
Spinal cord tumors usually are diagnosed through the use of a spinal MRI (magnetic resonance imaging). The MRI scan can distinguish between tumors and other problems in this area. Spinal fluid also may need to be analyzed for tumor cells and tumor markers.

What kind of tumors are found in the spinal cord?
The primary tumors found in the spinal cord, spinal nerves, and spinal meninges are identical to those found in the brain. They include astrocytomas, ependymomas, meningiomas, chordomas, as well as less common types. Some tumors of the spinal cord are benign.

How are primary spinal cord tumors treated?
Surgery is the usual treatment for spinal cord tumors. Surgeons, using new techniques in anesthesia, microsurgery, and ultrasound can operate successfully on the spinal cord. If the tumor cannot be completely taken out, external radiation and chemotherapy may be used.

How are spinal cord tumors that have metastasized from somewhere else treated?
Radiation treatment is sometimes used for metastasized spinal cord tumors.

PITUITARY GLAND

What is the pituitary gland?
The pituitary gland is a small organ, about the size of a pea, in the center of the brain just above the back of the nose. It is sometimes referred to as the master gland because it makes hormones that influence body growth, metabolism, and the functions of other glands in the body. Most tumors found in the pituitary gland are not cancerous. They are slow growing and do not usually spread.

What are the symptoms of cancer of the pituitary gland?
Some tumors, called functioning tumors, make too many hormones. Depending upon where the tumor is growing, different hormones may be affected. ACTH-producing tumors can result in a fat buildup in the face, back and chest with the arms and legs becoming very thin—sometimes referred to as Cushing's disease. High blood pressure, weakness in muscles and bones, and high blood sugar are other symptoms. Prolactin-producing tumors of the pituitary gland cause the breasts to produce milk and menstrual periods to stop when a woman is not pregnant and cause impotence in men. Another type causes the hands, face, and feet to grow bigger than is normal. There also are non-functioning tumors that do not make hormones. Nausea and vomiting, trouble with eyesight, or headaches are other symptoms that need to be checked.

How are tumors of the pituitary glands treated?
The most common treatment is surgery. The doctor will take out the tumor, either by cutting through the passage of the nose to do a transphenoidal hypophysectomy or cut in the front of the skull doing a craniotomy. Radiation or chemotherapy may also be used in addition to the surgery.

Web Pages to Check Out

www.cancer.gov: For general up-to-date information, and for clinical trials.

www.cancer.org: For general up-to-date information and community resources.

www.abta.org: American Brain Tumor Association.

www.braintumor.org: National Brain Tumor Foundation.

request.medacc.tmc.edu/~cspencer/brain.html: Brain Tumor Registry to identify families at high risk for brain cancer.

www.cancer.duke.edu/btc: Information on new treatments.

Also see Chapter 2, Searching for Answers on the Web, for more information.

Twenty-three

HEAD AND NECK CANCERS

There have been significant advances in the treatment of head and neck cancers using combinations of radiation and surgery, laser surgery, chemotherapy, and a variety of new reconstructive procedures. Because head and neck cancers can be disfiguring, it is important to look for a doctor who is committed to providing *the best possible treatment that causes the least functional and cosmetic disability.* While cure of the cancer is the primary goal, preserving appearance, the ability to function normally and maintaining quality of life, must also be considered. A comprehensive team approach, which includes the expertise of numerous specialists, makes it possible to be assured of the best possible results. Don't hesitate to explore all your options before committing to any treatment.

CANCER CAN AFFECT any part of the head and neck area—from the *oral cavity,* which includes the lips, hard and soft palate, tongue, gums, and tonsils to the *nasal* area, which includes the nose, nasal cavity, and sinuses, as well as the *upper respiratory area,* which includes the larynx, trachea, and muscles in the neck and upper back. In addition, the *ear* and the *thyroid areas* also are susceptible to cancerous growths. Although these cancers account for very small percentages of the total number of cancers each year, since they affect such vulnerable and visible parts of the body, it is important that possible suggested treatments be fully understood before they are undertaken.

What is head and neck cancer?

Cancer of the head and neck is a catchall phrase for an assortment of cancers that occur in the parts of our bodies that are responsible for speech, chewing, swallowing, seeing, and hearing. Some of the most common areas affected are:

- Thyroid.
- Mouth and oral cavity (tongue, gums, floor of mouth, lip, cheek, oropharynx, soft palate, tonsils, walls of pharynx, and back of tongue).
- Larynx (glottic, supraglottic, pharynx).
- Nose (nasopharynx, nasal cavity, paranasal sinus).
- Salivary gland (parotid gland).

Are most of these cancers difficult to treat?

Depending on the type of cancer and where it is located, you may be facing a simple operation or one that is quite complex. It is important to know before you begin any kind of treatment, exactly what you are dealing with.

What kind of doctor should I go to for treatment for head and neck cancers?

Careful examination and diagnosis is essential before any treatment is agreed upon for cancers of the head and neck. A multidisciplinary team approach is important since this is such a specialized area. Your treatment team may include a head and neck surgeon (also called an otolaryngologist), radiation oncologist, medical oncologist, oral surgeon, plastic surgeon, dentist, speech therapist and psychological counselor. Most of the major cancer centers around the country specialize in treating these cancers. See Chapter 28, Where to Get Help, for more information.

What new techniques are being used in diagnosing head and neck cancer?

Sentinel node radiolocalization is being used in some centers for some head and neck cancers. A radioactive tracer is injected around the tumor. The tracer goes into the lymphatics that drain from the tumor and travel to the first draining lymph nodes. After the tracer accumulates in these nodes, the doctor, using a hand held detector, can see a radioactive "hot spot" on the surface of the skin. If the hot spot can be seen, a biopsy can be done.

Are there hospitals that specialize in doing reconstructive work in the head and neck areas?
Some centers specialize in the delicate reconstructive work that may be necessary treating unusual cancers in the head and neck area that require extensive surgery. Some of the centers with special expertise include: Memorial Sloan-Kettering Cancer Center in New York, Roswell Park Cancer Institute in Buffalo, Indiana University in Indianapolis, the University of Chicago, University of California at Los Angeles, the University of Michigan, the University of Texas M.D. Anderson Cancer Center, and the Mayo Comprehensive Cancer Center in Rochester.

Questions to Ask Your Doctor About Treatment

- **What are my treatment choices?**
- **What are the risks and side effects I can expect?**
- **Will surgery be necessary?**
- **What other alternatives are there?**
- **Can radiation be used instead of surgery?**
- **Where is the best place to get treatment?**
- **Where would I have to go to have intensity modulated radiation therapy (IMRT)?**
- **Who will be doing the surgery?**
- **Can I have laser treatment?**
- **Where will the incision be and what will the scar look like?**
- **Will it be necessary for me to have a functional or radical neck dissection?**
- **How will the surgery affect the way I eat, talk and swallow after the surgery?**
- **Can radiation or radium implants be used instead of surgery? Is laser surgery an option?**
- **Will radiation or chemotherapy be used in addition to surgery?**
- **What kind of reconstructive surgery can be done?**
- **How many operations will that entail?**
- **What are the after effects?**
- **How long will it all take?**
- **Will it cure me?**
- **How expensive will it be?**

- Who else will be on my treatment team?
- When can I meet with them to discuss my operation?
- Will I be hospitalized? For how long?
- How many patients with head and neck cancer are you treating?
- Can you put me in touch with a support group?
- Do you know anyone who has had this treatment who I can talk with about it?

What are the most common types of cancers that occur in the head and neck area of the body?

The most common sites of head and neck cancer are those that occur in the thyroid, mouth (oral cavity), pharynx (throat), larynx (voice box), and sinuses.

What is a functional neck dissection?

A functional neck dissection removes the cancer and the lymph glands from the neck, but does not remove the arteries, nerves, and muscles from the neck. You can continue to move, speak, breathe, and eat normally. In many cases, a functional neck dissection now takes place of the radical neck dissection.

What is a radical neck dissection?

Between 150 and 350 lymph nodes can be found in the head and neck above the collarbone, which is nearly one-third of the total number of lymph nodes in the body. A radical neck dissection is performed along with the removal of the cancer, to remove the lymph nodes in the neck when cancers in the head and neck are found to have spread to the area. The operation is a major one and may require up to five or six hours to perform, when it is done along with the removal of the primary cancer. The surgery is done on one or on both sides of your neck depending on where the cancer has spread. You should know that in a radical neck dissection, the nerves and muscles that serve your neck and upper back and are responsible for arm motion are involved. For some time after surgery, you may find it difficult to raise your arms and to keep your shoulders from falling forward. Sometimes your ability to swallow is impaired. Special exercises will be prescribed by the doctor or hospital therapist to help you regain your strength in these muscles.

What kinds of facial changes might a patient with head and neck cancer have?

Because of the delicate areas where surgery is needed for head and neck cancers, changes in various facial structures including mouth, lips, cheek, neck, ears, nose, and eyes, may be necessary.

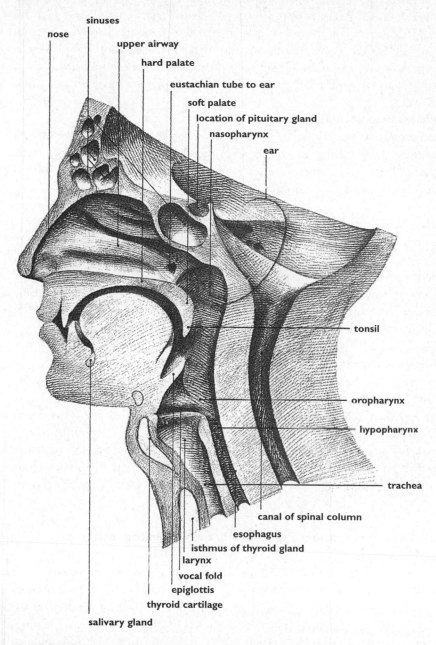

sinuses

nose

upper airway

hard palate

eustachian tube to ear

soft palate

location of pituitary gland

nasopharynx

ear

tonsil

oropharynx

hypopharynx

trachea

canal of spinal column

esophagus

isthmus of thyroid gland

larynx

vocal fold

epiglottis

thyroid cartilage

salivary gland

Head and neck

What is done to help correct these changes?

Reconstructive surgery is often done to minimize the effects of the drastic surgery needed. Another option may be maxillofacial prosthetics, which are sculpted silicone, urethane and acrylic artificial parts, used to restore facial features changed by cancer surgery. You may need a maxillofacial prosthesis to speak or eat or swallow. Or such a prosthesis may be necessary because you have lost an eye, your nose, or a portion of your face, jaw, or teeth and gums.

What is reconstructive surgery?

Reconstructive surgery is the reconstruction of features from the patient's own tissue. The reconstructive surgeon is familiar with the use of skin, cartilage, and bone grafts, and plays a key role in planning, initiating, and coordinating the process of rehabilitation.

What kind of doctors create maxillofacial prosthetics?

Doctors who specialize in restoring facial and oral features following surgery belong to the American Academy of Maxillofacial Prosthetics. A maxillofacial prosthodontist is a dentist who specializes in facial and oral restoration following surgery. These doctors are required to be skilled in restructuring the face, both from a cosmetic and functional point of view. See Chapter 28, Where to Get Help.

How expensive is it to have a prosthetic device made?

Prices vary, of course. An external facial prosthetic device, such as to replace a jaw, ranges between $1800 and $2500. Plastic and reconstructive surgery can cost three to four times as much and require multiple operations. There are, of course, pros and cons for either choice. There are still problems with matching color tone of the prostheses to skin color and the self-adhesives used in prosthetic devices may not be totally satisfactory. But advances are constantly being made and there are talented and devoted doctors who are dedicated to this field and their patients.

Are there organizations that can help me with information and resources?

Let's Face It is an international information and support organization for people with facial reconstruction needs and their families. It provides mutual support, educational services and an annual resource listing for individuals who are facially disfigured. The National Oral Health Information Clearinghouse, a service of the National Institute of Dental Research, is a resource for patients, health professionals, and the public seeking information on the health of people with oral health problems. For addresses and telephone numbers, see Chapter 28, Where to Get Help.

POSSIBLE SIDE EFFECTS

LOCATION OF CANCER	POTENTIAL PROBLEMS
Thyroid	Usually few side effects. However, it is extensive surgery, voice problems, muscle removal can cause one shoulder to be lower than the other; men taking large doses of I–131 may become sterile.
Larynx	If radiation used, voice may change. If whole voice box removed, must learn to speak through stoma.
Larynx, trachea	Breathing, feeding tube.
Jaw, salivary glands, muscles	Chewing, drooling problems.
Tongue, palate, pharynx, salivary glands	Swallowing, speech problems, indistinct speech, drooling problems.
General	Appearance, nutrition.

Do most people who have head and neck cancers have surgery?

Surgery is the mainstay of treatment for most cancers of the head and neck. Continual advances in surgical techniques, now allow more patients to preserve normal functions.

Is laser treatment ever used for head and neck cancer?

Yes, laser treatment may be used for head and neck cancer. In some cases, doctors can insert an endoscope and remove the cancer cells using laser resection. This treatment is faster, leaves no scars, and has fewer side effects, all without invasive surgery.

Can internal and external radiation be used together in treating head and neck cancer?

It depends on the site and the stage of your cancer. Internal radiation (brachytherapy) and external radiation therapy can be used together to locally cure cancers of the head and neck without surgery. Tiny metallic seeds containing radioactive isotopes, usually palladium or iodine, are implanted in the tumor.

Is high-dose brachytherapy used in the treatment of head and neck cancers?

It may be used in cancers of the tongue, cheek, floor of mouth, oropharynx, palate, tonsil, parotid gland, nasopharynx, and lymph nodes in the neck.

TYPES OF OPERATIONS USED FOR HEAD AND NECK CANCERS

NAME	WHAT IT MEANS
Lobectomy (hemithyroidectomy)	One lobe of thyroid, sometimes isthmus, tissue connecting lobes also removed.
Near-total thyroidectomy	Removal of parts of both lobes of thyroid and isthmus of thyroid tissue **or** removal of whole lobe and part of another.
Total thyroidectomy	Removal of all thyroid tissue.
Hemilaryngectomy (also called partial laryngectomy)	Part of larynx is removed.
Total laryngectomy	Entire larynx removed. Permanent hole in front of neck, called a tracheostomy, for breathing.
Laryngopharyngectomy or **partial laryngopharyngectomy** (partial may leave some voice use)	Larynx and all or part of hypopharynx removed. Since hypopharynx is involved with breathing, eating, and talking mechanisms, all may be affected. Plastic surgery may be needed.
Radical or modified neck dissection	Lymph nodes removed on one or both sides of neck, back and arm. Movement may be affected.

Most of the time an interstitial implant will be used. Rows of thin hollow tubes, called treatment catheters, are placed in the area around the tumor. The tubes are attached to the treatment unit, called an afterloader. Depending on the type of cancer and the stage, one to ten treatments will be done.

Is intensity modulated radiation therapy used for head and neck cancers?

This three-dimensional method of delivering external beam radiation, called intensity modulated radiation therapy, allows the radiation oncologist to "mold" the dose of radiation to encompass the tumor and spare the surrounding area. It helps avoid damage to healthy tissues, reduces side effects, and makes it possible to use higher, more effective doses of radiation.

Is chemotherapy used for head and neck cancers?

Chemotherapy is being used in many cases of head and neck cancers, especially in cases that previously would have been considered untreatable. Chemotherapy is often used to enhance the response of cancer cells to radiation and often makes it possible to preserve organs, such as the larynx, that once would have been removed.

**What kind of follow-up checkups are needed for those
who have had cancer of the head and neck?**

Monthly checkups are usually recommended for the first year; every two months the second year, and every three months the third year. After that, you should continue to see the doctor every six months. Usually, the doctor will do a careful physical checkup of the head and neck area and cervical nodes. A chest x-ray and barium swallow will be ordered on a yearly basis and, if needed, a CT scan may be done as well.

THYROID CANCER

The most common cancer in the head and neck area is thyroid cancer. Most lumps or nodules in the thyroid are NOT cancerous. In fact, studies show that in 75 percent of cases, the lump will be benign. Only four to seven percent of lumps will be determined to be malignant. Ten to 15 percent of the time, there will be an inconclusive result, and one to ten percent of the time, there will be an unsatisfactory diagnosis, which means that there were not enough cells gathered to make a diagnosis. In the last two instances, the fine needle biopsy will have to be repeated. If this happens, it is probably wise to seek a second opinion or to consult an endocrinologist.

What is thyroid cancer?

This cancer occurs in this ductless gland located in the front of the throat, below the Adam's apple and just above the breastbone. It is U-shaped and has two lobes—one on each side of the windpipe. Cancer of the thyroid accounts for less than one percent of all cancers. It is also one of the least frequent causes of death from cancer.

What are the symptoms of thyroid cancer?

You may become aware of a growth in the neck—or a growth may be discovered during a regular examination. There may also be enlargement of one or a number of nearby lymph nodes either above or below the thyroid nodule. The lump usually is not painful or tender. A hard, irregular lump that does not seem to move is the most suspicious. Softness, mobility, the indication of more than one lump, and slow growth usually indicate a benign tumor. Only a small percentage of thyroid lumps prove to be cancerous.

Is a goiter likely to turn into thyroid cancer?
A goiter is an enlarged thyroid. It may be caused by too little iodine in the diet or by other conditions. Most goiters are not cancerous.

Who usually gets thyroid cancer?
Cancer of the thyroid is found twice as often in women as in men and more often in whites than in blacks. It is frequently found in young adults and occasionally in teenagers. Interestingly, thyroid cancers have been found on autopsy in large numbers of people who never were aware of having cancer. Adults who were **treated** with x-ray (**not** those who had x-rays for diagnostic purposes) for conditions such as ringworm of the scalp, enlargement of the thymus glands in infants, various types of ear inflammations, deafness due to overgrowth of lymphoid tissue, enlargement or inflammation of tonsils and adenoids and acne, should have this fact noted on their permanent medical records, since these cancers may not occur until 20 years or longer after the treatment. They are at slightly higher risk for thyroid cancers, but only a small percentage of the people irradiated at an early age develop thyroid tumors.

How is the thyroid scan performed?
After you swallow radioactive iodine, a probe is used to determine how actively your thyroid tissue is absorbing the substance. If it is quite active, the lump is called "hot." If it does not absorb the substance, the lump is called "cold." Cold lumps may be cancerous, slow growing, and slow to spread. Hot spots usually indicate a benign growth. Even if your scan shows that you have a cold spot, you should not worry, because about 80 percent of the time, cold spots, upon biopsy, prove **not** to be cancerous. Sometimes two thyroid scan readings are taken—usually at two and 24 hours after administration of the radioactive material.

What are the different kinds of thyroid cancers?
There are a number of thyroid cancers that grow and spread in different ways. Well differentiated papillary cancers are very curable, but they can recur and grow rapidly, so follow-up is important. Follicular and medullary cancers are slow growing. Poorly differentiated or anaplastic thyroid cancers grow rapidly and may spread.

How is cancer of the thyroid treated?

Surgery is the most common treatment for cancers of the thyroid, although radioactive thyroid therapy (I–131) radiation, hormone therapy and chemotherapy are also used.

What are the operations performed for thyroid cancer?

Lobectomy (or hemithyroidectomy) means that one lobe of the thyroid (and sometimes the isthmus, or tissue connecting the two lobes) has been removed. Lymph nodes in the area may be removed and biopsied. A near-total thyroidectomy removes all of the thyroid except for a small part. The total thyroidectomy includes removal of both lobes. Because anaplastic thyroid cancer (unlike follicular and medullary thyroid cancer) often spreads very quickly to other tissues, it may be necessary to also remove the trachea (the breathing tube). A tracheostomy will be done so that there is a permanent airway in the throat for breathing.

How is radioactive iodine used in treating thyroid cancer?

When radioactive iodine is used for imagining tests, a small amount is taken by mouth and it collects in the thyroid. A probe is used to scan the thyroid. For treatment, the patient is given a larger dose, which kills the thyroid cells.

How is radioactive thyroid therapy done?

This treatment is used to destroy all the cells not removed by surgery or to treat thyroid cancer that has spread to lymph nodes and other parts of the body. The radioactive I–131 is usually given by mouth in liquid or capsule form. The intestine absorbs the I–131, which flows through the bloodstream and collects in thyroid cells. Thyroid cancer cells remaining in the neck and those that have spread to other parts of the body are killed when they absorb I–131.

Will I be radioactive if I take I–131?

If the dose of I–131 is low enough, you will usually be given the hormones to be taken at home. If a high dose is needed, the doctor will arrange for you to remain in the hospital for one or more days after receiving your dose. Any radioactive iodine not used by the thyroid gland will be eliminated during the first two days through urine, feces, saliva, and sweat. You will be in an isolation room and will be given special instructions on showering, using the toilet facilities, etc.

Is hormone treatment usually given after surgery?

Usually, patients who have had papillary or follicular thyroid cancer will, following surgery, be put on a regimen of hormone pills to replace the natural thyroid hormone.

TREATMENT CHOICES FOR THYROID CANCER

STAGE	PAPILLARY	FOLLICULAR	MEDULLARY*	ANAPLASTIC*
I	Surgery—Lobectomy and exogenous thyroid hormone treatment. (Radioactive iodine I-131 may be given after surgery) or total thyroidectomy	Surgery—Total thyroidectomy or lobectomy followed by exogenous thyroid hormone therapy. (Radioactive iodine may be given after surgery.) Regional lymph nodes biopsied.	Surgery—Total thyroidectomy and biopsy of tissues around thyroid to see if they contain cancer. If cancerous, lymph node dissection. Radioactive iodine should NOT be used. If spread to other parts of body, external radiation or chemotherapy. NOTE: Family members should be tested.	Surgery to remove thyroid and tissues around it; trachea may be removed. Airway in throat may be needed (tracheostomy) or external radiation or chemotherapy. Check clinical trials.
II	Same as above but cancerous lymph nodes removed.			
III	Total thyroidectomy plus removal of lymph nodes and tissues around thyroid where cancer has spread or Total thyroidectomy plus radiation with iodine or external radiation.			

IV   Radioactive iodine **or** External radiation **or**
      Hormone therapy **or** *Clinical trials:* chemotherapy.

      *There is no staging system for Medullary and
      Anaplastic thyroid cancers.

Recurrent Surgery effective 50 percent of the time for local recurrence. External radiation, intraoperative radiation, or
chemotherapy. Check clinical trials.

What kind of follow-up checkups do I need after being treated for cancer of the thyroid?

You should see your doctor every six months for the first and second year, and every twelve months thereafter.

What are the parathyroid glands?

The parathyroids are four small glands that are attached to the thyroid gland. They secrete a hormone, parathormone, which is involved with the balance of the body and the excretion of calcium and phosphorus necessary for bone growth and maintenance. They are part of the endocrine system.

What are other parts of the endocrine system?

Other parts include the adrenal glands and the pituitary glands.

Can cancer grow in any of the parts of the endocrine system?

It is possible to have cancer of the parathyroid glands, the adrenal glands, or the pituitary glands. Cancer of the endocrine system is relatively rare and is complex to diagnose.

LARYNX

What is the larynx?

The larynx is the voice box. It is the upper part of the windpipe above the trachea. The esophagus is just behind the trachea and the larynx. The openings of the esophagus and the larynx are very close together in the throat. The larynx forms the Adam's apple in the neck. Air coming in passes through the larynx to the lungs. In front of the larynx are the vocal cords. Muscles move the vocal cords, which are made to vibrate by air exhaled from the lungs.

Who is most likely to get cancer of the larynx?

Men are almost nine times more likely to develop cancer of the larynx than women, although the incidence in females is now rising, possibly due to increased smoking among women. Cancer of the larynx occurs most often in people over the age of 55. It is more common among African-Americans than among whites. One known cause of cancer of the larynx is cigarette smoking. The risk is even higher for smokers who drink to excess as well as for asbestos workers or those who have been exposed to nickel or mustard gas.

What are symptoms of cancer of the larynx?

The symptoms of cancer of the larynx depend on the size and location of the tumor. Since most tumors begin on the vocal cords, they almost always cause hoarseness or other changes in the voice. Tumors in the area above the vocal cords may cause a lump in the throat, difficult or painful swallowing, a cough that persists, a sore throat, or an earache. Tumors that begin in the area below the vocal cords, which are rare, can cause shortness of breath or harsh, noisy breathing. Larger tumors may cause swollen neck glands, pain, weight loss, bad breath, and frequent choking on food. Hoarseness that lasts for more than three weeks should be checked by a doctor.

Are all growths on the larynx cancerous?

No. Most tumors of the larynx are benign. Noncancerous growths may be caused by allergy, irritation, infection or overuse of the voice. They can be removed and the voice restored to normal. Sometimes, especially if the growths are wart-like, they may recur and will be operated on again. Cancer of the larynx can be removed by surgery when found early, and the voice may be saved.

Where does cancer of the larynx occur?

Cancer of the larynx cannot be considered one disease but rather three different, distinct types, depending upon where the cancer is. The three main parts of the larynx are the glottis (true vocal cords), the supraglottis (area above the vocal cords) and the subglottis (the area below the vocal cords). Cancers in each region involve different symptoms, treatments, and rehabilitation methods.

What is the meaning of the different stages of cancer of the larynx?

If your cancer is Stage I, this means that the cancer is confined to the area where it started and that the vocal cords can move normally. In Stage II, the cancer is only in the larynx and has not spread to lymph nodes in the area or to other parts of the body. Stage III means that the cancer has not spread outside the larynx, but the vocal cords cannot move normally, or that the cancer has spread to the tissues next to the larynx. Also included in Stage III are those larynx cancers where the cancer has spread to one lymph node on the same side of the neck as the cancer. The lymph node measures no more than three centimeters, or just a little over one inch. In Stage IV, the cancer has spread to tissues around the larynx, such as the pharynx or the tissues in the neck. The lymph nodes in the area may or may not contain cancer. Also considered Stage IV is cancer that has spread to more than one lymph node on the same side of the neck as the cancer, to lymph nodes on one or both sides of the neck, or to any lymph node that measures more than six centimeters (over two inches). If cancer has spread to any other part of the body, it will also be Stage IV.

TREATMENT CHOICES FOR CANCER OF THE LARYNX

LOCATION	STAGE I	STAGE II	STAGE III	STAGE IV
Supraglottis	External radiation or Surgery to remove supraglottis or Total laryngectomy.	External radiation or Surgery to remove supraglottis or Total laryngectomy. Possibly lymph node dissection or Radiation. *Clinical trials:* Hyperfractionated radiation or chemoprevention therapy.	Surgery with or without radiation or Radiation followed by surgery if not needed. *Clinical trials:* Hyperfractionated radiation or chemotherapy followed by radiation. (laryngectomy reserved for those who do not respond.) or chemotherapy combined with radiation or chemotherapy with radiation sensitizers or chemoprevention.	Total laryngectomy followed by radiation or Radiation followed by surgery. *Clinical trials:* Hyperfractionated radiation or induction chemotherapy followed by radiation or chemotherapy, radiation sensitizers or new forms of radiation or chemoprevention.
Glottis	Radiation or Surgery to remove vocal cord or	Radiation or Surgery to remove part of larynx or total	Same as Stage II.	Total laryngectomy followed by radiation or see Stage II.

	Surgery to remove part or all of larynx or Laser surgery.	laryngectomy or Laser surgery. *Clinical trials:* Hyper-fractionated radiation or chemoprevention.	Total laryngectomy plus total thyroidectomy and radical lymph node dissection usually followed by radiation or Radiation alone. *Clinical trials:* Hyperfrac-tionated radiation or simultaneous chemother-apy and hyperfractionated radiation or chemother-apy, radiation sensitizers or other new forms of radiation or chemopre-vention.
		Surgery to remove larynx, surrounding tissue and lymph nodes in neck usually followed by radiation or Radiation if surgery not possible. *Clinical trials:* chemotherapy with radiosensitizers or chemoprevention.	
Subglottis	Radiation or Hemilaryngectomy or Total laryngectomy. *Clinical trials:* Hyper-fractionated radia-tion.	Same as Stage I. *Clinical trials:* Hyper-fractionated radiation or chemoprevention.	

Recurrent cancers of the larynx: Treatment will depend on previous treatment. If surgery was used alone, you may have surgery again or radiation treatment. If you had radiation alone, surgery may be used. If you had surgery and radiation therapy, *Clinical trials:* New chemotherapy drugs.

Does the fact that I have cancer of the larynx mean that I will lose my ability to speak?

Loss of speech was once common after head and neck surgery. However, continual advances in surgical techniques, allow more patients to preserve their voices. Surgeons have perfected techniques that remove only part of the larynx instead of the entire organ. Larynx-preserving surgery is possible in more than half of the cases that once would have required the larynx to be removed.

What factors are considered in treating cancer of the larynx?

The doctor will try to prescribe treatment that will preserve the voice. Many small cancers of the larynx are successfully treated by radiation or surgery, including laser excision surgery. Some doctors reserve surgery for secondary treatment in the event that radiation is not successful. More advanced stages of cancer of the larynx are treated by combining radiation and surgery.

Is it important for a patient to stop smoking during treatment for cancer of the larynx?

Studies have shown that patients who smoke while receiving radiation for cancers of the larynx do not respond as well to the treatment and therefore do not live as long as those who stop smoking. Persons who wish to get help in stopping smoking can call the Cancer Information Service at 1–800–4–CANCER. A trained person will talk with you about ways you might use to quit.

Do cancers of the larynx recur?

Sometimes they do. The most likely time of recurrence is in the first two to three years. Recurrences after five years are quite rare.

Is there a change in the voice when radiation is used for treating cancer of the larynx?

In all probability you will be able to continue talking in much the same way as before radiation treatment. The treatment may change the way your voice sounds. Your voice may be weaker at the end of the day and may be affected by changes in the weather.

Will my voice change as a result of a *partial laryngectomy*?

Sometimes a change in voice occurs. Usually it sounds like you are slightly hoarse. However, most people are able to continue talking as they did before the operation.

What changes occur as the result of a *total laryngectomy*?

A total laryngectomy is a major operation. The entire larynx is removed. Before the operation, breathing and food passages had a common opening in the throat. Farther down, they divided into the windpipe for breathing and the esophagus for carrying food to the stomach. The voice box controlled the entry of air and guarded against the entry of food particles. When the voice box or larynx is removed, the end of the air passage is relocated as an opening at the front of the neck. This is called a stoma. It is a permanent opening in the front of the neck. You will breathe, cough, and "sneeze" through the stoma.

How are people who have had a laryngectomy able to communicate?

A speech pathologist usually meets with the patient before surgery to explain the various methods that can be used. There are a number of methods that are available. Esophageal speech instruction may begin before you leave the hospital. You will be taught to use air forced into the esophagus to produce your new voice. The sound may be low-pitched and gruff. It takes practice and patience to learn to speak understandably. A mechanical larynx may be used until you are able to learn esophageal speech or if esophageal speech is too difficult. The device may be powered by batteries (electrolarynx) or by air (pneumatic larynx). The speech pathologist can help you determine what method is best for you.

What is a tracheoesophageal puncture (TEP)?

A tracheoesophageal puncture is one-day surgery that can be done as long as ten years after larynx surgery. Its purpose is to give people who find it difficult to learn esophageal speech an opportunity to regain the use of their voices. The operation is performed to provide an opening. A small plastic or silicone valve is inserted to provide a source of air. The patient diverts air into the esophagus and uses it to resonate in the pharynx. Careful training is given by a speech pathologist to help the patient regain good speech.

Where can I get more information about living without my larynx?

You can call the nearest office of the American Cancer Society at 1–800–ACS–2345. They can direct you to literature and groups that can be of help to you. In some areas, the American Cancer Society sponsors Lost Cord Clubs, sometimes called New Voice Clubs, which are groups of laryngectomees and their families dedicated to helping new members get used to the same physical and emotional changes they have experienced. The International Association of Laryngectomees is another organization with excellent resources. Many of the groups offer speech therapy as part of scheduled meetings. It is reassuring to participate with others who have had the same experience. See Chapter 28, Where to Get Help, for more information.

PHARYNX

What is the pharynx?
The pharynx is the passage between the larynx and the esophagus. It is subdivided into the nasopharynx, oropharynx, and hypopharynx. Air and food pass through the pharynx on the way to the windpipe (trachea) or the esophagus.

What is the hypopharynx?
The hypopharynx is the bottom part of the throat. It is a hollow tube about 5 inches long that starts behind the nose and goes down to the neck to become part of the esophagus. The pyriform sinuses are part of this structure.

What are the symptoms of cancer of the hypopharynx?
Symptoms of cancer of the hypopharynx usually include difficulty swallowing and pain on swallowing, a sore throat that does not go away, a lump in the neck, a change in your voice or pain in your ear.

How is cancer of the hypopharynx treated?
Since this is a very difficult cancer to treat, it is most important that you be treated by a surgeon and/or radiation oncologist who is highly skilled in the multiple procedures and techniques available and who is actively and frequently treating patients who have this type of cancer. If the cancer has not spread to the lymph nodes, the larynx, and the pharynx will usually be surgically removed in an operation called a laryngopharyngectomy, often followed by radiation. Unless a partial laryngopharyngectomy can be performed with some vocal function being preserved, this means that speech as well as eating and breathing may all be affected by the operation. Some clinical trials are testing the use of chemotherapy to shrink tumors as the initial treatment so that the tumor can be more treatable with either surgery or radiation. Cancers of the oropharyngeal wall are similar to those of the hypopharynx.

What is the oropharynx?
The oropharynx is the middle part of the throat, also called the pharynx. It is a hollow tube about 5 inches long that starts behind the nose and goes down to the neck to become part of the esophagus which connects to the stomach. Cancer in the oropharynx is usually a squamous cell type cancer that starts in the cells that line this tube. If your cancer starts in the lymph cells of the oropharynx, it is considered to be non-Hodgkin's lymphoma. See Chapter 19, Hodgkin's Disease, Non-Hodgkin's Lymphoma, and Multiple Myeloma.

How is cancer of the oropharynx treated?

Managing oropharyngeal cancer is very complex and, especially if the tumor is more than four centimeters (about two inches) requires a highly skilled multidisciplinary team. Where radiation is to be the treatment, it is essential that it be done by a radiotherapist who is experienced in treating head and neck cancers. Treatment depends on where the cancer is in the oropharynx—whether it is in the back of the tongue, tonsil, posterior pharynx, or soft palate—as well as your age and state of health. Both surgery and external and internal implant radiation are used. In treating the tongue base, radiation may be preferred because it allows more function to be preserved. New surgical techniques developed in the last ten years, including micrographic surgery, make it possible for the cancer to be removed with the least possible tissue being lost. Often, surgery is combined with radiation therapy. Clinical trials are underway to test these various methods.

ORAL CAVITY

Cancers of the oral cavity (the area that includes the mouth) include the lips, the front two-thirds of the tongue, the membrane lining the inside of the cheeks and lips (buccal mucosa), the gums (gingivae), the hard palate, the floor of the mouth, and the small area behind the wisdom teeth (retromotor trigone).

Who is likely to get cancer of the mouth?

Cancers of the lip and oral cavity are more common in men than in women. It usually is found in people over the age of 45. People with light-colored skin who have been exposed to the sun are more susceptible to cancers of the mouth. It is also more common in people who chew tobacco or smoke pipes. Early cancers of the lip and oral cavity are highly curable by surgery or by radiation.

What are the symptoms of cancer of the mouth?

A lump in the lip, mouth or gums or a sore in the mouth that does not heal should be checked by the doctor. Bleeding or pain in the mouth or dentures that no longer fit may signal the need to have the mouth checked. Many times, cancers of the lip and oral cavity are found by dentists when they examine the teeth.

TREATMENT CHOICES FOR LIP AND ORAL

LOCATION	STAGE I	STAGE II	STAGE III	STAGE IV
Oral cavity stages	No larger than two centimeters, about one inch; no spread to lymph nodes.	Larger than two centimeters but less than four centimeters, about two inches; no spread to lymph nodes.	No larger than four centimeters or any size which has spread to one lymph node no more than three centimeters, on same side as cancer. NOTE: micrographic surgery followed by radiation being tested in clinical trials for all Stage III oral cancer locations.	Spread to tissues around lip and oral cavity. Lymph nodes may or may not be affected or any size cancer spread to lymph nodes on one or both sides of neck or any lymph node that measures more than six centimeters or over two inches or if spread to other parts.
Lip	Surgery or Radiation.	Surgery or External and/or internal radiation.	Surgery plus internal or external radiation or Radiation. *Clinical trials:* Chemotherapy followed by surgery or radiation or surgery	Surgery plus internal or external radiation. *Clinical trials:* Radiation or Chemotherapy combined with radiation or fractionated radiation therapy.

followed by chemotherapy, **or** surgery, radiation and chemotherapy **or** Superfractionated radiation **or** Chemotherapy plus radiation. NOTE: Additional radiation will be given to neck with or without surgery to remove lymph nodes in the neck.

Tongue			
Surgery **or** Surgery followed by radiation to neck **or** Radiation to mouth and neck.	Radiation **or** Surgery plus radiation.	External radiation with or without internal radiation **or** Surgery followed by radiation. *Clinical trials:* Chemotherapy plus radiation.	Surgery to remove tongue and voicebox (larynx) followed by radiation **or** Radiation to relieve symptoms. *Clinical trials:* Chemotherapy followed radiation **or** fractionated radiation.

(continued)

TREATMENT CHOICES FOR LIP AND ORAL CANCERS *(continued)*

LOCATION	STAGE I	STAGE II	STAGE III	STAGE IV
Buccal mucosa (lining inside cheek and lips)	Surgery **or** Radiation.	Radiation **or** Surgery **or** Surgery plus radiation.	Surgery **or** Radiation **or** Surgery plus radiation. *Clinical trials:* Chemotherapy followed by surgery or radiation **or** surgery followed by chemotherapy **or** surgery, radiation and chemotherapy **or** chemotherapy plus radiation.	Surgery to remove cancer and tissue around it **or** Radiation **or** Surgery plus radiation. *Clinical trials:* Chemotherapy combined with radiation **or** fractionated radiation.
Floor of the mouth	Surgery **or** Radiation.	Surgery **or** Radiation **or** Surgery followed by internal or external radiation	Surgery to remove cancer and lymph nodes in neck as well as part of jawbone if needed **or** External radiation with or without internal radiation.	Surgery followed by radiation **or** Radiation followed by surgery. *Clinical trials:* Chemotherapy combined with radiation **or** fractionated radiation.

Lower gum (gingiva)	Surgery **or** Radiation.	Surgery **or** Radiation. *Clinical trials:* Chemotherapy followed by surgery and radiation **or** fractionated radiation therapy **or** chemotherapy plus radiation.	Surgery **or** Radiation.	Radiation given before or after surgery to remove cancer. *Clinical trials:* Chemotherapy plus radiation.	Surgery and/or radiation. *Clinical trials:* chemotherapy combined with radiation **or** fractionated radiation therapy.
Retromolar trigone (behind wisdom teeth)	Surgery to remove part of jawbone **or** radiation followed, if needed by surgery.	Surgery to remove part of jawbone **or** radiation followed, if needed by surgery.	Surgery followed by radiation. *Clinical trials:* Chemotherapy followed by surgery or radiation **or** surgery followed by chemotherapy **or** fractionated radiation therapy **or** chemotherapy plus radiation.	Surgery followed by	Surgery followed by radiation. *Clinical trials:* Chemotherapy combined with radiation **or** fractionated radiation.

(continued)

TREATMENT CHOICES FOR LIP AND ORAL CANCERS (continued)

LOCATION	STAGE I	STAGE II	STAGE III	STAGE IV
Upper gums and hard palate	Surgery **or** Surgery followed by radiation.	radiation.	Radiation **or** Surgery and radiation. *Clinical trials:* Chemotherapy plus radiation.	Surgery plus radiation. *Clinical trials:* Chemotherapy combined with radiation **or** fractionated radiation.

Recurrent: If previous treatment was radiation, surgery may be tried. If surgery, more surgery, radiation therapy, or both. *Clinical Trials:* New chemotherapy drugs, chemotherapy plus additional radiation therapy, or hyperthermia.

NASAL AREA

To the layman, the nose is what protrudes from the middle of the face. To the medical expert, it is known as the nasopharyngeal area, a very complex structure that lies within the facial cavity and extends to the ears and neck. It reaches from the back of the nose and upper throat to just below the base of the skull and just above the soft palate. The area is divided into two parts, the nasopharynx and the nasal cavity. Cancers in the two areas are treated differently, so it is important to know exactly what kind of cancer you have so you can understand what treatment will involve.

What are symptoms of cancer of the nasopharynx?
The most common symptom is painless, enlarged lymph nodes in the neck. Other symptoms include trouble in breathing or speaking, frequent headaches, a lump in the nose or neck, pain or ringing in the ear (tinnitus), or hearing problems.

What kinds of tests are used to find nasopharyngeal cancer?
The doctor will usually first do a physical examination of the throat, feeling for swollen lymph nodes in the neck, examining the throat with a long-handled mirror. A nasoscope, a thin, lighted tube, will be used to check the nose for abnormal areas. Hearing and nerve function will be examined. MRI, CT scans, and other laboratory tests such as blood tests will be needed. A biopsy will be done to determine the exact type of cancer. Benign tumors of the nasopharynx are relatively rare, but they can include angiofibromas and hemangiomas. Benign tumors are also found in the minor salivary glands in the lining of the nasopharynx. It is a good idea to have thyroid function tests done before treatment so that thyroid function can be compared and monitored after treatment.

Who is most likely to have nasopharyngeal cancer?
- People who have been exposed to the Epstein-Barr virus.
- People of Chinese or Asian background. Interestingly enough, there does not seem to be any connection between nasopharyngeal cancer and excess use of tobacco or alcohol.

Where does nasopharyngeal cancer occur?
Cancer of the nasopharynx occurs in the area behind the nose and in the upper part of the throat, called the pharynx. The holes in the nose through which you breathe lead into the nasopharynx and two openings on the side of the nasopharynx lead into the ear.

What kinds of cancer occur in the nasopharynx?
Several types of cancers can occur in the nasopharyngeal area. The most common types are squamous cell tumors although other types are possible. Nasopharyngeal cancers are usually found to be keratinizing squamous cell, non-keratinizing squamous cell, or undifferentiated cancers. Cancers with excess keratin (karatinizing squamous cell) tend to be more aggressive. Lymphomas can also be found in the immune system cells normally found in the nasopharynx. See Chapter 19, Hodgkin's Disease, Non-Hodgkin's Lymphoma, and Multiple Myeloma.

What kind of treatment is usually recommended for nasopharyngeal cancer?
High dose external radiation to the cancer and the lymph nodes in the neck, sometimes boosted with internal implants, is the usual treatment for Stage I cancers. Surgery is usually reserved for later treatment in the event that lymph nodes fail to respond or for nodes that reappear after treatment. It has been found, through clinical studies, that chemotherapy given early, along with radiation—a one-two punch treatment—has increased survival rates dramatically. So chemotherapy, combined with radiation therapy is the usual treatment for Stage II, III, and IV nasopharyngeal cancers. Surgery to remove lymph nodes in the neck may be done for Stage III and IV cancers. Clinical trials of chemotherapy before, combined with or after radiation are being done for Stage III and IV cancers. If the cancer recurs, external radiation plus internal radiation is recommended, with surgery and/or chemotherapy if needed. Clinical trials of biological therapy and/or chemotherapy are being done.

NASAL AND SINUS CANCERS

The nasal cavity is the area where the nose opens into the nasal passageway. This cavity runs along the top of the palate and turns downward to join the passage from the mouth to the throat. The sinuses are small cavities or tunnels that are around or near the nose (sometimes referred to as paranasal) and they help filter, warm, and humidify the air you breathe. They also help give your voice resonance.

What are the different kinds of sinuses?
There are a whole network of paired sinuses including maxillary sinuses in the cheek area and on either side of the nose; frontal sinuses, above the inner eye and eyebrow area; sphenoid sinuses which are back behind the nose and between the eyes and ethrmoid sinuses located above the nose, between the eyes. The nasal cavity and sinuses are lined with mucosa, a mucous-producing tissue.

Where does cancer usually grow in the nose and sinus area?
All of the cells that make up the lining cells can become cancerous and each type behaves and grows differently. About 70 to 75 percent of cancer in the nasal cavity and paranasal sinuses is squamous cell cancer. Adenocarcinoma that arises from gland cells accounts for about 10 to 15 percent of these cancers. Malignant lymphomas make up about 5 percent of this type of cancer and melanoma is found in about 1 percent of cases.

What are the symptoms of cancer of the paranasal sinus and nasal cavity?
The symptoms can vary depending on which sinuses are affected. The symptoms are vague.

- Sinuses that are blocked and don't clear
- Pain in your upper teeth
- Swelling around the eyes
- Sinus infection
- Lump or sore in your nose that doesn't heal
- Headaches or pain in the sinus area
- Numbness in your cheek, upper lip, upper teeth, or side of nose
- Double vision

Having these symptoms does not mean that you have cancer in this area. But it is wise to check with your doctor in case any of these symptoms last more than a couple of weeks.

What kind of treatment is usually recommended for cancers in the nasal area?
Treatments vary depending upon where the cancer is located and what type of cancer is involved. For cancers of the nasopharyngeal cancer, high-dose external radiation to the cancer and the lymph nodes in the neck, sometimes boosted with internal implants, is the common treatment. Surgery is usually reserved for later treatment in the event that lymph nodes fail to respond or for nodes that reappear after treatment. For cancers in the paranasal sinus and nasal cavity, treatment varies considerably, depending on the type of cancer and where it is found. The chart on the next pages shows the various therapies.

Are warts in the nasal area usually cancerous?
Papillomas, which are wart-like growths, are not considered to be cancer but they do have a small chance of developing into squamous cell cancer. Inverting or sunken papilloma has a tendency to recur.

TREATMENT CHOICES FOR CANCERS OF THE PARANASAL SINUS AND NASAL CAVITY

LOCATION	STAGE I	STAGE II	STAGE III	STAGE IV	RECURRENT
Stage description	Cancer only in maxillary sinus.	Cancer has started to destroy bone around sinus.	Cancer has spread to one lymph node on same side of neck (3 centimeters or less), or cancer has spread to cheek, back of sinus, eyesocket, or ethmoid sinus.	Cancer has spread to eye or other sinuses, or cancer is only in sinuses or has spread to lymph nodes on one or both sides of neck, or cancer has spread to other parts of body.	Cancer has come back, either in paranasal sinuses, nasal cavity, or another part of the body, after it has been treated.
Maxillary sinus	Surgery; may be followed by radiation.	Surgery; radiation may be given before or after surgery.	Surgery; radiation may be given before or after surgery. *Clinical trials:* special radiation before or after surgery; chemotherapy combined with radiation.	Radiation. *Clinical trials:* chemotherapy before surgery or radiation; chemotherapy following radiation; chemotherapy combined with radiation.	If surgery was done before, more extensive surgery followed by radiation. If radiation was given, surgery. Chemotherapy may be used. *Clinical trials:* New chemotherapy drugs.

Ethmoid sinus	Radiation if cancer cannot be removed, or surgery followed by radiation.	Radiation or surgery followed by radiation.	Surgery; followed by radiation. *Clinical trials:* chemotherapy before surgery or radiation; chemotherapy following surgery with or without radiation; chemotherapy combined with radiation.	Surgery, followed by radiation; radiation followed by surgery. *Clinical trials:* chemotherapy before surgery or radiation; chemotherapy following surgery with or without radiation; chemotherapy combined with radiation.	If surgery was done, more surgery followed by radiation. If radiation was given before, surgery. Chemotherapy may be used. *Clinical trials:* new chemotherapy drugs.
Sphenoid sinus	Radiation	Radiation	Radiation	Radiation	Radiation. Chemotherapy if radiation not successful.

(continued)

TREATMENT CHOICES FOR CANCERS OF THE PARANASAL SINUS AND NASAL CAVITY *(continued)*

LOCATION	STAGE I	STAGE II	STAGE III	STAGE IV	RECURRENT
Nasal cavity	Surgery, radiation, or both.		Surgery or radiation; surgery plus radiation. *Clinical trials:* chemotherapy before surgery or radiation; chemotherapy following surgery with or without radiation; chemotherapy combined with radiation.	Surgery or radiation; surgery plus radiation. *Clinical trials:* chemotherapy before surgery or radiation; chemotherapy following surgery with or without radiation; chemotherapy combined with radiation.	If surgery was done before, radiation alone or more extensive surgery followed by radiation. If radiation was given before, chemotherapy may be used.
Inverting papilloma	Surgery.	Surgery.	If cancer comes back after surgery; radiation may be used.		
Melanoma or sarcoma	Surgery. For some sarcomas, surgery, radiation, and chemotherapy may be used.		Surgery. Radiation may be given if cancer cannot be removed by surgery. For some sarcomas, surgery, radiation, and chemotherapy may be used.	Surgery if possible. Radiation or chemotherapy if cancer cannot be removed by surgery.	Surgery or chemotherapy.

Midline granuloma	Radiation.	Radiation.	Radiation.	Radiation.
Nose (nasal vestibule)	Surgery or radiation.	External or internal radiation. Surgery if cancer comes back following treatment. *Clinical trials:* chemotherapy before surgery or radiation; chemotherapy following surgery with or without radiation; chemotherapy combined with radiation.	Radiation.	If radiation was given before, surgery. If surgery was done before, radiation alone or with more extensive surgery. Chemotherapy. *Clinical trials:* New chemotherapy drugs.

SALIVARY GLAND CANCERS

Where are the salivary glands located?

Major clusters of salivary glands are found just below your tongue, on the side of the face just in front of the ear, and under the jawbone. Smaller clusters are found in other parts of the upper digestive tract.

What are the symptoms of cancer in the salivary glands?

Any swelling around or under the chin or around the jawbone, facial numbness, muscles in the face that seem "frozen," or pain that does not go away in your face, chin, or neck should be checked by a physician.

What are the causes of salivary gland cancers?

One of the major risk factors involved with salivary gland cancer is exposure to radiation, either from diagnostic x-rays or from radiation therapy for cancerous or noncancerous conditions. It is also believed that the use of tobacco has a role in this type of cancer.

Are most tumors in the salivary glands cancerous?

Many growths in the salivary glands are not cancerous. Only about one-quarter of parotid gland tumors are found to be cancerous. Thirty-five to 40 percent of submandibular tumors are cancerous, while 50 percent of palate tumors and 95 percent of tumors of the sublingual gland are found to be malignant.

How is cancer of the salivary glands treated?

Treatment for cancer of the salivary glands depends upon the size of the cancer and upon whether it is a fast or slow growing type. Surgery is usually the treatment, with or without radiation following the surgery. Neutron radiation and radiosensitization are being tested in clinical trials. New chemotherapy drugs are also being tested. Because salivary glands help digest your food and are close to your jaw, treatment may require that plastic surgery be done if a large amount of tissue or bone is removed around the salivary glands.

Where is the incision made for salivary gland tumors?

The incision placement depends upon which glands are affected. For the parotid gland, the incision is usually in front of the ear and along the angle of the jaw. For sublingual gland tumors, the incision will usually be in the mouth or in the skin just below the chin.

OCCULT NECK CANCER

What is metastatic squamous neck cancer with occult primary?

Sometimes cancer starts in other parts of the body and spreads to the lymph nodes in the neck. When the cells are studied, the pathologist can determine whether these cells are from another part of the body. Sometimes, even with this information, it is impossible for the doctor to find the source of the original cancer. When this happens, the cancer is called metastatic squamous neck cancer with occult primary. Occult means unseen and primary refers to the original cancer. In other words, the source of the original cancer cannot be found, but the lymph nodes cells are cancerous. The doctor will continue to try to determine where the original cancer is, but meanwhile, treatment may be started. It is imperative that long-term repeat examinations be made so that the primary tumor can be found and treated. The neck should not be biopsied until the possibility of a primary cancer in the head and neck area has been excluded. Fine needle aspiration may be done for early diagnosis.

Web Pages to Check Out

www.cancer.gov: For general up-to-date information, and for clinical trials.
www.cancer.org: For general up-to-date information and community resources.
www.entnet.org: To find an otolaryngologist (head and neck specialist).
www.faceit.org: Resource for people with facial difficulties.
www.larynx.link: International Association of Laryngectomees.
www.asha.org: American Speech-Language-Hearing Association.
www.webwhispers.org: Patient-run site.

Also see Chapter 2, Searching for Answers on the Web, for more information.

Twenty-four

WHEN A CHILD HAS CANCER

Learning that your child has cancer is devastating. It is one of the greatest challenges any parent can face, laden with intense emotions and intensified by fear. However, you can take comfort in the fact that in the last thirty years, the statistics on children's cancers have been reversed—from 70 percent of children who *didn't* survive, to nearly 80 percent who *do*. There are better treatments and drugs and better methods to help deal with side effects. Children with cancer have a better quality of life through childhood as well as into adulthood with fewer long-term ill effects.

IN THE UNITED STATES, over 12,000 children and teenagers, between the ages of one and 19, will be diagnosed with cancers. Almost one quarter of these cancers are leukemias. The remaining are divided among several cancers, including brain tumors, childhood lymphomas, Hodgkin's disease, Wilms' tumor, neuroblastoma, osteogenic sarcomas, Ewing's sarcoma, retinoblastomas, and rhabdomyosarcomas.

One of the hardest things to comprehend, when your child is diagnosed with cancer, is that something like this can actually happen to your family. The depth of pain is indescribable. But reality must be faced. It is important for you and your family to take charge of the situation. You will find that children can cope and accept illness as well as adults can, sometimes better. Try to channel your anxiety to fuel your quest to understand the nature of the child's specific illness so that your family can deal with it in the most effective way.

What you need to know about childhood cancers

- Treatment at a major medical center where a team approach, using the skills of radiation therapists, pediatric medical oncologists or hematologists, pediatric surgeons, radiation therapists, rehabilitation specialists, and social workers is essential to ensure that your child receives the best treatment.

- In almost all cases of childhood cancer, its appearance in one child does not mean that a brother or sister is more likely to develop it.

- Diagnosis of pediatric cancers can be difficult due to the rarity of the diseases and the complexity of making a diagnosis.

- Acute lymphocytic leukemia accounts for 80 to 85 percent of childhood leukemia. Thirty years ago, the survival of newly diagnosed children was about 5 percent. Today, nearly 75 percent of these children can be expected to be cured.

- Even children who are diagnosed with unusually high white blood cell counts are often found to have something other than cancer.

- Young children, especially girls in their eighth year, may develop a mildly tender swelling in one or both breasts with an underlying mass. This need not alarm you. The mass usually regresses and disappears within six to 12 months. Breast malignancies are rare in children. The enlargement should be observed by a physician. Biopsies or surgical intervention should be postponed and the mass should be removed only if significant enlargement or symptoms occur.

- The possibility of entering your child into a clinical trial through a major medical center or of getting a second opinion or treatment from the National Cancer Institute in Bethesda, Maryland, should be explored.

What type of doctor should be treating my child?

Ideally, an oncological pediatrician should be responsible for coordinating your child's treatment. Pediatricians who do not specialize in childhood cancer and family practitioners may see fewer than half a dozen cases of a specific type of childhood cancer in their careers. Therefore, your own physician will usually refer you to an oncologist, who may suggest that you take your child to one of the major medical centers for treatment. If you decide you will take this treatment route, you will find that total patient care—all of the disciplines, including medical and other subspecialties, nursing, and social service—are orchestrated and individualized for the child's care. It may also be possible to arrange to have some of the treatment closer to home. Specialists from many of the Comprehensive Cancer Centers designated by the National Cancer Institute work with local physicians in planning and coordinating follow-up treatment. Or you may wish to have a second opinion, or possible treatment at one of the Comprehensive Cancer Centers. These centers of excellence, reviewed and selected by the National Cancer Institute, offer the most up-to-date diagnosis and treatment. You need to assess your own situation and decide what will work best for you and your family. However, implementing the latest treatment methods requires teamwork among medical oncologists, pediatric oncologists, surgeons, radiologists, hematologists, physiotherapists, nurses, and social workers.

Where should my 15-year-old son be treated?

You are right to be concerned about where a teenager is treated. It is difficult for adolescents with cancer because pediatric oncologists normally treat younger children and medical oncologists usually treat adults. In addition, adolescents have the many problems associated with growing up—becoming independent, fitting in with a group, how they look—all of which become more difficult when a cancer diagnosis is added. Since some cancers of adolescence are pediatric and some are adult cancers, you and your son need to look at medical centers that treat both children and adults, discuss the treatment alternatives with both pediatric and adult oncologists, and then decide where he would be most comfortable being treated.

Can I get a confirming second opinion on my child's treatment from the National Cancer Institute?

You can call the National Cancer Institute's Pediatric Oncology Branch (1–877–624–4878) yourself and request a second opinion appointment or your doctor can call.

Is it possible for my child to be treated at the National Cancer Institute?

The Pediatric Oncology Branch of the National Cancer Institute also offers treatment at the National Institutes of Health in Bethesda, Maryland. Your doctor needs to call (1–877–624–4878) to discuss the case with the attending physician to see if there is treatment available for the specific kind of cancer. The clinical center provides nursing and medical care without charge for children who have been diagnosed as having a particular kind or stage of cancer being studied in its clinical research programs. There is a hotel facility, the Children's Inn, which provides housing for children and their parents who are being treated at the Center.

Should I consider entering my child in a clinical trial?

This is something you should discuss with your doctor. Cooperative groups in the United States that organize clinical trials for childhood cancers include the Children's Cancer Study Group, Pediatric Brain Tumor Consortium, and Neuroblastoma Therapy Consortium. Doctors who belong to these groups or who take part in clinical trials can be found by calling the National Cancer Institute's Cancer Information Service (1–800–4–CANCER) or on the Internet. About two-thirds of children with cancer in the United States are treated on a clinical trial at some point in their illness.

Can my teenager participate in a clinical trial?

It depends on the age of your teenager. This is another question you need to discuss with your doctors. Some pediatric trials are open to an older group and some adult trials are open to younger patients. The National Cancer Institute is sponsoring an effort to focus on the special needs of cancer patients ages 15 to 30.

Where can I get help if I need to travel by air to get to a major cancer center?

There are several organizations that can help with air flights. The best overall source to check is the Web site of the Patient Air Transport Helpline (www.patienttravel.org.) where you can find information on all forms of charitable long-distance air transportation and referrals to appropriate sources of help available in a national charitable medical air transportation network. They also have a toll-free line: 1–800–296–1217.

Should children be told they have cancer?

Openness and honesty are usually the best approach, depending, naturally, upon the age and understanding of the child. Toddlers can be told that they are sick and need to take medicine to get better. Terms such as "bad cells" for a tumor should be avoided since a child may consider the tumor a punishment for bad behavior. Older children need to know that cancer is a serious but treatable illness. Many of them may have the mistaken impression from watching television that everyone who has cancer dies. They need reassurance that there are successful treatments and that new treatments are being used with very hopeful results. Do not avoid the subject for fear of saying something wrong. As awkward as your response may be, it is better to deal with the question in a matter-of-fact and honest manner so that you keep communication open. The NCI booklet, *Young People with Cancer: A Handbook for Parents* offers good advice, including how to talk with your child about the diagnosis. It's available on-line or with a toll-free call.

Should the other children in the family be told when a brother or sister has cancer?

Other children in the family can't help but be worried and concerned about the disruption in their sibling's and their lives. Naturally, the age of the child dictates how much needs to be told. A three or four-year-old can be told that his brother is sick, needs to go to the hospital and will be taking medicine for a long time. Older children can be given more detailed information. Young children may feel guilty and need to be reassured that they are not responsible for the illness. Children also worry that they may also become ill. Be aware of the many fears and jealousies that are awakened. Talking about them will help keep the sibling from becoming resentful about the time you must spend with your sick child. Most children's hospitals have liberal visitation policies for siblings of children with cancer so it is often possible for brothers and sisters to participate in their sibling's hospital life.

Is it normal for my child to be angry over the inconveniences that the treatments impose?

Anger is a very normal reaction—and the child should be allowed to vent some of it. You can let the child know that you understand the feelings but that the treatment is essential to lead a normal life.

How do you keep from overprotecting a child with cancer?

Finding a balance for your child's life at this time is a daily challenge. You will need to assess the question regularly, because cancer cannot be ignored, but neither can other important aspects of the young person's life. Special treatment at home or in the classroom can create resentment among peers. Although the diagnosis of cancer will change your child's life for a time, over-protection encourages dependency that prevents children from learning how to use their own resources. Learning the boundaries for behavior and activity is a valuable part of growing up and is doubly important for the child who may be faced with more uncertainty in the future.

Where can I get more information about childhood cancer?

The Cancer Information Service 1–800–4–CANCER phone service can provide you with information about the specific type of cancer which has been diagnosed, can tell you what hospitals in your local area are participating in the latest treatments, and can send you booklets and specific printed information on the subject. There is a wealth of information available for parents of children with cancer.

Questions to Ask Your Doctor About Your Child's Cancer and Treatment

- Exactly what kind of cancer does my child have and what stage is it in?
- Has this diagnosis been confirmed by other experts?
- Have you treated other children with this type of cancer? How many?
- What kind of treatment are you advising?
- Is it possible to receive treatments locally?
- Is it advisable to go to a cancer center or specialized hospital for a second opinion? For treatment? If no, why not?
- Where, in your opinion, is the best place for my child to be treated?
- Can you help me check out clinical trials that might be appropriate?
- Do you have the latest clinical trials information on my child's cancer?
- Will you help me get a second opinion from the National Cancer Institute?
- How long do you think my child will be hospitalized?
- What treatment choices are there and what have past results been?
- How long will my child be out of school? Do you have special information I can give to the school system while my child is being treated?
- What are the long-term effects of treatment?

LEUKEMIA

What is leukemia?

Leukemia is a form of cancer of the blood. Malignant cells are found in the blood and bone marrow. Normally, the bone marrow makes cells called blasts that mature into several different types of blood cells. In leukemia, the blood cells do not mature, are released into the circulatory system, crowding out normal white cells, platelets and red blood cells and are found in the blood and bone marrow. Leukemia is found in both children and adults. It can be acute, progressing quickly with many immature cancer cells, or chronic, progressing slowly with more mature-looking leukemia cells.

What kind of doctor is best for dealing with a child with leukemia?

To maximize the chance of cure, the first treatment your child receives must be the best available to totally eradicate his leukemia. Cancer centers designated by the National Cancer Institute and major medical institutions have teams that specialize in treating cancer in children. A team approach, incorporating the skills of the family physician, radiation therapists, pediatric medical oncologists and hematologists, rehabilitation specialists and social workers, ensures the best treatment. For information on cancer centers, see Chapter 28, Where to Get Help.

Are electromagnetic fields the cause of leukemia?

The cause of leukemia is unknown. Electromagnetic fields are routinely produced when electrical current passes through a wire or common household appliance. A large study of residential magnetic field exposures and childhood ALL was conducted by the NCI and the Children's Cancer Group. There was little evidence of a relationship between the risk for ALL in children and exposure to magnetic fields. The scientists also concluded that magnetic fields from electrical appliances were unlikely to increase the risk of childhood ALL.

What is the difference between acute and chronic leukemia?

If leukemia affects a young person suddenly, it is called acute because it comes on quickly and progresses rapidly unless it is treated. Almost all childhood leukemias are acute, but the disease may sometimes be of the chronic type. In chronic leukemia, the bone marrow is able to produce a good number of normal cells as well as leukemic cells so that, compared to acute leukemia, the actual course of the disease is milder for a period of time.

Are there different types of leukemia that affect children?

Leukemia is not just one disease. There is actually a type of leukemia for each of the three major kinds of white blood cells—neutrophils, lymphocytes, and monocytes. Leukemia in any one person can affect only one kind of blood cell. There are two major types of leukemia that are found in children—acute lymphocytic leukemia and acute myeloid leukemia. Acute lymphocytic leukemia, also called ALL and sometimes referred to as lymphoblastic or lymphoid, accounts for about 75 percent of all childhood leukemia. Acute myeloid leukemia (also called AML and ANLL as well as myelogenous, granulocytic, myelocytic and myeloblastic), accounts for the remainder of childhood leukemias but is primarily seen in adults. Other kinds of leukemia such as chronic lymphocytic leukemia (CLL), chronic myelogenous leukemia (CML), monocytic, myelomonocytic, progranulocytic, erythroleukemia and hairy cell leukemia are very rare, but still behave similarly to the more common kinds. For more information on leukemias also see Chapter 18, Adult Leukemia.

SYMPTOMS OF ACUTE LYMPHOBLASTIC LEUKEMIA (ALL) AND ACUTE MYELOID LEUKEMIA (AML)

- Fever.
- Tendency to bleed or bruise easily.
- Shortness of breath.
- Listlessness.
- Lack of appetite.
- Intermittent or low-grade fever, cough.
- Bone or joint pain.
- Abdominal pain or swelling.
- Frequent infections.
- Tiny red dots or purple spots on skin.

Who usually gets ALL?

Most children who have ALL are between two and six years of age when diagnosed, but ALL can also occur in people in their twenties and thirties. For reasons yet to be understood, slightly more boys get ALL than girls, and it occurs more frequently among white children than black children. Great strides have been made in the treatment of ALL in children. Where once it was considered a death sentence, it is now considered one of the most curable forms of cancer.

What tests are used to diagnose ALL?

The diagnosis of leukemia requires blood tests and examination of the cells in the bone marrow. Early symptoms can mimic diseases such as mononucleosis, anemia from other causes, tonsillitis, rheumatic conditions, meningitis, mumps, or other kinds of cancer. In order to examine the cells, a bone marrow aspiration is usually done. This test requires that a needle be inserted into a bone in the hip so that a small amount of bone marrow can be withdrawn for inspection under the microscope. Spinal taps are done to remove fluid surrounding the child's brain and spine to see if leukemia cells are present. X-rays may also be needed.

Why are so many tests needed?

In any acute leukemia, it is necessary to determine which type of white blood cell has become leukemic, since treatment and response are different for each kind. If the type of leukemic cell cannot be determined from microscopic inspection, special tests of the chromosomes and DNA (cytogenetics and molecular genetic tests) and cell chemistry (flow cytometry) are needed before treatment can begin. Most cases of childhood ALL are of the pre-B cell type. In rare instances, the cells are too young to be classified. Such cases are called acute stem cell leukemia or acute undifferentiated leukemia.

How is ALL staged by doctors?

Unlike most other cancers, there is no staging system for acute lymphocytic leukemia. Treatment is based on whether your child falls in the low, standard, or high risk group. The groupings depend on the cell type involved, age of the child, white blood count at diagnosis, chromosome abnormality and early response to treatment.

How is ALL usually treated?

The primary treatment for ALL is chemotherapy. Radiation therapy to the brain may also be used in certain cases where there is evidence that the leukemia cells have spread to the brain. Several types of bone marrow transplants are also being used. (For complete information on bone marrow transplants, see Chapter 11, New Advances and Investigational Treatments.)

Does it make a difference where my child is treated?

Where the child is treated is important as is the kind of treatment given. Much research and many trials have been done to determine the best treatments for the various types of leukemia. There are numerous different protocols that must be carefully selected and coordinated to achieve control of the disease. The treatments are intense. The larger cancer centers have well-trained, fully integrated staffs on hand to help with all aspects of dealing with the medical and emotional crisis of leukemia.

What are the phases of treatment?

There are three phases of treatment: induction (or remission induction), consolidation/intensification (with central nervous system sanctuary therapy), and maintenance.

What can I expect to happen during the initial treatment period?

The first phase of treatment is called induction therapy and uses several chemotherapy drugs. The purpose of induction therapy is to kill as many of the leukemia cells as possible. The initial treatment is designed to make all signs of leukemia disappear. Most children go into complete remission—that is all leukemic cells have disappeared—within the first four weeks. Treatment, of course, will vary with the severity of symptoms, the treatment plan, the doctor, and the hospital. Since the child may be anemic, susceptible to infection and at risk of bleeding, the period of initial treatment can be very difficult.

Does remission mean that the leukemia is cured?

A remission means that the leukemia is being controlled. At this point, the second phase of treatment, called consolidation therapy, begins. The intensity of this chemotherapy treatment varies, depending on the risk category. It is used to try to kill any remaining leukemia cells in the body. In addition, a preventive treatment, called central nervous system sanctuary or CNS prophylaxis, gives chemotherapy to the cells in the central nervous system, even if no cancer cells have been found there. If the leukemia cells have spread to the brain, radiation therapy may also be used.

What is maintenance therapy?

This is long-term treatment following initial treatments. Chemotherapy is taken, usually by pill, daily or weekly for two or three years, to maintain the remission.

What is a relapse?

Relapse, or recurrence, occurs when leukemic cells reappear in the bone marrow, blood, central nervous system, or any other site. The symptoms of relapse are usually similar to those at the time the disease was first diagnosed. Children who relapse can usually be reinduced into remission. However, third and subsequent relapses are more difficult to control, because the cells become resistant to chemotherapy. Stem cell transplants may be used for children who relapse.

What is AML?

AML, acute myeloid leukemia, also known as acute nonlymphocytic leukemia or acute myelogenous leukemia, is a cancer of the blood-forming tissue, usually of the bone marrow and lymph nodes. It is less common in children than is ALL. Several years ago, children with AML almost always died. Today, it is a potentially curable cancer.

What are the symptoms of AML?

The child will complain of feeling weak or tired all the time, with aching joints and bones. Fever, chills, bleeding or bruising easily; swollen lymph nodes may also be present.

How will it be diagnosed?

The testing will be similar to that for ALL. The doctor will be trying to distinguish it from other leukemias and to determine the subtype of cells.

How is AML treated?

Treatment is divided into two stages: induction and postremission intensification. The induction treatment for AML is high-dose chemotherapy, to achieve remission. Chemotherapy is also given to the central nervous system. After there are no remaining visible cancer cells in the bone marrow, chemotherapy or bone or stem cell transplants are used.

Do all cases of leukemia progress in the same way?

No two cases are alike—and exact predictions are impossible to make. A great deal depends on the type of leukemia, the treatment given and the way in which the individual body reacts to treatment.

Is it dangerous for my leukemic child to be vaccinated?

IMPORTANT: Your child **should not receive live-virus medicine**—such as that used in smallpox, mumps and measles vaccinations. In addition, brothers and sisters should not receive the live polio vaccine while their sibling is getting chemotherapy. Vaccines that are not live may be safe to give during cancer treatment (diphtheria, whooping cough, tetanus). Always check with the child's doctor before allowing any such procedures on a child with leukemia or the siblings. Some doctors do recommend chickenpox vaccine for both children with cancer and their siblings, even though it is a live vaccine. You should discuss this matter in detail with your doctor before any vaccines are given.

How can I help my child deal with hair loss and other changes in appearance?

Encourage your child and others in the family to ask questions and be prepared to answer them as honestly as possible. Siblings, as well as classmates, should be prepared for physical changes in the patient, such as hair loss. Many children and adolescents solve the hair loss problem with caps or more exotic headgear, instead of wigs. Sometimes, siblings or classmates will tease your child. It is best to prepare your child for such occasions. You may also wish to discuss these issues with the health care team. In some institutions there are programs in which classroom visits are made by hospital personnel. A social worker may also be available who can discuss the problems with the child.

Where can I get information and help about the medical aspects of leukemia, as well as the social and psychological issues?

Fortunately there is a great deal of help available on many different levels. An unusual amount of well-written literature is available free from the National

Cancer Institute, the American Cancer Society, Leukemia Society of America, and Candlelighters Foundation. You can get them either by calling their toll-free numbers or accessing the agencies on the Web. The NCI booklet *Young People With Cancer: A Handbook for Parents* is especially well done and answers many questions about talking with your child as well as giving practical advice for you to follow. See Chapter 28, Where to Get Help, for addresses and telephone numbers.

CHILDHOOD HODGKIN'S DISEASE

Hodgkin's disease in children under the age of 13, those who are still growing and have not attained sexual maturity, is quite rare and is treated differently than Hodgkin's disease which appears more commonly in young adults and adults over 65. Hodgkin's disease involves the lymph nodes near the surface of the body. These nodes can be felt as painless swelling in the neck, armpit, or groin. Children who have reached full growth will probably be treated according to the treatments set up for adults. See Chapter 19, Hodgkin's Disease, Non-Hodgkin's Lymphoma, and Multiple Myeloma, for more detailed background information on Hodgkin's disease and for treatments used for adults with Hodgkin's disease. More than 85 percent of all newly diagnosed children with childhood Hodgkin's disease are curable with modern radiation therapy and/or combination chemotherapy. The selection of treatment is influenced by the stage of the disease, the age of the child, and the potential long-term effects of treatments. Because the child is in the growing stage, every attempt is made in planning treatment to preserve the integrity of bone and connective tissues.

What kind of doctor should be treating a child with Hodgkin's disease?

Since it is so important to have treatment planned so that the child's growth is affected as little as possible, it is of primary importance that your child's treatment be overseen by a pediatric oncologist and a treatment team who understand childhood Hodgkin's disease. Radiation should be given by specialists in radiation oncology with experience in treating children with cancer. Check to see that modern megavoltage equipment will be used. Linear accelerators of 4 to 10 MV energy and treatment planning simulators will insure optimum treatment. Individually shaped blocks should be fabricated to shield normal tissues.

What kind of testing is needed to determine and stage childhood Hodgkin's disease?

Complete, careful clinical, laboratory and diagnostic imaging evaluations are needed to determine the extent of the disease. Lab studies should include a

SYMPTOMS OF CHILDHOOD HODGKIN'S DISEASE

- Fever.

- Weight loss. For young children, failure to gain weight may carry the same significance as weight loss. Teenagers may attribute weight loss to dieting without realizing that it was easier than usual for them to lose unwanted pounds.

- Night sweats that soak the body.

- Swollen glands that don't go away after a few weeks.

- Finding of Reed-Sternberg cells in blood.

complete blood count, sedimentation rate, routine liver and renal function tests, and bone marrow biopsy. CT scans and MRI may be used.

What are the stages of childhood Hodgkin's disease?

There are four stages, I, II, III, and IV, which are further divided into A or B categories. A means there are no symptoms. B means that symptoms include one or more of the following: loss of more than 10 percent of body weight in the previous six months (or for young children, failure to gain weight); fever without any other known cause; or night sweats that leave the child's body soaked.

Are there possible after effects to the treatments for childhood Hodgkin's disease?

With young children in the growing stages of their lives, the necessarily rigorous treatments can present problems for the future. Because of this, chemotherapy with low-dose radiation has become the main treatment for Hodgkin's disease in children who have not yet reached maturity. The risk of sterility and second cancers also are taken into consideration by the treatment team. This is why it is so important that the child be properly staged by an experienced team before any treatment is undertaken.

If my child has radiation and the Hodgkin's recurs, can chemotherapy then be used?

Chemotherapy is being used effectively for patients who have had radiation and then had the disease come back.

How are stem cell and bone marrow transplants used in treatment of Hodgkin's disease?

Stem cell and bone marrow transplants are sometimes used when Hodgkin's disease can no longer be treated with radiation therapy or chemotherapy. Because

TREATMENT FOR CHILDHOOD HODGKIN'S DISEASE

DESCRIPTION	STAGE	TREATMENT
Stage I Cancer found in only one lymph node area or in only one area or organ outside lymph nodes.	**Stage IA**—when cancer is above diaphragm and does not involve large part of chest.	Chemotherapy with low-dose radiation to areas that contain cancer. *Clinical trials*: chemotherapy with or without radiation **or** chemotherapy alone.
IA means there are no symptoms.	**Stage IA**—when cancer is above diaphragm but involves large part of chest.	Chemotherapy plus radiation therapy to chest or mantle field. *Clinical trials*: Chemotherapy plus low-dose radiation.
IB means there are symptoms.	**Stage IB**—when cancer is above diaphragm but does not involve large part of chest.	Radiation therapy to mantle field, lymph nodes in upper abdomen and spleen **or** Chemotherapy plus radiation to areas that contain cancer.
	Stage IB—when cancer is above diaphragm but involves large part of chest.	Chemotherapy plus radiation to chest or mantle field **or** radiation to mantle field, lymph nodes in upper abdomen and spleen. *Clinical trials*: Radiation therapy plus chemotherapy.
Stage II Cancer found in two or more lymph node areas on same side of diaphragm **or** cancer found in only one area or organ outside lymph nodes and in lymph nodes around it. Other lymph node areas on same side of diaphragm may also have cancer.	**Stage IIA or IIB**—when cancer is above diaphragm but does not involve large part of chest.	Chemotherapy plus low-dose radiation to areas that contain cancer. *Clinical trials*: Low-dose chemotherapy with or without radiation **or** chemotherapy alone.

(continued)

TREATMENT FOR CHILDHOOD HODGKIN'S DISEASE (continued)

DESCRIPTION	STAGE	TREATMENT
IIA means there are no symptoms **IIB** means there are symptoms.	**Stage IIA** or **IIB**—when cancer is located above diaphragm but involves large part of chest.	Chemotherapy plus radiation therapy to chest or mantle field. *Clinical trials*: Chemotherapy plus low-dose radiation.
Stage III Cancer found in lymph node areas on both sides of diaphragm. May have spread to areas near affected lymph nodes and/or to spleen.	**Stage IIIA**—no symptoms.	Chemotherapy **or** chemotherapy plus radiation. *Clinical trials*: chemotherapy with or without radiation.
	Stage IIIB—with symptoms.	Chemotherapy **or** chemotherapy plus radiation.
Stage IV Spread in more than one spot to organ or organs outside lymph system. Nearby lymph nodes may or may not be affected **or** Spread to one organ outside lymph system but distant lymph nodes involved.	**Stage IV**	Chemotherapy **or** chemotherapy plus radiation. *Clinical trials*: Chemotherapy with or without radiation to lymph nodes.
Recurrent	Cancer has recurred after treatment either in same area or another part of body.	If radiation given before, chemotherapy may be used; **or** if chemotherapy given before, different drugs. If cancer returns only in lymph nodes, radiation therapy **or** stem cell transplant with or without radiation. *Clinical trials*: Bone marrow transplantation.

very high doses of chemotherapy can destroy the bone marrow, marrow is taken from the bones before treatment. The marrow taken is frozen and high-dose chemotherapy with or without radiation therapy is given. The marrow that was removed is then thawed and returned to the body. This type of transplant is called autologous transplant. If the marrow given is taken from another person it is called an allogeneic transplant. For more information on bone marrow transplants, see Chapter 11, New Advances and Investigational Treatments.

CHILDHOOD NON-HODGKIN'S LYMPHOMA

It is important in the early stage of diagnosis that the child be referred to a treatment center with experience in this type of cancer. There, a multidisciplinary team can be certain that the diagnosis is correct before treatment begins.

How does non-Hodgkin's lymphoma differ from Hodgkin's disease?
The cells that are found in children with non-Hodgkin's lymphoma are different from those found in Hodgkin's disease. It develops in the lymph system but can spread to organs other than lymph nodes, such as the liver or the bones. There are three major types of childhood non-Hodgkin's lymphomas: small noncleaved cell lymphoma (Burkitt's and non-Burkitt's), lymphoblastic lymphoma, and large cell lymphoma. The type is determined by the way the cancer cells look under a microscope. This is known as the "histology" of the cancer. About 40 to 50 percent of non-Hodgkin's lymphoma in children is small noncleaved cell, about 30 percent is lymphoblastic and 20 to 25 percent is large cell. Although childhood non-Hodgkin's lymphomas are treated differently than adult non-Hodgkin's lymphomas, it will be helpful to read Chapter 19 which discusses adult lymphoma and gives additional general background information. There are high cure rates for children with non-Hodgkin's lymphoma, especially those who have limited disease when diagnosed.

What are the symptoms of childhood non-Hodgkin's lymphoma?
Abdominal pain or swelling, breathing and/or swallowing difficulties, as well as swelling of the face and neck are common symptoms. Swollen lymph nodes may appear in the head and neck as well as in the groin. They are usually painless and firm. If the tumor is in the chest area, difficulty in breathing may signal a medical emergency. Gastrointestinal tumors may produce symptoms similar to those of an obstruction or appendicitis.

Where do most small noncleaved lymphomas occur?
Small noncleaved cell lymphomas, the most common type of non-Hodgkin's lymphoma frequently occur in the stomach area, particularly in the area near

TREATMENTS FOR SMALL NONCLEAVED CELL CHILDHOOD NON-HODGKIN'S LYMPHOMA (BURKITT'S AND NONBURKITT'S)

STAGE	TREATMENT
Stage I Cancer found in only one area outside abdomen or chest.	Systemic chemotherapy with or without intrathecal chemotherapy.
Stage II Cancer found in only one area and in lymph nodes around it or in two or more lymph nodes or other areas on same side of diaphragm or cancer is found to have started in the digestive tract and lymph nodes may or may not be involved.	*Clinical trials*: New drug combinations.
Stage III Cancer found in tumors or lymph nodes on both sides of diaphragm or found to have started in chest or found in many places in abdomen or in area around spine, or outermost brain coverings. **Stage IV** Cancer spread to bone marrow, brain or to spinal cord.	Systemic chemotherapy plus intrathecal chemotherapy. *Clinical trials*: New drug combinations.
Recurrent Cancer has recurred either where it first started or in another part of the body.	Systemic chemotherapy with or without intrathecal chemotherapy **or** bone marrow transplant. *Clinical trials*: New treatments.

the appendix, and in the upper midsection of the chest. They are also found in the lymph nodes, liver, testicles, spleen, bone marrow, central nervous system, nasal sinuses, skin, and bones.

How is non-Hodgkin's lymphoma diagnosed?
The doctor will examine the child carefully and check for swelling or lumps in the neck, underarms, groin, and abdomen. If chest swelling is found, a chest x-ray will be required. If lymph nodes are abnormal or a lump is found in the chest or abdomen, a biopsy will be done to determine if there are any

TREATMENTS FOR LYMPHOBLASTIC CHILDHOOD NON-HODGKIN'S LYMPHOMA

STAGE	TREATMENT
Stage I Cancer found in only one area outside abdomen or chest. **Stage II** Cancer found in only one area and in lymph nodes around it or in two or more lymph nodes or other areas on same side of diaphragm or cancer is found to have started in the digestive tract and lymph nodes may or may not be involved.	Systemic chemotherapy plus intrathecal chemotherapy.
Stage III Cancer found in tumors or lymph nodes on both sides of diaphragm or found to have started in chest or found in many places in abdomen or in area around spine, or outermost brain coverings. **Stage IV** Cancer spread to bone marrow, brain or to spinal cord.	Same as above. Radiation also may be given if large mass in chest. *Clinical trials*: New drug combinations.
Recurrent Cancer has recurred either where it first started or in another part of the body.	Allogeneic bone marrow transplant **or** stem cell transplant **or** systemic chemotherapy with different drugs. *Clinical trials*: New treatments.

cancer cells. Before starting therapy, a complete staging workup should be done including a careful physical examination, a complete blood count, urine and liver testing, chest x-ray, CT scan, examinations of bone marrow and spinal fluid, and a bone scan to determine the disease extent.

Are childhood non-Hodgkin's lymphomas difficult to diagnose?

Especially if there is bone marrow involvement, there may be a question about whether the child has lymphoblastic lymphoma with bone marrow

TREATMENTS FOR CHILDHOOD LARGE CELL LYMPHOMA

STAGE	TREATMENT
Stage I Cancer found in only one area outside abdomen or chest. **Stage II** Cancer found in only one area and in lymph nodes around it or in two or more lymph nodes or other areas on same side of diaphragm or cancer is found to have started in the digestive tract and lymph nodes may or may not be involved.	Systemic chemotherapy with or without intrathecal chemotherapy.
Stage III Cancer found in tumors or lymph nodes on both sides of diaphragm or found to have started in chest or found in many places in abdomen or in area around spine, or outermost brain coverings. **Stage IV** Cancer spread to bone marrow, brain or to spinal cord.	Systemic chemotherapy with or without intrathecal chemotherapy. *Clinical trials*: New drug combinations.
Recurrent Cancer has recurred either where it first started or in another part of the body.	Allogeneic or autologous bone marrow transplant **or** systemic chemotherapy with or without intrathecal chemothrapy. *Clinical trials*: New treatments.

involvement or leukemia. Usually, if less than 25 percent of the cells are lymphoblasts, the child will be treated for lymphoma rather than leukemia.

What kinds of treatments are recommended for non-Hodgkin's lymphoma?

Treatments differ for the three types—small noncleaved cell, lymphoblastic, and large cell. Treatments include chemotherapy, radiation and bone marrow transplants, which are being tested in clinical trials. There are treatments for all patients with this disease and a large percentage of children are cured. The tables detail staging and treatment choices.

CHILDHOOD BRAIN TUMORS

The next most common type of cancer in children, after leukemia and lymphoma, is cancer of the brain. There are many different types of brain tumors in children and the outlook for recovery varies according to the type of tumor and where it is located in the brain. For best results, you should seek out treatment at a large center with an experienced team of pediatric specialists in neurosurgery, radiation therapy, oncology, neuroradiology, neurology, and psychology. As a first step, review of the diagnostic tissue by a neuropathologist who has particular expertise in this area is strongly recommended. Also see Chapter 22, Cancer of the Brain and Spinal Cord.

How are childhood brain tumors classified?
Brain tumors are classified by their location within the brain and the appearance and behavior of the tumor tissue, rather than by stage. Infratentorial tumors are found in the lower part of the brain, usually the cerebellum or brainstem. The cerebellum is the most common site of brain tumors in children. Supratentorial tumors are found in the upper part of the brain. Even physicians agree that the terminology used in classifying brain tumors is confusing.

What lower brain cancers (infratentorial) are found in children?
Tumors found in the lower part of the brain include medulloblastoma, cerebellar astrocytoma, infratentorial ependymoma and brain stem glioma.

What upper brain cancers (supratentorial) are found in children?
Tumors in the upper part of the brain include cerebral astrocytoma, supratentorial ependymoma, craniopharyngioma, central nervous system germ cell tumors, supratentorial primitive neuroectodermal and pineal tumors, and visual pathway and hypothalamic glioma.

What is the most common type of childhood brain tumor?
Almost half of all brain tumors in children are found in the lower part of the brain (infratentorial), and about three-quarters of them are located in the cerebellum or fourth ventricle. The most common types of childhood brain tumors are astrocytomas and medulloblastomas.

What research is being conducted into childhood brain tumors?
The Pediatric Brain Tumor Consortium (www.pbtc.org) is a group of academic institutions with extensive experience in the design and conduct of clinical trials for children with cancer. The Consortium conducts Phase I and II studies of new drugs, agents injected into the spinal fluid, and biological and radiation treatments for children with cancers of the central nervous

SYMPTOMS OF CHILDHOOD BRAIN TUMORS

- Seizures.
- Morning headaches.
- Vomiting.
- Irritability.
- Behavior problems.
- Changes in eating or sleeping habits.
- Lethargy.
- Vision changes.
- Changes in muscular coordination.

system. Their studies can be found on the clinical trials site of the National Cancer Institute (www.cancer.gov/clinical trials).

Why is there such concern about giving radiation to children under three years of age?
Doctors try to avoid giving radiation to children under three because it is during the first few years of life that a child's brain cells develop most rapidly. It is feared that radiation may cause some damage in the brain's growth that would be detrimental to the child's learning abilities in the future. Sometimes chemotherapy is used instead. There are clinical trials underway studying using chemotherapy to shrink the tumor in order to delay the use of radiation.

WILMS' TUMOR (NEPHROBLASTOMA)

Wilms' tumor, a cancerous kidney tumor, sometimes referred to as nephroblastoma, is usually found in children between the ages of one and four, and rarely after age seven. It is curable in the majority of children who are affected, if found in its early stages. Two cell types—anaplastic cells and sarcomatous cells—found in a small proportion of childhood kidney tumors, are more difficult to cure.

What you should know about Wilms' tumor

- Wilms' tumor has both hereditary and nonhereditary forms. The hereditary type usually appears at an earlier age, and it is likely to affect both kidneys or several sites in one kidney.
- It has been found that gene mutations on the short arm of chromosome 11 are associated with Wilms' tumor as well as with other mutations that

CHILDHOOD BRAIN TUMORS

TYPE	CHARACTERISTICS	POSSIBLE TREATMENT
Medulloblastoma	Fast-growing, found almost exclusively in children, tendency to spread to other parts of nervous system.	**Average risk:** Surgery **or** radiation with or without chemotherapy. **Poor risk:** Surgery **or** radiation **or** chemotherapy. **Under age 3:** Surgery, **or** chemotherapy **or** radiation with or without chemotherapy. *Clinical trials:* Chemotherapy to delay or reduce need for radiation.
Cerebellar astrocytoma	Slow growing; does not usually spread.	Surgery to remove all or part of tumor. Possible radiation if all not removed. Chemotherapy may be used to delay radiation in very young children if tumor progresses and further surgery not possible.
Infratentorial ependymoma	Arises from lining of lower part of brain. May spread to other parts of brain or spinal cord.	Radiotherapy **or** surgery to remove as much of tumor as possible. **Under age 3:** Chemotherapy to delay radiation. Surgery plus radiation being studied.
Brainstem glioma	May grow rapidly or slowly but rarely spreads. Focal or low grade is found only in one area of brain stem. Diffuse intrinsic glioma has spread widely throughout brain stem.	**Focal/low grade:** Surgery **or** cerebrospinal fluid diversion followed by watchful waiting observation. **Intrinsic:** Radiation therapy. *Clinical trials:* Chemotherapy and radiation **or** chemotherapy to delay use of radiation.

(continued)

CHILDHOOD BRAIN TUMORS (continued)

TYPE	CHARACTERISTICS	POSSIBLE TREATMENT
Low grade cerebral astrocytoma	Slow growing tumor found in upper part of brain. Cells look similar to normal astrocyte cells. Does not usually spread from site of origin to other parts of the brain.	Surgery or surgery and radiation or surgery with radiation delayed until tumor progresses or chemotherapy. **Under age 5:** Chemotherapy being evaluated.
High grade cerebral astrocytoma	Fast growing tumor found in upper part of brain. Cells do not look much like normal astrocyte cells. Can spread from site of origin to other parts of the brain.	Surgery, radiation and/or chemotherapy. *Clinical trials:* Postoperative chemotherapy with or without radiation. **Under age 3:** Chemotherapy after surgery to delay or modify radiation.
Supratentorial ependymoma	Tumor in lining of upper part of brain. May grow rapidly or slowly.	Surgery followed by radiation. **Under age 3:** Chemotherapy to delay or modify radiation. *Clinical trials:* Radiation with or without chemotherapy.
Cranio-pharyngioma	Located in pituitary region. Often curable. Doesn't spread but may cause pressure on nearby structures.	Surgery and/or radiation.
Central nervous system germ cell tumor	Tumors in center of brain, tend to be malignant, usually cannot be totally removed; can spread.	Surgery performed for biopsy purposes. Radiation usually given, with or without chemotherapy.
Visual pathway and hypotha-lamic glioma	Slow-growing tumor in optic nerve or optic tract.	If no symptoms, may be observed. If growing: surgery or radiation or chemotherapy. *Clinical trials:* Chemotherapy to shrink tumor and delay radiation.

CHILDHOOD BRAIN TUMORS (continued)

Type	Characteristics	Possible treatment
Pineal parncymal tumor	Found in center of brain near pineal gland, can be slow growing or fast growing and can spread to other parts of central nervous system.	Biopsy recommended. Surgical removal is controversial. Radiation. **Young children:** *Clinical trials*: Chemotherapy to delay radiation.
Supratentorial primitive neuroectodermal tumor. Sometimes called cerebral neuroblastoma	Found in upper part of brain, can spread to other parts of central nervous system.	Surgery with or without radiation or chemotherapy. **Under age 3:** *Clinical trials*: Chemotherapy to delay or reduce radiation.
Recurrent Cerebellar astrocytoma Medulloblastoma, ependymoma, brainstem glioma, cerebral astrocytoma, intracranial or germ cell tumors.	Tumor has come back after being treated. May be at the same place or in other parts of the brain and spinal cord.	Further surgery or radiotherapy. Chemotherapy.

sometimes occur in Wilms' tumor patients. A gene that causes a child to be born without an iris in the eye (aniridia) is located nearby.

- The risk of Wilms' tumor among offspring of persons who have had unilateral Wilms' tumor is quite low.

- Siblings of children with Wilms' tumor have little likelihood of developing Wilms' tumor.

- Wilms' tumor is one of modern medicine's success stories. Experience has shown that children treated for Wilms' tumor can be considered cured if they survive for two years without any signs that the disease has returned. Up until the early 1960s, almost all children with Wilms' tumor died of the disease. Now almost 90 percent are cured.

SYMPTOMS OF WILMS' TUMOR

- A swelling on one side of the upper abdomen.
- Blood in the urine.
- Stomach pain.
- Low-grade fever, loss of appetite, paleness, weight loss, and lethargy.
- The absence of the iris of the eye (the colored portion of the eye) called aniridia.
- A condition called hemihypertrophy, which means the abnormal enlargement of a part of the body—often in the development of the genitals or the urinary system.

- It is wise to take advantage of clinical trials at a major medical center to assure the best possible treatment.

How is Wilms' tumor diagnosed?

The diagnosis is usually made through the use of ultrasound, MRI or CT scan. These studies are able to outline the tumor as well as clarify whether there is regional spread or whether the opposite kidney is involved.

What are the stages of Wilms' tumor?

The staging indicates whether the tumor is confined to the kidney or has spread to other parts of the body and the other kidney. In addition, the pathologist will designate whether the tumor has favorable histology (FH) or unfavorable histology (UH). While all cancer cells lack the orderly arrangement of normal cells, those designated UH are especially primitive and lacking in organized microscopic structure. The vast majority of children with kidney cancer (about 95 percent) have cell types described as favorable. Kidney tumors that contain elements of sarcoma—cancer that arises from supportive or connective tissue rather than from lining tissue—are also designated UH, although most specialists believe that these cancers are another disease rather than Wilms' tumor.

Are there other kinds of kidney cancers that affect children?

Other kidney cancers—clear cell sarcoma of the kidney, rhabdoid tumor of the kidney, and neuroepithelial tumor of the kidney—are also childhood cancers but are treated differently from Wilms' tumor.

STAGES OF WILMS' TUMOR

STAGE	DESCRIPTION
Stage I (UH and FH)	Limited to kidney and can be completely removed by surgery.
Stage II (UH and FH)	Extends beyond kidney to fat or soft tissue or blood vessels but can be completely removed by surgery.
Stage III (UH and FH)	Cancer has spread to abdomen and cannot be completely removed during surgery; may have spread to nearby lymph nodes.
Stage IV (UH and FH)	Spread from kidney to bones, lungs, liver, brain, or other parts.
Stage V (UH and FH)	Cancer involves both kidneys.

What kinds of treatments are usually undertaken for Wilms' tumor?

The first order of business is usually surgery to remove the kidney, if possible. This operation is called a radical nephrectomy, taking out the whole kidney, ureter, and adrenal gland. Nearby lymph nodes may also be removed. Then, depending upon the type of cells found in the tumor, the treatment will depend upon whether the histology (cell type) is considered favorable or unfavorable, referred to as FH for favorable histology and UH for unfavorable histology.

How is clear cell sarcoma of the kidney treated?

This is a cancer that can spread to the lung, bone, brain, and soft tissue. The usual treatment is surgery to remove the kidney, followed by chemotherapy.

What kind of treatment will be given to a child who has rhabdoid tumor of the kidney?

Most rhabdoid tumors of the kidney are found in babies, usually under one year of age. It can grow and spread quickly. Treatment will probably be surgery to remove the kidney, followed by chemotherapy.

What is the treatment used for neuroepithelial tumor of the kidney?

Neuroepithelial tumor of the kidney is a tumor that grows and spreads quickly. Many times it will have spread to the outer layer of the kidney and other parts of the body before it is diagnosed. If your child has this tumor,

TREATMENTS FOR WILMS' TUMOR

STAGE	TREATMENT
Stage I (FH and UH)	Surgery plus chemotherapy.
Stage II (FH)	Surgery plus chemotherapy.
Stage II (UH)	Surgery, radiation, and chemotherapy.
Stage III (FH and UH) If very large tumor or tumors located near large blood vessels	Surgery, radiation, and chemotherapy. Chemotherapy or radiation to shrink tumor followed by surgery plus radiation.
Stage IV (FH and UH)	Surgery, radiation, and chemotherapy.
Stage V (FH)	Surgery and chemotherapy **or** surgery plus radiation plus chemotherapy.
Stage V (UH)	Surgery, radiation, if indicated, plus chemotherapy.

you should consider treatment on a clinical trial for Ewing's PNET (primitive neuroectoderm or peripheral neuroepithelioma).

NEUROBLASTOMA

Neuroblastoma is a cancer of the nervous system, usually found in certain nerve fibers of the body. These very young nerve cells, for unknown reasons, develop abnormally. Neuroblastoma usually affects infants and children under the age of five and is the third-most common cancer in children. A swelling can appear anywhere but is most commonly found in the abdomen, adrenal gland, chest, or eye. The older the child, the more difficult the disease is to treat. Neuroblastomas sometimes disappear spontaneously or may revert to a benign state.

What is the meaning of the staging used for neuroblastoma?
The staging for neuroblastoma is complex. It may be both difficult and confusing to sort out exactly what stage your child's cancer is in, since a number of different staging methods are used by different groups. The International Neuroblastoma Staging System (INSS) has combined elements from the previous Children's Cancer Group and Pediatric Oncology Group staging system and has come up with a system that uses Stages I–IV.

SYMPTOMS OF NEUROBLASTOMA

- Lump or mass in abdomen, adrenal gland, chest, or eye.
- Protruding eyes, black and blue or dark circles around the eyes.
- Listlessness, fever.
- Persistent diarrhea.
- Pain in the abdomen or elsewhere.
- Leg weakness.

What does the Children's Oncology Group's neuroblastoma risk grouping mean?

For your own information in trying to understand your child's cancer, the Children's Oncology Group (COG), uses the INSS system as well as age and tumor biology to assign risk groups—low, intermediate and high risk—to allow doctors to properly plan treatment. However, you may find that your own doctors are still using five groups for staging: "localized resectable," "localized unresectable," "regional," "disseminated," and "special." The COG uses a low, intermediate, and high risk stage for each of these five groups. As we said, much of this can be confusing, but it is helpful to understand what group your child's tumor is in so that you can unscramble some of the mystery of how your child's treatment is being staged.

Is Accutane being used in treating neuroblastoma?

Accutane, also known as isotretinoin, 13-*cis*-retinoic acid and 13-*cis*-RA, is normally used for treating severe acne. Recent research studies have found that it is effective in stopping the growth of neuroblastoma. It is being used for high risk neuroblastomas after treatment and recovery and for neuroblastomas that have been treated after recurring. Use of Accutane is usually prescribed for six months. It comes in capsule form and some children are resistant to taking the capsules. Some parents have resorted to squeezing out the contents of each capsule or removing the liquid from each capsule with a syringe. The manufacturers of Accutane advise against this because exposure to light causes Accutane, which is related to Vitamin A, to revert to an inactive form. Try to teach your child to take the capsule whole or squirt the contents directly into the child's mouth. If this is not possible, you can squeeze the contents directly into peanut butter or some other opaque food that will be eaten immediately. Removing Accutane from its capsule before giving it means that you run the risk of giving an inactive dose. You should be aware that Accutane could cause

INTERNATIONAL NEUROBLASTOMA STAGING SYSTEM

Stage I Localized resectable.	Cancer can be taken out by surgery and has not spread from where it started.
Stage IIA Localized unresectable.	Cancer has not spread from where it started but cannot be completely removed.
Stage IIB Regional.	Cancer has spread from where it started to nearby lymph nodes.
Stage III	Cancer cannot be taken out, has spread across midline (vertebral column) or to nearby lymph nodes.
Stage IV	Cancer has spread to distant lymph nodes, bone, bone marrow, liver, skin, and/or other organs (except as defined in IVS).
Stage IV S	*Special*: cancer is local with spread only to liver, skin, or to a limited degree, bone marrow.
Recurrent	Cancer has come back after treatment.

dry skin and dry mucous membranes. Some children experience peeling of the skin on the palms of the hands and soles of the feet.

Do adults ever get neuroblastoma?
Less than 10 percent of neuroblastomas are diagnosed in patients older than ten years of age. Adult neuroblastoma usually has a slower rate of growth but is more resistant to chemotherapy. Treatment usually includes surgery, chemotherapy, radiation therapy, and autologous bone marrow transplantation.

SOFT-TISSUE SARCOMA (RHABDOMYOSARCOMA AND NON-RHABDOMYOSARCOMA)

Rhabdomyosarcoma is the most common soft-tissue sarcoma in children. There also are a number of other soft-tissue sarcomas, known as non-rhabdomyosarcomas, which include: fibrosarcoma, synovial sarcoma, hemangiopericytoma, mesenchymal tumors, neurofibrosarcoma, leiomyosarcoma, liposarcoma, alveolar soft part sarcoma, and malignant fibrous histiocytoma. In young children, these soft-tissue sarcomas are more curable than in adults. Treatments are similar to those for rhabdomyosarcomas. Fibrosarcoma and hemangiopericytoma in infants and young children are less aggressive cancers

TREATMENT CHOICES FOR NEUROBLASTOMA

CHILDREN'S ONCOLOGY GROUP RISK GROUP	TREATMENT
Low Risk	Surgery to remove cancer **or** surgery plus adjuvant chemotherapy.
Intermediate Risk	Surgery to remove as much of the cancer as possible followed by chemotherapy.
High Risk	Chemotherapy followed by surgery to remove tumor followed by chemotherapy. Total-body irradiation and autologous stem cell transplant may be used. Radiation often done before, during, and after second chemotherapy.
Special Cancer is local with spread only to liver, skin or to a limited degree, bone marrow.	Depending on risk group treatment will differ. May require little or no therapy unless early complications develop.
Recurrent Cancer has come back after treatment.	Depends upon site, previous treatment, and extent of recurrence or progression.

than the others and can usually be cured with surgical removal. See Chapter 21, Bone and Soft-Tissue Sacromas, for other information.

RHABDOMYOSARCOMA

Rhabdomyosarcoma, where cancer cells begin growing in the soft tissues of muscle called striated muscle, is the most common type of soft-tissue sarcoma found in children. It can occur anywhere in the body but is most frequently found in the head, neck, bladder, vagina, prostate, testes, arms, legs, and chest. It occurs most frequently between the ages of two and six and in the teens. It is considered to be curable in the majority of children who are treated according to the latest methods. As with most cancers, the spread to lymph nodes and other parts of the body makes it more difficult to cure.

Are there different types of rhabdomyosarcoma?

This cancer can be divided into several types, according to the type of cancer cell that is found. These types include embryonal, alveolar, pleomorphic, and mixed. The embryonic type is the most common. These tumors usually grow

SYMPTOMS OF RHABDOMYOSARCOMA

- Swelling in the eye.
- Ear pain or discharge from ear.
- Bloody nasal discharge.
- Unexplained swelling or lump.
- Enlarged lymph nodes.
- Vaginal bleeding.
- Difficulty urinating or defecating.
- Bone pain.
- Tiredness.

in the head and neck or genitourinary tract but can also be found at other sites in the body.

What is the treatment for rhabdomyosarcoma?

Surgery is the first step for all children with rhabdomyosarcoma. It is essential to take out as much of the cancer as possible, leaving wide margins of cancer-free tissue. Chemotherapy is then given, followed by radiation if there is any cancer left after the surgery. If the cancer cannot be taken out by surgery, chemotherapy plus radiation will be used, followed by surgery. Clinical trials are testing new chemotherapy drugs, new ways of giving radiation, and bone marrow transplant. See Chapter 11, New Advances and Investigational Treatments, for more information on bone marrow transplants.

What is the treatment for rhabdomyosarcoma that has spread?

Surgery with or without chemotherapy will probably be the treatment, depending on how much of the cancer can be taken out, where it is, and what treatment your child originally had. New kinds of chemotherapy drugs followed by bone marrow transplant are being studied for those with metastatic disease. Clinical investigations are also being done with the use of intracavitary or interstitial radiation implants for girls with vaginal or vulval rhabdomyosarcomas.

Is rhabdomyosarcoma genetic?

Research has found damage to chromosomes in children with rhabdomyosarcoma. Patients with rhabdomyosarcoma also are often found in cancer-prone

STAGES OF RHABDOMYOSARCOMA

STAGE	DESCRIPTION
Stage I	Found in the eye, head, or neck or near sex organs and bladder.
Stage II	Found only in one area (but not the areas in Stage I), smaller than five centimeters (two inches), has not spread to lymph nodes.
Stage III	Found only in one area (but not the areas in Stage I), larger than five centimeters (two inches), may have spread to nearby lymph nodes.
Stage IV	Cancer has spread and found in more than one place when diagnosed.
Recurrent	Cancer has come back.

families who have the Li-Fraumeni syndrome or Beckwith-Wiedemann syndrome. However, the number of cases that can be tracked to inherited conditions is very small.

RETINOBLASTOMA

Retinoblastoma is an eye cancer that affects children, most of whom are under the age of five. The identification of the retinoblastoma gene now makes it possible for physicians to study the differences between hereditary and nonhereditary retinoblastoma. About 40 percent of retinoblastoma is of the hereditary type. Retinoblastoma is curable in most children and eyesight can usually be saved. Brothers and sisters of children with retinoblastoma should be checked to see if they have a tendency to develop the disease.

Where does retinoblastoma start?
Retinoblastoma is a tumor that starts in the retina, the thin nerve tissue at the back of the eye. Cells, instead of developing normally into those that can detect light and form images, become cancerous and can fill much of the eyeball. Retinoblastoma usually does not spread to nearby tissues or other parts of the body, unless the disease is advanced.

What is hereditary retinoblastoma?
Hereditary retinoblastoma is due to a genetic problem inherited from one parent. It is found in one or both eyes. It affects younger children, usually under the age of one. A rare brain cancer, trilateral retinoblastoma, may develop while treatment is being given. Secondary cancers may occur (primarily bone

SYMPTOMS OF RETINOBLASTOMA

- White light detected in the pupil behind the lens of the eye.
- Eye may appear to have a "cast" or squint.
- Eye pain.
- Redness in eye.
- Loss of vision. (Since young children usually are not aware of vision changes, this symptom is hard to identify.)

and soft-tissue sarcomas) sometimes many years after diagnosis and treatment, so consistent follow-up is important.

How does nonhereditary retinoblastoma differ from the hereditary type?

Children who develop nonhereditary retinoblastoma are a little older and the cancer is usually found only in one eye.

Can retinoblastoma be detected in the fetus?

It is possible to predict the possibility of retinoblastoma in pregnant women where there is a family history of this cancer. The infant's eyesight can be saved by prompt use of radiation on tumors that would not ordinarily be detected at an early age.

Who is best qualified to treat retinoblastoma?

Since this is an unusual cancer, treatment planning should be done by a multidisciplinary team of cancer specialists with experience in treating eye tumors in childhood. Especially important is the need to seek out expertise in pediatric radiation therapy and ophthalmology. The treatment should be planned after the extent of the tumor within and outside the eye is known.

What staging systems are used for retinoblastoma?

There are a number of staging systems but the one most often used is Reese and Ellsworth. However, for the purposes of treatment, the most reliable system is the categorization of intraocular or extraocular disease, which is listed in the following chart.

How is retinoblastoma treated?

There are treatments for all children and most can be cured. Treatment depends on the extent of the disease, whether it is in one or both eyes and

TREATMENT CHOICES FOR RETINOBLASTOMA

TYPE	TREATMENT
Intraocular: one eye (unilateral), has not spread into tissue around the eye or other parts of body.	Surgery to remove the eye **or** internal or external beam radiation **or** photocoagulation, with or without radiation **or** cryosurgery **or** thermotherapy. *Clinical trials*: Chemotherapy with or without other treatments.
Intraocular: both eyes (bilateral), has not spread into tissue around the eye or other parts of body.	Surgery to remove eye with most cancer, with or without radiation to remaining eye **or** radiation therapy to both eyes. *Clinical trials*: New combinations of chemotherapy drugs with or without stem cell transplants or different ways of administering chemotherapy drugs.
Extraocular: spread beyond the eye or other parts of body.	Radiation to eye with or without intrathecal chemotherapy **or** intrathecal chemotherapy alone. *Clinical trials*: New combinations of chemotherapy drugs with or without stem cell transplants or different ways of administering chemotherapy drugs.
Recurrent	If cancer returns in eye, surgery or radiation. If appears in other part of body, chemotherapy.

whether it has spread beyond the eye. Surgery is the most common treatment. If retinoblastoma is found in only one eye and the other eye has normal sight, the diseased eye may be removed (enucleation). Cryosurgery is sometimes used for very small cancers. Photocoagulation uses a beam of very strong light to destroy blood vessels that feed the tumor. Thermotherapy uses heat to destroy cancer cells. Radiation, either external or internal, and chemotherapy are also used.

OSTEOSARCOMA

Osteogenic sarcoma, sometimes called osteosarcoma, is the most common type of bone cancer in children. The bones most frequently involved are the large bones of the upper arm (humerus) and the leg (femur and tibia). This type of cancer is more common among boys than girls and usually occurs between the ages of ten and 25, although it is also seen in people in their 60s and 70s. Pain and swelling are the most common symptoms—and because they are such everyday complaints, they may be ignored. Diagnosis can be difficult because the symptoms can suggest injury, local infection, glandular deficiencies, arthritis, vitamin deficiencies, or benign tumors. The final diagnosis needs a biopsy to confirm the presence of cancer, and since osteogenic sarcoma spreads to other parts of the body, chest x-rays and CAT scans as well as bone scans are usually necessary before treatment is staged.

What You Need to Know About Osteosarcoma

- In general, more than 80 percent of patients can have limb-sparing surgery.
- Children with osteosarcoma should be thoroughly evaluated by an orthopedic surgical oncologist before biopsy.
- If saving a limb is a possibility, the biopsy should be performed by the surgeon who will do the future bone tumor removal, since placement of the incision is crucial.
- Studies have shown that there is no difference in survival between people who have had limb-sparing surgery and those who have had amputation.

How is osteosarcoma staged?

There are several different categories of osteosarcoma. The types are divided into high, intermediate, and low. There also are different cell types that are divided into central (medullary) and surface (peripheral) tumors. The most common type is conventional central osteosarcoma. The treatment stages are identified as localized, metastatic, and recurrent.

What treatment is usually used for localized osteogenic sarcoma?

Localized osteosarcoma is a highly treatable, often curable disease, although a great deal depends on where the tumor is located. Usually chemotherapy is given before the operation. The operation involves taking out the cancer without removing the arm or leg (limb-sparing) or, if necessary, removing all or part of an arm or leg (amputation) in order to remove all of the cancerous area.

What treatment is prescribed for metastatic osteogenic sarcoma?

Metastatic osteosarcoma, which means the disease has spread beyond the bone, is treatable and can sometimes be cured when a combination of therapies is used.

TREATMENT CHOICES FOR OSTEOSARCOMA

STAGE	TREATMENT
Localized Limited to the bone where cancer is found.	Preoperative chemotherapy followed by surgery to remove tumor, either limb-sparing, amputation or rotationplasty, with or without postoperative chemotherapy. *Clinical trials*: new ways of giving chemotherapy **or** new schedules of treatment **or** radiation therapy.
Metastatic osteosarcoma Cancer has spread to lung, other bones or other parts of the body.	Surgery to remove primary tumor and if possible, metastases followed by combination chemotherapy **or** Preoperative chemotherapy followed by surgery to remove primary tumor and metastases, followed by postoperative chemotherapy. *If in lungs*, surgery to take out tumors may be done in each lung separately.

Is it sometimes possible to save the child's limb and spare his having amputation?

The question of avoiding amputation is always a major one when making decisions about treatment for osteogenic sarcomas. Clinical studies have shown that there is no difference in overall survival between patients who have had an amputation and those treated with a limb-sparing procedure. However, before surgery it is necessary to determine if it is possible to save the limb and to take out the tumor with wide margins around it that are cancer-free. The amount of surgery required to remove the entire tumor is a major consideration. If saving of the limb is a possibility, the biopsy should be performed by the surgeon who will do the future bone tumor removal, since the placement of the incision is crucial.

What is rotationplasty?

This is a complex operation used to preserve as much movement of the arm or leg as possible. It may be done if the leg or arm needs to be removed. If it is the leg, it is amputated mid-thigh, and the lower leg and foot are rotated and attached to the thighbone where the ankle becomes the knee joint. If the cancer is in the upper arm, the tumor is taken out and the lower area reattached so that the arm is shorter but still is usable.

Is chemotherapy ever given before surgery?

Chemotherapy is often given before surgery. This is done to try to increase the possibility of limb-sparing surgery. Clinical trials are now in follow-up to determine the effectiveness of this treatment.

Are some tumors of the bone not really bone tumors at all?

Malignant tumors in other parts of the body sometimes metastasize to the bone. In some cases, the metastases are discovered before the primary tumor is found. A biopsy can often give a clue to the source of the metastasis. Before treatment begins, it is important to be positive about the origin of the cancer.

EWING'S FAMILY OF TUMORS

Ewing's family of tumors include Ewing's sarcoma of the bone, extraosseus Ewing's (tumor growing outside the bone), primitive neuroetodermal tumor (also known as PNET and peripheral neuroepthelioma or as Askin's tumor when it is in the chest wall). These are called Ewing's family of tumors because they have the same type of "mistakes" in their chromosomes. For many years Ewing's family of tumors were considered fatal, but with present treatment methods they are highly treatable and when found early can be curable.

What is Ewing's tumor of the bone?

It is a cancerous tumor of the bone that affects children and young adults. It differs from osteosarcoma in that it tends to be found in flat bones, such as the ribs, rather than the long bones of the arm and leg. It is uncommon before age five and after age 30 and is most commonly found between the ages of ten and 20. Black and Asian children rarely have Ewing's tumor of the bone. It may involve almost any part of the bony skeleton and may extend into the soft tissue around the bones. It may metastasize to the lungs or other bones.

What is extraosseus Ewing's tumor?

Extraosseous or "soft-tissue Ewing's sarcoma" is found outside the bones. This type of Ewing's sarcoma is usually treated like rhabdomyosarcoma.

Are the different types of Ewing's family of tumors difficult to diagnose?

They can be difficult to diagnose because the small, round cells resemble those in other cancers such as neuroblastoma, non-Hodgkin's lymphoma, or rhabdomyosarcoma. Any diagnosis for Ewing's sarcoma should be carefully checked by a pathologist with experience in the diagnosis of what is known as the "small round blue cell tumors of childhood." Evaluation of fresh tissue

SYMPTOMS OF EWING'S FAMILY OF TUMORS

- Bone pain.
- Swelling or lump, may be warm, red or tender.
- Fever.
- Limping.
- Back pain.
- Trouble breathing.
- Stiffness.
- Tenderness in bone.
- Tiredness.

by electron microscopy and immunohistochemistry make it possible for the pathologist to recognize features that lead to an accurate diagnosis. Every effort should be made at the start to be certain that it is correctly identified. As with other childhood cancers, this should be treated at a major medical center that specializes in treating cancer in children, since it will need the attention of a sophisticated multidisciplinary team, consisting of radiation therapist, medical oncologist, pathologist, surgeon, or orthopedic surgeon, who understand the Ewing's family of tumors.

How is Ewing's sarcoma staged?
The two most important factors to be identified are the location of the primary site of the tumor and whether the disease has spread. Localized Ewing's sarcoma is a tumor that has not spread beyond the original site. The tumor may have gone into nearby tissues or have spread to nearby lymph nodes and still be considered a localized Ewing's sarcoma.

What kind of treatment is usually recommended for Ewing's family of tumors?
Most patients with this disease are treated within clinical trials. Studies show that the addition of chemotherapy to surgery and radiation has markedly improved survival and cure rates. The way in which the various treatments are used depends upon the location of the tumor and whether the disease has metastasized to other parts of the body. Chemotherapy is usually given before surgery or radiation treatment and then is given again after the other treatment has been completed. Depending on the location of the tumor, limb-sparing surgery may be possible. When Ewing's sarcoma is found in a

POSSIBLE TESTS FOR DIAGNOSING THE EWING'S FAMILY OF TUMORS

- MRI.
- CT and bone scan.
- X-ray.
- Immunohistochemistry and cytogenetics to find errors in cells and chromosomes.
- Bone marrow biopsy.

very young child, surgery may be preferred over radiation therapy because of the side effect—retardation of bone growth—caused by radiation. If radiation is used, it should be done in a hospital which uses stringent planning techniques and by a physician who is experienced in the treatment of Ewing's family of tumors.

CHILDHOOD LIVER CANCER

Cancers that start in the liver (which are different from those that have spread to the liver from some other location) can occur in both infants and older children. There are two general types—hepatocellular, which is similar to the adult version of liver cancer, and hepatoblastoma, which is most frequently found in children. There is more information on liver cancer in Chapter 16, Gastrointestinal and Urinary Cancers.

What You Need to Know About Childhood Liver Cancer

- Liver cancers classified as hepatoblastomas usually occur before three years of age. Babies with a high cholesterol level in the first year of life may be at high risk for hepatoblastoma.
- Hepatocellular cancers most often occur between the ages of newborn to four or at the later ages of 12 to 15.
- When the tumor is totally confined to the liver and can be removed with surgery, it is highly curable.
- Many children with liver cancer have a tumor marker (serum alpha-fetoprotein) in their serum that indicates the presence of the disease.

TREATMENTS FOR CHILDHOOD CANCER OF THE LIVER

TYPE	TREATMENT
Stage I Tumor removable by surgery.	Surgery followed by chemotherapy.
Stage II Most cancer can be taken out by surgery; small amounts remain.	Surgery followed by chemotherapy.
Stage III Some cancer can be taken out by surgery but some tumor remains in abdomen or lymph nodes.	*Hepatoblastoma—one or more of following*: Chemotherapy followed by surgery **or** chemotherapy **or** radiation **or** chemotherapy put directly into liver **or** liver transplant. *Hepatocellular*: Chemotherapy followed by surgery.
Stage IV Tumor has spread to other parts of the body.	*Hepatoblastoma—one or more of following*: Chemotherapy followed by surgery followed by chemotherapy **or** surgery to take out cancer in lungs **or** chemotherapy put directly into liver **or** chemotherapy with substances that block or slow flow of blood **or** liver transplant. *Clinical trials*. *Hepatocellular*: Chemotherapy followed by surgery.

TREATMENT SIDE EFFECTS IN CHILDREN WITH CANCER

While my child is on treatment what symptoms are important enough for me to call the doctor?

- Fever over 100.4 degrees or other signs of infection, especially if the doctor has told you platelet counts are low.

- Mouth sores or difficulty in chewing that keep the child from eating.

- Vomiting not associated with the treatment.

- Painful urination or bowel movement.

- Trouble walking, bending, or talking.

- Dizziness, blurred or double vision.

- Sudden change in behavior, depression.

- Nosebleeds, red or black bowel movements, pink, red, or brown urine or many bruises.

- Severe or continuing headaches.

- Red or swollen areas or pain anywhere in body.

There is more information about dealing with general side effects in Chapter 9, Radiation, Chapter 10, Chemotherapy, and Chapter 27, Living with Cancer.

Do children sometimes encounter other health problems after being successfully treated for cancer?

There are now about 250,000 children in the United States who have had childhood cancer and are alive due to the great strides that have been made in treating these cancers. However, as the survivors become older, the long-term lingering effects of some of the aggressive treatments that have cured many childhood cancers are becoming evident. Studies are showing that chemotherapy and radiation, when they are given early in life, can have side effects on both the body and the mind. The physical problems can range from stunted growth, infertility, lung and heart problems, and the risk of a second cancer.

What kind of mental side effects are being seen?

Learning disorders, such as problems concentrating and perception problems, are among the major side effects. In addition, the trauma of cancer and its treatments can also cause post-traumatic stress.

Do all children get these side effects?

No. It depends on age, type of cancer, and type and amount of treatment. Children who are younger than five, who have brain tumors, or who have had radiation directed at the head and spinal cord seem to be at greater risk. Children who have chemotherapy injected into the space containing the brain and spinal cord may have some problems although not as severe. Radiation and chemotherapy can affect the cells of the brain involved in attention functions

TREATMENT SIDE EFFECTS IN CHILDHOOD CANCER

CONDITION	TREATMENT BELIEVED RESPONSIBLE
Late or early puberty	Cranial radiation.
Scoliosis	Spinal radiation (current radiation practices which include whole vertebral body in radiation have decreased, but still not eliminated, incidence).
Abnormal testosterone levels and sperm counts; ovarian damage; infertility	Chemotherapy and radiation. Ability to have normal sex life not affected. Most go on to have normal fertility and healthy offspring.
Thyroid dysfunction (laboratory values may normalize over time)	Radiation to the neck and chest, total body radiation before bone marrow transplant.
Growth problems such as delayed, slow, or stopped growth.	Cranial spinal radiation. Total body radiation before bone marrow transplant.
Learning disabilities, including poor performance in math, spatial relationships, problem solving, attention span, and concentration skills. Severity varies.	Cranial radiation therapy and chemotherapy.
Heart damage, including heart muscle injury, chronic heart failure	Chemotherapy—anthracyclines, high-dose cyclophosphamide, mitoxantrone—and chest radiation.
Pulmonary function abnormalities, lung scarring, reduced exercise tolerance	Whole lung or thoracic radiation, bone marrow transplants.
Kidney problems	Abdominal radiation, chemotherapy, antibiotic therapy.
Gastric or duodonal ulcers, small bowel obstruction, severe gastritis	Radiation, laparotomy.

(continued)

TREATMENT SIDE EFFECTS IN CHILDHOOD CANCER (continued)

CONDITION	TREATMENT BELIEVED RESPONSIBLE
Liver damage	Low-dose methotrexate and 6-mercaptopurine therapy.
Eye problems, including cataracts	Cranial radiation.
Dental problems, including failure of teeth to develop, arrested root development, unusually small teeth, enamel abnormalities	Head and neck radiation, chemotherapy.
Second cancers	Radiation and chemotherapy—mainly alkylating agents.
Weight gain after treatment	Reason is poorly understood. May be psychological but appears to have other explanations.

(basal ganglia). However, children who have not had cancer also may have learning and concentration problems, so all may not be due to treatment.

**How soon after treatment do the problems with
learning disorders appear?**
Brain cells die off slowly, so it may take up to three years for the problems to be seen.

**Are there any special programs that can help children who
have learning disabilities as a result of their cancer treatment?**
Dr. Robert Butler, a psychologist at the Oregon Health and Science University has created a program that is being tested through a grant from the NCI. The program, which consists of 20 two-hour sessions, teaches techniques for focusing and organizing thoughts—techniques that have been used to help people who have had strokes or other brain injuries. Activities such as practicing concentration techniques, learning memory strategies, number problems, word puzzles, and games that require concentration and memory skills, such as UNO and Mastermind are used. Seven hospitals across the country are involved in this research: The Children's Hospital of Philadelphia, University of Texas M.D. Anderson Cancer Center, University of Rochester,

Children's Hospital at Los Angeles, St. Jude's Children's Research Hospital, Children's Hospital Medical Center at Cincinnati, and the AMC Cancer Research Center.

Do cancer treatments have an effect on the children of adults who had cancer as children?

Studies to determine complete answers to this question are ongoing. However, one recent study showed that there was no evidence of increased risk of abnormalities in the children of adults who had childhood cancer and had received therapy that was potentially mutagenic. There was a very small increase in miscarriages in women treated with radiation.

How can I insure that my child gets the best care after treatment has been completed?

- You need to be aware that your child will need careful monitoring in the future.

- Talk to the doctor about follow-up. Usually at the beginning, the doctor will want to see the child every three months; then every six months, and finally every year. Make sure you talk with the doctor about when the exams will be and what tests will be done when you come for the exam.

- Understand what you need to look for. Ask about the signs and symptoms you should be checking to determine if the cancer should return.

- Look for signs of long-term aftereffects. Some cancer treatments have long-term side effects. They may affect how your child grows and learns. Make sure you have talked to the healthcare team about these side effects and keep alert for any problems, even long after treatment has ended.

- Listen to your child. Be aware of how the child and siblings are dealing with their feelings. They may need to talk with you or may need the help of a counselor or a social worker.

- Look at the picture over time. Studies have shown that many adult survivors of childhood cancer are not being followed on a regular basis. Over 50 percent of long-term survivors had not been seen by a doctor in the previous two years for evaluation of cancer-related problems.

Questions to Ask Your Doctor About Your Child's Follow-up

- **Who will be doing the main follow-up for my child?**
- **Will I also need to see any of our other doctors?**

- How often will we need to see you?
- What tests will you be doing during our follow-up exam?
- What will you be looking for?
- What are the long-term side effects I should be checking?
- What should I be watching for between our visits with you?
- What symptoms should I report? To whom?
- If I have concerns, how can I talk with you? Do I need to make a special appointment?

Do children who have had cancer need to have special follow-ups for the rest of their lives?

Children who have had cancer need to have follow-ups, both short-term and long-term. Many long-term survivors of childhood cancer remain dangerously ignorant of their need to take preventive measures such as having regular checkups. It is important to keep a complete record of treatments so that any child who has had cancer is fully informed of the original diagnosis, surgery, radiation site, specific types of chemotherapy drugs, and any other treatment information that may be helpful in the future.

What is Candlelighters?

The Candlelighters Childhood Cancer Foundation, which is the oldest and largest of the networking organizations for families with children who have cancer, has established links with 250 family support groups nationally and internationally. The self-help groups share practical information and ways of dealing with common problems, provide an outlet for the frustrations of those under stress, offer a social outlet for parents and siblings, and offer information through meetings featuring medical speakers, psychologists, or insurers. Candlelighters also has a Web site (www.candlelighters.org), publishes newsletters, operates a telephone hotline, provides training materials for long-term survivor and youth leadership groups and is involved in advocacy issues like education, medical leave policies, employment, and insurance. (Not all groups are called Candlelighters. The Wisconsin group is LODAT (Living One Day at a Time). For information about groups in your area contact: Candlelighters Childhood Cancer Foundation, 1312 18th Street, NW, Suite 200, Washington, DC 20036. 202–659–5136 or 1–800–366–CCCF.

What is the Ronald McDonald House?

The Ronald McDonald House facilities provide comfortable, accessible quarters for families of children undergoing treatment with long hospital stays away from the family's home. See Chapter 28, Where to Get Help, for information on where these are located and how they operate.

What is Children's Hospice International?

Although treatment is successful for many children with cancer, sometimes cancer cannot be cured. When this happens, some parents wish to have their child die at home rather than in the hospital. Information on home care is available from Children's Hospice International, which provides referrals for home and hospice care in your area. In addition, most pediatric oncology programs provide hospice-type support for their patients. For information contact Children's Hospice International at 330 North Washington Street, Suite 3, Alexandria, VA 22314. Telephone: 703–684–0330 or 1–800–242–4453.

Where can I get information on the organizations that make wishes come true for children with cancer?

There are a number of organizations across the country that make it possible for children's wishes to be fulfilled. For a listing, see Chapter 28, Where to Get Help.

Where can I get information about summer camps for children with cancer?

There are a growing number of summer camps for children with cancer. The camps are medically staffed, and many of the programs are free. See Chapter 28, Where to Get Help, for a listing of camps. For further information about camps in your locality, contact the Cancer Information Service, Candlelighters, or the American Cancer Society.

Web Pages to Check Out

www.cancer.gov: For general up-to-date information, and for clinical trials.

www.cancer.org: For general up-to-date information and community resources.

www.childrensoncologygroup.org: Children's Oncology Group—supported by the National Cancer Institute to conduct clinical trials devoted exclusively to children and adolescents with cancer at more than 200 member institutions in the United States Canada, Europe, and Australia.

www.pbtc.org: Pediatric Brain Tumor Consortium—includes nine institutions with extensive experience in treating children with brain tumors.

www.nant.org: Neuroblastoma Therapy Consortium—consortium of university and children's hospitals funded by the NCI to test promising new therapies for neuroblastoma.

www.cancer.umn.edu/ltfu#CCSS: Childhood Cancer Survivor Study—major component of NCI survivorship research effort, to learn about long-term effects of cancer and its therapy on childhood cancer survivors.

www.candlelighters.org: Information on how cancer affects children and where to find information and support.

www.chionline.org: Childrens Hospice, international site with database of resources.

Also see Chapter 2, Searching for Answers on the Web, for more information.

Twenty-five

DICTIONARY OF UNUSUAL CANCERS

SO OFTEN, IN talking with physicians and other health professionals, we, as laymen, stumble upon words that we do not understand. This is particularly true when unusual types of cancer, or unusual subtypes of cancer, are being discussed. It's frustrating to have your cancer described, and then not be able to find any information about it in the normal texts. To help gain a little perspective and shed a little light, this chapter seeks to further define, in the most basic manner, some of the less common types and designations of cancers and to give you clues that will help you to seek out further information.

If you have access to the Internet, you can find much more information by entering the word into a site like Google and asking for a search (see Chapter 2, Searching for Answers on the Web).

Acinar cell cancer: A form of exocrine pancreatic cancer.

Acral-lentiginous melanoma: A type of melanoma that appears as a dark spot on palms, soles, or nails.

Acute erythroleukemia: A form of acute myologenous leukemia (AML) characterized by overproduction of immature red cells mixed with a variety of immature white cells.

Acute promyelocytic leukemia: A subtype of acute nonlymphocytic leukemia (ANLL) characterized by the overproduction of primitive granulocytes.

Adamantinoma: Cancer of the long bones in the body, usually the shinbones.

Adenoid cystic carcinoma: Cancer of one of the minor salivary glands.

Adrenal cancer: Cancer of the adrenal glands located above the kidneys.

Adrenocortical cancer: Cancer of the outer shell of the adrenal glands, located above the kidneys.

Alveolar cell lung cancer: See *bronchioalveolar lung cancer*.

Alveolar soft part sarcoma: A soft tissue sarcoma that occurs primarily in thighs of adults and neck area of children.

Anaplastic thyroid cancer: An aggressive, difficult to treat, thyroid cancer.

Angiosarcoma: A soft tissue sarcoma originating in a blood vessel.

B-Cell acute lymphocytic leukemia: A type of ALL that affects immature stem cells that have started to mature along the B-cell line of development.

Basaloid cancer: Type of anal cancer.

Bile duct cancer: Cancer in the tube system that drains bile from the liver to the intestine. May be distal or proximal.

Bowen's disease: Skin cancer that occurs on areas unexposed to sun. Sometimes considered a precancerous condition.

Bowenoid papulosis: A variant of squamous cell cancer *in situ*.

Bronchioloalveolar lung cancer: A type of adenocarcinoma of the lung, not associated with smoking, affects bronchioles and alveolar walls of the lung.

Bronchogenic cancer: Type of lung cancer that starts in the bronchial tubes.

Burkitt cell acute lymphocytic leukemia: See *B-Cell acute lymphocytic leukemia*.

Burkitt's lymphoma: Fast-growing form of non-Hodgkin's lymphoma. Seen in children as well as AIDS patients.

CGL (See CML): Another name for chronic myelogenous leukemia. Stands for chronic granulocytic leukemia.

Cancer en cuirasse: A cancer of the skin of the chest, also called corset cancer or jacket cancer.

Carcinoma mucocellulare: See *Krukenberg tumor*.

Cholesteatoma: See *congenital brain tumor*.

Chordoma: A bone cancer that usually grows in the spinal column, most often at the ends of the spine or the base of the skull.

Choroid plexus tumor: Brain tumor originating in choroid plexus epithelial cells. More benign form is called choroid plexus papilloma. More malignant form is called anaplastic choroid plexus papilloma.

Cloacogenic cancer: See *basaloid cancer*.

Congenital brain tumor: a tumor that has existed in the brain since birth. Includes dermoids or cystic teratomas, cholesteatomas, and craniopharyngiomas.

Connective tissue cancer: See *soft-tissue sarcoma* (see Chapter 21).

Craniophaynglioma: See *congenital brain tumor*.

Cushing syndrome: See *pituitary tumor* (see Chapter 22).

Dedifferentiated chondrosarcoma: A type of malignant chondrogenic bone tumor.

Desmoplastic fibroma: A primary fibrosarcoma of bone.

Diffuse large cell lymphoma of bone: Usually a sign of disease that has spread but sometimes may be a solitary lesion.

DiGugliemo's syndrome: See *erythroleukemia*.

Eaton Lambert syndrome: See *myasthenic syndrome*.

Eosinophilic granuloma: See *histiocytosis X*.

Eosinophilic leukemia: A form of leukemia affecting the eosinophils or granular leukocytes.

Ependemoblastoma or Ependymoma: A tumor composed of differentiated ependymal cells.

Epidermoid cancer: Any tumor appearing in a part of the body other than the skin that is made up of skin-like elements.

Erythroleukemia: Type of acute nonlymphocytic leukemia (ANLL) affecting both red and white cells.

Erythroplasia of Queyrat: A variant of squamous cell cancer *in situ*.

Fibrosarcoma of bone: Bone tumor, most often found in long bones, sometimes found in head and neck. Usually appears in middle age, characterized by interlacing, herringbone-patterned bundles of collagen fibers.

Fibrosarcoma of soft tissue: Sarcoma derived from fibroblasts that produce collagen.

Fibrous histiocytoma: See *malignant fibrous histiocytoma*.

Giant cell tumor of bone (GCT): An aggressive bone tumor that may recur locally but has a low potential for metastasizing.

Glomus tumor: A noncancerous small tumor of the neural tissue usually occurring in the head and neck.

Glucagonoma: A cancer of the endocrine pancreas.

Grawitz's tumor: A type of kidney cancer known as cancer of the renal parenchyma.

Hashimoto's thyroiditis: A type of lymphoma that develops in the thyroid glands of people who have chronic lymphocytic thyroiditis.

Hemangiopericytoma: A type of soft-tissue sarcoma originating in the blood vessels of arms, legs, and trunk.

Hepatoblastoma: A type of liver cancer that consists chiefly of embryonic hepatic tissue. Occurs in infants and young children.

Histiocytosis X: A generic term that includes three related disorders, eosinophilic granuloma, Letterer-Siwe disease and Hand-Schuller-Christian disease, characterized by large histiocytes (macrophages).

Indolent non-Hodgkin's lymphoma: A group of slow growing non-Hodgkin's lymphomas.

Infantile hermangiopericytoma: A type of soft-tissue sarcoma originating in the blood vessels in the arms, legs, trunk, head, and neck of infants up to age one.

Islet cell cancer: A form of pancreatic cancer that originates in the endocrine glands that produce hormones.

Juxtacortical osteosarcoma: See *parosteal osteogenic sarcoma.*

Krukenberg tumor: Also called *carcinoma mucocellulare.* A type of cancer of the ovary that has usually metastasized from the gastrointestinal tract.

Lacrimal gland tumor: A growth in the tear gland that may be malignant.

Lentigo maligna melanoma: Also known as *melanotic freckle of Hutchinson.* A brownish pigmented spot on the skin that is considered to be noninvasive.

Leptomeningeal cancer: Cancer that has metastasized from another part of the body to the tissue lining the spinal canal.

Leukemic reticuloendotheliosis: Hairy-cell leukemia.

Macroglobulinemia: A condition characterized by increase in macroglobulins in the blood.

Malignant fibrous histiocytoma (MPH): A high grade bone tumor usually found in adult long bones, especially around the knee.

Medulloblastoma: A brain tumor composed of undifferentiated neuroepithelial cells.

Melanoma sarcoma: Rare clear cell sarcoma sometimes referred to as malignant melanoma of soft parts.

Meningeal carcinomatosis: Cancer that has spread over the surface of the brain and its lining.

Merkel cell tumor of the skin: A type of primary skin cancer characterized by peculiar distinctive granules. Appears in elderly persons.

Mesenchymoma: Soft tissue, mixed cell sarcoma.

Mucinous breast carcinoma: Slow growing breast cancer that appears in ducts and produces mucus.

Mullerian tumor: A cancer of the uterus, ovary or fallopian tubes that arises from remnants of embryonic tissue. Occurs usually in women ages 55 to 60.

Multiple endocrine neoplasia (MEN): An endocrine system cancer that may be inherited.

Myasthenic syndrome: A condition, with symptoms similar to myasthenia gravis, associated with small cell lung cancer.

Null cell acute lymphocytic leukemia: An undifferentiated form of ALL in which grossly immature stem cells that exhibit no differentiation are affected.

Osteochondroma: Cartilage tumor, usually benign.

Pancoast tumor: A form of small cell lung cancer in which a slow growing tumor is found in the groove along the top edge of the lung.

Parosteal osteogenic sarcoma: Also called juxtacortical osteosarcoma. A slow growing sarcoma that involves the midshaft of the long bones.

Periosteal osteosarcoma: A type of osteosarcoma that grows on the cortex of the bone, usually the tibia.

Peripheral neuroepithelioma: A noncentral nervous system sarcoma found in children and young adults. Treated like Ewing's sarcoma.

Pheochromocytoma: Cancer of the inner core of the adrenal glands.

Pineal gland tumor: A benign tumor located near center of brain. Occurs most often in children and young adults.

Plasmacytoma: A tumor of the plasma cells, multiple myeloma.

Reticulum cell sarcoma of bone: See *diffuse large cell lymphoma of bone.*

Round-cell sarcomas: Two most common types of round-cell sarcomas are Ewing's sarcoma and non-Hodgkin's lymphoma.

Small cell osteosarcoma: A variant of round-cell osteosarcoma that resembles Ewing's sarcoma, but may be treated differently.

Schminke tumor: lymphoepithelioma found in the nasopharynx.

Spindle cell lung cancer: Terminology used for squamous cell lung cancer, also called epidermoid.

Sterloi-Lydig tumor: A cancer of the ovary. Also called androma, arrhenoblastoma, andreioma, and arrhenoma.

Superior sulcus tumor: See *pancoast tumor.*

Thymoma: A cancer of the tissues of the thymus.

von Hippel Lindau syndrome (VHL): Rare familial disorder that can result in cancer in patients who have vixceral lesions. (For further information, contact VHL Family Alliance, 171 Clinton Road, Brookline, MA 02445–5815. Telephone: 1–800–767–4845. Fax: 617–734–8233. E-mail: info@vhl.org.)

Waldenstrom's macroglobulinemia: A cancer of the white blood cells that behaves like myeloma. Most often seen in males over 50.

Twenty-six

WHEN CANCERS RECUR OR METASTASIZE

The first question many people ask their doctors after cancer surgery is, "Did you get it all?" assuming that surgical removal of a cancer is a guarantee of cure. "Getting it all" may be impossible if cancer cells have already started their journey in the body. That's why many treatments and strategies have been developed that include chemotherapy and other measures that try to destroy all cancer cells at the original site, as well as trying to stem the movement of cancer cells to other parts of the body. Cancer can recur, that is, it can come back again. It might come back in the same place as before (local recurrence), somewhere close to the first area (regional recurrence), or it may spread far from where it was first found. When cancer cells spread, it is referred to as metastasis or metastatic cancer.

IF IT SHOULD happen in your case that some cells were able to escape and do their damage elsewhere in your body, you are faced with the fact that the cancer which you hoped had been cured, has recurred or spread, and you must be prepared to deal with it as a chronic disease.

THINGS TO REMEMBER:

- **A recurrence is not a death sentence. It is a crisis to be faced.**

- Many of your concerns may be unfounded, so rather than worry unnecessarily, ask your doctor exactly what he thinks the recurrence means and whether this is a chronic problem that can be treated. Medical skills and advances now make it possible to deal with many problems and crises in very positive ways.

- There are many appropriate treatments available. You may want to investigate a clinical trial—many are designed especially for people with cancer that has recurred or spread.

- Some recurrences are inherently less a cause for alarm than others.

- Cancer that recurs is very much like the first cancer in the way that it starts. If not stopped, cancer cells will continue to replace normal cells. Cancer that has metastasized may be found in places far from the original site.

- Not every cancer cell that breaks away is able to start a growth elsewhere. Most are stopped by the body's natural defenses or can be destroyed by treatment.

- Be sure to use the resources discussed in Chapter 7, Treatment, to make certain you are getting the very newest treatment. Renew your use of the toll-free 1–800–4–CANCER number so that you will have the latest information and help in dealing with your present problems. Your past knowledge, your familiarity with the medical system, and your ability in dealing with the original cancer give you an advantage in this area.

> Don't hesitate to call
> 1–800–4–CANCER
> for the latest information on treatment

Is it normal to think that every ache and pain is a sign that my cancer has recurred?

This is a perfectly normal reaction. Many people who have had cancer have gone through the routine of fearing every cough, every bone ache, every headache, every change, thinking it might be a sign that they might have a recurrence. Since about 50 percent of all cancers are cured with the first treatment, you may be worrying without reason. To help you to deal with this, you should talk over your fears with your physician. Though no one, not even your doctor, can predict your future, you may find it helpful to ask if there is very little chance of recurrence with your kind of cancer, where metastases might occur, and what symptoms you should watch for.

Does having a recurrence mean there's no hope for me?

Some people make that assumption—and they couldn't be further from the truth. Don't try to make any assumptions about the meaning of the recurrence until you have had plenty of time to have all the tests that need to be run completed and analyzed. So many people, during this crisis time, assume that nothing can be done. Many people try to make critical family and personal decisions during an emotionally charged period. Families often are even more discouraged than the patient and mistakenly begin to prepare themselves mentally for a future without their loved one. This can be disastrous for everyone concerned. If you are faced with a recurrence, though it is difficult to do, take time to wait for a full diagnosis. Discuss the situation fully with your doctor. Check out all the newest treatments. Ask enough questions to make sure you are getting clear information.

What if I just can't face the thought of going back through treatment again?

This is a normal reaction. It is certainly easy to understand your reluctance to undergo further discomfort and disability. You need to ask your doctor for a frank assessment of the possible outcome of the treatment. Arrange for a second opinion from another doctor. In many cases, the treatment will be successful. Your attitude toward the treatment is an important factor in a return to health. If it is possible for you to think of cancer as a chronic disease, much as you would if you had diabetes or heart disease, it is easier to deal with facing what is happening to you.

Isn't it true that sometimes the risks and side effects of further treatment aren't worth the benefits?

The point at which this begins to be true is always debatable. Some people feel that once they've been through the initial treatment, that is all they care to deal with. Of course, with the fast-moving progress of medicine, it's important not to come to this conclusion too hastily. It is up to each patient to weigh the pros and cons, the side effects and aftereffects, to determine what is right in each case. In this highly personal area of decision making, it is possible only to suggest some avenues that should be considered.

Questions to Ask Yourself

- **Have I gotten another opinion so that I am certain that what has been found is indeed a recurrence?**

- Have I checked out what other treatments might be available?

- Have I been to a major cancer center for information and consultation?

- Have I checked the PDQ (you can do this by calling the toll-free 1–800–4–CANCER information service phone number or by getting on the Internet) to see what investigational treatments are available?

- Am I most interested in the *quality* or *quantity* of my life at this point, or am I looking for a compromise of the two?

- Have I asked my doctor what benefits are expected from the treatment? What side effects? What risks? What will happen if I choose not to have further treatment?

- Am I ready to stop treatments altogether?

- What is it that I am most afraid of?

Try to isolate what your biggest fears are—pain, isolation, leaving things undone, being unable to take care of yourself, dying—and discuss them with your doctor, your family and other competent counselors for advice and guidance.

Is it unusual for me to be angry with my doctor?
Most of us have expectations for our doctors that can be quite unreasonable and impossible. Quite frankly, we expect our doctors to cure us. When cancer recurs, we often feel that it's the doctor's fault. We know it's irrational, but sometimes we just need to blame someone or something for our illness. This anger is rooted in our mistaken feelings about a doctor's infallibility. Doctors do not have all the answers. Cancer is a very elusive disease and even with all the advances, it can still be very unpredictable. If you find yourself with angry feelings about your doctor, you should examine the reasons for your feelings and discuss them with your doctor. Schedule an extra 15 minutes at your next appointment to talk over the problems as you see them. Discussion will help to dissipate some of the frustration and anger, and should make communication easier. The doctor's business is to help you. This cannot be done unless the doctor knows what is bothering you. Clear the air. Be honest and share your feelings. If that doesn't help, then perhaps it's time for you to make the break and start using another physician. After all, you need someone who is supportive and willing to communicate with you so you can approach your problems in a positive fashion.

Questions to Ask Your Doctor if a Recurrence Is Suspected

- Is it possible that my symptoms could be caused by some other medical problem?

- **What tests will you perform to find out?**
- **When will the tests be done?**
- **When will I get a decision and if necessary, a recommendation for treatment?**
- **If it is cancer, is it a recurrence or a new type of cancer?**
- **If it is a recurrence, where has it spread?**

Why does cancer recur?

When cancer recurs it means that disease that was thought to be cured, or was at least inactive for a period of time, has become active again. Sometimes cancer recurs after several months, sometimes it may remain dormant for many years. It is always hoped that the original treatment will destroy the original cancer and any of the cells that may have become detached from it. Sometimes, however, microscopic cells, too small to be detected, may survive and eventually start to grow in the same or in another location.

What is a local recurrence?

Local recurrence means that the cancer has come back in the same place as the original cancer. The term local also means that there is no sign of cancer in nearby lymph nodes or other tissues. For example, someone who has had breast cancer could later have a local recurrence in or around the area of the original surgery. The same is true of colon or bowel cancer, where sometimes recurrences occur in the scar area of nearby tissues.

What is a regional recurrence?

A regional recurrence involves growth of a new tumor in lymph nodes or tissues near the original site, but with no evidence of growth at distant sites. A woman treated for cervical or ovarian cancer may have a regional recurrence in the abdomen.

What is a metastatic recurrence?

In the case of a metastatic recurrence, cancer has spread to organs or tissue at some distance from the original site, such as in the lung, bone, liver, or brain.

How does metastasis occur?

Metastasis is a complex course of events that is still not completely understood. However, the term "metastasis" or "metastatic" means that the cancer has spread from one part of the body to another, from the primary or original site to another part of the body. Under the microscope, the metastatic cancer cells usually resemble the cancer cells from your original disease.

Metastases start from cells that break away from the original tumor and travel through the lymph system or bloodstream to start new cancer growths.

If I had breast cancer and it metastasizes to my lungs, do I have lung cancer?

The cancer that reappears is the same type as the original cancer—no matter where it appears. This means if your breast cancer recurs in the lung, it is not lung cancer, it is breast cancer that has spread to the lung. The physician might refer to it as "breast metastasis in the lung." In other words, what you have is not a second cancer, not lung cancer, but a recurrence of the breast cancer you had before. You will not be treated for lung cancer, but for breast cancer that has spread to the lungs.

How do cells become metastatic?

The avenues leading to uncontrolled growth of a cell are varied and distinctive and not fully understood even by the scientists. All cancer involves changes in genetic information—the DNA—but damage in some cases is a mere blip and in others involves a total reshuffling of the information. Some cells become malignant by losing the function of tumor suppressor genes, while others do it by turning on cancer-causing genes. The cancer cells are influenced by the organs in which the original tumors occur. There is more detailed information on how cancer starts in Chapter 4, What Is Cancer?

Why is it that the first treatment sometimes fails to kill all the cancer cells?

If only the answer to that was known, we wouldn't have to deal with metastasis. The goal of treatment is always to remove all of the cancer cells. However, a single cancerous tumor might itself be composed of a mixture of cells having different properties. Cell subpopulations can vary in their ability to spread to other sites in the body, as well as in their susceptibility to treatment. They also vary in the ease with which they provoke or avoid an immune attack and in their ability to produce chemical markers that are used to detect the presence of particular cancers. It is no wonder that sometimes a few cells escape from the original tumor and form new tumors at other sites in the body without medical science presently being able to forecast or circumvent their spread.

Are there places where specific cancers commonly spread?

Some primary cancers have a tendency to spread more often in specific places. The most common locations for distant metastases to occur are in the lungs, bones, liver, and brain.

COMMON AREAS OF DISTANT SPREAD

ORIGINAL SITE	WHERE IT USUALLY SPREADS
Bladder	Bone, lung, liver, brain
Breast	Bone, lung, brain, liver, adrenal gland, ovary, other breast
Bone	Lung
Colon/rectal	Lung, liver, ovary
Eye	Liver
Head and Neck	Lung, liver, brain, bones
Kidney	Bone, lung, liver
Leukemia/lymphoma	Liver, lung, membranes of brain and spine
Lung	Brain, liver, bone, adrenal glands
Melanoma	Brain, liver, bowel
Prostate	Bone
Sarcomas	Lung
Stomach	Liver, lung
Testicle	Liver, lung
Thyroid	Bone
Uterus	Lung, liver

Are there cancers that are more unpredictable in their ability to spread?

There is a large group of common cancers that show a great deal of variation from one person to another. These include cancers of the breast, lung, bowel, stomach, and melanoma of the skin.

What tests are used to detect recurrence?

The testing will be similar to those you went through for the original cancer. Discussion of your symptoms, physical exam, blood tests, CT scans, MRI, bone scans, tests for tumor markers, ultrasound or biological markers and a biopsy might be needed. Go back to Chapter 6, How Cancers Are Diagnosed, for descriptions of the tests that might be used.

Should I get a second opinion?

As it was with the original diagnosis, it is important that you are carefully evaluated to make sure that there is a problem before any treatment is started. We feel that it is always worthwhile to have a second opinion at a comprehensive cancer center or at a major medical center to assure that the diagnosis is correct and complete and that the treatment program is the best for your type of recurrence.

Questions to Ask Before Starting Treatment for a Recurrence

- **What will this treatment do?**
- **Why do you think it is the best for me?**
- **Will the treatment cure the cancer? If not, what is your goal in giving it to me?**
- **Is there a clinical trial for my type of recurrence?**
- **Where is the best place for me to get treated for this problem?**
- **What are the risks in taking this treatment? The benefits?**
- **What will happen if I don't get treated at all?**
- **How long will the treatment last? How many treatments will I need?**
- **Will I need to be in the hospital to get them?**
- **What are the side effects of the treatment?**
- **How much will the treatment cost? Will my health plan or insurance cover it?**
- **Is this treatment different from the last treatment I had?**

What treatments are used for cancers that have recurred or metastasized?

Your treatment will depend upon what kind of cancer you have and where it has spread. There are many treatments now available for cancer that has spread. They range from chemotherapy to radiation, from hormonal treatment to monoclonal antibodies. Many of the new and investigational treatments (discussed in Chapter 11, New Advances and Investigational Treatments) are available for metastatic cancer. Do not be discouraged. There are many roads that you can take during this next cancer journey.

What kinds of cancer are likely to spread to the lung?

Spread of cancer to the lung is quite common in breast, colon, ovary, stomach, kidney, bladder, uterus, melanoma, sarcomas, lymphomas, leukemias, and germ cell tumors. A few tumors, like sarcomas, metastasize almost exclusively to the lung and can, in some cases, be cured with surgery. Others, like testicular cancer, for which chemotherapy is used to eradicate the original cancer, can be surgically removed. Some tumors, like kidney cancers, metastasize to the lungs with a few slow-growing spots that can be surgically removed. Most of the metastasized tumors that grow in the lung are quite small, round, and sharply demarcated. Usually if there is an irregular border, this indicates a primary lung cancer or infection.

What are the symptoms when cancer has spread to the lung?
Though many people who have cancer that has spread to the lung have no symptoms, shortness of breath may be a sign that there is some involvement in the lung.

What is the treatment for cancers that have spread to the lung?
Treatment will depend on a number of factors including the tumor type, the length of time from treatment of the primary tumor to lung metastases, how quickly the tumor is growing, whether there are other metastatic growths in other parts of the body, and, of course, your own health status. Chemotherapy, hormone therapy, external beam radiation, and surgery are all treatments that can be used for lung metastases. Clinical trials include new drugs, immunotherapy, gene therapy, and new radiation techniques.

What kinds of cancers are most likely to metastasize to the bone?
Metastases to the bone are seen most often in patients with breast, lung, kidney, bladder, or prostate cancer. Metastatic bone cancer rarely is life threatening, and many patients live for years after the discovery of bone metastases. However, pain from these cancers sometimes can be debilitating and fractures can make it difficult for you to move, walk, and work.

Where are the bone metastases found?
They are most often found in the spine. The pelvis, hips, upper leg bones and the skull are other areas of bone metastasis. Some metastases occur singly, some are multiple. They are usually small and well defined, though tumors in the hip and pelvis may be larger. It has been found that the denser the pattern, the slower the growth.

What kind of treatment is used for bone metastases?
It depends on where the original cancer is and which bones it has spread to. The treatment could include chemotherapy, hormone or immunotherapy, and external or internal radiation. Clinical trials are underway using neutron/photon radiation, chemotherapy, hormonal treatments, bone-seeking

radioisotopes, and radioactive monoclonal antibodies. Surgery might be used to put in a rod to strengthen a bone or, if bones have been broken, to repair them.

What is Strontium-89 (Metastron)?

Strontium-89 (often referred to as Metastron) is a radiopharmaceutical, a radioactive agent used for cancers that metastasize to the bone. It is used to help relieve pain of multiple bone metastases. It can only be given by or under the direct supervision of a doctor who has specialized training in nuclear medicine or radiation oncology. It is injected and goes directly to the sites of metastatic bone disease where, like calcium, it is absorbed in the bones. The injection contains small amounts of a specially selected form of radioactive strontium, chosen because almost all of its radiation is given to the area where it is absorbed, allowing it to deliver therapy precisely where it is needed. A single out-patient injection generally provides pain relief for an average of six months, and has minimal effect on normal bone and sur-rounding tissues. The effects of Strontium-89 are confined within your body, which means that other people cannot receive the effects of radiation through bodily contact with you. However, for the first week after injection, Strontium-89 will be present in your blood and urine and your doctor will discuss simple precautions that should be taken.

What are the side effects of Strontium-89 (Metastron)?

Some people experience a mild facial flushing immediately after injection. This may happen when the medication is administered too quickly (in 30 seconds rather than in a one or two minute time frame). Some people have a mild but temporary increase in pain several days after the injection that may last for two or three days. Doctors usually prescribe an increase in painkillers until the pain is under control. After one or two weeks, sometimes a little longer, the pain begins to diminish and continues to diminish, with effects lasting for up to six months. You may be advised to reduce the dose of other pain medications gradually. Eventually, you may not need painkillers at all. You can eat and drink normally. There may be a slight fall in your blood cell count. Your doctor will probably ask you to have routine periodic blood tests. Repeated dosages can be given if the doctor feels this is the most appropriate treatment.

What are bisphosphonates?

In some cancers, the level of calcium in the blood is high. Bisphosphonates are a group of drugs that lower calcium, used to prevent pain or to prevent bones from breaking. Two bisphosphonates, zoledronic acid (Aredia) and pamidronate (Zometa) have been approved by the FDA for treatment of bone metastases, in conjunction with chemotherapy drugs. These drugs have been used for breast and prostate cancer and multiple myeloma.

Are bone fractures from metastasized bone cancer hard to heal?

Fractures and forced immobility are two of the most difficult side effects of metastatic bone cancer. Bone metastases from breast cancers and multiple myelomas are known to have the highest rate of healing. Metastases from lung and colorectal cancers and melanomas have been found to be more difficult to heal following bone fractures. It has also been shown that patients who have had high dose postoperative radiation (greater than 3,000–3,500 rads) may have greater difficulty in healing. Cryosurgery is useful for metastasized bone tumors that have recurred and those in difficult anatomic locations.

What kinds of cancers metastasize to the liver?

Liver metastases occur in many kinds of cancer. Tumors of the colon, rectum, stomach, testes, pancreas, bladder, kidney, ovary, and uterus often metastasize to the liver. Breast and lung cancers and lymphomas are often less found to have metastasized to the liver.

What are the symptoms when cancer spreads to the liver?

An enlarged or tender liver is an indication that there may be metastases in the liver. Symptoms may include weight loss, abdominal swelling, a yellowish tinge to the skin (jaundice), a fever or a buildup of fluid in the abdominal cavity (ascites).

What treatment is used when cancer spreads to the liver?

Treatment depends on a number of factors, including the number of metastases, their location in the liver, and the primary site of the cancer. Chemotherapy with or without hormonal therapy, surgery, and internal radiation can all be used. When the entire tumor can be removed, chances of recovery are excellent. The recuperative powers of the liver are amazing, and many people live perfectly normal lives after surgery has removed as much as 80 percent of their livers. Metastasis may sometimes return again in the liver and may be operated on a second time. In cases where surgery of the liver is not possible, regional treatment of the liver with the use of an implantable pump may be used. New techniques using pumps and chemotherapy regimens designed to take advantage of daily variations in chemotherapy metabolism are being evaluated, as are biological response modifiers, palliative radiation, cryotherapy, hyperthermia, and embolization.

What is the outlook for cancer that has spread to the brain?

Today's expectations for patients with cerebral metastatic cancer have gradually improved with modest benefits for the majority of patients and guarded optimism for selected patients. Sometimes cancer spreads to the brain after it has already spread to another organ, such as the lung or the liver. Melanomas are the most likely cancers to spread to the brain, followed by lung and breast. Lung, melanoma, and renal tumors tend to spread more quickly following initial diagnosis. Breast and colon cancers and sarcomas seem to take longer to metastasize.

What are symptoms of metastatic brain cancer?

Headache, usually occurring in the morning or early hours and gradually increasing in duration and frequency, is a common symptom. Focal weakness, seizures, loss of sensation or difficulties with gait or balance may be other symptoms. Many times, family members or friends will notice lethargy, emotional instability, or personality changes.

How are brain metastases diagnosed?

CT and MRI scanning are the most specific and sensitive for evaluating brain metastases. Other conditions can mimic brain metastases, so it is important that careful evaluation be conducted to avoid inappropriate or dangerous and unnecessary treatment.

What treatment is most common for brain metastases?

Chemotherapy, hormone treatment, external or internal radiation therapy, laser-assisted surgery, immunotherapy, and gene therapy are all used in treating brain metastases. Sometimes two of the treatments are used together, such as surgery combined with radiation therapy. Steroids may be used along with radiotherapy. Interstitial radiation to increase the dose without damaging any more tissue than is necessary is also being studied.

What are the symptoms of heart involvement due to metastasis?

Symptoms can be quite vague and include labored breathing, difficult breathing except when upright, cough, palpitations, weakness, fatigue, dizziness, and chest pain.

What is the treatment for pericardial effusion?

Some patients whose echocardiograms or CT scans show effusions do not require any specific therapy. However, if the heart becomes compressed (*tamponade* is the medical term) an emergency situation exists and pericardiocentesis (needle used to remove fluid for examination) may be done for diagnosis. Treatment can include drainage followed by chemotherapy, radiation or surgical procedures, depending on many factors. Being clinically evaluated is sequential intrapericardial chemotherapy.

What causes severe swelling of the abdomen (ascites)?

Ascites is a medical term for severe swelling of the abdomen. It is not unusual for fluid containing cancer cells to be found in the lining of the wall of the abdomen in advanced cancers.

What types of cancers metastasize and cause ascites?

Malignant ascites is seen most commonly in patients with ovarian, endometrial, colon, gastric, and pancreatic cancer.

What treatments are used for malignant ascites?

A variety of treatments may be used. Intraperioteneal chemotherapy, delivered through a surgically implanted catheter makes it possible for higher doses of some drugs to be delivered to the tumor than other methods.

Do some cancers regress spontaneously?

There are a few kinds of cancer that are known sometimes to disappear spontaneously. These include low grade lymphomas, melanomas, and kidney cancer. How that happens is a mystery.

Can you have a metastasis without ever having had cancer?

Sometimes a metastasis is discovered first, such as when pain is experienced in the bone before any symptoms of a primary cancer are seen. If the original site of the cancer cannot be found, it is known as "cancer of unknown primary."

What if the primary tumor can't be found?

A small number of cancer patients have tumors that clinically and pathologically can be proven to be cancer metastases, yet tests and examinations do not reveal where the first cancer is located. Even after extensive diagnostic studies, some of these primary cancers are impossible to detect. There are a number of ways in which such cases are managed, depending on the history, the site of the metastatic cancer, and where the doctor suspects the primary cancer might be located. In such cases, it is especially important that your pathology be completely reviewed by a skilled pathologist and a doctor who understand cancers of unknown primary. Be sure to report any previous problems with what were thought to be harmless symptoms. Such information includes skin tumors that were removed, benign polyps of the colon, D&C or conization procedures, biopsies of the prostate, etc. The tissue that was removed may have been considered benign, but could explain the location of the original tumor. Think carefully about your past medical history—changes in bowel habits or voiding pattern, vaginal or other unusual bleeding, pelvic discomfort, or pain—that might give the doctor clues that will help determine where the original cancer is located. It is sometimes necessary to start treatment before the original cancer is found—and many times the original site is never pinpointed.

What are some of the medical emergencies that can occur as the result of metastasized cancers or their treatments?

There are a number of medical emergencies that can occur as the result of metastasized cancer or treatment for it. As more effective and aggressive treatments are used, patients live longer and have a greater likelihood of encountering complications. Awareness of symptoms, prompt reporting, and diagnosis of the problems allow for appropriate treatment. Some of the medical emergencies include:

- **Blood clotting problems** may occur that cause chronic problems such as bleeding gums and mild to moderate urinary or gastrointestinal bleeding, phlebitis, or pulmonary embolism. These are most often seen in patients with gastrointestinal, pancreas, prostate, lung, breast and ovarian cancers, melanoma, acute leukemia, and myeloma. Any early signs of bleeding should be reported so that underlying causes can be treated.

- **Bowel obstruction** resulting in loss of function requires immediate attention. Bowel obstruction may be due to a number of causes—impacted fecal matter, lesions, bands of adhesions or scar tissue from past surgery or spread of cancer to the bowel wall. Abdominal and pelvic radiation can also cause tissue changes, sometimes as long as 20 years after treatment. Many times, fluid and electrolyte imbalances are identified and corrected. Symptoms of bowel problems such as vomiting, abdominal distension, and constipation should be reported to the doctor promptly so that measures can be taken to help prevent complications. Following careful investigation and observation, surgery may be required.

- **Superior vena cava syndrome** is the result of a tumor compressing the vena cava (the vein that drains blood from the head, neck, upper extremities, and chest). Airway obstruction, cough, neck vein distention, shortness of breath, and facial swelling are most common symptoms. Radiation and chemotherapy are the common treatments.

- **Pericarditis** or pericardial effusion is caused by the accumulation of fluid in the pericardial space, the sac that surrounds the heart. It can be the result of radiation to the chest area or the spread of cancer to the area. The most common symptom is chest pain that can be somewhat relieved by leaning forward but is more severe when the patient is lying down. Other symptoms are shortness of breath, cough, abdominal tenderness, and nausea. It may occur in patients with lung cancer, breast cancer, leukemia, Hodgkin's disease, lymphoma, melanoma, gastrointestinal tumors, and sarcomas. Pericardial fluid is withdrawn and treatment is given to prevent reaccumulation of fluid.

- **Septic shock** may be caused by infections resulting from corticosteroids and chemotherapy, or by the tumor itself. Because cancer patients are often vulnerable to infections, microorganisms, either bacterial or fungal, may cause toxic blood conditions. Symptoms of early septic shock include: fever, shaking, and chills, followed by stiffening of muscles, rapid cardiac rate, confusion, and hypotension. Any such symptoms should be reported to the doctor immediately so that immediate treatment can be given.

- **Hypercalcemia,** an excess of calcium in the blood, can cause weakness, depression, anorexia, nausea, and constipation. It occurs most frequently in patients with multiple myeloma and breast cancer and less frequently in patients with lung cancer. Bone metastases from a wide variety of cancers are also a cause of hypercalcemia. Reduction of the tumor burden or control of the tumor is necessary to reverse hypercalcemia. However, since hypercalcemia sometimes occurs in patients whose cancer is advanced and has not responded to treatment, this is not always possible. Treatment is generally nonspecific and based on a many factors including the condition of the patient and the degree of severity of the hypercalcemia. Attempts are made to increase the elimination of calcium through urination. If the hypercalcemia is severe, hospitalization will be required so that intravenous methods can be used.

- **Tumor lysis syndrome** is a side effect that can occur as a result of the administration of chemotherapy to certain very bulky tumors. It may occur in patients with high grade lymphoma or acute lymphoblastic leukemia when abnormally high levels of potassium and phosphorus are released. A large amount of tumor may shrink in days as chemotherapeutic agents destroy tumor cells while the cells are dividing, causing the patient's system to deal with massive tumor burdens. Symptoms include weakness, muscle cramps, nausea, vomiting, diarrhea, and lethargy.

- **Spinal cord compression** may occur as the result of a metastasis in the spinal cord. Since the spinal cord contains motor and sensory elements, the severity of the problem depends upon the tumor location within the spinal cord. Symptoms can include back pain from pressure on the spinal cord, foot drop, weakness, balance disturbances, and locomotion impairment. Again, depending upon the location of the tumor, other symptoms such as sensory impairment, incontinence, bowel problems, loss of feeling, etc. can occur. The goal of treatment is to relieve the compression as rapidly as possible to prevent further damage to the spinal cord.

Will I have pain as a result of my recurrent or advanced cancer?
Many people, when their cancer recurs or metastasizes, are afraid that they will have pain. However, some cancer patients, even those with advanced disease, have little or no pain. For those who do have pain problems, new pain therapies are being explored with good results. The many ways of dealing with pain are described in Chapter 27, Living with Cancer.

Web Pages to Check Out

www.cancer.gov: For general up-to-date information, and for clinical trials.
www.cancer.org: For general up-to-date information and community resources.
www.cancerlinks.com/metastatic.html: Links to information on metastatic cancer.

Also see Chapter 2, Searching for Answers on the Web, for more information.

Twenty-seven

LIVING WITH CANCER

Dealing with cancer isn't easy. But there are lots of practical tips that can help, and a great deal of advice from others who have been through it, to guide you along the way.

THIS CHAPTER DEALS with the many practical aspects of living with cancer on a day-to-day basis—both during treatment and after treatment is completed. It also covers information on feelings and the emotions that you are likely to encounter. Some of the questions apply to all patients, while some may be relevant to only a few. You'll find helpful information about complementary methods you may want to incorporate into your routine. There is information about nutrition, exercise, sexual problems that may arise, dealing with pain, as well as practical advice on money matters and insurance. Since dying is part of living, this chapter deals frankly with that subject and includes some information on wills, care at home, hospice care, euthanasia, dying, death, and autopsies. Much of the information should be of interest to the healthy as well as to those who are ill.

EATING WELL

Can I go to my doctor for information about what diet is best for me?
Many doctors, realizing the heightened public interest in nutrition as it relates to health, are advising patients to seek nutritional help. Many traditional doctors still are not educated in nutrition and some can be quite antagonistic about the whole subject. Although you will want to let your cancer specialists know your concerns about improving your diet, don't be surprised if your request is met in a noncommittal, half-hearted or even hostile way. However, you can ask the doctor or nurse to arrange for you to consult with a dietician at the hospital where you have been treated or find a nutritionist who can help you.

Is it a problem if I gain weight during cancer treatment?
During treatment, you should try to achieve and maintain a healthy weight. So whether it is good or bad to gain at this time depends on what your weight was before you started. If you were at a normal weight for your frame and height, you should try to maintain that weight during cancer treatment. If you had been losing a lot of weight, you should try to get back to the normal weight, because further loss of weight can interfere with completing your treatment, delay healing, and increase complications. However, if you were overweight or obese, you should be careful not to add weight during treatment. Some dietitians feel that it might be helpful for those who are overweight or obese to lose weight during this time, using a healthful, well-balanced diet with physical activity tailored to your specific needs. Obesity is a risk factor for some cancers, such as postmenopausal breast cancer and colorectal cancer, so the issue of weight is an important one. Changes in weight need to be discussed with your healthcare team, since your body size and weight can affect planned chemotherapy and radiation treatments.

Are there special nutrition requirements for people undergoing treatment?
Good nourishment is essential for healing and building new tissues. People who eat well during treatment, especially foods high in protein and calories, are better able to stand the side effects of treatment. Some researchers feel it may even be possible for these patients to withstand higher doses of certain treatments. There are nutrition experts who believe that during chemotherapy, for example, you may need as much as 50 percent more protein than usual and 20 percent more calories.

What happens when you don't feel like eating?
When a person eats less, for whatever reason, the body uses its own stored fat, protein, and other nutrients, such as iron. When this happens, your natural

defenses are weakened and your body cannot fight infection as well. It is not unusual to lose interest in food during treatment, but you must try to eat a diet that is high enough in calories to keep up your normal weight, if at all possible. Eat any time you are hungry. Try to keep a supply of nutritious, caloric, high protein foods on hand. Protein can help repair the body if the body is getting enough calories. If it is not, the body will use the protein for energy instead of repair.

What kind of nutritional supplements can I use to boost my diet?

Many people find, when they cannot get enough calories and protein from their diets, that it is helpful to add commercial nutrition supplements, such as formulas and instant breakfast powders that are available in supermarkets and drugstores, to their diets. These supplements are high in protein and calories and have extra vitamins and minerals. They come in liquid, pudding, and powder forms. Since these products need no refrigeration until after they are opened, they're easy to have on hand. They can be carried with you so they can be used when you feel hungry or thirsty. They make a good between-meal or bedtime snack and they require no preparation.

Is it unusual to have weight gain as a result of treatment?

Breast cancer patients may gain extra weight during and after treatment even though they are not adding extra calories. In addition, some chemotherapy drugs, such as prednisone, can cause the body to hold on to fluids and thus, add extra weight. You need to discuss any weight gain with your doctor. If your weight gain is from the chemotherapy, the extra weight may be water retention rather than the result of overeating. It is important not to go on a diet at this point without discussing it with your healthcare team. If the extra weight is due to the drugs, you may be advised to limit the salt you eat because salt can cause your body to retain water. Diuretic drugs may be prescribed to help reduce water retention.

How can I find a good nutritionist?

Since most states do not license or certify nutritionists, finding a good one on your own can be difficult. Most of the legitimate ones are registered dietitians (RDs), which means they have been certified by the American Dietetic Association. There are nearly 50,000 registered dietitians in the United States, some of whom are employed by hospitals, clinics, and beauty spas. There are also MDs with postgraduate training and clinicians with PhDs in nutrition. They are usually members of the American Society of Clinical Nutrition and certified by the American Board of Nutrition. A lack of registered credentials does not necessarily mean a lack of competence. It does mean you should check out reputation by other means.

- Check the Web site of the American Dietetic Association (www.eatright.org). Their "Find a Dietitian" database lists professionals who can provide nutrition information. The directory is searchable by type of service, area of expertise, and location and provides names, addresses, phone numbers, and e-mails for the professionals.

- Ask a doctor, nurse, or local hospital for a recommendation. Many food counselors work in conjunction with the medical profession. If you have been a patient at the hospital, you can get a referral to a dietitian there.

- Look in the Yellow Pages of your telephone directory under Nutrition. Listed there, you will probably find a number of names, only a few of whom will be PhDs or registered dietitians. Some counselors will have MS after their names, indicating an advanced degree in science. Nutrition counselors and clinical nutritionists are common listings, but do not give you information as to qualifications—except by omission.

- Questionable credentials include a degree in nutrition counseling from unaccredited correspondence schools or degree initials such as CH, Certified Herbologist; or RH, Registered Healthologist. Listings offering nutritional and metabolic evaluation services such as hair analyses and cytotoxic blood tests for determining food sensitivities are questionable.

- You can learn a great deal quickly by making telephone calls to those listed. Ask questions about qualifications and background, how long they have been counseling, what types of patients they usually work with, what kind of treatment and testing, if any, is used. Be sure to ask what the charges will be and how many visits most patients average. Usually two visits are sufficient for nutrition counseling. Few people need more than six sessions unless there are complex problems. Services may vary from $30 to $100 an hour.

- Be wary of counselors who suggest megadoses of vitamins and minerals or who sell the remedies they prescribe. Most reputable nutritionists prescribe vitamins and minerals sparingly, concentrating on sharpening your nutritional skills instead.

Where can I get additional information about what to eat while I'm under treatment?

The one best source is a brochure published by the National Cancer Institute entitled "Eating Hints for Cancer Patients: Before, During, and After Treatment." You can order it by calling 1–800–4–CANCER. You also can access it on the NCI Web site (www.cancer.gov).

What can be done about sore mouth or a sore throat that is a side effect of treatment?

First of all, check with your doctor to be sure the soreness is a treatment side effect and not an unrelated problem. The doctor or dentist can give you medication that will help ease throat and mouth pain. Foods that are difficult to chew can irritate a tender mouth or throat. Try eating soft foods that are easy to chew and swallow such as soups, cottage cheese, pastas, pureed meats and vegetables, mashed potatoes, eggs, milkshakes, bananas, applesauce, fruit nectars, watermelon, oatmeal, custards, puddings, and gelatins. Mix food with butter, thin gravies, and sauces to make them easier to swallow. Avoid foods that can irritate your throat such as citrus fruit or fruit juices, spicy or salty foods, rough, coarse, or dry foods such as raw vegetables, granola and toast. Rinse your mouth with water often to remove food and bacteria and to promote healing. If swallowing is difficult, you may find it helpful to tilt your head back or move it forward to change the position of the swallowing mechanism to make it more comfortable.

Do treatments sometimes change your sense of taste?

Many people find that chemotherapy, radiation or the cancer itself can alter taste sensations. Sometimes called mouth blindness, or taste blindness, this side effect can leave you with a sense that food is tasteless or with a bitter, metallic taste in your mouth, especially when eating meat or other protein foods. Usually, this is a short-term problem that eventually resolves itself. To help make foods taste better, you may find that adding flavorings to meats such as bacon, onions, lemon, basil, oregano, or rosemary helps. If red meat is a particular problem, you may want to switch to chicken, turkey, eggs, dairy products, or bland fish for a while. If you don't have a sore mouth or throat, you may find that tart foods such as oranges, lemons, limes, and grapefruit help to bolster your taste buds.

What can be done to relieve a dry mouth or a lack of saliva?

Chemotherapy and radiation therapy in the head or neck area can reduce the flow of saliva and cause you to feel that your mouth is very dry. To help combat this feeling you may find it helpful to suck on hard candy or lollipops (there are many sugar-free types on the market) or chew sugar-free chewing gum. Popsicles are handy to have on hand to help produce more saliva. Keeping a glass of water close by that you can sip every few minutes helps you to swallow and talk more easily. Lip salves help to moisten your lips. If they can be tolerated, very sweet, as well as hot, spicy or tart and sour foods and beverages may help encourage the production of saliva. Lemonade works well but is not advised if you are also suffering from a tender mouth and sore throat. If the problem is very severe, you can ask your doctor or dentist to prescribe products now on the market that coat and protect your mouth and throat.

What can I eat when my mouth and throat are sore from treatment?

Many people who are having chemotherapy or radiation treatments complain of soreness that makes eating difficult.

- Be sure to have the doctor examine the area to see whether or not special medication will help.
- If you have sores under your dentures, remove them and do not wear them when you do not need them for eating.
- Make sure to see your dentist for special care during this period.
- Put your cooked food into a blender so that it is easier to eat.
- Cold foods can sometimes help to soothe the soreness. Add ice to milk and milkshakes.
- Stews and casseroles can be softened with extra liquids and longer cooking times.
- Mashed potatoes, scrambled and poached eggs, egg custards, ricotta cheese, puddings, gelatins, creamy cereals, all kinds of pastas and milkshakes are easy to eat and good for you.
- Stay away from foods that sting and burn such as citrus fruits and tomatoes; hot spicy foods with pepper, chili powder, nutmeg, and cloves; rough and coarse foods such as raw vegetables and bran, and dry foods like toast and hard bread.
- Do not use hot water or commercial mouthwash to rinse your mouth. A mixture of one teaspoon salt or baking soda to a quart of water or equal parts of glycerin and warm water can be soothing. Rinsing with club soda can relieve dry mouth or thick saliva. Oragel, available at the pharmacy, can help deaden the pain.
- If your problem is severe, your doctor can prescribe medication to numb your gums and tongue. Artificial saliva is also available.

Are there ways to help control nausea caused by treatments?

Nausea, with or without vomiting, can be a side effect of surgery, chemotherapy, radiation therapy, and immunotherapy, although today antinausea medications taken before or during treatment usually help to prevent or control it. If you do have nausea, it can be a serious problem because it keeps you from getting the nutrients you need. Foods that are fatty, greasy or fried or hot and spicy, as well as sweet foods such as candy, cookies or cake should be avoided. Foods like toast and crackers, yogurt, sherbet, pretzels, angel food cake, oatmeal, skinned baked or broiled chicken, ice chips, and soft, bland fruits and vegetables usually can be most easily tolerated. Drink or sip liquids through a straw throughout the day, except at mealtimes. Eat small amounts of food often and slowly. Some people find that hot foods can add to nausea, so eat foods at room temperature or cooler. Try to rest after meals. Rest sitting up, if possible, for about an hour after meals. If nausea is a problem in the morning, try eating dry toast or crackers before getting out of bed.

What are some ideas for how to deal with vomiting?
Vomiting may be brought on by treatment, food odors, motion, or gas in the stomach or bowel. You should let your doctor know if vomiting is severe or lasts for more then a few days. Some people find that certain situations or surroundings (such as the hospital setting) may trigger vomiting. Very often, if nausea is controlled, vomiting may be prevented. To help you deal with vomiting, you should not drink or eat until you have the vomiting under control. Once your stomach seems to have settled down, try taking small amounts of clear liquids. Begin with a teaspoonful every 10 minutes, gradually increasing the amount to a tablespoonful every 20 minutes. Then, try two tablespoonfuls every 30 minutes. Once you are able to keep down clear liquids, you can slowly begin to try a full-liquid diet. Continue taking small amounts as often as feels comfortable. Once you are functioning on a full-liquid diet, you can start returning to a regular diet, starting with soft, bland foods. Be sure to discuss any vomiting problems with your doctor and if it cannot be brought under control, ask about medications designed to deal with the problem.

**Is acupuncture ever used as a treatment for nausea
and vomiting caused by chemotherapy?**
Acupuncture, a part of traditional Chinese medicine that is still in use today, has been found, through several clinical studies, to be effective in easing the nausea and vomiting caused by chemotherapy. There also is evidence that it can be used to help control pain, which is discussed later in this chapter. You can find an acupuncturist through the American Academy of Medical Acupuncture, 323–937–5514 (www.medicalacupuncture.org).

**Are there guidelines on amounts of protein and
calories required during recuperation?**
During illness, treatment and recovery, it is estimated that women need about 80 grams of protein (compared to a normal daily need of 44 grams) and men require 90 grams (compared to a normal daily need of 46 grams). An additional 200 to 300 calories should also be added to the diet. Of course,

if your weight is stable, you probably will not need to increase your intake. If you are losing weight, you should definitely try to add extra nourishment.

How can I add protein to my diet?

You can add protein to the diet in several ways without increasing the amount of food you eat. (Some of these are a dieter's dream come true.) For example:

- Add grated cheese, chunks of cheese or melted cheese to sauces, vegetables, soups, sandwiches, and casseroles.

- Add cottage cheese or ricotta cheese to vegetables, fruits, eggs, and desserts.

- Add diced or ground meat or fish to soups, salads, omelets, sauces, and casseroles. Calf or chicken livers are good sources of protein, vitamins and minerals and are a good addition to your diet.

- Cook and use dried peas and beans and bean curd (tofu) in soups, casseroles, pastas, and grain dishes that also contain cheese or meat.

- Add cream cheese or peanut butter as well as butter to your bread.

- Choose dessert recipes that contain eggs—custards, bread puddings, or rice puddings.

- Use milk in beverages and in cooking. Add skim milk powder to your regular milk.

- Use peanut butter—on crackers, waffles or celery sticks—or eat it out of the jar.

- Add ice cream, yogurt, and frozen yogurt to other beverages such as ginger ale and milkshakes, as well as to cereals, fruits, and pies.

- Increase your nut, seed, and wheat germ intake by adding to casseroles, breads, pancakes, waffles, or anywhere a crunchy topping would taste good.

How can I add calories?

- Add butter and margarine to soups, potatoes, hot cereals, rice, noodles, cooked vegetables, sauces, and gravies.

- Use mayonnaise instead of salad dressing on salads or sandwiches. Mayonnaise adds 100 calories per tablespoon.

- Use peanut butter on fruits, vegetables, and sandwiches. One tablespoon of peanut butter has 90 calories and is also rich in protein.

- Use sour cream for vegetable dip and on vegetables. Add to gravy, soups, casseroles, sauces, and salad dressings. One tablespoon of sour cream has 70 calories.

- Add whipping cream to pies, fruit, puddings, hot chocolate, Jell-O, or other desserts. One tablespoon adds 60 calories.

- Add raisins, dates, or chopped nuts and brown sugar to hot cereals or to cold cereals for a snack.

- Have nuts, dried fruits, popcorn, crackers and cheese, and ice cream on hand so you can have a quick snack whenever you feel hungry.

- Add jam, honey, and sugar to bread, cereal, and milk drinks.

- Milkshakes add calories and are easy to make with a blender.

- In food preparation, sauté and fry foods when possible because these methods add more calories than baking or broiling.

Should I worry about how much fat I am eating?
Fats are the most concentrated source of energy. They give about twice the number of calories as do an equal weight of protein or carbohydrates. Therefore, nutritionists believe that if you need additional calories, the most efficient way to get them is by adding fat to the diet.

Doesn't fat cause cancer?
Some research shows that eating too much fat may increase your chance of getting cancers of the colon, prostate, and endometrium. However, you need to look at the requirements your body has while you are undergoing treatment versus the diet you might want to follow for the rest of your life. You need to consider the importance of making sure your body is receiving enough nourishment during treatment.

Is it a good idea for me to go on the higher-fiber, lower-fat diet recommended by the National Cancer Institute for preventing cancer while I am having treatment?
No. For individuals under treatment for cancer, the highest priority is a diet adequate in calories, protein, and vitamins. After you complete treatment, you can modify your diet in order to lower fat intake and raise fiber levels.

Should I also be taking extra vitamins and minerals?
Some researchers suggest adding vitamins and minerals to the nutritional regimen to help protect the body during and following surgery and while taking chemotherapy, to help improve the functioning of the immune system. It's important to distinguish between reasonably large doses of vitamins and vitamin megadosing. Injectable vitamins are another way of boosting vitamin efficiency.

What vitamins and minerals and in what amounts are best for you?

Though the government has come up with a set of standards, the role of many vitamins and minerals is still not fully understood. However, it is known that people recovering from injuries or surgery have greatly increased requirements for certain vitamins. People who smoke, drink moderate amounts of alcohol, or take oral contraceptives also need more vitamins than they otherwise would and may undergo vitamin depletion even when their vitamin intake is normal. The B-complex vitamins are essential in the process by which food is used for energy, cell repair, and all the other essentials of life. Vitamin C is necessary, among other things, for the body to make collagen, a major component of skin, tendons, and bones. The body depends on Vitamin A for healthy epithelial tissue—that is, the tissue that forms the covering or lining of all body surfaces, including the lining of the digestive tract, lungs and blood vessels. Vitamin E is an antioxidant. It protects lipids (water soluble fats) from the attack of oxidizing agents. Potassium deficiencies can result from diarrhea or vomiting. Attention should be paid to increasing potassium either through supplements or by adding potassium-rich foods like potatoes, molasses, apricots, raisins or bananas to the daily diet. However, you should be aware that some vitamins and herbs might affect your treatment negatively. Folic acid, for instance, can interfere with the chemotherapy drug methotrexate. St. John's Wort also has been shown to have adverse interactions with some drugs. Just because a substance is natural doesn't mean it's safe. You should talk with your doctor before you take dietary supplements.

Is there a difference in nutritional needs once treatment is completed?

During treatment, your body needs extra protein and calories to help in the healing process. Once that is all behind you, you'll want to learn about diet and nutrition as it relates to cancer prevention. Although there is little research on whether or not nutrition can prevent recurrence, more and more evidence is being gathered through animal studies and studies of large population groups that correlates lifestyles with cancer, showing that there is a strong connection between good nutrition and good health. Both the American Cancer Society and the National Cancer Institute recommend a diet low in fat and high in fiber. Checking through your nutritional needs with a qualified nutritionist is important since self-prescribing of vitamins or diets can be dangerous. The American Cancer Society has guidelines for Diet, Nutrition and Cancer Prevention for those who are on or have completed treatment.

What can I do about diarrhea problems?

Some kinds of cancers and some kind of treatments can cause diarrhea, excessive gas, or a bloated feeling.

- Drink liquids between meals instead of with them. Liquids are important since diarrhea causes loss of fluids and salts that must be replaced.

- Eat small amounts of food more often. Applesauce, bananas, white rice, tapioca, and plain tea are helpful. Fatty foods and foods which are highly spiced should be avoided.

- If your intestines are irritated, lower the amount of fiber, using only cooked fruits and vegetables and avoiding those with tough skins and seeds such as beans, broccoli, corn, onions and garlic.

- Be aware of your potassium and salt intake. These important elements are lost in great quantities when you have diarrhea, and the result is that you may feel weak. Add foods that are high in potassium but won't worsen diarrhea. Bouillon and fat-free broth are good liquid choices. Bananas, apricot, or peach nectar, and potatoes are all good sources of potassium and don't cause diarrhea.

- Limit foods and beverages that contain caffeine, such as coffee, strong tea, some sodas, and chocolate.

- Diarrhea may be caused by lactose intolerance, which means you have problems digesting the lactose in milk or milk products. Buttermilk, sour cream, and yogurt may be easier for your body to handle.

- If you have cramps, stay away from foods that may encourage gas or cramping, such as carbonated drinks, beer, beans, cabbage, broccoli, cauliflower, and highly spiced foods.

- If your diarrhea is persistent or has blood in it, or if you start to lose weight, see your doctor.

What can be done about constipation?

Constipation may result from treatment with some drugs.

- Make sure your regular diet includes a variety of fruits and vegetables, breads, cereals, bran, dried fruits, and nuts. If you cannot chew or swallow these, grate them or put them in a blender to make them easier to eat.

- Drink plenty of liquids—eight or ten glasses each day.

- Drink prune juice, heated, to stimulate bowel activity.

- Add extra bran to other foods such as cooked cereals or casseroles.

- Eat high-fiber snack foods such as sesame sticks, date-nut or prune bread, oatmeal cookies, Fig Newtons, dried pineapple, date or raisin bars, and granola.

- Try doing some light exercise daily.

- Schedule time to concentrate on bowel movements each day.

- Check with the doctor or nurse before taking a laxative or stool softener.

OUTSIDE HELP

Many kinds of services are available to help you deal with some of the problems that you are likely to face. There are homemaker services, nurses, therapists, and support groups—a whole battery of people who have specialized training to help you through difficult times and specific problems.

What do homemaker services provide?

Homemaker services provide well-trained, adaptable, mature people to help keep a household running. Homemaker services may be available in your area through a community health or welfare agency, a church, a club or some other nonprofit organization. Look in the yellow pages under Homemaker Services.

How can visiting nurses help?

Visiting nurse associations or city health departments provide part-time nursing help to patients at home and offer advice and guidance to help the family and others with care. A visiting nurse will give health instructions and referrals to other agencies that may be of help. You can contact the visiting nurses either directly or through your doctor. If you have health insurance which covers nursing care, the charges (which are adjusted to the patient's ability to pay) may be payable under the policy. Medicare covers some part-time public health nursing in the home if it is ordered by your doctor. Many public health nursing organizations use practical nurses, who attend to all general health needs of the patient and work under the direction of a professional nurse.

Should I schedule extra visits with my dentist?

Cancer and cancer treatment may cause tooth decay and other problems with your teeth and gums, so be sure to schedule follow-up visits with your dentist. Patients who are receiving treatment that affects the mouth, such as those who are having radiation to the head and neck, may need to see the dentist more often than usual. If your gums are very sensitive, clean your teeth with a very soft toothbrush, cotton swabs or mouth swabs made especially for this purpose. Rinse your mouth with warm water to sooth sore gums and mouth.

How can I find a professional sex therapist or counselor?

Many people have sexuality problems following cancer surgery or treatment. Some doctors find it uncomfortable to discuss this subject. However, it is reasonable for you to explain to your doctor that you have concerns about the sexual part of your life. If the doctor is unable to help you with your problem, ask for a recommendation of someone else to help you. You also could ask a nurse or another health professional or minister to make a referral. (See section on Sexuality in this chapter for more information.)

How do I find appropriate support groups?

Today, there are many different kinds of groups, from those that you go to in person and are locally run to chatrooms on the Internet to telephone support groups. Some groups offer support, some education, some are for patients, some for family members and some for both. Some are less traditional and focus on complementary techniques such as visualization, relaxation, and meditation. All offer encouragement, information, strategies for coping and a wonderful place to form friendships with others who understand your problems. The American Cancer Society's I Can Cope program, for instance, addresses the educational and psychological needs of people with cancer and their families. A series of classes are set up to discuss cancer, how to cope with daily health problems, how to express feelings, living with limitations and available local resources. Your nurse, social worker, or the American Cancer Society can assist you with finding a group. The Web site for Cancer Care has a nationwide listing of support groups (www.cancercare.org). It also runs telephone and on-line support groups for various audiences and cancer types. Chapter 28, Where to Get Help, lists other support group information.

Is rehabilitation help available for cancer patients?

Until about ten years ago, most rehabilitation services were prescribed for persons with physical handicaps. Today emotional assistance as part of rehabilitation efforts has been extended to patients with cancer and heart disease. Nearly all cancer patients can benefit from rehabilitation services. The focus is on physical, social, psychological, and vocational needs. It has been found that about 30 percent of people recovering from cancer need assistance with activities involved in daily living and in coping with pain. About 15 percent are deeply concerned about their physical appearance. Arm and leg swelling or breathing problems are of concern to about 10 percent, and about 7 percent have needs in communication and transportation.

What kinds of help are available from a rehabilitation team or physiatrist?

Depending on the needs, team members will vary but the goal is to help you to readapt and to live as normal and full a life as possible. In some cases, a *physiatrist —a doctor who specializes in rehabilitation techniques,* including the strengthening of muscles, the use of artificial limbs, and retraining in day-to-day activities—may be required. Physical therapists or occupational therapists often work together to teach patients the skills needed to allow them to perform their daily tasks. For mastectomy patients, the physical and occupational therapists sometimes work together to teach arm exercises that will help overcome swelling and weakness. Oncology nurses are often helpful in assisting the family to support the patient in becoming more independent.

Social workers, members of the clergy, and lay volunteers can be called upon to provide assistance and advice in both personal and religious matters. Psychologists and other mental health professionals, speech pathologists, dietitians, and pharmacists, all play a role in helping with readjustment.

Is individual therapy a good idea to help me adjust to my cancer diagnosis?

A growing number of psychologists, psychiatrists or licensed clinical social workers specialize in counseling people affected by cancer. Many people find it helpful to explore feelings with a professional who, without judging them, will help them to find ways to deal with the upset in their lives.

What is family counseling?

Family counseling can be valuable if the family group is having problems in dealing with feelings. It can be difficult to discuss the many emotions that changes have brought about. Major shifts in family responsibilities can cause resentment within a family. The loss of accustomed responsibility or authority can cause misunderstandings mingled with anxiety over a loss of power. Children are especially vulnerable as they find their usual roles no longer are defined clearly. If a family has trouble discussing its problems, talking them through in the nonjudgmental atmosphere offered by a professional counselor can be helpful. Besides private counseling services, there are many county health departments and neighborhood or community mental health clinics.

What if I need oxygen to help my breathing problems?

If you need oxygen therapy outside the hospital, your doctor will write a prescription for it, spelling out the flow rate, how much oxygen you need per minute and when you need to use it. Some people use oxygen therapy only while exercising, others only while sleeping and still others need oxygen continuously. There are several different ways oxygen therapy is given. You will be provided with a system that is suitable for your needs. Most systems are set up so that you will have the ability to carry the oxygen with you. If you are using an electrically powered device, you must have a cylinder of oxygen as a backup in the event of a power failure. You should advise your electric power company so that priority service can be given in case of an emergency. You should never change the flow of oxygen unless directed by your physician. Avoid using alcohol or taking any other sedating drugs because they will slow your breathing rate. Be sure to warn visitors not to smoke near you when you are using oxygen. Stay at least five feet away from gas stoves, candles, lighted fireplaces, or other heat sources.

How do I go about getting help for my problems?

Though help is available, it can only come to you at your request and with your consent. Many people suffer needlessly because they are afraid to ask for the help they need. Home healthcare agencies and services such as the American Cancer Society, Visiting Nurses, and public health departments are helpful in pinpointing the specific services that can be utilized. Many county health departments include psychological services, and neighborhood or community mental health clinics are becoming common in cities. Community service organizations such as the United Way usually support mental health facilities. Most of them can be reached with a simple phone call and most of them are more than willing to help you determine what help you need and who is best to call to obtain help.

COMPLEMENTARY THERAPIES

Complementary therapies that include relaxation techniques and other coping strategies are being used in many different ways by many different people. The various techniques embrace the entire field of biofeedback, relaxation, visualization, and meditation. Each method uses its own formula to expand the mind and allow the body to enter a new dimension. We will cover only the basic information needed for you to begin to try the various methods to see if they appeal to you. There are many books, videotapes and cassettes that deal specifically with each technique.

Some of the most common techniques used include:

- Relaxation
- Spirituality and prayer
- Imagery
- Visualization
- Meditation
- Ayurveda
- Yoga
- Biofeedback
- Hypnosis
- Verbal therapy
- Therapeutic touch
- Qigong
- Reiki
- Massage

- Myotherapy
- Polarity therapy
- Laughter

Most of these techniques involve a creative growth process, not a rigid or formal therapy, and you must involve yourself to make them work. At first, you may find the experience confusing and frustrating. But once you learn to concentrate, you may find the whole experience relaxing and rewarding.

What are the basic steps in learning simple relaxation techniques?
Relaxation techniques can be very helpful in daily life, but many people with cancer have found them particularly helpful in dealing with the stresses of treatment and daily living with cancer. There are several simple methods that you can learn quickly.

- **Inhale/tense, exhale/relax.** Breathe in deeply. At the same time, tense all your muscles or a group of muscles of your choice. For example, you can squeeze your eyes shut or you can frown, or clench your teeth, or make a fist, or stiffen your arms or legs, or draw up your arms and legs as tightly as you can. After doing any of these, hold your breath and keep the muscles tensed for a second or two. Then let go and breathe out. Let your body go totally limp. Then relax.

- **Slow rhythmic breathing.** Stare at an object, or close your eyes and concentrate on your breathing or on a peaceful scene. Take a slow, deep breath and, as you breathe in, tense a set of muscles (your arms, for example). As you breathe out, relax and feel the tension draining. Now, remain relaxed and begin breathing slowly and comfortably, concentrating on your breathing. Take about six to nine breaths a minute. Do not breathe too deeply. To maintain a slow, even rhythm as you breathe out, you can say silently to yourself, "IN, one, two, OUT, one, two." If you feel out of breath, take a deep breath and then continue the slow-breathing exercise. Each time you breathe out, feel yourself relaxing and going limp. Try doing a different set of muscles each time. If you feel that some muscles are not relaxed, tense them as you breathe in and relax them as you breathe out. Continue slow rhythmic breathing for a few seconds or up to ten minutes, depending on your need. To end, count silently and slowly to three. As you open your eyes, say silently to yourself: "I feel alert and relaxed."

What can I do if I find it hard to get into a relaxed state?
Learning to relax yourself completely may be hard at first. Practice the simple forms of relaxation several times during the day. You may try doing relaxation

exercises sitting up in a comfortable chair or lying down. Try to choose a quiet spot where you will not be disturbed. Do not cross your arms and legs because that may cut your circulation and cause numbness or tingling. If you are lying down, be sure you are comfortable. Place small pillows under your neck and under your knees, if you find that comfortable.

Is there a quick relaxation theme that I can try?

One that has been found to be almost universally helpful is the beach scene. Think of your favorite beach spot. Recall the pleasant warmth of the sun and the tranquilizing sound of the waves. Imagine yourself basking in the warmth and let the sound of the waves lull you into relaxation. Always try to put yourself inside the scene, rather than being on the outside looking in.

What's the best way to decide which relaxation technique is best for me?

- Try all the different methods, then use the one that suits you best on a regular basis, once or twice a day for five or ten minutes at a time until it becomes easy and routine.

- You should not use these techniques for more than one hour a day.

- Remember that your ability to use relaxation techniques may vary from day to day.

- Take a deep breath if you have a sensation of shortness of breath or of suffocation. Sometimes, however, this feeling may be caused by breathing too deeply. If this is the problem, take shallower breaths and breathe more slowly.

- If the technique puts you to sleep and you don't want to go to sleep, try sitting in a hard chair. You can also set a timer or alarm as insurance. *Spirituality and Health* (www.spiritualityhealth.com) offers its e-mail magazine.

Do many people find spirituality helpful in coping with cancer?

Many people find that their religious beliefs, faith, and prayer are a great comfort, especially during times of crisis. A study of 50 patients at the University of Alabama Comprehensive Cancer Center found that 80 percent felt their religious beliefs helped them in coping with their cancer. This same study also noted that half felt the overall quality of their lives was better after cancer than before their diagnosis. They worried less about material things, they appreciated friends and family more, and their religious beliefs became clearer. These people were realistic yet hopeful, and were combining this hope with renewed interest in their daily lives and involvement with people. *Spirituality and Health*'s (www.spiritualityhealth.com) e-mail magazine offers articles, self-tests, discussion groups, articles, daily thoughts, and e-courses.

What is imagery and how does it work?

Imagery means using your imagination to create mental pictures of situations. There are many different imagery techniques and, though there is no evidence that imagery or visualization can influence the development or progression of cancer, it can help create feelings of being in control. It is like deliberate daydreaming that uses all your senses—sight, touch, hearing, smell and taste. Some believe that imagery is a form of self-hypnosis. To practice the technique, close your eyes. Breathe slowly until you feel relaxed. Then imagine a ball of healing energy forming in your lungs or on your chest. You might imagine it as a white light. Watch it form and take shape. When you are ready, imagine that the air you breathe in blows this healing ball of energy to the area where you have cancer. Once there it heals and relaxes you. When you breathe out, imagine that the air is blowing the ball away from your body, taking the cancer cells with it. Continue to breathe in, bringing the ball of energy to the spot. Breathe out and watch the ball of energy take the cancer cells away. To end this exercise, count slowly to three, breathe in deeply, open your eyes, and say silently to yourself: "I feel alert and relaxed."

What is visualization?

Visualization is a technique in which the mind is given a strong mental experience that it almost cannot distinguish from an actual physical experience. It has been used in a variety of ways over the last few decades. Carl and Stephanie Simonton adopted some of the techniques used by Silva Mind Control after learning that users of biofeedback often were able to communicate with their bodies more effectively by means of an image than by directly trying to influence a certain organ or function. Dr. Bernie S. Siegel has used a similar technique with his patients and has written several books on the subject.

How does visualization work?

No one understands precisely how it works, but psychologist Charles Garfield studied cancer patients who had recovered at the University of California Medical Center in San Francisco. He concluded that most of them had the ability to enter states of mind that enabled their bodies to perform at extraordinary levels—much as trained athletes do. Garfield found similarities between their behavior and the behavior of athletes who had used visualization techniques.

How is visualization taught to athletes?

It is instructive to know how this technique is used in the sports field, because it gives you insights into how you might adapt it for your own use. Most athletes are taught to visualize in a step-by-step process. First they are instructed to write down the entire process in three different ways. They write about preparing to compete, about the actual competition, and about their actions and feelings when they win. Goals are set for each part, focusing on what the person wants to achieve and the end result. The athletes are told to describe as vividly as possible the details of each phase of their participation—the excitement of being part of the event, the crowds, the weather, the sounds and smells. The written description includes feelings of being in control of their physical and mental state, imagining relaxation, and detailing smooth performance at each point in the match or event. Next, they are taught how to review their written material, looking for flaws and making changes until it satisfies them. They are then instructed in relaxation techniques and in the use of visualization of what they have written. This step-by-step process allows the athletes to make the program a part of themselves, feeling it, seeing it in written form and internalizing it. Some athletes report they actually see the movements and all that goes along with them in their minds. Others say they "see" only through strong feelings in their bodies, while still others may hear only the sounds or the rhythms. However, in rigorous athletic training, visualization tries to use all the senses, concentrating them in the brain to foster confidence and achievement. Many do a final visualization before they go to sleep and the next day "play the film back" as they get ready to compete.

How can I make visualization work for me?
The first step is to learn the art of relaxation. Then you can start perfecting the mental picture that addresses your problem in your way. You can imagine your brain turning off the valve that directs the flow of blood to your tumor. Some people picture the cancer cells as crabs. One person said he could imagine a fisherman scooping them up in the net. Another pictured the crabs shriveling up and disappearing. You might choose to think in more medical terms—of your white cells attacking cancer cells and destroying them. The important point, in visualization, is to learn to focus your attention on directing your body to do something positive about changing your cancer situation. Many patients make a point of spending some quiet time each day facilitating the healing process by concentrating on the healing energy in their bodies.

Are there any techniques for making me relaxed enough to do visualization?
Some people find it hard to learn the techniques for reaching relaxation. You may find it helpful to use a tape recorder with a relaxation tape you've bought or made yourself. Making your own tape can be helpful. You may want to ask a friend to help you investigate the technique. It's important, in making your own tape, to go at your own speed. Give yourself images that you enjoy, talking slowly and in a relaxed manner. Repeated use of the technique will make the images more and more vivid. You can do this several times, each time

telling yourself that you'll be even more relaxed when you close your eyes again. Use the tape recorder as long as you feel comfortable with it. Once you've learned the techniques, you may find that the tape is confining and that you can be more creative and relaxed without it. Relaxation becomes easier each time you practice.

How are pictures or drawings used in visualization?

The technique of using drawings was first used successfully with children with leukemia. Many therapists are using the technique to identify conflicts and then using visualization techniques to reprogram the unconscious. Dr. Siegel explains that the most common conflict is in the patient's attitude toward treatment. The patient often says, "I know this treatment is good for me," but unconsciously feels, "This stuff is poison." Dr. Siegel has worked with patients to change the attitude through visualization—making the patient conscious on an intellectual level that this is what may be blocking his progress. He feels that the drawings are a way to get people to open up and think and talk about things they would otherwise conceal, even from themselves.

Where can I find more information on relaxation, imagery and visualization?

There are many books on the subject: *Love, Medicine & Miracles* by Bernie S. Siegel, MD (HarperPerennial, 1998), *Getting Well Again* by O. Carl, MD, et al. (Bantam Books, 1992), and *The Path to Love, Spiritual Strategies for Healing* by Deepak Chopra (Three River Press, 1998).

How is meditation used by cancer patients?

Meditation, like relaxation and self-hypnosis techniques, is another way of disengaging your mind from everyday thoughts and focusing it in a different direction. This mind–body process uses concentration, or reflection to relax the body and calm the mind. It is one of several relaxation methods cited by the National Institutes of Health as having been assimilated into general medical practice as a complementary therapy for improving the quality of life and for treating chronic pain.

What is Ayurveda?

This is a technique developed thousands of years ago in India. Today Ayurveda practitioners are trained in India by institutions in state-recognized programs. There are numerous Ayurveda clinics in the United States. The belief is that all diseases result from imbalances in the body's fundamental forces and disharmony with the environment. Practitioners combine dietary programs, herbal remedies, intestinal cleansing preparations, yoga, meditation, massage, breathing exercises and imagery to treat their patients. Induced vomiting and bloodletting are sometimes recommended. Since many people with cancer already have low blood cell counts because of their disease, these practices can cause imbalances in the blood. Some of the herbal preparations can have interactions with conventional drugs. Two of the herbal preparations used by Ayurveda (called MAK-4 and MAK-5) are being studied by the National Cancer Institutes of Health for their anticancer potential.

How is yoga being used for cancer patients?

You will find a growing number of medical and cancer centers adding yoga as a way for some patients to cope with cancer. Yoga can help improve muscle tone, increase energy, reduce fatigue, and enhance well-being. It also can decrease pain and anxiety and allow patients to better tolerate their chemotherapy. Low impact yoga, known as Kripalu, is the form most often recommended for cancer patients.

How does biofeedback work?

Biofeedback uses electronic signals to help you control your body's automatic functions, such as heartbeat, blood pressure, and muscle tension. The electronic machinery is wired to you and your involuntary functions are monitored and reported through light or sound signals. Through observation of the results, you learn to regulate your body. In learning how to relax muscles, for example, patients are wired to a machine that picks up the electrical current produced by a muscle when it contracts. The machine converts this signal to a light or sound. The person learns how to turn off the signal by relaxing the muscle. With practice, muscle relaxation can then become a conscious action.

Can you do biofeedback on your own?

Biofeedback is best taught with professional supervision. If you want to continue biofeedback on your own once you have learned the technique, several home devices are available. Biofeedback is a tool. You train your body to achieve the relaxation results that the device is measuring. The device serves as a graphic demonstration that you can regulate your hand temperature or your pulse rate. To locate people in your area who are working with biofeedback, look under Biofeedback in the Yellow Pages of your telephone directory, or you can locate a practitioner near you on the Web.

Is hypnosis helpful?

Hypnosis is one of several relaxation methods being studied by the National Institutes of Health as a complementary therapy for treating fear, anxiety, nausea, and chronic pain. You can find hypnotherapists in the yellow pages of your phone book or you can train yourself to use hypnotic techniques. Besides looking in the yellow pages under "hypnotherapists" you can call your county medical society or one of the following organizations to locate a qualified hypnotist: National Board of Clinical Certified Hypnotherapists, Inc., 1110 Fidler Lane, Suite L1, Silver Springs, Maryland 20910 (1–800–449–8144); American Association of Professional Hypnotherapy, 4149-A El Camino Way, Palo Alto, California, 94306 (650–323–3224) or the American Board of Hypnotherapy, 2002 E. McFadden Ave., Suite 100, Santa Ana, California 92705 (1–800–872–9996). See Web page listings at end of chapter. Using these Web pages, you can search for the names of therapists in your area.

How is hypnosis used in healing?

When we hear the word hypnosis, many of us think of hypnosis that is performed on the stage—where an otherwise inhibited, reserved person changes character and behaves in an out-of-character manner. The American Medical Association approved hypnosis as a tool in 1957 and it is being taught to students as a technique in medical schools. Your local medical center may be able to provide you with referrals. Many medical centers are using hypnosis for treatment of pain and many people have used it successfully to help stop smoking. You might consult a doctor, a psychologist, or a hospital-affiliated social worker who has experience with hypnosis rather than going to someone who is simply billed as a hypnotist. Many people start out by going to a qualified hypnotherapist before they try self-hypnosis.

Can I practice self-hypnosis?

There are many different ways of achieving a self-hypnotic state and there are numerous books that cover these methods. We will outline one basic way in which you can achieve a state of relaxation to induce self-hypnosis:

Stage 1

Sit comfortably with your feet on the floor or lie down on a couch or mat. You can direct yourself to relax, or you can repeat a prayer or phrase, you can fix your eyes on one spot or object or listen to a monotonous sound, such as the ticking of a clock or dripping water. Any of these can be used to prepare you so you are ready to progress to the next state. Once you feel ready to relax fully through one of these methods, close your eyes, breathe deeply, and feel your muscles becoming loose, limp, and relaxed.

Stage 2

Some people can become profoundly relaxed with one of the Stage 1 self-hypnosis methods. For most people, however, a second stage of relaxation is necessary to go deeper. You can use any or several of these methods to help you sink into deep relaxation:

- **Deep-breathing method**: Start breathing deeply, counting slowly from one to ten, feeling yourself becoming more and more relaxed. Suggest to yourself that by the time you reach 20, you'll be in a state of deep relaxation.

- **Staircase or elevator method**: Imagine yourself standing barefoot at the top of a beautiful staircase or in a plushly lined elevator that leads down, down, down. The stairs are covered with a thick, luxurious carpet that gets thicker and more luxurious as you go down the stairs. You begin thinking of yourself walking down the carpeted steps, one step at a time, moving slowly. Each step down makes you feel more and more relaxed. Suspended above the stairs as you descend are numbers from one to five. As you pass each number, you feel more and more relaxed and you know that when you reach number five, you will feel completely relaxed.

Stage 3

Now you are ready to take yourself into the third stage, from the staircase or elevator in Stage 2 into your own special environment. Imagine a comfortable space that is your very own. It is furnished to your own taste. It could be a beautiful room, an exquisite garden, a spot by a babbling brook. Make it a safe, neutral spot where you can pause and luxuriate. After experiencing the quiet for a few moments, find a place where you can sit or lie down. Now you can begin to focus on your visualization, seeing your treatment and your immune system removing cancer cells from your body. Try to form active pictures of how this happens. Tell yourself how wonderful you will feel, how well you will be as the cancer disappears from your body.

Stage 4

When you feel ready, you can gradually begin to return from your hideaway, walking to the stairs, climbing the stairway upward, passing level five, then four, then three, then two, and finally one. Take some deep breaths, each breath making you feel better and more alert. Realize that when you open your eyes, you'll feel wonderful and refreshed.

After doing these exercises several times a day, you'll be able to do them more quickly and easily each time. No two people do them in exactly the same way, but it can be satisfying and productive.

Are there any benefits to hypnosis over other kinds of complementary treatments?

Hypnosis seems to offer many benefits and few drawbacks, mainly because hypnosis does not usually have any unpleasant side effects. Some doctors have found that hypnosis is so effective that some patients are able to give up painkilling drugs.

How does hypnosis work?

It depends upon the techniques being used. Hypnosis has been used to block awareness of pain, to substitute another feeling for the pain, to move the pain to a smaller or less significant area of the body, to change the sensation to one that is not painful, and in extreme cases to dissociate the body from the awareness of the pain. Although no one knows exactly how hypnosis works to control real physical pain, there are many who feel they have been helped by this treatment.

What is verbal therapy?

Verbal therapy is the use of words and voice to effect changes. We've all talked to ourselves at one time or another and we all know that talking to ourselves is a way of preparing ourselves mentally, physically, and emotionally for some event. We tell ourselves to slow down or hurry up. We admonish ourselves to calm down when we're about to lose our temper. We all do it, and we do it because it works. You can try this technique concentrating it on a specific part of your body, or on the whole body. Think of your mind and body as a computer that needs positive commands given to it. One helpful exercise calls for programming a statement that represents what you wish to happen, such as "I feel better and better every day." Take a few minutes to repeat it over and over, imagining how good you will feel and the positive results of the improvement. Do this whenever you have a few spare minutes—while waiting in line, driving to work, folding the laundry, mowing the lawn. Get into the habit of verbally giving yourself positive suggestions when talking with others. Listen to how you answer when people ask how you are doing. Do you describe yourself as sick, weak, tired? These words can act as self-suggestions, which can react internally. There are positive affirmation or motivational tapes that can be used to help you in perfecting the technique.

How is therapeutic touch used in healing?

Everyone has the latent ability to use his own natural energy in healing. Scientifically, it is believed that electron-transfer resonance explains what happens when hands are used to transfer energy to another part of the body. Some people unconsciously are able to focus their natural bioenergy field and become known as "healers." The technique is being taught at many nursing schools across the country. But most people can learn the technique and use it on themselves.

- Start by taking three deep breaths to relax your muscles.
- Rub your hands together in a circular, clockwise motion for 15 to 30 seconds.
- Hold your palms six inches to a foot apart for a few seconds and imagine there is an energy field between them, growing stronger and stronger.
- Cup your fingers inward, place your hands just above the area to be treated, and imagine the energy entering the area and healing. It may help to imagine the energy as a bright color.
- Rub your hands again and repeat.

What is qigong?

Qigong, sometimes called chikung, is another form of touch therapy. *Qi* or *chi* = energy and *gong* or *kung* = skill. So qigong is the skill of attracting vital energy. A self-healing art that combines movement and meditation, qigong comes from China and is part of its traditional medicine. Slow, deliberate movements, meditation, and breathing are used to enhance the flow of the body's vital energy that is believed to be disrupted by disease, injury, and stress. Visualizations are used to enhance the mind/body connection and assist healing. Qigong is said to improve blood circulation, reduce stress, establish balance, integrate the mind, body, and spirit and enhance the immune system.

What is the meaning behind Reiki?

Reiki, a Japanese word that represents Universal Life Energy, is also a form of touch therapy. It is a hands-on treatment that realigns fields of energy that are blocked or disturbed. You lie down with your clothes on and the Reiki practitioner places her hands on various parts of your body to adjust the flow of energy.

What is myotherapy?

Myotherapy, sometimes called trigger point therapy, or pressure point therapy, is a form of massage using trigger points in soft tissues of the body to relieve pain and muscle tension. A therapist trained in this method probes muscles to find active trigger points. Direct, firm pressure is applied using a variety of techniques such as direct pressure applied to irritable points along a muscle, massage, and corrective stretching. Many myotherapists are licensed massage therapists and many nurses have learned the techniques. This is a technique that can be used by the caregiver to give relief to a patient who is suffering from muscle pain.

What is polarity therapy?

Polarity therapy is a massage/relaxation technique that is based on the theory that a natural flow of energy through the body maintains health and disruptions of that flow caused by trauma, stress, and other factors, leads to energy imbalances. According to this theory, the top and right side of the body have a positive charge. The feet and left side of the body have a negative charge. The stomach is considered neutral. Practitioners of polarity therapy believe they can identify the sources of energy blockages and disruptions and by applying a variety of hands-on techniques, they can balance and clear the energy field. Some of the techniques used include spinal realignment, rocking motions, deep breathing exercises, stretching, yoga, and using crystals to emit vibrations along the natural energy pathways.

Can laughter help make me feel more relaxed?

It might. Some psychologists are using laughter to help patients who are anxious and depressed. It has been shown to boost your immune system, increase your ability to withstand pain and reduce stress hormones. There are all kinds of ways you can try, such as reading the comics or a humorous book, looking at a funny movie, or listening to an amusing record.

Is holistic medicine a good idea for someone who has cancer?

Holistic medicine covers a whole spectrum of physical, mental, emotional, and spiritual elements. The treatment usually concentrates on the whole body rather than focusing specifically on treating cancer. Practitioners usually recommend changing diet and behavior, and suggest botanical supplements and complementary therapies. While adopting healthy lifestyle habits is considered important, relying on this type of treatment alone, and avoiding conventional medicine, is not a good idea when you are dealing with a cancer problem.

EXERCISE

Should I exercise while I am having cancer treatment?

There are a growing number of studies, especially in breast cancer, that show the value of exercise during cancer treatment. Not only is there evidence that exercise is safe and feasible, but it can also help control side effects such as fatigue, pain, and nausea, increase your physical well-being, and improve how you feel. Even if you are confined to bed, doing some exercise is helpful in counteracting fatigue and depression. If you were exercising before you started treatment, try to maintain that level of activity as much as possible. If you were not, start slowly and continue to add as time goes on. If you feel unsteady, have someone around to help you when you exercise, or do exercises sitting or lying down.

What kind of exercise should I consider doing?

There are many kinds of exercise that you can practice depending upon your energy level. Choose a way of exercising that is something you enjoy. Do it until you are relaxed and pleasantly tired. Don't turn it into another stress in your life. Many people find that walking is one of the best ways to exercise. Consider, if it's convenient, doing your walking in an indoor shopping mall. Many people find it a perfect place to walk because you don't have to worry about the traffic, the weather, or ruts or holes. Any kind of repetitive exercise, such as walking, running, swimming, rowing, or dancing, gives you a chance to relax, meditate or visualize, because you don't have to think about what you are doing.

What if exercise seems like it's too much for me?

Of course you must pace yourself and listen to your body. What's important is finding things to do that you enjoy. Relaxation means different things to different people. People who are physical become filled with tension unless they are active. Aerobics, swimming, bicycle riding, rowing, sailing, tennis, racquetball, golf or volleyball are all ways of relieving physical tension. Or yoga and massage may be your idea of pleasure. Someone else may find relaxation in meditation, mental relaxation techniques, reading, doing crossword or jigsaw puzzles, playing chess or card games, watching TV, or playing computer games. Or perhaps knitting, needlepointing, carpentry, or some other craft activity is your idea of a good escape. Try to give yourself the time to do whatever it is that makes you happy. Pleasure is a powerful prescription for health.

Is it a good idea to combine meditation and exercise?

Studies show that the effects of meditation are multiplied when combined with exercise. Meditation also has physical effects on the body. Like exercise, it tends to lower blood pressure and pulse rates. Brain wave patterns change, showing less excitement. The blood has few stress hormones in it. There is even some indication that there is a connection between meditation and the immune response.

FEELINGS

People deal with their feelings in many different ways. Some people find that talking about their feelings with others is a good way for them to cope. Others find that discussing their disease only with those closest to them works best for them. Normal is what feels right for you. But there are many feelings that are expressed over and over again by people who have been through cancer and it is reassuring to know that you are not alone in your emotional responses.

What should I do if I feel that the treatment is worse than the disease?

In the midst of treatments, many people feel like giving up. You would be wise to voice this feeling to your doctor or nurse. Don't discontinue taking your treatments without a frank discussion with your doctor. They can explain the pros and cons and alternatives for you to think through the reasoning and you can then make the decision about how you wish to proceed.

Why should I stick with a treatment that is difficult and depressing?

Treatments like chemotherapy or radiation are extremely difficult, drawn out and depressing. However, in most cases, they are set up so that you know when they begin and when they end. If you skip out on treatments, you are cutting yourself off from the full benefits of the treatment. You'll increase your chances of being cured if you can keep your sights on the future. Counting down the treatments, and being especially good to yourself while they are going on, can help to make it easier for you to deal with the day-to-day difficulties.

What if I decide to refuse further treatment?

It is your right to refuse further treatment. If you make this decision, treatment will be given only to relieve pain and other symptoms and to keep you as comfortable as possible. If your condition stabilizes, treatment can always be started again. Your doctors will be able to advise you, but they cannot act against your wishes. You are entitled to have complete information about your illness and prognosis, as well as to withhold this information from others if you wish. A federal law requires all medical facilities receiving Medicare and Medicaid payments to inform patients of rights and options about type and extent of medical care. This law, The Patient Self-Determination Act, also requires medical care facilities to provide information about wills and power of attorney.

How can I deal with the idea that I might be dying?

A serious illness like cancer makes you examine your own mortality. There are no simple ways to deal with the question of dying except to try to put it into perspective. Simplistic as it sounds, everyone is one day closer to dying every day of life. You may find it helpful to talk with a good friend, a clergyman, or someone in your family about your fears.

What should I tell relatives, friends, neighbors and others about my cancer illness?

Deciding what to tell others, and how much, is something that each patient or family must deal with. Experience indicates that it is better to discuss the subject than to try to hide it. However, the way in which this is done depends upon your own lifestyle. You may prefer to share problems with those around you fully or it may suit you better to keep discussions about your cancer to a minimum.

Shouldn't children be protected from knowing that a parent has cancer?

It really is best not to try to hide the illness from children. You'll find that intuitively they know what is happening. It is frightening and confusing for them not to be told the reason for the concerns within the household. Children need support and reassurance that whatever happens, they will continue to be loved and nurtured. It is better to tell them only as much as they are able to understand and give them a chance to share and to help. It is a good idea to stay in contact with the child's teacher, coach, Scout leader or school to get more insight into how they are coping with the illness in the family.

Are there special things I should be sure to tell my children?

There are a few things that are useful to remember when you talk with your children. Tell them that they cannot "catch" cancer from you, either by being close to you or by touching you. Be sure they understand that they did not cause you to get the cancer—that it is not their fault. Explain that you are going to be treated and that things may change around the house but that there will be people to take care of them and their needs. Ask if they have any questions—and answer them as honestly as you can.

Is it common for cancer patients to have a hard time concentrating?

You may have heard the term "chemo brain" or "chemo fog." Researchers, who have just begun to study this problem, are finding that one out of every four people with cancer reports to have some memory and attention problems after undergoing chemotherapy. Add to that fact that most cancer patients are older—and people often have memory loss as they get older. In addition, anxieties can create mental disorganization, confusion, and memory disturbances, and give you a feeling of being constantly distracted. You may experience a general feeling of loss of motivation. Even simple tasks like writing a check, dealing with routine business tasks, cooking a meal, or making necessary phone calls can seem overwhelming. Once you concentrate on the fact that the reason for the feeling is because of your underlying health conditions and concerns, you can begin to focus your energy on finding ways to cope with these problems.

What can I do to help with my memory and concentration problems?

The NCI booklet, *Facing Forward: Life After Cancer Treatment*, has several good suggestions:

- Use a pocket notebook to plan out your day, writing down tasks, how long they will take and where you need to go.

- Put small signs around the house to remind you of a couple of the recurring small tasks you need to do, such as taking out the trash or locking up the house.

- Talk yourself though a task with a number of steps. That can help you stay focused.

- Learn relaxation skills.

- Before you go to a party or a work function, practice the information you need to remember—names, dates, etc.

- Repeat what you want to remember so that it can get stored in your memory.

How should I deal with postconvalescence letdown?

The time immediately following the end of treatments can be difficult because it is a cutoff point that leaves you without the routine that had occupied you following diagnosis. In addition, you are no longer seeing your treatment team. This may increase worrying and anxiety levels. You need to be thinking about what you want your new life to be like and get back into a routine as quickly as possible. Taking up a new hobby, starting a new class, getting involved in something that allows you to be completely absorbed will help you to feel alive again. The numbness gradually disappears as you invest yourself in living.

How long does it take for energy level to return to normal?

Many people report that they feel their energy level takes a long time to return to normal—often a year or two after treatment. Studies have shown that some people are still struggling with feeling worn out two or three years after treatment has ended. They explain it as different from being tired because it doesn't seem to get better with resting. Just understanding that it is a side effect and that you are not the only one who has it can be helpful. You should talk with your doctor to make sure that some of the medicines you are taking aren't adding to your fatigue.

How can I describe fatigue to my doctor or nurse?

As with other symptoms, it is very helpful if you can be specific. That means you will have to keep a log or a daily journal so you will have proper information. Keep track of items like:

- When did you first feel it (hours, days, weeks)?
- How long does it last? Do you feel it all the time?

- How does it interfere with your everyday living?
- How many hours are you sleeping at night?
- How do you feel after you sleep? Are you rested?
- Are you cold? Dizzy? Short of breath? Do you have a headache?
- What have you tried? Exercise? Planning activities around resting?
- When were your last treatments? What were they?
- What medicine are you taking?
- What are you eating?
- How much liquid are you drinking?

What can be done about fatigue?

In the past ten years, there has been increasing interest and study in this area. There are a few findings that might help:

- **Exercise:** This area has been studied especially in women with breast cancer. There is strong evidence that aerobic exercise, such as walking or swimming, can decrease fatigue.

- **Improving hemoglobin levels:** For people who have anemia as a result of chemotherapy, the use of erythropoietin (a colony-stimulating factor that stimulates the production of red blood cells) has helped to improve energy levels.

- **Antidepressants:** Although antidepressants can improve moods, it has not yet been shown that they improve fatigue.

There are studies underway in several other areas, such as sleep and rest, stress management, nutritional support and energy conservation that will give additional information on this important subject.

Is it a good idea to plan for a vacation while I'm still under treatment?

We know many people who have chosen to go off on extended trips—sailing, touring, archeological digs, or just beach sitting—and regained a sense of themselves. The first step is to talk with your doctor to find out whether there is a time during treatment that you could get away, perhaps transferring treatment to another location, if necessary. You will need to know:

- How to get in touch with the doctor if there are problems.
- The name, address and phone numbers of doctors who can help you in areas where you will be traveling.

- How to register in advance at an out-of-town hospital or office, what their routine is, how the treatment will be done.

- What arrangements need to be made to pay for treatment, whether the vacation location will accept your insurance, etc.

- The kinds of medications that you should bring with you, possible problems and side effects. Be sure to get your medical records and full information on treatment protocols.

Is it unusual to feel that the loss of a part of my body is more difficult to accept than having cancer?

Many people, especially women who have lost their breasts express this feeling. Any loss of a part of the body, even the extraction of a tooth, is likely to bring about such feelings. Therefore, it's not surprising that the loss of a major body part or function may be more devastating than the fear of cancer. It takes time for these feelings to diminish. Awareness of them can be the first step in developing acceptance.

Are most co-workers supportive of a person with cancer?

Attitudes naturally vary. Some studies have found that coworkers can be among the strongest support networks. However, blue-collar workers were less supportive than white-collar workers. Those people who had cancers that were most visible, such as on the face or neck, had more problems with co-workers than did those whose cancer was not as easily seen. People who had long absences, took off many extra days, or were tired and weak and unable to complete their work had more work-related problems. On the other hand, in the study of white-collar workers, it was found that co-workers willingly took on extra duties and gave moral support and encouragement.

SEXUALITY

Why does the anger I feel at having cancer affect my most personal relationships?

It is not unusual for deep feelings of anger to surface after cancer diagnosis and treatment. Most people feel some form of anger at having a disease over which they feel they have no control. The feeling of helplessness about the situation, the indignities and difficulties of treatment all combine to bring about feelings of anger. Those who are close to you also may have these feelings. Because there is a close connection between anger and sexual feelings, problems in sexual expression may result. Though anger reactions may be different for each partner and each couple, they often exist and are sometimes repressed. An important part of the healing process is to allow these feelings to be expressed. Once the anger has been confronted and understood, steps can be taken toward accepting it and other emotions triggered by a cancer diagnosis.

Is it common for couples who never had sexual problems to develop problems when one of them has cancer?

Since 50 percent of the general population has sexual problems caused by stress, it's certainly understandable why cancer and cancer treatments may put stress on sexual relationships. In addition, as people age, changes take place in response and performance as well as in attitudes toward sexuality. These changes may not be noticed until a crisis occurs. Open, honest communication between partners is essential. Try to express your feelings and concerns honestly.

Why is it that since I've had cancer I have little or no sex drive?

The way you feel is quite normal and can be an expected change as stress decreases. There can be physical reasons, such as decreased desire caused by treatments. Lessening of sex drive can occur during many different stages of the disease: during diagnosis, at various times during treatment, when new treatments need to be undertaken, or when you feel ill or in pain. At these times, there is a great need for physical contact, though not necessarily for sexual intercourse. Partners should be aware that the special warmth of a loving touch conveys feelings in a very direct way. Sitting or lying together, holding each other, cuddling, giving a warm, spontaneous hug, a kiss on the cheek, gentle stroking of hair, or a relaxing back rub are all ways of being sexual and fulfilling the need to be physically close. You need to tell your partner how important it is to you to be touched and held even if you do not want to have intercourse. Try not to make your partner guess at your feelings.

Is it possible that my partner thinks my cancer could be contagious?

There is a great deal of anxiety about sexual transmission of disease, due largely to herpes and AIDS. However, there is no evidence to show that cancer is contagious. Sexual contact will not cause your partner to "catch" your cancer or to develop cancer of the sexual organs, mouth, or any other body part. Nor will you develop a recurrence or spread your cancer as a result of having sexual intercourse. If this is a problem, you need to talk openly with your partner about this fear.

Will my body responses ever be the way they once were?

Some people complain that they feel sad and frightened because their body does not respond as it once did. By accepting the lonely and fearful feelings, acknowledging them to someone else and having your feelings accepted, you begin an important process. Try giving yourself the freedom to explore and perhaps to define what gives you sexual pleasure. You can help bring new closeness by talking about the changes with people you love. Examining alternatives is, in itself, an important step.

Can I have children after I have had treatment for cancer?

If you wish to have children after you've had cancer treatment, you need to discuss this with your doctor before you start treatment. Whether or not you will be able to get pregnant or father a child depends on the type of cancer you have and the kind of treatment you are going to undergo and where that treatment will be given to your body. The good news is that many people have had children after being treated for cancer. Also there doesn't seem to be any increased risk of damage to the chromosomes (which result in birth defects) in children born to parents who have had cancer treatment.

Can surgery be done in a manner so that I can have children?

Yes. For instance, you can have surgery for cancer of the cervix that takes out only the cervix and leaves the neck of the uterus. The doctor will be able to use purse-string sutures at the end of the uterus to improve the chances of holding on to a pregnancy. However, some surgeries will affect your ovaries, vagina, or other reproductive organs that make it impossible to get pregnant. It is important to discuss this question thoroughly with your doctor.

Does the fact that I had chemotherapy affect my ability to have children?

Many of today's chemotherapy drugs are less damaging to the reproductive system and do not cause permanent infertility. Your fertility may return months or even years after treatment ends. However, some chemotherapy drugs can damage the heart or lungs. Women need to be tested to see if they can withstand the demand of being pregnant.

Can radiation treatment cause problems with my ability to become pregnant?

Radiation in the abdomen area might cause thinning of the uterus lining that may result in premature birth or low birth weight. If your radiation is in the abdomen or pelvic area you might lose your ovarian function. However, it is often possible to protect reproductive organs from radiation damage. It is possible to have an oophoropexy (an operation to move the ovaries behind the uterus) before beginning radiation therapy. This helps preserve ovarian function by shielding the ovaries from exposure to radiation during treatment. At some research centers, ovarian tissue is being frozen for future egg development, but the technology is at a very basic stage.

Can I get pregnant soon after I finish treatment?

Most doctors advise women to look at the normal time for recurrence, if any, of their individual cancers. They urge women to wait until after that time has passed before getting pregnant. This is another subject that you need to discuss with your doctor in-depth because it not only depends on the type of cancer you have had and the treatment you received but also on your own attitudes and needs. (There is more information about pregnancy and cancer in Chapters 13, 14, and 20.)

Why is it so hard for me to talk to my doctor about intimacy and sexual feelings?

Many people tend to be afraid that others will be shocked or embarrassed if we bring up sex when they feel we should be concentrating on our health and well-being, as though sex weren't a natural part of well-being. Fortunately, an increasing number of people (doctors included) will respond to direct questions about sexual function without embarrassment or shock. And if you make it a habit to try to have a continuing dialogue with your partner, you will be keeping communication lines open so that you can continue to express yourself and your needs.

If my doctor won't discuss my sexual problems with me, who should I see?

It's reasonable for you to say to your doctor, "I have concerns about sex. Is this something you can help me with, or can you refer me to someone else?" Some doctors are uncomfortable with questions that pertain to personal relationships. It may be tempting to give up when you've been rebuffed, but remember that your concerns are legitimate and that support and information are available. There are many people trained to deal with the problems you are experiencing.

What does a sex therapist do?

Usually, a sex therapist wants to hear from both partners about problems and how each partner views them. Just bringing problems into the open and discussing them with a professional can be a big help.

How do I find a professional sex therapist or counselor?

The professionals most qualified to deal with your sexuality problems include psychiatrists (medical doctors who specialize in mental health), psychologists (people with a PhD or master's degree in psychology), licensed marriage and family therapists, and social workers. Those who specialize in marriage or family counseling usually are best qualified to deal with the kinds of problems you may be experiencing. Those who are most highly trained usually belong to one or more of the following organizations:

- American Association of Sex Educators, Counselors and Therapists
- American Association for Marriage and Family Therapy
- Association of Oncology Social Workers

Two of the organizations—the American Association for Marriage and Family Therapy (www.aamft.org) and the American Association of Sex Educators, Counselors and Therapists (www.aasect.org)—have searchable Web sites that provide names of therapists with information on education, professional licenses, practice description, and health plan participation. If your physician or other health professional or minister cannot make a referral, you also can locate members of these organizations by looking in the yellow pages under Marriage and Family Counseling or by consulting the American Cancer Society, Cancer Information Service, local Family Service, or United Way agencies.

What questions should I ask the therapist before starting therapy?
Some questions you might want answered include:

- What is your professional training?
- Have you had training and experience in dealing with sexual problems relating to cancer?
- Do you usually see partners together or as individuals? (It is advisable if both partners are together when advice is given.)
- How frequently will we meet?
- How long are the sessions?
- What does each session cost?
- Does insurance cover the cost?

Why is it so difficult to start an intimate relationship after cancer surgery?
Before you can expect someone else to become accustomed to the changes in your body due to cancer surgery, you must come to grips with your own feelings of self-rejection. These very normal feelings hamper your self-image and make it hard for you to move into new intimacies. You may find it necessary to risk rejection as part of your emotional healing process. You will learn, through this risk, that you are still desirable and attractive. Take time to become accustomed to the way your changed body looks. It is helpful to study yourself nude in front of a mirror. Once you become more comfortable

with the way you look, you'll be able to move toward a new intimate relationship with more confidence.

How can a single person deal with telling a potential partner about a cancer history?

This is a difficult question with different answers for different people. Much, of course, depends upon your own medical situation. To help you with your perspective, try to think about how you would tell someone about yourself if you had heart disease or diabetes rather than cancer. Usually, discussing the subject in an honest and open manner is best. This does not mean that you need to discuss your problems with everyone you meet in a casual way. If the subject should arise in the course of conversation, then you can contribute insights from your own personal experience. This question is one that is often discussed in support groups. It might be possible for you to find a group in your area where there are other people with the same concerns with whom you could share your thoughts.

How can a single person without a partner fulfill needs to be touched and held?

It is difficult to be alone during times of stress, and the need to have real contact with others is one that needs to be recognized and fulfilled. It is important, especially in time of crisis, to have the support of friends, neighbors, family, and religious or social groups.

- Reach out to friends, coworkers and neighbors, letting them know your needs. Greet them with a warm embrace. Take the time to include them in your life.

- Find a cancer support group where you can discuss your problems with others who understand.

- Massage can give real relief from depression, stress, anxiety and pain. Perhaps a friend can give you a simple back rub. Or you might treat yourself to the services of a massage therapist. Check with local YMCAs, health clubs, or beauty salons for names of qualified massage therapists.

- Giving pleasure to yourself, through masturbation, is a possible avenue for some to explore.

How can I get my partner to start talking about sexual feelings?

Sometimes it's hard to discuss intimate feelings. Yet it can be dangerous to second-guess what your partner is thinking. The questionnaire on pages 975–976 was designed so that each partner could fill it out separately. Make a second copy for your partner. You can then compare notes and use what you learn about each other to gain greater understanding. This is not a test. There are no passing or failing scores. The statements merely highlight what is happening in your sexual life and may help you to understand each other better.

After you have discussed your checklists together, you may want to talk about the following questions:

- How satisfied are you with the quality of closeness you share?
- How important is sexual intercourse to you as an expression of intimacy?
- How important are other means of physical interaction to you?
- What makes you feel most loved and appreciated?
- What was one recent circumstance that made you feel close?
- What keeps you from becoming closer?
- What would make you happier?
- What does your partner think makes you happiest in your physical relationship?

What does the doctor mean when he tells me to find "other means of sexual expression"?

Genital intercourse is only one way of expressing physical love. If your cancer problems no longer make this possible, there are other alternatives. People find that using hands, thumbs, fingers, tongues, lips, and mouths can provide exciting and pleasurable alternatives to "normal" intercourse. A sexual therapist can help you and your partner to explore possibilities.

Is masturbation a solution?

If your religious, social and cultural background permits it, masturbation is a form of sexual activity that can be a satisfactory form of gratification when sexual intercourse is not possible or not desired. Some people have found that mechanical vibrators can be used, either alone or along with other sexual activities, with their partners.

PAIN

People who have cancer may have pain for a number of reasons. It may be due to the cancer itself or may be the result of treatment. It can depend on the type of cancer, the stage of cancer, and personal tolerance for pain. Many people put up with pain, thinking that nothing can be done. Some people have concerns about side effects of pain medications because they think they can become addicted. As a matter of fact, addiction is extremely rare in people

PUTTING YOUR RELATIONSHIP INTO PERSPECTIVE

	TRUE OR FALSE	DON'T WANT TO DISCUSS	DOES NOT APPLY
I want to share intimacy but am not up to sexual intercourse.			
She/he doesn't seem interested in sex.			
I don't seem to get sexually aroused.			
I'm afraid it will hurt.			
I'm not interested anymore.			
I purposely avoid sex.			
Sex is unsatisfying for me.			
I'm satisfied just being held and cuddled.			
I feel failure and inadequacy about sex.			
I wish we could be more open and frank.			
I get excited but don't reach a climax.			
I'm getting too old to enjoy sex.			
I can't seem to get an erection/climax so I avoid sex.			
My partner won't try anything different.			
My illness has changed the way I see myself as a person.			
I'm not sure whether he/she is avoiding me, doesn't feel up to it, or just isn't interested.			
I think it's time we faced the fact that we cannot have intercourse and should discuss other means of physical interaction.			
I would be happy if he/she would talk with me honestly about how he/she feels about making love.			
He/she is afraid of catching cancer.			
I'm embarrassed about the changes in my body.			

(continued)

PUTTING YOUR RELATIONSHIP INTO PERSPECTIVE (continued)

	TRUE OR FALSE	DON'T WANT TO DISCUSS	DOES NOT APPLY
I think my partner is unfair to want sex when I'm so ill.			
I think it's inappropriate to be thinking about sex in the midst of a life-threatening illness.			
I'm ready to give up the sexual factor in our relationship, but I'd like to talk about it.			
I've never tried masturbation.			
I find self-stimulation is a good sexual outlet for me.			
I'm turned off by changes in his/her body.			
I think masturbation is abnormal.			
Sex is still good, even though we have problems.			
I'd be willing to try some different ways of making love.			
Our love has developed into deeper love.			

taking medication for cancer pain. Pain is a separate medical condition that requires separate treatment. When pain is not well controlled, it can lead to depression, fatigue, anger, or isolation. Almost all pain caused by cancer can be relieved. However, a team effort is important when managing cancer pain. Patients and families need to talk with doctors, nurses, and pharmacists about pain and its treatment. Information in this chapter under "Relaxation Techniques" has been helpful in reducing pain for many people.

Is it true that most cancer patients do not experience a great deal of pain?

Most people think of cancer as a painful disease. The truth is that many cancers cause little or no pain in their early stages. Therefore, the people whose cancers are found and treated in an early stage usually have only the pain and discomfort that is part of any operation or treatment. This pain is temporary and can be easily tolerated and controlled with medication.

What can be done for pain that is caused by cancer?

The best way to manage pain is to treat the cause. If you have a cancer that has spread, then your doctor will probably recommend surgery, radiation therapy, or chemotherapy to remove the tumor or decrease its size. When none of these procedures can be done, or when the cause of the pain is not known, then other pain-relief measures are needed—and there are many available. Together, you, your doctor and nurse, can decide which methods are best for you.

Is it important to treat pain a patient has as a result of surgery?

There are some new studies that indicate that it is important to treat pain aggressively before, during, and after surgery, especially during the first 48 to 72 hours. Pretreatment with pain medication before surgery can decrease the dose needed after the operation.

Is pain more of a problem with advanced cancers?

Pain occurs more often in people with advanced cancers. But even among people with advanced disease, more than half have little or no pain or discomfort. Some advanced patients require light medication. For those who experience severe pain, there are excellent methods of pain relief that can be prescribed.

Is cancer pain different from pain of other illnesses?

Some recent studies seem to indicate that when cancer pain occurs, it has different characteristics, since it may be both severe and of long duration. And since it is a reminder of the disease, the pain of cancer patients is also believed to have some psychological aspects.

Do some people feel more pain than others?

Some people are more sensitive to pain than others. Response to pain depends upon a number of factors: a person's general makeup, whether there are especially sensitive nerves at the point of pain, how long the pain has persisted and how much pain can be endured (called pain tolerance or threshold of pain).

Can worry, unhappiness, or fear intensify pain?

Studies have shown that worry, unhappiness, or fear can make pain feel more intense. This does not mean that the pain does not exist—it means that if you can learn how to keep yourself from worrying about it, it can be lessened and tolerated more easily.

What are the main causes of pain for patients with advanced cancer?
Pain can result from any of the following causes:

- Pressure on a nerve caused by a tumor.
- Infection or inflammation.
- Poor blood circulation because of blocked blood vessels.
- Blockage of an organ or tube in the body.
- Bone fractures caused by cancer cells that have spread to the bone.
- Aftereffects of surgery, stiffness from inactivity, or side effects from medications.
- Nonphysical responses to illness—such as tension, depression, or anxiety.

What methods are available for controlling pain?
There are a variety of methods available for helping to control pain. There are many drugs that can be used to help reduce pain as well as other methods that you can use.

How do doctors decide how much pain medication to give me?
Physicians who treat cancer pain use a three-step ladder, developed by the World Health Organization, for cancer pain management. Treatment usually begins as low as possible on the ladder, working up gradually until control of the pain is achieved.

- The first step deals with mild pain. Analgesics such as acetaminophen (Tylenol) may be used. Or nonsteroidal, anti-inflammatory drugs such as aspirin or ibuprofen (Motrin or Advil) may be ordered. Other types for specific pain or other types of symptoms may require antidepressants such as Elavil; anticonvulsants like Tegretol or Dilantin; antinausea medication and antianxiety medicines such as Xanax, Valium, Ativan, Atarax or Vistaril.
- The second step, for moderate pain, includes weak narcotics, which may be prescribed for use along with some of the medications listed above. Codeine, Darvon or Darvocet, Empracet and Wygesic may be used for short-term help since they cause side effects when used over a long period. Tylox, Percocet, and Percodan are stronger medications that are also used for moderate pain.
- The third step is reserved for severe pain. These strong narcotics may be either short-acting or long-acting. Morphine, Dilaudid, and Numorphan are strong narcotics that last from three to four hours. Methadone, another strong narcotic, gives four to six hours of relief. Many of these medicines are available in 12-hour time-released pills.

What other methods can be used for pain relief?
Several other procedures can be used:

- Medication can be combined with a number of methods such as skin stimulation, distraction, relaxation, acupressure or acupuncture, biofeedback, and imagery.

- Nerve blocks or neurological pain relief can be used to block pain messages that are sent by nerves to the brain.

- Surgery or injection of a local anesthetic into the nerve sometimes works.

- Radiation therapy is often used to relieve pain when cancer has spread to other sites.

Is it wise to do something about pain as soon as it begins?
It is important to try to prevent pain from becoming chronic. Don't wait for pain to get worse before doing something about it. Learn which methods of pain relief work best for you. Plan on varying and combining pain-relief methods. Try each method more than once. If it doesn't work the first time, try again before giving up on it.

What if my doctor says nothing more can be done to help relieve my pain?
Cancer pain almost always can be lessened or relieved. And, it is important to remember that it takes less pain medication to keep pain away than to break an acute, established pain cycle. If your doctor feels that nothing more can be done, ask about a referral to a pain clinic or specialist in pain management. The following sources can help you locate a pain program or specialist:

- Call the Cancer Information Service at 1–800–4–CANCER. They will be able to help you find pain-related services in your area. Ask them specifically about "Cancer Pain Initiatives" in your state.

- The American Cancer Society is another source of information about pain specialists. For more information you may call the American Cancer Society at 1–800–ACS–2345.

- There are a number of associations of physicians who deal with pain. The American Academy of Pain Medicine, 4700 W. Lake, Glenview, IL 60025, telephone 847–375–4731 is a good place to start. You can also bring up names of pain specialists in your area by using the Web sites listed at the end of this chapter.

- There are pain clinics in all parts of the country that specialize in dealing with pain. Check the Web sites at the end of this chapter for how to find a pain clinic.

What if the medication isn't working, or if there are side effects caused by the medication?

If there is still significant pain, ask the doctor about other medicines or ways of taking them.

- Ask about increasing the amount of medicine by small amounts until the dose works.
- Ask about shortening the time between doses.
- Ask about taking short-acting or immediate-release narcotics in between long-acting medications.
- Ask if there is another way to give the medication if taking pills is difficult:
  - Skin patches, which are placed on the body, can deliver medication through the skin to give pain relief for up to 72 hours.
  - Pain medicine sometimes comes in suppository form, liquid form, or can be given by injection.
  - Subcutaneous needles can be placed by a nurse, with medicine injected through the line every few hours. These lines can also be hooked to pumps or simple battery devices that deliver the medicine at regular times.
  - Larger intravenous lines called Hickmans, Broviacs, or catheters can be placed into large veins.
  - Small portable pumps with IV lines can be worn on the body. They can deliver medicine evenly during the day and night.

Don't give up looking for ways to relieve pain. If pain persists, the patient, caregiver, and health care staff should discuss what can be done to bring about relief.

Is it a good idea to save the pain medicine until the pain is severe?

Taking pain medicine for mild discomfort does not affect how well it will work when the pain is more severe. Do not hold back on taking pain medicine. Take it as prescribed. It takes more medicine to treat pain that is uncontrolled than it does to prevent the pain. You may need more pain medicine in the future because the pain has changed. If the pain is controlled now, you know that the medicine works.

Questions to Ask the Doctor About Pain Medication

- **What do I do if the medicine wears off and the pain returns but it is too early for the next dose?**
- **What do I do if the pain causes insomnia?**
- **What do I do if I accidentally skip a dose of medicine?**
- **Can the pills be crushed by the pharmacist or mixed in a liquid so they're easier to swallow?**

What is breakthrough pain?

Breakthrough pain is a sudden flare-up of pain that breaks through the medication you take for your persistent pain. It may last a few minutes or for 30 minutes before it subsides. Eighty-six percent of patients report this type of pain. The treatment for breakthrough pain is different than for the pain you normally feel. A short-acting opioid, such as immediate release oral morphine, can be used. It will relieve breakthrough pain quickly, with a long-acting opioid added for persistent pain. You should discuss this type of pain with your doctor. Do not assume that what you're doing is all that is available. Keep track of when the breakthrough pain occurs, how long it lasts and how intense it is. Ask for a quick-working medication you can keep on hand that will help to alleviate the problem.

Is it a good idea for me to keep a record of my pain?

Keeping a record of when you have pain and how bad the pain is, is the first step in dealing with it.

How can I describe how intense the pain is?

A pain scale has been devised to assign a number to the intensity of the pain:

0 = no pain

1 = discomfort

2 = mild pain

3 = distress

4 = severe pain

5 = the worst pain

What should a record of my pain include?

Included should be: The number on the rating scale that describes your pain before and after using a pain-relief medication or technique; the time you take medication; any activity that seems to increase or decrease pain; any

SOME POSSIBLE SIDE EFFECTS OF PAIN MEDICINES

Call the doctor or nurse if any of the following symptoms occur:

- Hallucinations (hearing or seeing things that are not there).
- Ringing or buzzing in ears.
- Sudden confusion.
- Severe trembling or convulsions.
- Numbness or tingling in feet or lower legs.
- Inability to hold urine or stool when this was not a problem before.
- Inability to urinate even though feeling the need.
- Inability to have a bowel movement for a number of days.
- Nausea or vomiting without relief.
- Hives, skin rash, itching or swelling of face.

If you are bothered by side effects from one medication, ask the doctor about other medicines or ways of taking them that might be more effective.

activity that you cannot do because of pain; the name of the pain medicine taken and dose; how long the medication works; any other techniques used besides pain medication. The chart shows you one way of organizing your pain diary.

DAILY PAIN DIARY FOR _____ (NAME)

DATE: _____

TIME	PAIN RATING	MEDICATION USED	OTHER PAIN RELIEF METHODS TRIED	ACTIVITY
Set up hour by hour or for specific times of day	Use scale numbers 1–5 as suggested or set up your own scale	List type of medication taken and dosage	List anything tried— relaxation, etc. and success rating	List whether resting, sitting, standing, walking, etc.

What do I need to tell the doctor or nurse about my pain?

There is specific information you can tell your doctor and others who are helping you with pain, such as:

- Where do you feel the most pain?

- What does it feel like? Is it sharp, dull, throbbing, or steady?

- When did it begin?

- Does it keep you from doing your daily activities? Which ones?

- What relieves the pain?

- What makes it worse?

- What have you tried for relief?

- What helped? What did not help?

- Have you been successful in the past in relieving pain? How?

- Is the pain constant? If not, how many times a day (or week) does it occur? Does it occur when you are lying down, standing, walking, etc.?

- How long does it usually last?

- Does it interfere with sleeping?

- Does it interfere with eating?

- Does it affect you emotionally?

Only when health professionals know exactly how pain is affecting you can they help you to find the right type of pain control.

What are the usual nonprescription pain relievers used?

These include **aspirin** sold under brand names like: Bufferin, Ascriptin, Ecotrin, etc.; **acetaminophen** sold over-the-counter as: Anacin-3, Tylenol, Datril, etc.; and **ibuprofen** such as: Advil, Motrin, Nuprin, etc. Other brand names also contain one of these three medicines, which are effective for relief of moderate and mild pain. You can check the labels, or your druggist can help you to find a generic product that may be less expensive than the brand name ones. (Be sure to check with your doctor or nurse to be certain they are safe to take along with your other medications.)

Do aspirin, acetaminophen, and ibuprofen help solve different problems?

- Aspirin and ibuprofen are often used to reduce the pain of swollen joints and other inflamed areas. Acetaminophen is not.

- Acetaminophen does not irritate the stomach. Aspirin and ibuprofen can irritate and cause stomach bleeding.

- Acetaminophen has no effect on blood clotting. But kidney or liver damage may result from use of large daily doses or drinking large amounts of alcohol with the usual dose. Aspirin and ibuprofen can affect blood clotting and cause bleeding.

- Ibuprofen can make existing kidney problems worse. In normal doses, aspirin and acetaminophen usually do not cause kidney problems. It may be dangerous for patients with low platelet counts to take these drugs because they can interfere with the ability of blood to clot.

- Aspirin, when used to treat children with viral diseases such as the flu or chicken pox, may cause Reye's syndrome, a rare brain and liver disease. Acetaminophen and ibuprofen can be used to treat viral diseases without causing Reye's syndrome.

- Aspirin should be avoided by people who are on anticancer drugs that may cause bleeding and steroid medicines such as prednisone, are taking blood-thinning medicine, have stomach ulcers, are taking prescription drugs for arthritis or are taking oral medicines for diabetes or gout.

- Some nonprescription drugs also contain aspirin—such as Excedrin, Coricidin and Alka-Seltzer.

- Be sure to check with your pharmacist to be certain there is no aspirin in prescription pain relievers.

What are safe daily dosages of aspirin, acetaminophen and ibuprofen?

You should always check with your doctor, nurse or pharmacist about taking any medication because doses of these pain relievers are different for different people. However, in general, here are some guidelines.

Aspirin: The usual safe dose is two to three tablets (325 mg or five grains each) taken three or four times a day. Eight aspirins a day is the average dose, but many adults can take 12 a day. Any higher dose should be taken only if prescribed.

Acetaminophen: The same as aspirin. Extra-strength formulas, such as extra-strength Tylenol, which are 500 mg or seven and a half grains, should be limited to eight tablets over 24 hours.

Ibuprofen: One 200 mg tablet every four to six hours is the usual dose. No more than six tablets should be taken in 24 hours. Larger doses should be taken only if they are prescribed by the doctor.

Aren't prescription medications stronger and more effective than nonprescription pain relievers?

Many nonprescription medicines are stronger analgesics than people realize. Research has shown that for most people the usual dose of nonprescription pain relievers provides as much pain relief as prescription medications such as codeine or Darvon—and with fewer side effects.

What are some of the prescription non-narcotic, drugs used for pain relief?

There are many prescription non-narcotic drugs. They include celecoxib, choline magnesium trisalicylate, diclofenac, etodolac, fenoprofen calcium, endomethacin, ketorolac, meclofenamic acid, meclofenamate sodium, nabumetone, naproxen, oxaprozin, piroxicam, rofecoxib, sulindac, and tolmetin sodium.

Are both nonprescription and prescription drugs sometimes ordered?

Many doctors find that patients who need prescription pain medicine also can benefit from continuing to take regular doses of nonprescription drugs. The two types relieve pain in different ways, attacking pain on two levels. It is a good idea to discuss with your doctor whether you should continue taking aspirin, acetaminophen, or ibuprofen in addition to prescribed drugs.

What are the different kinds of high-powered pain relievers?

There are a number of different kinds. Narcotics, also called opioids or opiates, may be natural or synthetic products. They may be taken by mouth, intramuscularly by injection, through a vein, through a skin patch or by rectal suppository (not all are available in each of these forms). Among those more commonly used are:

- Codeine
- Hydromorphone
- Hydrocodone
- Levorphanol Methadone
- Meperidine
- Morphine
- Fentanyl (available as a skin patch)
- Oxycodone
- Oxymorphone

Won't I become addicted if I use narcotics for pain relief?

Narcotic addiction means that you depend on the regular use of narcotics to satisfy physical, emotional and psychological needs rather than for medical reasons. Drug addiction in cancer patients is rare. Addiction is a common fear of people who take narcotics for pain relief. If narcotics are the only effective way to relieve pain, your comfort is more important than a remote possibility of addiction. If you have concerns about addiction, share them with your doctor or those who are caring for you. Remind yourself that other people's concerns about pain relief addiction are often due to lack of information.

Isn't morphine given only to patients who are dying?
Morphine is not reserved for those who are dying. It is an effective medicine for many types of cancer pain and taking it does not mean that you are dying. It is a drug commonly used at the time of a major surgery. Some people go back to work and resume their regular activities because the morphine is so effective in preventing pain.

If pain becomes severe, will I need shots for pain relief?
Probably not. Intramuscular injections or "shots" are rarely used for relieving cancer pain. Narcotic rectal suppositories can be effective, and new methods of giving narcotic pain relievers have been developed. Long-acting morphine tablets are now available and some narcotics provide quick pain relief when they are given under the tongue (sublingually). One narcotic drug, fentanyl, is now available as a skin patch which continuously releases the medicine through the skin for 48 to 72 hours.

What is patient-controlled intravenous medication?
With this method, a portable computerized pump containing the medication is attached to a needle that is placed in a vein, just under the skin or in the spinal area. You control the pain medication. When you press a button on the pump, a preset dose of pain medicine is delivered.

How is the skin patch used?
A patch that looks much like a bandage is put on the skin. The medicine in the patch releases slowly through the skin for two to three days.

Isn't there a method that dispenses the medication under the skin?
A simple, safe and effective method, called continuous subcutaneous infusion, uses a small electronic pump to dispense the drug automatically through a small needle placed under the skin.

How does an ambulatory infusion pump work for relieving pain?
An ambulatory infusion pump makes it possible to have medication, such as continuous morphine infusions, away from a hospital setting, and while continuing usual activity. The pump operates on a seven-day rechargeable power pack. It fits into a pocket so that continuous medication and ongoing pain relief are possible.

What about medication injected into the spine?
Another way of treating cancer pain is to inject the pain medicine into the space around the spine, called intrathecal drug delivery. Because the medicine goes directly to the cells in the spinal cord, less is needed to relieve pain. You also may be able to have a programmable pump implanted under the skin, around your waist area, to deliver the medicine at a set rate into the intrathecal space.

What is the injectable radioactive medication for bone metastases?
Strontium-89 (Metastron) is sometimes used in treating the pain of bone metastases. More information on this medication is found in Chapter 26, When Cancers Recur or Metastasize.

Is heroin available for pain relief?
Heroin is not legally available in the United States. Strong narcotics like morphine and Dilaudid usually relieve very severe pain. In fact, the body converts heroin to morphine. Even in England, where heroin is available, morphine is being used routinely because it has been shown to be just as effective as heroin.

Are there other drugs that can be used along with narcotics to relieve cancer pain?
There are several classes of drugs that are used along with—or instead of—narcotics to relieve cancer pain.

- Antidepressants, such as amitriptyline, nortriptyline, desipramine, and antiseizure drugs, such as carbamazepine and phenytoin, are used to control burning and tingling pain.

- Antihistamines, such as hydroxyzine or diphenhydramine, relieve pain, help control nausea, and help with sleeping problems.

- Antianxiety drugs, such as Diazepam and Lorazepam, may be used to treat muscle spasms that may go along with severe pain. They are also helpful in treating anxiety.

- Steroids, such as prednisone or dexamethasone can be used to lessen swelling that can cause both chronic and acute cancer pain.

- Nonsteroidal anti-inflammatory drugs, such as Motrin, decrease inflammation and lessen pain from bone metastases.

Are prescription drugs available free to patients who are unable to pay for them?
Many prescription drug manufacturers make their medications available free of charge to patients that do not have the means to pay for them. Call the Cancer Information Service, 1–800–4–CANCER or check www.phrma.org

for further information. Usually the physician must certify that you are unable to afford the cost of the drug and are unable to obtain assistance elsewhere.

Can nerves be severed to relieve pain?

A neurosurgeon can cut nerves close to or in the spinal cord to block the pain impulses to the brain. A *rhizotomy* means that a nerve close to the spinal cord has been cut. A *cordotomy* means that bundles of nerves in the spinal cord itself have been severed. When the nerves that transmit pain are destroyed, the sensations of pressure and temperature can no longer be felt. For this reason, after such an operation, patients can be injured easily as they no longer have the protective reflexes of pain, pressure, or temperature.

What are nerve blocks?

Local anesthetics, sometimes combined with cortisone can be injected into or around a nerve to stop pain. For longer lasting pain relief, phenol or alcohol may be used. There can be side effects to nerve blocks. Muscle paralysis may result or the affected area may lose all feeling.

What is electric nerve stimulation?

Sometimes called TENS, for Transcutaneous Electric Nerve Stimulation, this is a technique that uses mild electric current, which seems to interfere with pain sensations. A small power pack connected to two electrodes is applied. The current can be adjusted so that the sensation is pleasant. It is sometimes described as a buzzing, tingling feeling. Pain relief lasts beyond the treatment. Your doctor or physical therapist should be able to tell you where to get a TENS unit.

What is acupuncture?

This ancient Chinese method of treatment has been used in Asia for thousands of years. To perform the treatment, special needles are inserted into the body at certain points and at various depths and angles. Particular groups of acupuncture points are believed to control specific areas of pain sensation. The patient usually feels no pain from the insertion of needles. Treatments are generally given in a series—sometimes every day for a week or more. Acupuncture has been studied in clinical trials and has been proven as a useful treatment for chemotherapy-induced nausea and vomiting. Many major cancer centers, including the National Institutes of Health Clinical Center, have acupuncturists on their staffs. Acupuncturists are usually listed in the yellow pages of the telephone directory.

What is electro-acupuncture?

Electro-acupuncture is the use of pulsating electrical current instead of or in addition to hand needles. In some practices, the needle is inserted as it would normally be by the practitioner, then an electrode is attached to the needle to give continued stimulation. Others find the acupuncture points, then, without inserting a needle, stimulate the pain away electronically.

What is acupressure?

Acupressure is based on principles similar to those of acupuncture, but it can be performed by anyone or on yourself without using anything except fingertip pressure. A group of therapists called myotherapists practice pressure point or trigger point therapy and are often licensed massage therapists. They use a variety of massage techniques but the basic method concentrates on stimulating trigger points in the body. To test the technique you can try the following. The most popular pressure point is above the thumb, in the fleshy area between the thumb and the first finger. The technique is simple and involves probing deeply with the tip of the forefinger or thumb until a sharp twinge is felt, and then stimulating as deeply as possible for from a few seconds to a few minutes. The same spot on the opposite side of the body is then given the same treatment for the same amount of time. Applying steady circular motion pressure appears to relax the tenseness and relieve the pain. It is worth trying, since it is free of any harm and you can do it yourself. There are a number of books that detail this method. It is a technique that has been used in China for centuries, and is taught to Chinese children by their mothers.

Is marijuana helpful?

Because marijuana is not legally available in most states, the quality of marijuana varies a great deal, and there is still controversy over its use and effectiveness. Though marijuana has been reported to reduce anxiety or control nausea, some patients have reported that, rather than decreasing pain, smoking marijuana increased pain. (There is a prescription drug, called Marinol, which is a synthetic form of the active marijuana constituent THC that is available and is sometimes prescribed to reduce nausea and vomiting.)

Is a drink before dinner or with meals a good idea?

Drinking small amounts of alcoholic beverages with meals or in the evening may help you to relax. However, check with your doctor to make certain that the combination of alcohol with other pain-relieving drugs, chemotherapy, or other medications you are taking is not dangerous to you, since many drugs have serious effects when combined with alcohol.

What options do I have if pain is not relieved?

You can ask for a consultation with a pain specialist. Many of the larger hospitals now have pain clinics, devoted to helping patients cope with pain. There are many different techniques being used to relieve pain and many professionals feel that much suffering can be eliminated through the use of proper pain control techniques. If your doctor is not able to refer you, here are some other ways to find a pain specialist or treatment center:

- Access the Web site of the American Alliance of Cancer Pain Initiatives (www.aacpi.org). This national organization is dedicated to promoting cancer pain relief nationwide by supporting the efforts of state and regional Pain Initiatives. It lists people in each state who are involved in the Initiative locally. Call the person located closest to you to ask for a referral.

- Call your local hospital. Ask for the Department of Anesthesiology. They may have pain specialists on staff or can tell you about a pain treatment center or clinic nearby.

- Contact the nearest medical school or teaching hospital (the Association of American Medical Colleges Web site www.aamc.org has a searchable geographic listing of both medical schools and teaching hospitals) to see if they offer pain treatment or can refer you to a pain specialist.

Are there additional written materials on pain control?

There are several good booklets that discuss pain control in cancer patients. *Pain Control: A Guide for Patients and Their Families,* published by the National Cancer Institute, is available by calling 1–800–4–CANCER or on-line at www.cancer.gov. The American Cancer Society's booklet *Cancer Pain, Treatment Guidelines for Patients,* includes guidelines for assessing and treating pain (1–800–ACS– 2345 or www.cancer.org). The federal Agency for Healthcare Research and Quality (AHRQ) also offers written material (1–800–358–9295 or www. ahrq.gov3).

MONEY MATTERS

Bills, insurance forms, and money matters are part of all our lives. But they are especially important when they involve hospitalization and medications. If you are like most cancer survivors, the cost of initial treatment and continuing care are a major concern. What happens to insurance coverage and costs during and after treatment for cancer is something you can't help worrying about. Hopefully new national initiatives will help to ease some of the burden. But meanwhile, the problems of the present must be addressed. People who had life and health insurance before treatment are usually able to keep it, although costs and benefits may change. However, those who change jobs or apply for new policies may find it more difficult. Understanding your rights and how the system works can help you to get the most out of your coverage.

What is the best way to set up my records concerning doctor visits, hospitalizations, medications, etc.?

The most efficient way seems to be with a loose-leaf notebook divided into sections. A sheet at the beginning of the book can be used to keep an ongoing record of every visit to a doctor or hospital. Another section in the notebook can be set up for each doctor, for hospital information and for insurance information. In the section under each doctor, you may want to have a sheet that is divided to list the date, the reason for the visit, treatment recommended, complications, prescriptions, cost of visit, how paid, and reimbursement information. You should add copies of any bills received from the doctor in the same section. You may even wish to add a sheet with the date of visit, the questions asked and the answers given. You can set up the rest of the notebook in the same manner. Keep a chart of your insurance claims. This information will also be helpful in determining if you can deduct medical expenses on your tax returns. You will find that if you keep all of the information about your case in one spot, you'll have everything you need when a new bill or reimbursement statement arrives. There are commercially produced books that are extremely helpful, such as *The Cancer Patient's Workbook* by Joanie Willis, DK Publishing, 2001.

What kinds of items and services should my insurance cover?

Health insurance policies differ in what they cover, so it's a good idea to check your policy before a procedure, test or treatment, to see what items and services will be reimbursed and what the deductible is. Have the customer insurance representative tell you what is covered. And ask that it be put in writing. Also ask who will be the contact person who can assist you with problems when you call. Without that information, you may be cheating yourself because you are unaware of what can be claimed. If you are in a managed care plan, check to see what you will pay for each appointment and treatment. In addition, you will need to know whether the doctors and health care facility where you will get your treatment are covered or whether you can get part of the cost with out-of-network treatment coverage. This is discussed more fully in Chapter 3, Choosing Your Doctor and Hospital.

What does Medicare cover?

Medicare, the health insurance program of the federal government provided through Social Security or Railroad Retirement, comes in two parts: Medicare

Hospital Insurance, Part A, covers room and board in a semiprivate room, nursing care, supplies and equipment, x-ray, radiology, operating room, medical supplies and lab tests. Part B, which must be applied for separately and is an optional plan, covers 80 percent of the allowable charges. It is intended to fill some of the gaps left in medical insurance coverage under Part A. The major benefit under Part B is payment for physician's services. Covered by Part B are: medical and surgical services of physician, in the hospital, nursing home, office, clinic, or patient's home. (Part B, for example, covers the administration of chemotherapy by a nurse at a physician's office.) It covers radiology and pathology costs as well as services prescribed by the physician in connection with diagnosis and treatment. Emergency room and clinic services, physical therapy, lab tests, radiology services, casts, surgical dressings and rental or purchase of medical equipment such as oxygen, wheelchairs, and colostomy equipment are covered. Medicare will also help pay for transportation by an approved ambulance service to a hospital or skilled nursing facility if used to avoid endangering the patient's health. Some items not covered are: prescription drugs not covered by changes in Medicare, routine physical checkups, custodial care, eyeglasses, hearing aids, cosmetic or dental services.

Is insurance to supplement the Medicare A and B plans available?

Some companies offer plans (sometimes referred to as Medigap plans) with an annual premium based on age, sex, and number in the family. Most of these are guaranteed renewable and offer hospital benefits. These are in addition to Medicare benefits.

If I have Medicare do I need any other insurance?

As good as Medicare is, it was never meant to cover all the healthcare expenses of older people. Medicare, Plan B, helps to cover major medical expenses. However, as with all healthcare insurance, there are deductible amounts and percentages of charges for various services that you must pay before becoming eligible for payment. Whatever type of basic health insurance you have—Medicare or other—adding some supplemental protection is a good idea. Some companies offer special Medicare supplemental insurance that fills the gaps in Medicare A and B. Medicare does not cover costs of long-term nursing home care.

Is Medicaid different than Medicare?

Yes. Medicaid is a federally sponsored plan that is administered by the state, with each state setting its own rules of eligibility and coverage. It is a *public assistance program based on financial need* for people of all ages and usually pays hospital and doctor bills, prescription drugs, home care and many other services.

Will I have any special insurance benefits if I am a veteran?

If you or your spouse are, or have been a member of the Armed Forces you might be able to get help from the Veterans Administration. What you will receive depends on many factors, but can include:

- Hospital care in Veterans Administration hospitals
- CHAMPVA (The Civilian Health and Medical Program of the Veterans Administration) that may pay for medical services and supplies
- Prescription drugs (disabled veterans) with copay

For additional information, call 1–800–827–1000 or www.va.gov.

Is cancer insurance a good buy?

Most insurance experts feel that good general medical and surgical policies are a better investment than specialized cancer insurance. Cancer insurance, as a supplement to existing health insurance, is available in most states. Many of the benefits offered are similar to those available through most major medical plans. The regular plans, however, cover the family in other medical emergencies and usually give more economical coverage. Cancer insurers require buyers to sign a pledge that they do not have cancer and have never had it. Payments are made in addition to claims paid by basic health insurance. Some of the policies specifically state that they do not cover diagnostic x-ray and laboratory examinations.

Should I consider buying a mail order insurance policy?

As with every other type of product, there are good and poor buys in mail order policies. Check the company and policy carefully before buying. Buyers should bear in mind that any omission of pertinent health information will be held against them when they try to collect. At claim time, some companies have been known to find some preexisting condition to justify nonpayment of claims. Furthermore, the benefits in some policies are based on the number of days of hospitalization. Usually they are advertised as having a maximum payment of $400, $800 or $1000 a month. The payment is usually a direct cash payment. One thousand dollars a month breaks down to $33.33 a day, far less than daily hospital costs and far less coverage than most people require. This type of policy is a very inadequate one as a basic protection plan, but might be a useful supplement.

What about getting a loan against my insurance policy?

It may be possible to get a loan against your life insurance policy. In addition, check to see if your policy includes an accelerated benefits provision, where

INSURANCE POLICY CHECKLIST

ITEM OR FEATURE	COMMENTS	YOUR POLICY
Number of days of hospitalization	Least should be 30 days; many offer 90 days.	
Coinsurance/copayment	Check to see how much insurer pays and how much you pay— usually insurer pays 75–85 percent of covered cost, you pay rest.	
Outpatient services	Important since vital cancer treatments such as chemotherapy and radiation are given on outpatient basis.	
In-hospital services	Make sure anesthesia, x-rays, laboratory tests, drugs, CT scans, blood and blood components, nursing care are covered.	
Home health benefits	Check whether services of visiting nurses, homemakers, aides are covered.	
Deductibles	First $100, $500 or $1000 may not be covered. Many policies with higher deductibles give better long-range coverage. For long illnesses, like cancer, this type may be preferable.	
Who is covered	Wise to check especially if you have stepchildren or foster children.	
Retirement benefits	Check limitations regarding age or place of employment. Can benefits be converted to individual policy or Medicare supplement at retirement?	
Cancellation	Check to be sure you will be covered even if health deteriorates or you have severe or repeated need for treatment.	

(continued)

INSURANCE POLICY CHECKLIST *(continued)*

ITEM OR FEATURE	COMMENTS	YOUR POLICY
Maximum, lifetime or benefit limits	Check to see what maximum figure refers to. Is it paid in full for each illness or all illnesses in course of a year? Is it paid only once in life of policy?	
Stop loss provision	Many major medical plans provide that you share (with copayments) the cost of care up to a specified amount. After that, insurance pays full costs.	
Inside limits	This refers to payment of a fixed amount for hospital room or surgical conditions, etc., with the policyholder paying the difference.	
Preadmission certification	Some health plans require certification before procedures are performed and indicate maximum length of hospital stay. Stay can be extended only at direction of physician and will be paid for by insurance company only if company agrees that a longer stay is indicated.	
Elimination period	For disability policies. Specifies length of time at beginning of disability during which no benefits are available.	
Preexisting conditions	If there is an exclusion, should never go back longer than one year.	
Waiting period	If buying a new policy, check waiting period. The shorter the waiting period (30–60 days) the better.	

(continued)

INSURANCE POLICY CHECKLIST *(continued)*

ITEM OR FEATURE	COMMENTS	YOUR POLICY
Guaranteed renewable	Policy stays in effect up to specified age as long as premium is paid. Premium rate cannot be raised for any one individual, but only for all policyholders with same type of benefits.	
Noncancelable—guaranteed renewable	Safest type. Cannot be canceled and premium rate cannot be changed.	
Physician/surgeon services	Check to see if these are covered.	
Second opinions	Many policies cover these to insure against unnecessary surgery. May need referral from primary physician.	
Diagnostic tests	Check to see exactly what is covered.	
Physical therapy	Check to see if covered on an outpatient basis.	
Oxygen/oxygen supplies	Check to see if and how covered.	
Prescription drugs	Check type of coverage.	
Prosthetic devices	Check coverage.	
Rehabilitation services	Check coverage.	
Respiratory therapy	Check coverage.	
Ambulance services	Check coverage.	
Transfusions	Check coverage.	
Outpatient mental health services	Check coverage.	
Rental of hospital bed/wheelchair, etc.	Check coverage.	
Experimental treatment	Check to see if there is a specific exclusion.	
Nursing home care	Special insurance is now available to cover this, not usually part of regular policy.	

you can get anywhere from 25 to 100 percent of your death benefit as early payment. Call your State Insurance Commissioner (see Chapter 28, Where to Get Help) or your company's Claims Department to find out whether your life insurance policy allows for accelerated benefits or loans, and how much it will cost.

What does a viatical settlement mean?

Viatical settlement means selling your life insurance policy to a third party, or viaticating it as the insurance industry says. This is a complex transaction that may or may not be good for you. Usually you only get 50 percent of the value of your life insurance policy. In return, you will need to name the viatical company as your beneficiary and have a medical person estimate your life expectancy (it usually needs to be fewer than two to four years depending on the company). You will need to continue paying the premium on the policy. Before you decide to do this, make sure you've checked with more than one company, understand the process and what it will mean to you, have checked the background of the company you've chosen, understand what the exact amount of the settlement is, and when and how you will receive it. Discuss all the issues with your family. Ask your accountant or tax advisor whether you will have to pay federal, state or local taxes on the money you receive. Viaticating your policy may make you ineligible for public assistance programs, such as Medicaid. You may need to contact an attorney to help you understand all the options and ramifications and assure that the settlement money will be forthcoming.

What should I know about filing for insurance benefits?

In order to make the most of the insurance benefits you have paid for, it is important that you understand what benefits are covered. You need to read your policy and have a general record of what is covered. Many times because of lack of knowledge, items that are covered are not claimed. It's a good idea to have a family member or friend become familiar with your policies and records so that claims can be handled if you are unable to do so yourself.

- Understand the language insurance companies use. For example, if you ask your doctor to write a prescription for a hairpiece, be sure the prescription specifically uses the term "hair prosthesis," since this is what is reimbursable under many insurance policies. Be sure the receipt for the hairpiece also calls it a hair prosthesis rather than a wig. This is important, since this documentation will be the basis for your claim for reimbursement.

- Keep a chart of your claims. Accurate records are essential not only for insurance but for tax returns.

- Make copies of all bills and correspondence and use copies when filing claims or questioning charges. Never send original bills to the insurance company unless they insist on it. If you are required to send originals, make good copies to keep for your own records.

- Get all information in writing, if possible. Make notes concerning telephone conversations. Always get the names of people with whom you are talking. Follow up, if possible, with a written note confirming the conversation.

- Use the insurance company's claim forms and fill them out completely. Using the doctor's form, or failing to complete the insurer's form can delay payment.

- Submit your claims in the correct order. The patient's insurance should be filed first. Wait to receive payment and an Explanation of Benefits. Then, if you have a secondary policy, submit the claim to that insurer and include a copy of the Explanation of Benefits from the patient's insurer. The second insurer will pay only on the amount not covered by the first insurance company, not on the total original claim. This is called coordination of benefits and is designed to assure that the patient collects no more than 100 percent of the original claim.

- Read your Explanation of Benefits (called the EOB) carefully. Every medical treatment has a corresponding numerical code, which is filled in by your doctor. The wrong codes translate into incorrect reimbursements. Check this statement carefully to be certain that your care is recorded correctly.

- If your claim is denied for insufficient information reasons, submit additional information.

- If your claim is denied or you think the insurer should have paid more, ask to have the case reviewed and ask your doctor to supply additional information. If you are turned down again, check to see what the company's appeal process is.

- Don't hesitate to call the insurance company and talk to a supervisor in the claims department. Follow up any phone call with a letter recapping the conversation and restating your claim. Include background information, even if you have sent the same information before.

- Many policies have time limits on appeals—often six to 12 months—and the disputed amount must usually be over $100.

- If you still feel you have been treated unfairly by your insurance company, you can report the case to the state insurance commission. (See Chapter 28, Where to Get Help, for a list of state insurance commissions.) Send a copy of your letter to your state representative and senator.

What is involved in making an insurance appeal?

The first step is to notify the insurance company that you are dissatisfied with your reimbursement. If possible, make your appeal in person. Usually, however, it is more convenient to appeal by mail—and having a paper trail is always a good idea. Send the insurer:

- A short letter explaining why your claim should be covered.

- A copy of the doctor's bill you submitted with your original claim (always keep an extra copy in your files).

- A copy of the Explanation of Benefits (EOB).

- If a mistake by your doctor's office was responsible for the underpayment, you should also enclose a note from your doctor stating that your insurance claim was filled out incorrectly.

- If you do not receive a response within a month, call to ask what the status of your claim is.

Is there anywhere else to turn if the insurance company turns down my case?

If your appeal is denied you may want to bring your case to the attention of your state insurance commissioner. Many states now have a state review process. Each state's external review process is different but they do allow for independent medical review of disputes. (Alabama, Arkansas, Idaho, Nebraska, Nevada, North Dakota, South Dakota and Wyoming do not have review programs.) However, you are not eligible for a state review if your health plan is self-insured or if you depend on Medicare only for health benefits. If your complaint involves Medicare, contact your Social Security office or check your telephone book or your state information center to see if there is a state Medicare Advocate who can help you. Send copies to your state and U.S. senator and representatives. For more information about insurance complaints, you may wish to call the National Insurance Consumer Hotline at 1–800–942–4242.

How do you go about making an insurance appeal?

First of all, you must be familiar with your health insurance policy. If you're in a self-insured plan, you can't use your state's external review process. Ask your employee benefits office for a copy of the Evidence of Coverage document for your policy. Check your state's Insurance Commissioner or Bureau of Insurance Health Care Division for information on how to arrange for an Independent External Review. (Note: Some states charge a filing fee for arranging an External Review.) If you are eligible, you should put together an appeal packet that includes your health plan's denial letters, your doctor's or specialist's plan for care and your medical records, as well as any articles from professional journals that support your case. Be sure you have a copy of all the material for your own records. Send your packet of information by registered mail, return receipt requested. (See the end of this chapter for information on booklets available to help you understand your plan's coverage rules and how you can appeal denials.)

At what point should I consider hiring a lawyer?

If stalling a decision means that you and your doctor agree that you are jeopardizing your future, you may want to hire a lawyer immediately. Check with your state bar association for names of lawyers who specialize in health care law. Patient advocacy groups in your area may be useful in helping you find the right lawyer.

Should hospital bills for outpatient or inpatient services be checked and questioned?

One study showed that more than 90 percent of hospital bills have errors in them—and 75 percent of the errors are in favor of the hospital. One reason for this is that hospitals usually charge patients for goods and services when the physician orders them, rather than when they are received. To help you in checking your bill, request an itemized bill, which most hospitals provide only upon request. Ask for a bill you can understand, not one with indecipherable computer codes. If it is not ready when you leave the hospital, ask to have it sent to you. Check the bill carefully to make sure you were billed correctly for:

- The kind of room you used (private or semi-private).
- The correct number of days.
- The correct time spent in specialized units.
- Specific treatments (radiation, chemotherapy, inhalation, etc.).
- The x-rays and tests that were actually given.
- The medications, dressings, injections, etc. that you received.
- Make sure that any bedpans, humidifiers, thermometers, or other personal items listed were items you were allowed to take home.
- The correct number of daily hospital visits by your doctor.

If there is anything on the bill that you do not understand, ask for an explanation. Don't pay for any charge that is under dispute until the hospital has shown proof that the item or service was provided. If the bill is being paid by the insurance company and you feel that there are unexplained charges that cannot be justified, contact the fraud division of the insurance company.

Where can I get help in keeping track of my medical bills?

This can become almost a full-time job, and can be very draining if you are also trying to deal with treatments and recovery. Perhaps a family member or friend may be willing to take over this task. Sometimes help can come from an American Cancer Society volunteer (in some areas, volunteers are trained to help with insurance claims) or from your local American Association for Retired Persons chapter (which also trains volunteers in insurance claims). There are also medical claims companies that provide this service for a fee. You can find them in the yellow pages under Insurance Claim Processing Services.

Will insurance cover costs for legitimate clinical trials or investigational treatments?

Some insurers will not cover certain costs when a new treatment is under study. Although some clinical trials offer some care free of charge, there usually are other expenses involved. Before becoming involved in the treatment, be sure to check your insurance policy or health care provider to see if there is a specific exclusion for experimental or investigational treatment. Also ask your doctor:

- What has been the experience of other patients in the trial?
- Have insurers paid for their care?
- Have there been recurring problems with insurance payment?
- Is it possible to describe the procedure in a way that would increase the possibility of getting insurance coverage?

Does Medicare cover clinical trials treatments?

Medicare covers treatment in clinical trials. It will cover anything that is needed by the clinical trial. For example, Medicare will pay for the administration of a chemotherapy drug that is being tested in a trial, including the provision of antinausea drugs to prevent complications from the chemotherapy drug. It also covers anything normally covered even if it resulted from the clinical trial. For instance, if an adverse event requiring hospitalization or a diagnostic test that Medicare would ordinarily cover, it would do so, even if the adverse event occurred or the diagnostic test was used as a result of participating in a trial. To be sure, check with the doctor's or hospital's office to assure that what is being used is covered.

Where can someone who is hard to insure because of serious medical conditions go for health insurance coverage?

A number of states currently sell comprehensive health insurance to state residents with serious medical conditions who can't find a company to insure them. These are often referred to as "risk pools." A list of the states which offer these programs can be found in Chapter 28, Where to Get Help, under Difficult to Insure Health Insurance Coverage. If your state is not listed, you should contact your state department of insurance to find out if such programs are being made available in your state.

What costs are not covered?

Health insurance does not cover most of the nonmedical costs of cancer, such as transportation to and from treatment, childcare, home care, over-the-counter medicine, and many medical aids.

How do I deduct my medical expenses on my income tax?

If you spend more than 7.5 percent of your adjusted gross income on medical and dental expenses, you can have an income tax deduction. You will need to fill out a long form 1040. Deductions are available for the current tax year, as well as for the two previous years, if amended returns for those years are filed. For a complete explanation of what expenses are covered, ask for IRS Publication 502 by calling 1–800–TAX–FORM or by using the Web site, ww.irs.gov.

How does the Family and Medical Leave Act work?

If you are an eligible employee, this national law allows you to take up to 12 weeks of unpaid leave from your job each year to care for children, spouses, or parents who have serious health conditions or to recover from your own serious health condition. (It allows the same coverage for care of newborn or newly adopted babies.) After the leave, the law entitles you to return to your previous job or an equivalent job with the same pay, benefits, and other conditions. You are covered if you work for an employer that has 50 or more employees within 75 miles of the workplace, the federal government, or state or local government. You must have worked for your employer for one year, and at least 1,250 hours the previous year. Your employer must continue to pay health benefits at the same rate while you are on leave. But if you do not return to work, your employer may try to recover the cost of the premiums, unless the reason you didn't return was continuation of serious health conditions or other circumstances beyond your control.

Should I give up my company's group plan
when I leave for a new job?

Cancer patients are advised not to leave a job with insurance benefits until they have a new job with good coverage or have made other plans for insurance. Your partner, if you have one, should keep this in mind if you are covered under his or her policy. Consider continuing to take part in your current company's group plan after you leave. If a new job does not work out, you could be left with no coverage. Federal law (Public Law 99-272, COBRA or the Consolidated Omnibus Budget Reconciliation Act) requires many employers to allow employees who quit, are let go, or whose hours are reduced to pay their own premiums for the company's group plan. This protection lasts 18 months for employees (and up to 29 months if they lose their jobs due to disability and are eligible for Social Security disability benefits at the time they leave the job) and 36 months for their dependents. If an employee leaves a company and takes a new job, continuation coverage by the former company can be kept for up to 18 months if the new company's coverage is limited or excludes a preexisting condition, such as cancer. It pays to look for work in a large company whose group insurance plans rarely exclude employees with a history of illness.

What are other ways of qualifying for insurance when you have cancer?
Some people are able to obtain dependent coverage under a partner's insurance plan. Sometimes it is possible to join a plan during open enrollment periods when you may be accepted regardless of your health history. Professional, fraternal, membership and political organizations sometimes have group plans that you can join. An independent insurance broker can sometimes locate a reasonable insurance package for you. Seek out an agent who specializes in finding policies for high-risk individuals, but be sure to do your homework before you accept a policy, checking to make certain it is financially sound and has a reputable service record. When filling out an application, think about how much you need to divulge. Many cancer survivors divulge superfluous information that may wave a red flag unnecessarily. Unless you call attention to special circumstances regarding your health, your application is likely to go through in routine fashion.

**Are cancer patients discriminated against
when seeking employment?**
Having cancer can sometimes be a hurdle to returning to work. Although no comprehensive federal cancer survivor bill of rights has been passed, many national lawmakers understand the issues of discrimination based on cancer history. Federal and many state laws provide protection for those who are termed physically handicapped—a stereotype most cancer patients feel does not apply to them. Be that as it may, the laws that protect those who have had cancer from employment discrimination are most often contained in provisions protecting the physically handicapped. (These laws include The Rehabilitation Act of 1973—Sections 501, 503 and 504; The Americans with Disabilities Act of 1990, as well as state laws prohibiting employment discrimination.) For more information, you can contact the American Cancer

Society and the National Coalition for Cancer Survivorship, the two organizations who are taking leadership roles in organizing on behalf of those who are faced with discrimination because of cancer.

Why do employers discriminate against people who have had cancer?

Many discriminate because of their own fears and lack of information about cancer. They maintain that they are hesitant to invest in an employee who, in their minds, may die. They consider their judgments to be business ones, citing fears that insurance companies will increase their rates or refuse to insure them. They fear that the employee will become less and less productive because of medical problems. Of course, the facts all prove just the opposite. Half of all individuals in the United States diagnosed with cancer this year will overcome the disease. For people under the age of 55, survival rates are even higher. There are nine million cancer survivors in the United States. Decades of studies confirm that cancer survivors have the same productivity rates as other workers. Millions of individuals remain as productive or more productive after a cancer diagnosis than they were before. Furthermore, cancer accounts for only 20 percent of deaths in the United States. Cardiovascular disease incapacitates and kills twice as many people as cancer.

How honest should I be in filling out an application for a new job?

You can be honest without disclosing your entire health history. You should be aware that your employer needs to know your health history only as it affects your ability to do the job for which you are applying. Moreover, that knowledge is needed only after you have been given serious consideration as an applicant.

What can I say during a job interview if I am asked about my health?

Answer in a straightforward manner. Remember that it is not necessary to completely explain or dwell on your cancer history. Be positive and assertive. Stress your strengths and capabilities. Bring a letter from your doctor to the interview, attesting to your health status. Don't forget that you are selling the employer on your ability to do the job. You have no obligation to talk about your cancer unless it has some bearing on job performance. Leave the interviewer with the impression that you want the job and that you intend to be a faithful, hardworking employee. If you have had an attendance record at your last job that reflects the fact that you were absent because of your cancer experience, you can stress your attendance average in terms of how many days per month you were absent over the entire period of your last employment. Phrases like "I like to work and I give my best to every job I've ever done" can help present you in a positive way and change the focus of the question.

THINKING ABOUT DYING

We debated whether or not to include this whole subject in the book since so many people are living with cancer as a chronic disease for longer and longer periods of time. But we decided that this subject needed to be openly discussed, since it is a topic that is on the mind of every cancer patient. Besides, the time to face wills and living wills and the decisions about prolonging life is when you are still well enough to make those decisions in a rational way. So, we will share with you questions and insights we have gathered from the many people we know who have had to find answers to their questions on this very difficult subject.

Should I be thinking about writing a will?

Everyone should have a will. A lawyer can help you with all the intricacies of your own special situation. For a small set fee, you may have an initial office consultation to review your needs, discuss fees, and determine whether you wish to have the attorney draw up a will. If your will is a simple one, it can be drawn up for $100 or less. If you wish, you can call a lawyer on the phone, outline your needs, explaining your property worth and ask about the charge. Of course, the more complicated your situation, the higher the cost.

Can I write my own will?

If there are any complicated trust or tax situations, this can be risky. However, in every state, you can buy a standard will form from a stationery store. Many people have a will drawn up by a lawyer in addition to a handwritten will for their personal possessions. Some states will accept an unwitnessed will in the form of a letter or note written entirely in your own handwriting. However, most states require at least two witnesses, and some require three.

What is a Living Will?

A Living Will is a legal document that lets you specify exactly how much you want done to prolong your life. The Living Will is now valid in most states. The document is designed to permit you to specify in writing your wishes regarding the use of life support systems to keep you alive if you become terminally ill or enter a permanent coma or persistent vegetative state. The document takes effect only if you become incapacitated and can no longer actively decide and direct your physician as to the medical care you desire. In most states, a physician who is presented with a copy of your Living Will must either comply with your wishes or take all reasonable steps to transfer your medical care to another physician or health care provider who is willing to comply with your wishes. As a practical matter, you may want to inform your regular physician, while you are in good health, that you have completed a Living Will and provide your physician with a copy of it. Even with a Living Will, there are no guarantees that it will be followed should you be taken to the hospital under emergency circumstances. You should be aware that ambulance crews are bound by law to give aggressive treatment such as trying to start the heart if it has stopped, inserting tubes for fluids and attempting to restore life. You should make it very clear to everyone around you what your wishes are so that there are no misunderstandings about your care. You can get a copy of the Living Will, in the form preferred in your state, from Partnership for Caring, 1620 Eye Street NW , Suite 202, Washington, DC 20006; telephone: 1–800–989–9455.

What other legal documents are recommended?

In addition to a will and a Living Will, you may want to discuss with your attorney the advisability of appointing someone as your Health Care Agent. This person is empowered to convey your decisions about withholding or withdrawal of life support systems, Power of Attorney for Health Care Decisions (which allows the appointed to make a wide variety of health care decisions but does not extend to making decisions regarding the withholding or withdrawal of life support systems) as well as Power of Attorney for money matters. Some people also like to leave a document outlining their wishes for funeral arrangements and services.

What is a Medical Power of Attorney?

A Medical Power of Attorney is a document by which you appoint a trusted person, most often a partner, sibling or adult child. This person can act on your behalf in the event you are unable to act for yourself, regarding the hard decisions that must be made if you are terminally ill.

When does the Medical Power of Attorney become effective?

It is effective immediately after it is executed and delivered to the person chosen as your agent. It is effective indefinitely unless it contains a specific termination date. Your "agent" may make decisions only if the attending physician certifies in writing that you are incompetent to make your own decisions. Treatment may not be given or withheld if you object.

What is the difference between a Medical Power of Attorney and a Directive to Physicians?

The Directive to Physicians is a document that is limited in scope, addressing only the withholding or withdrawing of medical treatment for those persons having a terminal or irreversible condition. The Medical Power of Attorney is broader in scope and includes all health care decisions with only a few exceptions. The Medical Power of Attorney does not require that the patient

MEDICAL POWER OF ATTORNEY
FOR HEALTH CARE FORM

Medical Power of Attorney Designation of Health Care Agent.

I,_____(insert your name) appoint:

NAME _____

ADDRESS _____

PHONE _____

as my agent to make any and all health care decisions for me, except to the extent I state otherwise in this document. This medical power of attorney takes effect if I become unable to make my own health care decisions and this fact is certified in writing by my physician.

Limitations on the Decision-Making Authority of My Agent Are as Follows:

_____

_____

Designation of Alternate Agent.

(You are not required to designate an alternate agent but you may do so. An alternate agent may make the same health care decisions as the designated agent if the designated agent is unable or unwilling to act as your agent. If the agent designated is your spouse, the designation is automatically revoked by law if your marriage is dissolved.)

If the person designated as my agent is unable or unwilling to make health care decisions for me, I designate the following persons to serve as my agent to make health care decisions for me as authorized by this document, who serve in the following order:

A. First Alternate Agent

NAME _____

ADDRESS _____

PHONE _____

B. Second Alternate Agent

NAME _____

ADDRESS _____

PHONE _____

The original of this document is kept at:

_____

_____

_____

The following individuals or institutions have signed copies:

NAME _____

ADDRESS _____

_____

NAME _____

ADDRESS _____

_____

Duration.
I understand that this power of attorney exists indefinitely from the date I execute this document unless I establish a shorter time or revoke the power of attorney. If I am unable to make health care decisions for myself when this power of attorney expires, the authority I have granted my agent continues to exist until the time I become able to make health care decisions for myself.

(IF APPLICABLE) This power of attorney ends on the following date:_____

Prior Designations Revoked.
I revoke any prior medical power of attorney.

Acknowledgment of Disclosure Statement.
I have been provided with a disclosure statement explaining the effect of this document. I have read and understand that information contained in the disclosure statement.

(YOU MUST DATE AND SIGN THIS POWER OF ATTORNEY.)

I sign my name to this medical power of attorney on __day_____(month, year) at

_____
(CITY AND STATE)

_____
(SIGNATURE)

_____
(PRINT NAME)

Statement of First Witness.
I am not the person appointed as agent by this document. I am not related to the principal by blood or marriage. I would not be entitled to any portion of the principal's estate on the principal's death. I am not the attending physician of the principal or an employee of the attending physician. I have no claim against any portion of the principal's estate on the principal's death. Furthermore, if I am an employee of a health care facility in which the principal is a patient, I am not involved in providing direct patient care to the principal and am not an officer, director, partner, or business office employee of the health care facility or of any parent organization of the health care facility.

_____
SIGNATURE

_____   _____
PRINT NAME   **DATE**

_____
ADDRESS

SIGNATURE OF SECOND WITNESS

_____
SIGNATURE

_____   _____
PRINT NAME   **DATE**

_____
ADDRESS

be in a terminal or irreversible condition before the "agent" can make health care decisions on the patient's behalf.

Do you need a lawyer to execute a Medical Power of Attorney?
No. A lawyer is not necessary in order to execute a Medical Power of Attorney.

How can I arrange to donate my body or body organs?
A uniform anatomical gift act or similar law has been passed in all states. Persons can become donors by signing a card in the presence of two witnesses. The card allows the person to specify what donation is desired. You may contribute any organs or parts, restrict donation to certain organs or parts, or give the entire body for anatomical study. More information can be obtained from Living Bank, telephone: 1–800–528–2971, or www.livingbank.org.

Will I be allowed to make a decision about whether I plan to die at home or in the hospital?
It is important to let your feelings be known to your doctor so that everything possible can be done to see that your wishes are followed. For those who prefer to spend their last days at home, the Hospice program, which in most communities is run by the hospital, a skilled care facility or the visiting nurses association, has instituted home care programs, with medical supervision in the home under trained medical staff. Hospice emphasizes the management of pain and other comfort measures, providing help for the family as well as the patient. Hospice makes the family the unit of care, centering much of the caring process in the home with the support of a team of medical professionals and trained volunteers. It seeks to enable the patient to carry on an alert and pain-free existence. The decision of how your illness will be managed depends on many different factors, but if you feel strongly about your desire to die at home, you should discuss it with your family and doctor so that when the time comes, your wishes can be carried out.

Do doctors sometimes fail to respond to the right-to-die wishes of a patient who has advanced cancer?
According to a study of terminally ill patients, many doctors misunderstand or ignore requests from patients for compassionate end-of-life care. Large numbers of people still die alone, in pain and often tethered to mechanical ventilators in intensive care units. This is a sensitive topic but all should give serious thought to how they want this kind of situation to be handled. You need to be very clear about your wishes so that your doctor and your family are not forced to "second guess" your preferences.

FOR FAMILY, FRIENDS, AND CAREGIVERS

It's not easy to learn the news that someone you love has cancer. Many people have the idea that because a person has cancer, he or she is going to die—and very soon. Some people do die from cancer. But many people live a long time with the disease. If you hold on to the outdated thinking that there's no hope for someone who has cancer, you make it very hard for the person you love who has it—and very hard for yourself as well. So the first lesson is: Don't make any assumptions. Don't panic. Don't carry on in a hysterical fashion. Be honest about your own fears and encourage the same honesty from the patient. Facing up to reality won't make the problems go away, but it will make them easier to cope with.

Is it usual for the family as well as the patient to be in shock at first?
Accepting a cancer diagnosis, with all the fears that go with it, makes this a very difficult time for everyone. All of the testing and planning takes a great deal of time, leaving the patient and family "hanging" while decisions are made. To combat the feeling of helplessness, you may want to turn your attention to being the information source for the patient, researching doctors, hospitals and treatments so that you'll be able to help the patient make the best possible decisions.

What can I say to someone who I've just learned has cancer?
Being frightened by the image that someone we love is dying often leaves us silent, leaving a void that can be misinterpreted. One well-known newspaper columnist who wrote on the subject of her cancer said that the most remarkable statement ever made to her by a friend upon hearing her news was, "That's a tragedy." Another simply said, "Oh, dear friend" and reached for her hand. Another said, "Care to tell me more?" It isn't always what we say, but how we react. A hug says more than any words. Don't try to hide your feelings and turn away. Don't stop calling or visiting because you feel uncomfortable. If you feel uncomfortable, express that. It's okay to say you're scared too and don't know what to say or do.

How do you deal with a circumstance where you're told to prepare yourself for the death of a cancer patient and the patient recovers?
This happens more frequently than one would dare to imagine, particularly in families where the word cancer is still synonymous with death. When a family member has cancer, some people begin to prepare themselves for what they consider is the inevitable. In so doing, they may unconsciously begin excluding the patient from family life and decisions, in a way "practicing"

what it will be like when the person dies. When the patient continues to live, there can be unexpected resentment leading to feelings of guilt and remorse. Being aware that this can happen, you should discuss it with family members so that everyone is realistic about the patient's outlook.

Why is it that the whole family seems to be affected by the fact that one member has cancer?

It has been observed that cancer is a family disease because it does affect the whole family. To avoid negativeness, it is important for the family to realize that their own adjustments to cancer are as crucial as the patient's adjustment. Being able to say "I'm scared" and to get beyond empty talk, anger and falseness is what the whole family needs. When death threatens one person in the family—whether or not it is due to occur now or at a distant time is unimportant—it threatens all. Talking about the possibility of death and our feelings about it is the first step in coming to grips with the problem. Indeed, it is an important part of the recovery process as well.

Isn't it best if everyone just pretends that the patient isn't dying?

If you've been warned that death is imminent, pretending that a patient isn't dying is very difficult both for the patient and for family and friends. It puts a tremendous burden on the patient, who can be plunged into depression. It takes a great deal of energy, which is exhausting. By denying the truth, all parties have a harder time. The patient becomes isolated. The family is stranded with its denial. Friends are locked out. Anger is suppressed. True feelings of love and caring are blocked. Your initial reaction may be to protect the patient from facts that you feel the person cannot face. Experience has shown that, in almost every case, the patient knows anyway. Advice from every quarter is: don't try to keep the diagnosis a secret. Naturally, if stoicism is your family's way of life, they can deal with this in the accustomed way. But stoicism is not denial, and pretense really does not make it easier for the patient.

How do I handle the patient's depression at being sick and dependent?

Being cheerful and optimistic in front of a depressed patient creates an atmosphere that isn't normal. It leaves him alone with his feelings. It's better to say something like, "I'm sorry you're feeling so down but I certainly understand that being so sick is depressing." By acknowledging and accepting feelings, you can offer help in a way that makes the depressed person feel in control. Statements like, "I'm available to help you in any way I can," and "Tell me what I can do to help," leave openings for further discussion. Distracting

FOR FAMILY AND FRIENDS

Some suggestions on what to say:

- I love you because you're you.
- I'm here for you.
- I'll help in any way I can, any time, at your convenience.
- You can always count on me.
- I'll be thinking of you (and praying for you).
- It's hard, I know, but you're handling it like a pro.

and what NOT to say:

- I know exactly how you feel. (You don't!)
- I have a friend who's going through the same thing, only worse.
- I saw in the paper that they're curing cancer in Mexico (or Germany, etc.).
- I feel as bad about this as you do.
- I don't want to hear about cancer anymore. I've had too many friends die.
- It's just God's will.
- After all, we're all terminal.
- I could be run over by a bus tomorrow.
- You're going to be just fine.

the patient's attention away from himself by discussing what is happening outside the sickbed setting can be helpful. If the problem is persistent, there are numerous antidepressant drugs available. Discuss the problem with the doctor who may prescribe medication if it could be beneficial.

Should we tell people about the cancer diagnosis?

This is the hardest question for many people—and one that should be faced squarely. It was a more difficult question in the days when cancer was inevitably fatal. But even in those days, the truth was less painful to live with than denial. Today, with so many new treatments and choices it is imperative that honesty be used.

HOME CARE

Where can I look for information on the different kinds of health care services in my community?

Many communities, even small ones, have a directory of health agencies available in the community. Ask at the public library. You'll be amazed to find agencies you never knew existed. Other sources of information include the yellow pages, your doctor, the social services department at your hospital, the Cancer Information Service, the American Cancer Society and the local visiting nurse association.

What kind of help will be needed to care for a patient at home?

Often a patient can be cared for at home with little more professional assistance than a periodic visit by a nurse. If the patient is more seriously ill, part- or full-time nursing care may be necessary. If round-the-clock nursing care is performed by registered nurses, the cost can be almost as much as hospital care. Often, a nurse can be retained for a few hours a day or several days a week. Many tasks can be performed by licensed practical nurses (LPNs) or nurse's aides. If family members are willing and able to perform bedside duties, an agency-supplied part-time homemaker may be able to relieve the family of domestic duties so they can spend time with the patient.

Where can I get information about how I can learn to care for a patient at home?

The book *Caregiving: A Step-by-Step Resource for Caring for the Person with Cancer at Home* by Peter S. Houts and Julia A. Buchard, published by the American Cancer Society is a good resource. The American Red Cross offers a course that teaches home-nursing skills as well as first aid. Learning the basics and following the guidance of available health personnel can make it possible for you to bring comfort and peace to convalescence.

What are some guidelines for setting up a comfortable space for convalescence?

A restful, comfortable atmosphere is the goal.

- Make sure the room is near a bathroom.
- Give the patient a handbell or get a small intercom so that the patient can call when needed.
- A hospital bed is convenient if much time will be spent in bed. (Hospital beds may be rented and the monthly fee may be covered by your medical insurance or Medicare.)

- A low bed is best for someone who is not confined to the bed. Be sure the bed is firmly anchored and will not slip.

- Mattresses can be protected with a waterproof pad. Rubberized pads available in baby sections of stores work well, are inexpensive and can be reused and cleaned. Placing a dropsheet on the bed under the patient's hips provides added protection. Disposable waterproof bed pads are a great innovation.

- A visitor's chair encourages relaxed visiting.

- A bedside table with space for tissues, drinking water, a radio, telephone and reading and writing material should be provided.

- A good light, firmly attached and within easy reach, is a must.

- A pull-up device can be made to help if the patient has trouble rising from bed or changing position. A strong rope, tied to the end of the bed, knotted at intervals, is very useful.

- Other special items such as bathtub handrails, a commode or a raised seat in the bathroom, bed tables and such items available at surgical supply houses should be considered.

- Whenever possible, help the patient to enjoy a change of scenery by making it possible, through the use of a wheelchair or walker if necessary, to spend part of the day sitting up or resting in the family living room or kitchen, with the rest of the family.

How can I keep track of medicines that need to be taken?

Keep a daily written record of the type and amount of medicine and the time it was given, along with a record of the patient's temperature and pulse, etc., as recommended by the doctor. This is especially important if more than one person is helping care for the patient. Remember that you must give only the medications prescribed by the physician at the time and in the amounts specified. One helpful idea for pills is to set out the amount needed for the day. This makes it easy to check to see that all medications are taken each day. There are compartmentalized plastic containers available at pharmacies and by mail order for this purpose.

What do abbreviations mean on prescriptions?

The typical prescription gives the dosage strength in milligrams (mg), usually notes the type of medicine such as capsule or tablet, how many times a day it should be taken, and how much of the medicine is prescribed. How many times the prescription can be refilled is also noted. Some of the common terms used are:

- **A.C. (ANTE CIBOS):** before meals

- **AD LIB. (AD LIBITUM):** take drug freely as needed

- **D. (DIE):** day

- **DUR.: DOLOR (DURANTE DOLOR):** while the pain lasts

- **G:** gram

- **H. (HORA):** hour

- **H.D. OR H.S. (HORA SOMNI):** at bedtime

- **MG.:** milligrams

- **OMN. HOR. OR OMN. NOCT:** every hour or every night

- **P.C. (POST CIBOS):** after meals

- **P.O. (PER OS):** by mouth

- **P.R.N. (PRO RE NOTE):** whenever necessary

- **Q. (QUAQUE):** every

- **Q. 2 H (QUAQUE 2 HORA):** every two hours, etc.

- **Q.D. (QUAQUE DIE):** every day

What should I tell the doctor when I call to report a change in the patient's condition?

Always give your name and the patient's name, address and telephone number. Explain that you are calling because of changes in the patient's condition. Before calling, write down all the pertinent information, such as:

- What has happened to prompt you to call the doctor—rise in temperature, heavy breathing, weak pulse, bleeding, etc.

- The time when the changes took place and how the patient's condition has changed.

- If you want the doctor to visit the patient, be sure to say so.

- Listen carefully and write down any instructions you are given.

- If the doctor is not available and you are told to expect a call back, ask what time the doctor usually makes these calls so that you are certain that you or someone else will be available to give the information.

Is it possible to arrange for intravenous therapy at home?

Many visiting nurse associations and other nursing services now have programs that provide intravenous therapy to patients at home. The nurses' association will train patients and their families to administer the medication, but nurses are available for visits on a 24-hour-a-day basis.

Can tube feeding be done at home?

Tube feeding, called parenteral feeding, is used for patients who, as a consequence of surgical or radiation treatment are unable to eat normally or for patients who need to build up their bodies nutritionally before surgery, chemotherapy, or radiation treatments. A hollow plastic tube is inserted surgically into a central vein. The fluids, a mixture of amino acids, fat, sugar, vitamins and other essential nutrients, are slowly infused into the tube by means of a small pump that the patient operates. It takes 10 to 14 hours to infuse a full day's nourishment, but the patient can usually rest or sleep while the food is being injected. Any patient who requires parenteral feeding and who does not otherwise require being in a hospital can be cared for at home.

How can incontinence be handled in the home setting?

This problem often looms as a barrier to providing home care for a patient. The doctor and visiting nurse will be helpful in the decision as to how the patient can be handled. Incontinence is an embarrassment to the patient, and often comes as such a shock that the patient becomes depressed, and even may insist that he or she would rather die than be a bother. Organizing the changing process so that it is done quickly and simply helps to alleviate guilt feelings. The use of adult toss-away diapers, sanitary napkins, and bed pads makes it easier. In the case of the male patient, a plastic bag filled with absorbent toweling or tissues, secured to the patient with masking tape can be an easy solution. The visiting nurse can be most helpful in teaching techniques for handling this difficult job.

What is the best way to help the patient with bathing and keeping clean?

- The first rule is to allow the patient to do as much for himself or herself as possible.

- Shaving someone, if you've never done it before, takes skill. If the patient wears dentures, they should be worn for shaving. Use an electric razor if possible. If not, soften the whiskers by leaving a towel wrung out in hot water on the face for a few minutes. Stretch the patient's skin tightly to prevent cutting skin. Shave by stroking upward and returning downward over the same area.

- A shower is less strain on a patient than a tub bath. A shower chair, a small straight chair with locking wheels, works best. Soap on a string around the patient's neck is another convenience. It is helpful to arrange a ramp so that the shower chair can be wheeled into the shower. If a tub is the only facility available, there are chair/shelf type arrangements that make it possible for the person to enter the tub from a sitting position. Medical supply stores have many helpful items needed to care for the home patient.

- Be sure to check the strength, direction and temperature of the water before the patient enters. Aim the spray to reach below shoulder level.

- Never leave the patient alone in the shower or bath.

How can bedsores be prevented?

Bedsores often occur when a patient is bedridden or sitting in one position on a couch or recliner for a period of time. They can be prevented by changing the patient's position frequently. Pillows of various sizes, both hard and soft, can be used to change the patient's position. Rolled up pillows can also be used to keep the weight of bedclothes off the toes, knees or other parts of the body. Bed pads of real or synthetic sheepskin and eggcrate foam mattresses also help to deter bedsores. If you see a red spot or a bedsore developing, discuss it with the visiting nurse. There are special medications and medicated patches that can be used to treat bedsores. The sooner they are medicated, the better the chance for healing.

Is it a good idea to get a hospital bed for use at home?

Hospital beds are a wonderful help and may be purchased or rented (the monthly fee may be covered by your medical insurance or Medicare), or they may be borrowed from the various voluntary health agencies. A hospital bed makes it much easier for both the patient and those who are helping. An electric bed as opposed to a crank-type bed makes it is easy for both the patient and others to operate. Many find that setting the bed up on the first floor makes it convenient for those who are caring for the patient and for visitors as well.

What are some ideas for soothing the patient?

Back rubs or massages are wonderfully comforting. To give a back rub, heat body lotion by placing the container in a pan of warm water. Then, starting at the patient's neck, move gently with long, firm strokes down to the lower spine and buttocks and up again to the neck. Repeat several times. Circular motions can also be used. Back rubs are a wonderful way to promote relaxation, and to help stimulate circulation. Avoid skin lotions that contain alcohol. Gently rub lotion on the elbows, heels, back and spine. This helps to keep the skin supple on these areas that become very dry and can break down. Soaking the feet in warm water also can feel good to someone who can't take a bath or shower. Help the patient soak one foot at a time in a pan of warm water. Changing sheets and pillowcases often helps the patient to feel refreshed.

**Is it unusual for friends to stop visiting when
someone is very ill with cancer?**
Prolonged illness seems to have a profound effect on relationships. The fault
lies with society's being uncomfortable with the whole subject of dying—
which has been a taboo subject for so long. Coupled with what has always
been thought of as a dreaded disease, the idea of cancer sometimes makes
people withdraw because they cannot handle the situation emotionally. Even
doctors and nurses sometimes have a difficult time. The patient and family
can help by encouraging people to visit, by letting friends know the best
times to visit, by discussing the illness and by letting others share the concern
and the needs.

**Can't the doctor do more to help with the underlying
physical problems?**
Probably, at this point, there is not much that can be done to change the
prognosis, but it is possible to do many things to ease discomfort.

**What should I do if I cannot make the
patient comfortable?**
You can ask for help from hospice or home care staff or if home care nurses
or hospice staff is not available, you should call the doctor's office and
explain that you do not know how to make the person comfortable.

What does the word resuscitate mean?
As the body nears death, some of the body functions, including the heart,
may stop. Resuscitation means bringing someone back to consciousness after
the heart stops. The decision of whether or not to do this is a difficult one
to make. If you do not want to be resuscitated, it is important to tell your
caregivers.

**Should I call 911 or an emergency response team
if the patient is having trouble breathing?**
If the patient and the family have agreed that they wish to allow for a natural death, have a Living Will, and do not want to be resuscitated, you need to
be aware of how to proceed. If an emergency presents itself, you should
understand that when you or someone else calls 911 or the emergency number in your area, the crew will arrive prepared to save a life or give "aggressive treatment." Ambulance crews are bound by law to do this. Aggressive
treatment means inserting tubes, trying to start the heart if it has stopped
and attempting to move air into and out of the body. It is sometimes difficult to persuade the emergency crew that you simply want help controlling
a symptom, such as trouble with breathing or pain, and that you do not

necessarily want them to use life-saving procedures. Because the goal of the emergency team is life-saving action, they will probably move the patient from the home to the hospital. Once the person is in the hospital, the Living Will may be ignored until physicians there agree that the patient can be allowed to die a natural death. Some areas and certain states allow communication between home health agencies and hospices and local 911 and emergency response teams to prevent this problem. But many do not. So be sure to check with your doctor or hospice team about the best way for you to deal with an emergency before it occurs. Also be sure to have clear instructions for people who provide care for the patient about how you wish an emergency to be handled.

What are the physical signs that the end of life is growing close?
Most people spend more time in bed, they eat less food or no food at all, have difficulty swallowing, and so drink fewer liquids. They sleep for longer periods of time, lose weight and become visibly weaker, losing interest in the outside world. Some haziness or confusion about time may be noted as one day slips into the next.

What should I do if the patient is severely confused or overly anxious?
If the patient seems to be upset and confused, not knowing where he is or who he is with, seeing things that are not there and seeming visibly upset, you should ask for professional help. Sometimes these problems can be caused by medication. The medication can be changed and antianxiety medication can be prescribed. A visiting nurse or hospice staff can talk with the doctor and arrange for help.

What can I do if the patient slips in and out of a coma?
Even when people slip in and out of coma, they are aware. Touching, giving back rubs, holding hands and talking are important. Inviting close friends and relatives to sit with the patient, talking about old times may be welcomed. Soft music is comforting. The aim is to let the person know that he is not alone.

What if I am not able to care for the patient at home at the end even though the person wishes to be there?
Circumstances sometimes make it impossible to continue to give care at home. But there is no reason to feel guilty. This is not a failure on your part. Many people who have been able to take part in care during the course of the illness find that circumstances make it impossible to cope with the final stages of illness. This is a very painful time, and each family must find its own answers. Visiting nurse agencies or hospice can help you arrange for nurse's

aides to give baths, do light laundry, change the bed, etc. Registered nurses and other professionals can be called upon to help you manage. And family and friends can be asked to help. But sometimes it is necessary to have the patient hospitalized. Arrangements can usually be made for some member of the family to stay at the hospital, helping as much or as little as he or she chooses and giving comfort to the patient just as would be done if the patient were at home.

When should we contact Hospice?

It's a good idea to contact Hospice and understand their services before they are truly needed. The Hospice community says that the most persistent barriers to effective hospice care are late referrals and reluctance on the part of families to initiate this kind of care. Understanding how Hospice can be of help reduces the burden on both the patient and the family.

What services does Hospice offer?

The primary concern of hospice care is quality of life, not cure. Hospice seeks to prolong life, not prolong dying. The goal is to control pain and other symptoms so the patient can remain as alert and comfortable as possible. Hospice offers many kinds of care. Most will help with home care, some provide services in special hospice centers, others are located within a hospital or skilled nursing facility. Many Hospice programs offer a combination of these services, tailored to patient and family needs.

How can I find out about Hospice in my area?

For information on hospices, contact the National Hospice Organization (See Chapter 28, Where to Get Help). The Cancer Information Service (1–800–4–CANCER) or the American Cancer Society may also be able to guide you to Hospice service in your area. Also check the yellow pages under "Hospice."

Is it wise to encourage the patient to talk about dying?

Very often the inclination is to brush off an expression of fear of dying by assuring the patient that everything is going to be fine. Acknowledging that death is a possibility but that you'll do everything you can to help during his illness offers the kind of positive comfort every patient needs. Thoughts of death occur to almost every patient and it is wise to encourage the patient to discuss both his fears of dying and how he wishes to die openly.

Is it a good idea to give the patient permission to die?

Many patients feel entrapped by their families at the end of their lives and they desperately try to hold on to life. They don't want to do anything to hurt us—they don't want to distress us by dying. Those in the helping professions, who are skilled in the process of death, emphasize that it is important to allow patients to "finish their business." Those who are prepared for death, knowing their lives are in order, usually die in a serene manner, releasing their grip on the physical so that the final process is made easier. You can help this process by giving the person permission to die. Just saying "I'm here with you because I love you. I will always love you. So I am telling you that everything is all right with us. It's okay for you to let go."

How can a person be helped to die in comfort?

When it is determined that the patient is dying and there is no reasonable hope for recovery, the patient, family and doctor can make plans to help the patient die comfortably. Either at home with help from Hospice, or in the hospital, all testing, transfusions, etc., can cease. This means that temperature no longer needs to be taken at the usual intervals and the obtaining of blood samples etc. can be curtailed so that the patient will not be disturbed. Morphine, or whatever drugs are most effective, should be prescribed to be given continuously to relieve pain. Glucose and water can be given intravenously if the patient cannot eat or drink and complains of thirst. Oxygen may be used if there is shortness of breath. A catheter can be inserted in the bladder for comfort. Lips can be kept moist with Vaseline, ice chips or glycerin sponges. The important thing for everyone to keep in mind is that any measures that are taken are for the purpose of maintaining the patient's comfort.

What kind of care must be given to the dying patient?

Being with the patient as much as possible is the most important consideration. Remember that even if the patient does not seem to be able to hear what is happening, awareness may be very acute. Professionals say that it is helpful to give the dying person your permission to "let go." The patient may want to talk about dying, and those close to the patient can help him to do so. Do not be afraid if the patient seems to be in physical distress and frightened, restless, gasping for breath, and disoriented. Keep the patient warm. Most important, keep the mouth moist. Special oiled swabs that can be used to remove mucus from inside the mouth and which help keep the mouth and lips moist are most helpful. Placing the patient on his side helps drain mucus from mouth and nose. Every effort should be made to reduce irritating conditions, and provide an atmosphere that is peaceful and comfortable.

What are the specific signs of impending death?

People in the health-care field who see death almost every day tell us that although many people think of death as being a traumatic time for the patient, in reality, most people die very peacefully, in their sleep or while at rest. The signs of death will vary from patient to patient. It is very important to note changes in the patient's normal status. Some of the significant changes to be aware of include:

- Marked changes in breathing: labored, spasmodic, heavy breathing, followed by quiet or shallow breathing or a decreased number of breaths per minute (sometimes referred to as Cheyne-Stokes respiration).

- Heartbeat rate either faster or slower than usual.

- Change in skin texture and temperature; though the patient feels cold to the touch, there may be profuse perspiration.

- Lapsing in and out of consciousness, being confused, or going into a coma.

- Loss of sensation, power of motion, and/or loss of reflexes first in legs, then in arms.

- Tendency to turn the head toward the light as a result of failing sight and hearing.

Why are autopsies necessary?

Autopsies are not always necessary, but this final examination may be requested by the patient, family, or the physician to determine the cause of death, and to allow data to be gathered on the effects of the disease. By comparing findings, treatment for others with the same disease may be improved in the future. The medical profession treats an autopsy as a surgical procedure with full respect of the individual. However, if you do not wish to allow an autopsy, it is your right to withhold permission.

CARING FOR THE CAREGIVER

What can I do when I feel angry or depressed about dealing with a caregiving situation?

The first thing you need to understand is that it is normal to feel angry and frustrated from time to time. If at all possible, when the feeling overwhelms you, you should try to get out of the house, if only for ten minutes. A walk in the fresh air can be rejuvenating. If you can't get out of the house, remove yourself from the situation by just walking away, if only to another room.

As rewarding as caretaking can be, it can also lead to difficult situations when the patient or other family members take things out on you. Another great way to vent your feelings is to keep a daily journal. If the entire situation gets to be too much for you, remember that there is "respite" help available.

Why does the patient focus his anger on me?

It's hard to deal with a patient who is angry with you when you feel you've given up so much of yourself to caring for the patient. You can tell yourself that you're not the cause of the hostility—but when angry exchanges are made, it's hard not to return anger with anger. If at all possible, try to respond with compassion and understanding. Realize that even if you can't handle the situation as you might like, honest exchanges are valuable if they allow you to share feelings honestly. Research has confirmed that very often, in the course of an illness, there needs to be someone on whom anger can be directed. Very often it is the person who is nearest and dearest to the patient. Other times it is the doctor, the hospital, or other people who are part of the support care group. It's helpful if you can remember that this is the patient's way of releasing feelings of anger and rage at his illness and that the anger is not directed at you but at the illness itself.

How can I keep the patient from becoming demanding?

Many families complain, and feel guilty because they do, that the cancer patient becomes very self-centered and demanding. Isolating the patient and catering only to his schedule removes one whole aspect of a patient's life—the sharing, helping, giving side. This focuses his thinking on his problems, removing him from the need to feel useful. It shines attention on the negative aspects of illness. Strive for an honest relationship that encourages full expression and venting of emotions, but emphasizes the positive. Seek guidance from professionals, if needed. If everyone concerned does not agree to getting advice, by all means get help for yourself if you feel you need it.

What can I do to make it easier for myself?

There are many things that you can try:

- Talk about your feelings. Don't be afraid to say what's difficult for you to do to family and friends.
- Check around your community to find help. Look for home care service, transportation agencies, and support groups.

■ Schedule time for yourself, whether it be a quiet time at home, a walk on the beach, a concert or play or a shopping trip.

■ Stay organized with lists of things you need to do. Put the caregiving tasks into your list for the day along with your other chores.

■ Accept other people's help or ask them to do things for you. This pertains to both family and friends.

■ Take care of yourself. Don't skimp on your own needs. Don't skip your medical appointments, hairdressing appointments or other needs because you are the main caregiver.

How can I help friends to be helpful?

We've all heard the offer and made it ourselves: "Just let me know what I can do to help." You can help yourself as you help your friends, who truly are sincere about helping, by taking advantage of such an offer. Try to keep a list of needs at hand and accept the help that is offered. A specific chore or errand, no matter how simple, lets others feel useful. Make a list of tasks that others can help with—mowing the lawn, raking leaves, picking up the dry cleaning, shopping, taking children to lessons, providing transportation for treatments, walking the dog, relieving you for an hour. Listing specific assignments and needs allows others to choose what they can do within their own schedules.

How can I find respite help?

You can find respite help by calling a social worker, nurse or an agency such as your area Agency On Aging to find helpers to aid you when you feel worn out from extra responsibilities. Many times, a person with advanced cancer is eligible to have a visiting nurse come to the house to find out what your needs are. The nurses can send out a nurse's aide to help with bathing and bedmaking. Aides cannot stay longer than one or two hours and they usually cannot visit in the evening or at night. The local Agency On Aging can send out a social worker to assess the situation and help you find extra help. This agency can recommend workers who they know are reliable and they will explain your options and the costs involved. Sometimes, there are funds available from the county or state to help pay for respite care workers. Some areas also have volunteers who are experienced in helping families with cancer crises.

Why should I involve the patient in making plans for extra help?

Many times, patients are resistant to having extra help in the home. The person you are caring for may be more willing to accept help if you explain that you need help to keep giving care at home. Then, try using the helper a few times a week for a limited time—two or three weeks. Then both you and the patient can decide if you want to continue. If the first person does not work out, you may want to try with someone else, setting a new trial period.

What if we don't like the help we are sent?

Having helpers in your home requires some adjustments for everyone. However, most families find that they become very close to the helpers and look forward to seeing them. If one helper does not work out, you can try others. Agencies are accustomed to trying several people before the right one is found.

**What if the patient refuses to try respite care or is
unhappy with every helper we try?**

If this is the case, then it may be necessary to find other ways to get the rest you need. It may be that you will have to move the patient to a nursing home for a while. The patient can return when you are rested or when he or she decides that the extra home help is a better solution than staying in a nursing home.

**Why do I feel relief after the death of my loved
one who had a prolonged illness?**

When an illness is prolonged, often the grieving process is completed before the actual death. It is not uncommon for the family to feel relief that the pain, suffering, and uncertainty have ended. Some people may misinterpret this acceptance and think you are unfeeling. You must not feel guilty, for this has been found to be a perfectly normal reaction. People experience grief in different ways, and often the deepest grief may be that felt by those who do not show grief outwardly.

Web Pages to Check Out

www.cancer.gov: For general up-to-date information, and for clinical trials.
www.cancer.org: For general up-to-date information and community resources.

Nutrition
www.eatright.org: American Dietetic Association.

Hypnotherapy
www.natboard.com: National Board of Clinical Certified Hypnotherapists, Inc.
www.aaph.org: American Association of Professional Hypnotherapists.

Biofeedback

www.aapb.org: Association for Applied Psycophisiology and Biofeedback.

Pain Management

www.painmed.org
www.ampainsoc.org
www.abms.org
www.pain.com (also has listing of pain clinics)
www.aacpi.org: American Alliance of Cancer Pain Inititatives.
www.aamc.org: Geographical listing of medical schools and teaching hospitals.

Free Living Will and Power of Attorney Forms

www.partnershipforcaring.org: Living Will forms.
www.texmed.org: Medical Power of Attorney forms.

Insurance and Insurance Appeal Information

www.consumersunion.org

Caring for the Patient

www.patientadvocate.org
www.aarc.org: American Association for Respiratory Care.
www.hospicefoundation.org: Hospice Information.
www.nhpco.org: National Hospice and Palliative Care Organization.
www.hospiceweb.com: Links to other Hospice sites.
www.acponline.org: Information for caregivers.
www.cancer.gov/cancerinfo/support: General information on support groups.
www.cancercare.org: Local support groups.
www.acor.org: Online support groups (all types of cancer and cancer issues).
www.cms.hhs.gov/: Medicare questions.
www.holistic-online.com/guidedimagery.htm: Imagery and visualization.

Viatical Life Insurances

www.bbb.org/library/viatical.html: Better Business Bureau.
www.nationalviatical.org: National Viatical Association.
www.ftc.gov/bcp/conline/pubs/services/viatical.htm: Federal Trade
  Commission.

Books, Articles, and Other Resources
You May Want to Read

Facing Forward: Life After Cancer Treatment. A Guide for People Who Were Treated for Cancer. National Cancer Institute. #02-2424; 2002.
Consumer Guide to Handling Disputes with Your Private or Employer Health Plan, available through Consumer's Union and the Henry J. Kaiser Family Foundation.
The Cancer Patient's Workbook, Joanie Willis. New York: DK (Dorling Kindersley) Publishing, Inc., 2001.

Also see Chapter 2, Searching for Answers on the Web, for more information.

Twenty-eight

WHERE TO
GET HELP

QUICK REFERENCE FOR ESSENTIAL INFORMATION

Cancer Information Service
1–800–4–CANCER
www.cancer.gov/cancerinfo

American Cancer Society
1–800–ACS–2345
www.cancer.org

American Board of Medical Specialties
866–ASK–ABMS

NOTE: LISTINGS IN this chapter are focused on organizations that operate on a national level. Since there are many local or regional organizations that are too numerous to mention, these listings are just a starting point for your information seeking. The listings in this chapter are up-to-date at the time of publication. You may find that some of your inquiries will be routed to different organizations and individuals. Some organizations are available only through their Web site. Where appropriate, we have listed these Web pages at the end of the chapters in this book.

MAJOR INFORMATION SOURCES

National Cancer Institute's Cancer Information Service

Call 1–800–4–CANCER
(1–800–422–6237)
www.cancer.gov

The Cancer Information Service covers the entire United States. Based on the area code from which you are dialing, you will be connected to the regional center that covers your area.

The Cancer Information Service (CIS), a program of the National Cancer Institute (NCI) has a nationwide toll-free telephone service for cancer patients and their families, the public, and health care professionals. The CIS information specialists, who are experienced in providing medical information in easy-to-understand terms, give you rapid access to the latest information on cancer from the NCI on a range of cancer topics, including the most recent advances in cancer treatment. They take as much time as each caller needs, provide thorough and personalized attention and keep all calls confidential. They can:

- explain diagnostic procedures.
- tell you about standard treatments options, using PDQ, a computerized database of the National Cancer Institute.
- give information in layman's language that you will understand.
- help you form questions you wish to ask your doctor.
- conduct a computer search to give you information on where investigational treatment is being done.
- give you referrals to clinical trials and cancer-related services, such as treatment centers, mammography facilities, or other cancer organizations.
- send free printed material.
- discuss rehabilitation assistance and home-care assistance programs.
- help you find financial aid or emotional counseling services.
- discuss prevention.
- assist you in quitting smoking.

- give you information on causes of cancer.

- answer questions in English and Spanish.

- generally help you to get answers to any questions you might have.

CIS can tell you what hospitals and doctors in your area are involved in what kinds of investigational treatment. If, for instance, a relative lives in a different part of the country the staff can explore investigational treatments in that area. In many places, the Cancer Information Service offices are affiliated with Comprehensive Cancer Centers (specialized research and treatment centers designated by the National Cancer Institute).

What kind of questions should I ask when I call the Cancer Information Service?

The more specific you can be with your questions, the better the information you will receive. It is wise to think through what you want to know and to write down the questions you want to have answered before you call. You can call as many times as you wish. You do not have to give your name if you do not want to. All calls are kept confidential.

Can the Cancer Information Service tell me where different kinds of investigational treatments (clinical trials) are available in the United States? Overseas?

Yes, the Cancer Information Service, through the PDQ database, has information on the investigational treatments being conducted in the cancer centers and community hospitals around the country and overseas.

What is PDQ?

PDQ is a comprehensive data-based treatment information system supported by the National Cancer Institute. It offers cancer information summaries of the latest published information on cancer prevention, detection, genetics, treatment, supportive care, and complementary and alternative medicine. Most summaries are available in two versions, a patient version written in easy-to-understand, nontechnical language, and a health professional version that provides detailed information written in technical language. PDQ offers state-of-the art treatment statements, compiled and updated monthly by panels of experts in cancer and related specialties, giving the range of effective treatment options that represent the best available therapy for a specific type or stage of cancer. PDQ also gives the latest information on clinical treatment trials being offered around the country for each type and stage of cancer. It is a ready reference, with over 1,700 active trials, that is updated monthly by review boards composed of cancer specialists.

What do I need to know in order to have a PDQ search of clinical trials for my kind of cancer?

If you call the Cancer Information Service and request a PDQ search, you will be asked a series of questions to determine the information needed to complete the search for you:

- Whether or not you are currently receiving treatment. If you are already being treated, a search of potential clinical trials is not appropriate.
- Whether you (or the patient) is interested in participating in a clinical trial.
- Whether you are able, or willing, to travel to a participating center and how far you are willing to travel for treatment.
- The primary site of your cancer, the stage, and if possible cell type and grade; for breast cancer patients hormonal and menopausal status.
- The site of metastases, if any.
- What previous treatments you have had, type of treatment, when and where, including names of drugs previously received and when.
- Major medical conditions that might preclude participation.

What is LiveHelp?

CIS also provides live, online assistance to users of the NCI Web site through LiveHelp, an instant messaging service, that provides answers to questions about cancer and help in navigating the NCI Web site (www. cancer.gov).

What is CancerFax?

This is a service of the National Cancer Institute that allows you to get PDQ treatment information via a fax machine, 24 hours a day, seven days a week for the cost of your fax call. You first need to get instructions and a list of necessary codes (call 301–402–5874).

American Cancer Society

Call 1–800–ACS–2345
(1–800–227–2345)

www.cancer.org

Call this number anywhere in the country to get information from the American Cancer Society.

The American Cancer Society (ACS) is the nationwide, community-based, voluntary health organization dedicated to eliminating cancer as a major health problem through research, education and service. Its telephone service can do the following:

- answer all kinds of questions on all types of cancer and offer printed material on cancer free of charge.

- provide guidelines for treatment, drugs, and clinical trials.

- provide information and guidance concerning ACS services, community health services, and other resources, such as transportation to and from a doctor's office, clinic, or hospital for treatment.

- refer you to rehabilitation programs, including:

  - Cancer Survivors' Network: A telephone-based and online community for cancer survivors, friends and families (877–333–HOPE).

  - I Can Cope: Lecture, group discussion course.

  - Look Good, Feel Better: A free national public service program founded in partnership with the National Cosmetology Association and the Cosmetic, Toiletry, and Fragrance Association Foundation to help women with cancer restore self-image.

  - Man to Man: Information program for men and their partners about prostate cancer.

  - Reach to Recovery: Program featuring volunteers who have had breast cancer, designed to help new patients with breast cancer cope with their diagnosis, treatment and recovery.

  - Hope Lodges: Temporary residential facilities for patients and their families. Provide sleeping rooms and related facilities after approval from doctor or referring agency. (Available in Birmingham, Alabama; Little Rock, Arkansas; Gainesville, Florida; Decatur/Atlanta Georgia; Indianapolis, Indiana; Baltimore, Maryland; Worcester, Massachusetts; Rochester, Minnesota; St. Louis, Missouri; Buffalo and Rochester, New York; Cleveland, Ohio; Hershey, Pennsylvania; San Juan [children only], Puerto Rico; Charleston, South Carolina and Burlington, Vermont.)

National Office

American Cancer Society
1599 Clifton Road NE
Atlanta, GA 30329–4251
1–800–ACS–2345

Division Offices

California Division
California Division, Inc.
710 Webster Street, Suite 10
Oakland, CA 94612
510–893–7900

Eastern Division (New Jersey,
  New York)
Eastern Division, Inc. (Northern office)
6725 Lyons Street
East Syracuse, NY 13057
315–437–7025

**Eastern Division, Inc. (Southern
  office)**
2600 U.S. Highway 1
North Brunswick, NJ 08902–
  6001
732–297–8000

Florida Division (Florida, Puerto
  Rico)
Florida Division, Inc.
3709 West Jetton Avenue
Tampa, FL 33629–5146
813–253–0541

Puerto Rico Division, Inc.
Calle Alverio #577
Esquina Sargento Medina
Hato Rey, PR 00918
787–764–2295

Great Lakes Division (Indiana,
  Michigan)
Great Lakes Division, Inc.
1205 East Saginaw Street
Lansing, MI 48906
800–723–0360

Heartland Division
  (Kansas, Missouri, Nebraska,
  Oklahoma)
Heartland Division, Inc.
1100 Pennsylvania Avenue
Kansas City, MO 64105
816–842–7111

Illinois Division, Inc.
77 East Monroe Street, 13th Floor
Chicago, IL 60603–5795
312–641–6150

Mid-Atlantic Division (Delaware,
Maryland, Washington, DC, Virginia,
West Virginia)
Mid-Atlantic Division, Inc.
1875 Connecticut Avenue, N.W.
Washington, DC 20009
202–483–2600

Mid-South Division
  (Alabama, Arkansas,
  Kentucky, Louisiana,
  Mississippi, Tennessee)
Mid-South Division, Inc.
1100 Ireland Way, Suite 300
Birmingham, AL 35205
205–879–2242

Midwest Division
  (Iowa, Minnesota, South
  Dakota, Wisconsin)
Midwest Division, Inc.
3316 Sixty-sixth Street
Minneapolis, MN 55435
612–925–2772

New England Division
  (Connecticut, Maine,
  Massachusetts, New
  Hampshire, Rhode Island,
  Vermont)
New England Division, Inc.
  (Framingham)
30 Speen Street
Framingham, MA 01701–1800
508–270–4600

New England Division, Inc.
  (Meriden)
Meriden Executive Park
538 Preston Avenue
Meriden, CT 06450–1004
203–379–4700

Northwest Division
  (Alaska, Oregon,
  Washington, Montana)
2120 First Avenue North
Seattle, WA 98109–1140
206–283–1152

Ohio Division (Ohio)
5555 Frantz Road
Dublin, OH 43017
800–686–4357

Pennsylvania Division
  (Pennsylvania)
Route 422 and Sipe Avenue
Hershey, PA 17033–0897
717–533–6144

Rocky Mountain Division
  (Colorado, Idaho, North Dakota,
  Utah, Wyoming)
Rocky Mountain Division, Inc.
2255 South Oneida
Denver, CO 80224
303–758–2030

Southeast Division
  (Georgia, North Carolina,
  South Carolina)
Southeast Division, Inc.
2200 Lake Boulevard
Atlanta, GA 30319
404–816–4994

Southwest Division
  (Nevada, Arizona,
  New Mexico)
Southwest Division, Inc.
2929 East Thomas Road
Phoenix, AZ 85016
602–224–0524

Texas Division (Hawaii, Texas)
Hawaii Pacific Division, Inc.
2370 Nuuanu Avenue
Honolulu, HI 96817
808–595–7500

Texas Division, Inc.
2433 Ridgepoint Drive A
Austin, TX 78754
512–919–1800

PATIENT SERVICE ORGANIZATIONS

Air Care Alliance
1515 East 71st Street, Suite 312
Tulsa, OK 74136
Phone: 888–260–9707
Fax: 918–745–0879
E-mail: mail@aircarecall.org
www.aircarecall.org
National organization of volunteer
  pilots who arrange patient
  transportation. Web site offers
  central searchable source for all free

air transportation services provided
by volunteer pilots and charitable
aviation groups.

American Association of Tissue Banks
1350 Beverly Road, Suite 220-A
McLean, VA, 22101
800–635–2282
www.aatb.org
Maintains a registry of sperm banks in
  the United States.

(The) American Bone Marrow Donor Registry
Search Coordinating Center
University of Massachusetts Medical Center
55 Lake Avenue, North
Worcester, MA 01655
508–756–6444
Assists those with leukemia, aplastic anemia and other blood-related disorders in finding compatible bone marrow donors.

American Brain Tumor Association
(formerly Association for Brain Tumor Research)
2720 River Road Suite 146
Des Plaines, IL 60018
708–827–9910
800–886–ABTA (patient line)
Offers free services including publications about brain tumors, support group lists, referral information. Supports research.

American Self Help Clearinghouse
St. Clares-Riverside Medical Center
Denville, NJ 07834–2995
973–326–6789
Provides current information and contacts for national self-help groups. Gives information concerning any state or local self-help group that may exist. Supports caller in forming group if none exists. Publishes Self-Help Source Book.

Bone Marrow Foundation
70 East 55th Street, 20th floor
New York, NY 10022
800–3650–1336
www.bonemarrow.org
Mission is to improve quality of life for bone marrow patients and their families.

Bone Marrow Transplant Family Support Network
PO Box 845
Avon, CT 06001
800–826–9376
Offers support to families coping with decisions, daily routines prior to and following transplants, follow-up care.

Bone Marrow Transplant Newsletter
1985 Spruce Avenue
Highland Park, IL 60035
Newsletter and book on issues, attorney referrals for those having difficulty obtaining reimbursement for treatment.

Breast Cancer Alliance, Inc.
15 East Putnam Avenue, Box 414
Greenwich, CT 06830
203–861–0014
www.breastcanceralliance.org
Funds breast cancer research, promotes breast health through outreach and education.

National Breast Cancer Coalition
1797 L Street NW, Suite 1060
Washington, DC 20036
202–296–7477
www.natlbcc.org
A grassroots breast cancer advocacy organization. Seeks funding for research on breast cancer, better access to services for women, and influence by the breast cancer patient in decision making.

Breast Cancer Registries (Familial)
Metropolitan New York Registry of Breast Cancer
School of Public Health
Columbia University
New York, NY 10032
212–305–8856
www.metnyreg.org

Northern California Cooperative
  Family Registry
Northern California Cancer Center
Union City, CA 94587
510–429–2500
www.nccc.org

Ontario Registry for Studies of
  Familial Breast Cancer
Cancer Care Ontario
Toronto, ON M5G 2L7, Canada
416–971–9800
www.cancercare.on.ca

Philadelphia Familial Breast Cancer
  Registry
Fox Chase Cancer Center
Philadelphia, PA 19012
1–800–325–4145
www.fccc.edu

Utah Cooperative Breast Cancer
  Registry
University of Utah Health Sciences
  Center
Salt Lake City, UT 84112
800–936–6343
www.hci.utah.edu/5095.html

**Breast Implant Information Service
  (FDA)**
Food and Drug Administration
Office of Device Evaluation
Division of General, Restorative and
  Neurological Devices
9200 Corporate Boulevard, HFZ-410
Rockville, MD 20850
800–532–4440
www.fda.gov/cdrh/breastimplants/
Provides latest information on breast
  implants.

**CAN ACT (Cancer Patients Action
  Alliance)**
26 College Place
Brooklyn, NY 11201
718–522–4607

Addresses problems of access to
  advanced cancer treatments, barriers
  created by the FDA drug approval
  process and restrictive insurance
  reimbursement policies.

Cancer Care, Inc.
275 Seventh Avenue
New York, NY 10001
800–813–4673
www.cancercare.org
A nonprofit social service agency
  helping patients and families cope with
  emotional, financial, and psychological
  consequences of cancer. Services provided by oncology social workers in
  person, over the telephone and though
  the Web site. Financial counseling is
  also available, as is financial assistance
  for home care and transportation.

Cancer Genetics Network
Web page:
  www.epi.grants.cancer.gov/CGN/
Information on program, how to
  enroll, studies underway, participating
  institutions.

Participating institutions:
*Carolina-Georgia Center of the
  Cancer Genetics Network
Duke University Medical Center
cancer.duke.edu/CGN

*Lombardi Cancer Center Genetics
  Network
Georgetown University Lombardi
  Cancer Center
Washington, DC
lombardi.georgetown.edu/research/areas/
  cancercontrol/cgn

*Mid-Atlantic Cancer Genetics
  Network
Johns Hopkins University
Baltimore, MD
www.macgn.org

*Northwest Cancer Genetics Network
Fred Hutchinson Cancer Research
 Center
Seattle, WA
www.fhcrc.org/phs/cgn/index.htm

*Rocky Mountain Cancer Genetics
 Coalition
University of Utah
Salt Lake City, UT
www.hci.utah.edu/cgn

*Texas Cancer Genetics Consortium
University of Texas M.D. Anderson
 Cancer Center
Houston, TX
www.texas.cgnweb.org

*UCI-UCSD Cancer Genetics
 Network Center
University of California at Irvine and
 at San Diego

*University of Pennsylvania Cancer
 Genetics Network
University of Pennsylvania
Philadelphia, PA
www.oncolink.com

Cancer Information Service
(a program of the National Cancer
 Institute)
800–4–CANCER (800–422–6237)
www.cancer.gov/cancerinformation
Nationwide information service
 for cancer patients and their families,
 the public, and health care
 professionals. CIS information
 specialists have extensive training
 in providing up-to-date and
 understandable information about
 cancer. Can answer questions in
 English and Spanish and send free
 printed material. Web site gives
 information, including clinical trials
 available.

CANCERVIVE, Inc.
11636 Chayote Street
Los Angeles, CA 90049
1–800–486–2873
(800–4–TO–CURE)
A nationwide network that runs
 support groups to help with everyday
 concerns of survivors. Number given
 will put you in touch with group
 nearest you or advise you how to start
 a group of your own.

**Candlelighters Childhood Cancer
 Foundation**
PO Box 498
Kensington, MD 20895–0498
800–366–2223
www.candlelighters.org
An organization formed by parents of
 young cancer patients. An important
 goal of the organization is to help
 families cope with the emotional
 stresses of their experiences.

Center for Medical Consumers
237 Thompson Street
New York, NY 10012
212–674–7105
Provides information and referrals to
 national health organizations and
 maintains a medical consumers'
 public library.

ChemoCare
Scott Hamilton Initiative
Cleveland Clinic Taussig Cancer Center
Cleveland Clinic Foundation
Cleveland, OH
www.chemocare.com
Sponsored by drug companies but has
 important information about
 chemotherapy side effects.
 Excellent specific question and
 answer information. Especially
 helpful to young people.

Children's Hospice International
901 North Pitt Street, Suite 230
Alexandria, VA 22314
703–684–0330
800–242–4453
www.chionline.org
Non-profit agency that encourages use of hospices and home care programs for children.

Children's Oncology Camping Association of America
PO Box 35
Mountain Center, CA 92561
900–737–2667
Publishes international directory of children's oncology camps.

The Children's Organ Transplant Association
2501 COTA Drive
Bloomington, IN 47403
800–366–2682
www.cota.org
Helps families and communities raise funds for children needing transplants and transplant-related expenses.

Clinical Center of the National Institutes of Health
Patient Referral Service
Building 10, Room IC 255
9000 Rockville Pike
Bethesda, MD 20892
301–496–4891
See page 1058 for additional information.

Colon Cancer Alliance, Inc.
175 Ninth Avenue
New York, NY 10011
877–422–2030
Fax: 425–940–6147
www.ccalliance.org

Offers educational materials to help colorectal cancer survivors and their loved ones in their battle with colorectal cancer.

Corporate Angel Network, Inc.
Westchester County Airport
One Loop Road
White Plains, NY 10604–1215
914–328–1313
866–328–1313
Fax: 914–328–3938
E-mail: Info@corpangelnetwork.org
www.corpangelnetwork.org
A service that matches available space on corporate airplanes with cancer patients in need of transportation to recognized treatment centers.

DES
Registry for Research on Hormonal Transplacental Carcinogenesis
University of Chicago
Department of Obstetrics and Gynecology
5841 South Maryland Avenue MO2050
Chicago, IL 60637
773–702–6671
A worldwide registry for individuals who developed clear cell adenocarcinoma as a result of exposure to DES.

DES Action USA
610 16th St., Suite 301
Oakland, CA, 94612
510–465–4011
Provides counseling, educational materials, and a newsletter about diethylstilbesterol (DES), a synthetic hormone once given to pregnant women to prevent miscarriages.

DES Cancer Network
514 Tenth St. NW, Suite 400
Washington, DC 20004
800–DES–NET–4
(800–337–6384)
Provides information about
DES-related cancer.

Encore
YWCA of USA
For postoperative breast cancer
patients. Supportive discussion and
rehabilitative exercise. Call your local
YWCA branch.

Food and Drug Administration
Office of Consumer Affairs HFE-88
Rooms 16–63, 5600 Fishers Lane
Rockville, MD 20857
301–443–3170
MedWatch Program
800–332–1088
Provides information of federal
regulation of drugs.

**Gilda Radner Familial Ovarian
Cancer Registry**
Roswell Park Cancer Institute
New York Department of Health
Elm and Carlton Streets
Buffalo, NY 14263
800–685–6825, ext. 4503
Individuals can register; newsletter.

Hereditary Cancer Institute
Creighton University
Omaha, NE 68178
402–280–1746
Nonprofit organization devoted to the
study of the genetics of familial cancer.
Attempts to assess and verify the
nature of cancer patterns in families
and the simple or complex modes of
inheritance that may help in predicting cancer risk to family members
and their offspring. Maintains a

registry of families interested in
participating in its work.

Hospice
See National Hospice Organization.

Hospice Link
Hospice Education Institute
3 Unity Square, P.O. Box 98
Machiasport, ME 04655–0098
800–331–1630 or 207–255–8800
The institute offers information about
hospice care and can refer cancer
patients and their families to local
hospice programs.

I Can Cope
American Cancer Society
1–800–ACS–2345
A patient education program of the
American Cancer Society designed to
help patients, families, and friends
cope with the day-to-day issues of
living with cancer.

**International Association of
Laryngectomees**
8900 Thornton Road, Box 9931
Stockton, CA 95209
866–IAL–FORU
www.larynxlink.com
Voluntary organization composed of
190 member clubs. Assists people
who have lost their voices as a result
of cancer, provides education in skills
needed by laryngectomees, and works
toward total rehabilitation of patient.
Maintains registry of postlaryngecto-
my speech instructors, publishes educational materials, sponsors meetings
and other activities.

**International Bone Marrow
Transplant Registry**
Medical College of Wisconsin
870 Watertown Plank Road,

PO Box 26509
Milwaukee, WI 53226
414–456–6530
Collects and analyzes data about allogeneic bone marrow transplantations.
Most BMT teams throughout the
world participate in the registry. Staff
is available to answer questions about
the procedure. Donor matches are
not made by this registry. (See
National Marrow Donor Program.)

International Myeloma Foundation
13605 Riverside Drive, Suite 206
North Hollywood, CA 91607
800–452–CURE
818–487–7454
Promotes education and research,
informs patients about available treatments and provides support to community and patient support groups.

**Komen (Susan G.) Breast Cancer
Foundation**
PO Box 650309
Dallas, TX 75265–0309
800–IMA–WARE
Breast cancer organization dedicated
to eradicating breast cancer as a
life-threatening disease through
research, education, screening and
treatment.

Let's Face It USA
PO Box 29972
Bellingham, WA 98338–1972
360–676–7325
www.faceit.org
International information and support
organization for people with head
and neck cancer and others with
facial disfigurement.

Leukemia and Lymphoma Society
1311 Mamaroneck Avenue
White Plains, NY 10605

800–955–4LSA
914–949–5213
www.leukemia-lymphoma.org
Focuses on leukemia, the lymphomas,
and Hodgkin's disease. Provides referral services to other sources of help in
community. Offers financial assistance
for drugs used in care, treatment,
and/or control of disease; transfusing
of blood, transportation to and from a
doctor's office, hospital, or treatment
center and x-ray treatment. Supports
research and provides printed materials.

Living Bank
PO Box 6725
Houston, TX 77265–6725
713–961–0979
800–528–2971
www.livingbank.org
Information on donating body or
organ parts.

Look Good . . . Feel Better
American Cancer Society
800–395–LOOK
Program developed by the Cosmetic,
Toiletry, and Fragrance Association in
cooperation with the American Cancer
Society and the National Cosmetology
Association. It focuses on techniques
that can help people undergoing cancer
treatment improve their appearance.

**Lymphedema Network (see National
Lymphedema Network)**

**Multiple Myeloma Research
Foundation (MMRFO)**
3 Forest Street
New Canaan, CT 06840
203–972–1250
www.multiplemyeloma.org
Dedicated to accelerating the search for
a cure for multiple myeloma. Funds
research, provides information on

clinical trials, and offers information for patients and families on treatment options.

National Alliance of Breast Cancer Organizations (NABCO)
9 East 37 Street, Tenth Floor
New York, NY 10016
888–80–NABCO
www.nabco.org
212–719–0154
Advocates for needs and concerns of patients/survivors and all women at risk for breast cancer. Register here for mammography e-mail reminder.

National Brain Tumor Foundation
414 Thirteenth Street, Suite 700
Oakland, CA 94612–2603
800–934–CURE
510–939–9777
www.braintumor.org
Raises funds to support brain tumor research and provides information and support services to patients and families.

National Cancer Institute
www.cancer.gov
Federal government's principal agency for cancer research and treatment. See pages 1030 and 1053 in this chapter for more information.

National Coalition for Cancer Survivorship
1010 Wayne Avenue, Suite 770
Silver Spring, MD 20910
301–650–9127
877–NCCS–YES
www.canceradvocacy.org
Network of groups and individuals offering support to cancer survivors and families. Information and resources on life after a cancer diagnosis. Advocates for employment and legal rights of people with cancer.

National Colorectal Cancer Research Alliance
11132 Ventura Boulevard, Suite 401
Studio City, CA 91604–3156.
800–872–3000.
www.nccra.org
Promotes education, fundraising, research and early medical screening. Founded by Katie Couric, Lily Tartikoff and the Entertainment Industry Foundation.

National Consumers League
1701 K Street NW, Suite1200
Washington, DC 20006
202–835–3323
National nonprofit membership organization offering publications on a range of health issues such as hospice, home health care and insurance.

National Council Against Health Fraud
119 Foster Street
Peabody, MA 01960
800–821–6671
Provides information on questionable health practices and organizations.

National Hospice Organization
1700 Diagonal Road
Suite 300
Arlington, VA 22314
800–646–6460
703–837–1500
www.nhpco.org
Association of groups that provide hospice care. Designed to promote and maintain hospice care and to encourage support for patients and family members. Information about hospice concepts also available.

National Kidney Cancer Association
320 North Michigan Avenue, Suite 203

Chicago, IL 60601–1375
800–850–9132
847–332–1051
www.nkca.org
Provides information to patients and
physicians, sponsors research on kidney cancer and acts as an advocate on
behalf of patients.

National Lymphedema Network
Latham Square, 1611 Telegraph
Avenue, Suite 1111
Oakland, CA 94612
800–541–3259
510–208–3200
www.lymphnet.org
Nonprofit network provides information about prevention and treatment
of lymphoma and information about
support groups.

National Marrow Donor Program
3001 Broadway Street NE, Suite 500
Minneapolis, MN 55413
800–MARROW–2 (800–627–7692)
www.marrow.org
Funded by the Federal Government
and created to improve effectiveness
of search for bone marrow donors
so that a greater number of bone
marrow transplantations can be carried out. Maintains computer data
bank of available tissue-typed marrow donors.

**National Oral Health Information
Clearinghouse**
Box NOHIC
Bethesda, MD 20892–3500
301–402–7364
www.nohic.nider.nih.gov
Resource for patients, health professionals and public seeking information on oral health of special care
patients, such as those whose medical
treatment causes oral problems.

**National Organization for Rare
Disorders**
PO Box 8923
New Fairfield, CT 07812–1783
203–746–6518
www.rarediseases.org
Organization dedicated to the prevention, treatment and cure of rare diseases; alphabetical database and
informational material.

National Patient Travel Helpline
c/o Mercy Medical Airlift
4620 Haygood Rd. Ste.1
Virginia Beach, VA 23444
800–296–1217
Fax: 757–318–9107
www.patienttravel.org
Provides information about
long-distance medical air
transportation and referrals to
all help in the national charitable
medical air transportation network.

National Women's Health Network
514 10th Street NW, Suite 400
Washington, DC 20004
202–628–7814
Provides information on women's cancers and other issues related to
women's health.

Office of Rare Diseases
National Institutes of Health
6100 Executive Boulevard,
Room 3A07, MSC 7518
Bethesda, MD 20892–7518
301–402–4336
Fax: 301–480–9655
E-mail: ord@od.nih.gov
www.rarediseases.info.nih.gov
Office of the National Institutes of
Health that specializes in rare diseases.
Its Web page lists more than 6,000
rare diseases, including current
research, publications from scientific

and medical journals, completed research, ongoing studies, and patient support groups. Also can give you information on genes and genetic testing.

Partnership for Caring
1620 Eye Street NW
Washington, DC 20006
800–989–9455
Provides latest information on right-to-die, Living Wills, etc.

Patient Advocate Foundation
753 Thimble Shoals Blvd. Suite B
Newport News, VA 23606
800–532–5274
Fax: 757–873–8999
www.patientadvocate.org
Provides information, legal counseling, and referral concerning managed care, financial issues, job discrimination and debt crisis matters.

PDQ (Physician Data Query)
800–4–CANCER
www.nci.nih.gov/cancerinformation/pdq/
National Cancer Institute's computerized listing of up-to-date information for patients and health professionals on latest cancer treatments, research studies, clinical trials, promising cancer treatments and organizations and doctors involved with cancer.

Pharmaceutical Research and Manufacturers of America
1110 15th Street NW
Washington, DC 20005
www.phrma.org
Organization of companies that manufacture chemotherapy and other drugs. Web site lists programs offered by some pharmaceutical companies to help pay for medication and cancer treatment drugs.

Quality Care National Resource Center
2 Copley Place, Suite 200
Boston, MA 02116
800–645–3633
National provider of home nursing services. Operates toll-free telephone line that provides information about home care and related services such as home nursing services, hospices, skilled nursing, rehabilitation facilities and homemaker services throughout the United States. Two hundred-office network can provide referral information for these services and also for some specialty programs for cancer patients.

R.A. Bloch Cancer Foundation, Inc.
The Cancer Hotline
4400 Main Street
Kansas City, MO 64111
816–932–8453
www.blochcancer.org
Information for people diagnosed with cancer to help them find the best ways of treating it.

Reach to Recovery
c/o American Cancer Society
800–ACS–2345
Offers assistance to breast cancer patients. Trained volunteers who have had breast cancer lend emotional support and furnish information.

Ronald McDonald House
Kroc Drive
Oak Brook, IL 60521
630–623–7048
www.rmhc.com
Nonprofit organization offers home-away-from-home for parents and families of children being treated for serious illness. Found in US, Canada and Sydney, Australia. Each Ronald McDonald House is different,

created by a team of local citizens to meet needs of community. Each house is owned and operated by local not-for-profit organization comprised of volunteers and is primarily funded by local contributions. Call national coordinator for locations.

(The) Skin Cancer Foundation
245 Fifth Avenue Suite 1403
New York, NY 10016
800–SKIN–490
www.skincancer.org
National organization concerned exclusively with skin cancer. Conducts public and medical education programs to increase public awareness of importance of taking protective measures against damaging sun rays, and to teach people how to recognize early signs of skin cancer.

State Vocational Rehabilitation Service
c/o American Cancer Society
800–ACS–2345
Service offers training for another vocation for those physically unable to return to the same work performed prior to surgery. Check "State Services" in telephone directory.

United Ostomy Association
19772 MacArthur Blvd., Suite 200
Irvine, CA 92712–2405
800–826–0826
www.uoa.com
Provides education, information, support and advocacy to people who have had ostomies. Offers a variety of booklets compiled from the experiences of many hundreds of patients, nurses and doctors. Web site gives information from other patients, has discussion groups for various ages and a listserve. Local chapters are located

across the country and are listed on the Web site.

US-TOO, International
American Foundation of Urologic Diseases
930 North York Road, Suite 50
Hinsdale, IL 60521–2993
800–82–US–TOO
630–795–1002
www.ustoo.com
An international support network for prostate cancer survivors. Contact them for the chapter nearest you.

VHL Family Alliance
171 Clinton Road
Brookline, MA 02146
800–767–4VHL (800–767–4845)
Offers information and support to families with the rare familial disorder called Von Hipped Linda Syndrome (VHL) which can result in cancer in patients who have visceral lesions.

Well Spouse Foundation
63 West Main Street, Suite H
Reehold, NJ 07728
800–838–0879
www.wellspouse.org
Network of support groups and families that provide emotional support to spousal caregivers. Advocates for families of the chronically ill.

(The) Wellness Community
919 18th Street NW, Suite 54
Washington, DC 10006
33 E 7th Street
Cincinnati, OH 45202
888–793–WELL
www.thewellnesscommunity.org
Provides free psychosocial support to people fighting to recover from cancer, as an adjunct to conventional medical treatment. Has 23 worldwide locations.

Y-ME
212 W. Van Buren, Suite 500
Chicago, IL 60607
800–221–2141
www.Y-me.org
Twenty-four-hour hotline, manned by
breast cancer survivors, counseling,
educational programs and self-help
meetings for breast cancer patients,
family and friends.

Young Survival Coalition
Box 528
52A Carmine Street
New York, NY 10014
212–916–7667
www.youngsurvival.org
Focuses on issues and challenges faced
by women aged 40 and under diagnosed with breast cancer.

DOCTORS AND OTHER HEALTH PROFESSIONALS

**American Academy of
Dermatology**
PO Box 4014
Schaumburg, IL 60168–4014
708–330–0230
www.aad.org
Organization of doctors who specialize
in diagnosing and treating skin problems. Provides information and references to dermatologists in your area.

**American Association for Marriage
and Family Therapy**
112 S. Alfred Street
Alexandria, VA 22314–3016
703–838–9808
www.aamft.org
Provides names of therapists who are
Clinical Members of the American
Association for Marriage and Family
Therapy on searchable Web site. The
directory provides information on the
therapist's office locations and availability, practice description, education, professional licenses, health plan
participation, achievements and
awards and languages spoken.

**American Association of Sex
Educators, Counselors and
Therapists (ASECT)**
PO Box 5488
Richmond, VA 23220–0488

319–895–8407
Provides names of sex therapists in
your area.

**American Board of Medical
Specialties**
866–ASK–ABMS
www.ABMS.org
Toll-free telephone line provides
verification of physician's certification status. (See Chapter 2,
Choosing Your Doctor and
Hospital).

American Brachytherapy Society
1250 Roger Bacon Drive, Suite 8
Reston, VA 20190–5202
www.americanbrachytherapy.org
Promotes highest standards of practice
of brachytherapy and clinical and
laboratory research in this specialty.
Encourages continuing education for
radiation oncologists.

American College of Radiology
1891 Preston White Drive
Reston, VA 22091–4397
800–ACR–LINE
www.acr.org
Will provide updated information
concerning mammograms. ACR
voluntary program evaluates and
approves equipment, personnel,

procedures and facilities. ACR accredited facilities are staffed with doctors and personnel trained to perform and interpret mammograms.

American College of Surgeons
633 North St. Clair Street
Chicago, IL 60611–3211
312–664–5000
www.facs.org
Provides list of board-certified surgeons in all specialties. Maintains certification program for hospitals relating to quality of cancer care. Programs are surveyed at request of hospital administrators or medical staffs or both. Approved status is based on level of excellence in relation to standards established by the College of Surgeons. In order to be certified the hospital must have a cancer committee, a cancer registry, a clinical education program, and means for evaluating the quality of care in the hospital. Hospitals that have been given approved status are listed in the College of Surgeons Directory, published annually and updated twice a year.

American Foundation for Urologic Disease
1128 North Charles Street
Baltimore, MD 21201–2463
800–828–7866
www.afud.org
Provides educational opportunities for the public, patients and health care professionals about urologic diseases. Support groups: US TOO, Bladder Health Council and Prostate Health Council.

(The) American Society of Clinical Hypnosis
140 North Bloomingdale Road
Bloomingdale, IL 60108–1017
630–980–4740
www.asch.net
National organization for clinical hypnotists

American Society of Clinical Oncology
1900 Duke Street, Suite 200
Alexandria, VA 22314
703–299–0150
www.asco.org
Exchange and diffusion of information and ideas relating to human neoplastic diseases.

American Society of Plastic and Reconstructive Surgeons
444 East Algonquin Road
Arlington Heights, IL 60005
888–4–PLASTIC
Provides names of board-certified plastic surgeons in your area and free information regarding surgical procedures.

American Society for Therapeutic Radiology and Oncology
2500 Fair Lakes Circle, Suite 375
Fairfax, VA 22033–3882
800–962–7876
www.astro.org
Extends benefits of radiation therapy to patients with cancer or other disorders, advances scientific basis, provides education.

Armed Forces Institute of Pathology
6825 16th Street NW
Washington, DC 20306–6000
202–782–2100
www.afip.org

Specializes in pathology consultation, education and research. Second opinions on difficult, unusual or rare pathology. Over 100 pathologists on staff.

Association of Oncology Social Workers
1211 Locust Street
Philadelphia, PA 19107
215–599–6093
www.aosw.org
National organization of professional social workers in oncology.

Association of Pediatric Oncology Nurses (APON)
4700 W Lake Avenue
Glenview, IL 60025
847–375–4724
www.apon.org
Promotes highest standards in nursing care for children and adolescents with cancer and for their families.

International Union Against Cancer
Union Internationale Contre le Cancer (UICC)
Rue de Conseil-General 3
1205 Geneva
Switzerland
(41–22) 22–809–18–11
Nongovernmental, voluntary organization devoted solely to promoting research, therapeutic and preventive aspects of cancer throughout the world. Worldwide association with member organizations in 78 countries. Facilities exchange information among national cancer organizations. With NCI support, publishes International Directory of Specialized Cancer Research and Treatment Establishments.

Joint Commission on Accreditation of Healthcare Organizations (JCAHO)
1 Renaissance Boulevard
Oak Brook Terrace, IL 60181
800–994–6610
Hospital accrediting organization. Will tell you if health care facility has been accredited by JCAHO. Complaints about quality of care at health care organizations can be filed with them.

National Center for Cancer Complementary and Alternative Medicine
National Institutes of Health
Bethesda, MD 20892
888–644–6226
www.nccam.nih.gov
Established in 1992 to investigate complementary and alternative treatments using the same scientific methods used in conventional medicine. Funds research in five domains: mind-body medicine, biologically based therapies, alternative medical systems, manipulative and body-based energy therapies as they relate to many different diseases including cancer.

National Society of Genetic Counselors
233 Canterbury Drive
Wallingford, PA 19086–6617
610–872–7608
www.nsgc.org
Resource link for list of genetic counselors. Exchange of information on genetic diseases and training of counselors.

Oncology Nursing Society
125 Enterprise Drive
Pittsburgh, PA 15215–1214
866–257–4667
www.ons.org

Professional organization dedicated to providing optimal care to persons with an actual and/or potential diagnosis of cancer.

(The) Society for Clinical and Experimental Hypnosis
Washington State University
PO Box 642114
Pullman, WA 97164–2114
509–335–2097
www.sunsite.utk.edu/1JEC/scehmain.htm

Society of Gynecologic Oncologists
401 North Michigan Avenue
Chicago, IL 60611
312–644–6610
www.sgo.org
Professional organization dedicated to improving care of patients with gynecologic cancer, advancing knowledge and standards, encouraging research.

State Physician Licensing Boards

www. healthcare associates.org.

ALABAMA
Alabama State Board of Medical Examiners
PO Box 946
Montgomery, AL 36102
334–242–4116

ALASKA
Alaska State Medical Board
Division of Occupational Licensing
3601 C Street, No. 722
Anchorage, AK 99503
907–269–8260

ARIZONA
Arizona Board of Medical Examiners
2001 West Camelback Road
Suite 300
Phoenix, AZ 85015
602–255–3751

ARKANSAS
Arkansas State Medical Board
PO Box 102
Little Rock, AK 72202
501–296–1802

CALIFORNIA
California Board of Medical Quality Assurance
1430 Howe Avenue, Suite 56
Sacramento, CA 95825
916–920–2389

COLORADO
Board of Medical Examiners
132 State Services Building
1525 Sherman Street
Denver, CO 80203
303–894–7692

CONNECTICUT
Connecticut Department of Public Health
PO Box 340308
Hartford, CT 06134
860–509–7586

DELAWARE
Board of Medical Practice
861 Silver Lake Blvd.
Dover, DE 19903
302–736–4522 x229

DISTRICT OF COLUMBIA
Board of Medicine
614 H Street NW, Room 108

Washington, DC 20001
202–727–5365

FLORIDA
Board of Medicine
1940 N. Monroe Street
Tallahassee, FL 32399–0770
850–488–0595

GEORGIA
Composite State Board of Medical
Examiners
166 Pryor Street SW, Room 424
Atlanta, GA 30303
404–656–3913

HAWAII
Board of Medical Examiners
PO Box 3469
Honolulu, HI 96801
808–548–4100

IDAHO
State Board of Medicine
280 N. 8th Street, Suite 202
Boise, ID 83720
208–334–2822

ILLINOIS
Illinois Board of Medical
Examiners
320 W. Washington, 3rd Floor
Springfield, IL 62786
217–785–0820

INDIANA
Indiana Health Professionals Bureau
One American Square
Suite 1020, Box 82067
Indianapolis, IN 46282
317–232–2960

IOWA
Board of Medical Examiners
Capitol Complex Executive Hills West
1209 E. Court Avenue
Des Moines, IA 50319
515–281–5171

KANSAS
State Board of Healing Arts
253 SW Topeka Boulevard
Topeka, KS 66603
785–296–7413

KENTUCKY
Kentucky Board of Licensure
400 Sherburn Lane
Suite 333
Louisville, KY 40207
502–896–1516

LOUISIANA
Louisiana State Board of Medical
Examiners
PO Box 30250
630 Camp Street
New Orleans, LA 70130
504–524–6763

MAINE
Maine Board of Registration in
Medicine
137 House Station
2 Bangor Street
Augusta, ME 04333
207–289–6590

MARYLAND
Maryland Board of Physician Quality
Assurance
PO Box 2571
4201 Patterson Avenue
Baltimore, MD 21215–0002
410–764–4777

MASSACHUSETTS
Massachusetts Board of Registration in
Medicine
10 West Street, 3rd Floor
Boston, MA 02111
617–727–3086

MICHIGAN
Michigan Board of Medicine
PO Box 30670

611 W. Ottawa Street
Lansing, MI 48909
517–335–0918

MINNESOTA
Board of Medical Examiners
2829 University Avenue SE
No. 400
St. Paul, MN 55414
612–617–2166

MISSISSIPPI
Mississippi State Board of
  Medical Licensure
2688D Insurance Center
  Drive
Jackson, MS 39216
601–354–6645

MISSOURI
Missouri State Board of Reg. Healing
  Arts
PO Box 4
Jefferson City, MO 65102
573–751–0098

MONTANA
Montana State Board of Medical
  Examiners
PO Box 200513
Helena, MT 59620
406–444–1988

NEBRASKA
Nebraska State Board of Examiners in
  Medicine and Surgery
PO Box 95007
Lincoln, NE 68509–5007
406–471–2115

NEVADA
Nevada State Board of Medical
  Examiners
PO Box 94986
1105 Terminal Way, Suite 301
Reno, NV 89510
702–688–2559

NEW HAMPSHIRE
Board of Registration in Medicine
2 Industrial Park, Suite 8
Concord, NH 03301
603–271–1203

NEW JERSEY
New Jersey Board of Medical
  Examiners
140 East Front Street, 2nd Floor
Trenton, NH 08608
609–826–7100

NEW MEXICO
New Mexico State Board of Medical
  Examiners
491 Old Santa Fe Trail
Santa Fe, NM 87501
505–827–5022

NEW YORK
State Board for Medicine
Cultural Education Center, Room 3023
Empire State Plaza
Albany, NY 12230
518–486–2937

NORTH CAROLINA
North Carolina Board of Medical
  Examiners
PO Box 20007
Raleigh, NC 27619
919–876–3885

NORTH DAKOTA
North Dakota State Board of Medical
  Examiners
418 East Broadway Avenue
Suite 12
Bismarck, ND 58501
701–328–6500

OHIO
Ohio State Medical Board
77 S. High Street, 17th Floor
Columbus, OH 43266–0315
614–728–5946

OKLAHOMA
Oklahoma State Board of
  Licensure
PO Box 18256
Oklahoma City, OK 73154
405–848–2189

OREGON
Board of Medical Examiners
620 Crown Plaza
1500 SW 1st Avenue
Portland, OR 97201
503–229–5770

PENNSYLAVANIA
Pennsylvania State Board of
  Medicine
116 Pine Street
Harrisburg, PA 17105
717–787–2381

RHODE ISLAND
Board of Medical Licensure and
  Discipline
Cannon Building, Room 205
Three Capitol Hill
Providence, RI 02908
401–222–2158

SOUTH CAROLINA
South Carolina Board of Medical
  Examiners
PO Box 11289
110 Centerview Drive, Suite 202
PO Box 12245
Columbia, SC 29211
803–896–4500

SOUTH DAKOTA
South Dakota Department of Medical
  Examiners
1323 S. Minnesota Avenue
Sioux Falls, SD 57104
605–336–1965

TENNESSEE
Tennessee State Board of Medical
  Examiners
426 Fifth Avenue
Nashville, TN 37219
615–532–4348

TEXAS
Texas State Board of Medical
  Examiners
PO Box 2029
Austin, TX 78768
512–305–7010

UTAH
Utah Physicians Licensing Board
PO Box 146741
614 East 300 Street
Salt Lake City, UT 84145
801–530–6628

VERMONT
Vermont Board of Medical Practice
109 State Street
Montpelier, VT 05609
802–828–2673

VIRGINIA
Virginia State Board of Medicine
6606 W Broad Street, 4th floor
Richmond, VA 23230
804–662–9960

WASHINGTON
Washington State Department of
  Health
Division of Professional Licensing
PO Box 1099
Olympia, WA 98504
360–664–8480

WEST VIRGINIA
West Virginia Board of Medicine
101 Dee Drive
Charleston, WV 25311
304–348–2921

WISCONSIN
Wisconsin Board of Medical Examiners
PO Box 8935
1400 Washington Avenue
Madison, WI 53708
608–266–0483

WYOMING
Wyoming Board of Medical
   Examiners
211 West 19th Street
Cheyenne, WY 82002
307–778–2069

NATIONAL CANCER INSTITUTE CANCER CENTERS

National Cancer Institute
Andrew Von Eschenbach, MD, Director
National Cancer Institute
National Institutes of Health
Bethesda, Maryland, 20892

The National Cancer Institute (NCI) is the federal government's principal agency for research on cancer prevention, diagnosis, treatment, and rehabilitation, and for dissemination of information for the control of cancer. It is one of eleven research institutes and four divisions that form the National Institutes of Health (NIH), located in Bethesda, Maryland. As an agency of the Department of Health and Human Services, the NCI receives annual appropriations from Congress. These funds support cancer research in the Institute's Bethesda headquarters and in about 1,000 laboratories and medical centers throughout the United States.

The NCI also conducts research and treats a limited number of patients on specific research studies at the NIH Clinical Center located in Bethesda, Maryland.

NCI is responsible for the National Institute Cancer Centers Program that is made up of more than 60 NCI-designated Cancer Centers actively engaged in multidisciplinary research efforts to reduce cancer incidence, morbidity, and mortality. Within this program there are three tiers of cancer centers:

- **Comprehensive Cancer Centers** that conduct programs in all three areas of research: basic, clinical and cancer control and prevention. They also conduct programs in community outreach and education.
- **Clinical Cancer Centers** that focus mainly on clinical research but may have programs in other areas.
- **Cancer Centers** that engage in basic or cancer control research, but do not do clinical research.

Many people choose to go to one of these major centers either for treatment or for a second opinion. See Chapter 3, Choosing Your Doctor and Hospital.

Comprehensive Cancer Centers

The comprehensive cancer centers are designated as "centers of excellence," having met specific NCI criteria established for "comprehensiveness." It is the top designation given by the National Cancer Institute after vigorous peer review. The centers investigate and provide the latest scientific knowledge to doctors who are treating cancer patients. Comprehensive cancer centers have teams of experts working together on research, teaching and patient care. They are carrying out the newest investigational treatments for cancer, using clinical trials as described in Chapter 11, New Advances and Investigational Treatments.

ALABAMA
University of Alabama at Birmingham
  Comprehensive Cancer Center
1824 Sixth Avenue South
Birmingham, AL 35294
800–822–0933

ARIZONA
Mayo Clinic Cancer Center—
  Scottsdale
13400 East Shea Boulevard
Scottsdale, AZ 85259
480–301–8484

University of Arizona Cancer Center
1501 North Campbell Avenue
Tucson, AZ 85724
800–622–2673

CALIFORNIA
Chao Family Comprehensive
  Cancer Center
University of California at Irvine
101 The City Drive
Orange, CA 92868
714–456–8200

The City of Hope Cancer Center
1500 East Duarte Road
Duarte, CA 91010
800–826–4673

The Kenneth T. Norris Jr.
  Comprehensive Cancer Center,
University of Southern California
1441 Eastlake Avenue
Los Angeles, CA 90033–0804
880–872–2773

Jonsson Comprehensive Cancer Center,
  UCLA
8-684 Factor Building
Los Angeles, CA 90095
310–825–5268

University of California, San Diego
  Cancer Center
9500 Gilman Drive
La Jolla, CA 92093
858–534–7600

University of California, San
  Francisco
2340 Sutter Street
San Francisco, CA 94143
800–888–8664

COLORADO
University of Colorado
  Cancer Center
1665 North Ursula Street
Aurora, CO 80010
800–473–2288

CONNECTICUT
Yale Cancer Center, Yale University
  School of Medicine
333 Cedar Street
New Haven, CT 06510
203–785–4095

DISTRICT OF COLUMBIA
Lombardi Cancer Research Center,
Georgetown University Medical
  Center
3800 Reservoir Road NW
Washington, DC 20007
202–784–4000

FLORIDA
H. Lee Moffitt Cancer Center and
  Research Institute
12902 Magnolia Drive
Tampa, FL 33612
813–972–4673

Mayo Clinic Cancer Center—
  Jacksonville
4500 San Pablo Road
Jacksonville, FL 32224
904–953–2272

ILLINOIS
The Robert H. Lurie Comprehensive
  Cancer Center,
Northwestern University
710 North Fairbanks Court
Chicago, IL 60611
312–908–5250

IOWA
The Holden Comprehensive Cancer
  Center at the University of Iowa
200 Hawkins Drive
Iowa City, IA 52242
800–237–1225

MARYLAND
The Sidney Kimmell Comprehensive
  Cancer Center at Johns Hopkins
  Oncology Center

North Wolfe Street Rm 157
Baltimore, MD 21287
410–955–8822

MASSACHUSETTS
Dana-Farber Harvard Cancer Center
44 Binney Street
Boston, MA 02115
617–632–3000

MICHIGAN
Meyer L. Prentis Comprehensive
  Cancer Center of Metropolitan
  Detroit
4100 John R Street
Detroit, MI 48201
800–527–6266

University of Michigan Comprehensive
  Cancer Center
1500 East Medical Center Drive
Ann Arbor, MI 48109
800–856–1125

MINNESOTA
Mayo Comprehensive Cancer Center
200 First Street Southwest
Rochester, MN 55902
507–284–2111

University of Minnesota Cancer Center
420 Delaware Street SE
Minneapoli, MN 55455
612–624–8484

NEW HAMPSHIRE
Norris Cotton Cancer Center,
  Dartmouth-Hitchcock Medical Center
One Medical Center Drive
Hanover, NH 03756
603–650–6300

NEW JERSEY
The Cancer Institute of New Jersey,
  Robert Wood Johnson Medical
  School
195 Little Albany Avenue
New Brunswick, NJ 08901
732–235–2465

NEW YORK

Herbert Irving Comprehensive
Cancer Center
622 West 168th Street
New York, NY 10032
212–305–9327

Memorial Sloan-Kettering
Cancer Center
1275 York Avenue
New York, NY 10021
800–525–2225

NYU Cancer Center, New York
University Medical Center
550 First Avenue
New York, NY 10016
212–263–6485

Roswell Park Cancer Institute
Elm and Carlton Streets
Buffalo, NY 14263
800–767–9355

NORTH CAROLINA

Duke Comprehensive Cancer
Center
PO Box 3843, 301 MSRB
Durham, NC 27710
919–684–3377

Lineberger Comprehensive
Cancer Center
University of North Carolina
Chapel Hill, NC 27599
919–966–3036

Comprehensive Cancer Center of
Wake Forest University
Medical Center Boulevard
Winston-Salem, NC 27157
336–716–4464

OHIO

Ireland Cancer Center
11100 Euclid Avenue
Cleveland, OH 44106
216–844–5432

Ohio State University
Comprehensive Cancer
Center
300 West 10th Avenue
Columbus, OH 43210
800–293–5066

PENNSYLVANIA

Fox Chase Cancer Center
7701 Burholme Avenue
Philadelphia, PA 19111
800–728–2570

Abramson Cancer Center of
the University of
Pennsylvania
3400 Spruce Street
Philadelphia, PA 19104
215–728–2570, 800–789–7366

University of Pittsburgh
Cancer Institute
3600 Forbes Avenue
Pittsburgh, PA 15213
800–237–4724

TENNESSEE

The Vanderbilt-Ingram
Cancer Center
649 The Preston Building
Nashville, TN 37232
888–488–4089

TEXAS

The University of
Texas M.D. Anderson
Cancer Center
1515 Holcombe Boulevard
Houston, TX 78229
800–392–1611

VERMONT

Vermont Cancer Care, University of
Vermont
149 Beaumont Avenue
Burlington, VT 05401
802–656–4414

WASHINGTON

Fred Hutchinson Cancer Research
  Center
1100 Fairview Avenue North
Seattle, WA 98109
800–804–8824

WISCONSIN

University of Wisconsin
  Comprehensive Cancer Center
600 Highland Avenue
Madison, WI 53792
608–263–8600

Clinical Cancer Centers

The National Cancer Institute designated clinical cancer centers have active programs in clinical research. They also may have other programs such as basic or prevention research. Clinical cancer centers have also been given thorough review by the National Cancer Institute. Although they have not met all the criteria to qualify as comprehensive centers, they are well qualified to provide investigational treatments.

CALIFORNIA

University of California, Davis
4501 X Street
Sacramento, CA 95817
800–326–5566

HAWAII

Cancer Research Center of Hawaii
1236 Lauhala Street
Honolulu, HI 96813
808–586–3010

ILLINOIS

University of Chicago Cancer Research
  Center
5758 South Maryland Avenue
Chicago, IL 60637
888–824–0200

INDIANA

Indiana University Center
535 Barnhill Drive
Indianapolis, IN 46202–5288
317–278–0070

MISSOURI

Siteman Cancer Center
660 South Euclid St.
Saint Louis, MO 63110
800–600–3606

NEBRASKA

University of Nebraska
  Medical Center, Eppley
  Cancer Center
600 South 42nd Street
Omaha, NE 68198
402–559–4238

NEW YORK

Albert Einstein College of
  Medicine, Cancer Research
  Center
1300 Morris Park Avenue
Bronx, NY 10461
718–430–2302

OREGON

The Oregon Cancer Center
3181 Southwest Sam Jackson Park
  Road
Portland, OR 97201
503–494–1617

PENNSYLVANIA

Kimmel Cancer Center
T233 South 10th Street
Philadelphia, PA 19107
800–533–3669

TENNESSEE
St. Jude Children's Research
  Hospital
332 North Lauderdale Street
Memphis, TN 38105
910–495–3300

TEXAS
San Antonio Cancer Institute
8122 Datapoint Drive
San Antonio, TX 78229
210–616–5590

UTAH
Huntsman Cancer Institute, University
  of Utah

2000 Circle of Hope
Salt Lake City, UT 84112
801–585–0303 (1–877–585–0303)

VIRGINIA
Massey Cancer Center, Medical
  College of Virginia
401 College Street
Richmond, VA 23298
804–828–0450

Cancer Center, University of Virginia
  Jefferson Park Avenue
Charlottesville, VA 22906
434–924–5022

The last category of cancer centers designated by the National Cancer Institute, called cancer centers, refer to those organizations that have scientific disciplines outside the specific qualifications of a comprehensive or clinical center. They may concentrate on basic research, epidemiology and cancer control research or other research areas. They do not offer screening, diagnosis or treatment services and thus we have not listed them.

NIH Clinical Center

Warren Grant Magnuson Clinical Center

The National Institutes of Health has a medical research center and hospital— the Warren Grant Magnuson Clinical Center located in Bethesda, Maryland, just outside of Washington, DC. The hospital portion of the Clinical Center is especially designed for medical research. The number of beds available for a particular project and the length of the waiting list of qualified patients are important in determining whether and when you can be admitted. Research on a particular disease may allow only one or two patients to be studied at any given time. The Clinical Center provides nursing and medical care without charge for patients who are being studied in a clinical research program.

You can be treated at the Clinical Center only if your case fits into a research project. Each project is designed to answer scientific questions and has specific medical eligibility requirements. For this reason you must be referred by your own doctors, who can supply the Clinical Center with the needed medical information, such as your diagnosis and details of your medical history. You should first discuss your options with your doctor, and if a

clinical trial at the NIH Clinical Center is an option, here are the steps you
and your doctor need to take:

- To find out if there is a study available for a specific cancer you (and your
  doctor) can call the Clinical Trials Support Center at 1–888–624–1937
  weekdays between 9 a.m. and 5 p.m., Eastern Time. You can talk with an
  oncology nurse or an information specialist who can identify the trials
  that might be appropriate. Information, including the summaries of the trials can be sent to you.

- You should review the clinical trial summaries with your doctor to decide
  which study to consider further. The doctor should then contact the Clinical Studies Support Center and talk with the doctor in charge of the study.

- If you meet the initial medical eligibility requirements, you will be
  screened at the NIH Clinical Center. You may need to undergo some
  tests at that time.

- After you have heard all the information and agree to take part in the
  study, you will be asked to sign an informed consent form.

The Pediatric Branch of the Clinical Center conducts clinical trials for a
wide variety of childhood cancers at the NIH Clinical Center. The kinds of
cancers treated and the protocols change periodically. To refer a patient to the
pediatric branch, your doctor should call 877–624–4878 between 8:30 a.m.
and 5:00 p.m. The Pediatric Branch also provides second opinions. Also see
Chapter 24, When a Child Has Cancer.

MONEY MATTERS

Cancer can impose heavy economic burdens on both patients and their families. For many people, a portion of medical expenses is paid by their health
insurance plan. An employer's personnel office or an insurance company can
provide information about the types of medical costs covered by a particular
policy. Medical costs that are not covered by insurance policies sometimes
can be deducted from annual income before taxes.

For individuals who do not have health insurance or who need additional
financial assistance, several resources are available, including Government-
sponsored programs and services supported by voluntary organizations.

Before leaving the hospital, discuss any concerns you may have about
medical costs with a hospital social worker or patient accounts representative.
They often can help patients identify appropriate sources of aid and can also
help patients negotiate a payment plan.

- Medicare, a health insurance program that is administered by the Social Security Administration (SSA), is designed for people over 65 or who are permanently disabled. The telephone number of the closest Social Security office is listed in the telephone directory or can be obtained by calling 1–800–772–1213.

- Medicaid is a program for people who need financial assistance for medical expenses. It is coordinated by the Health Care Financing Administration of the Department of Health and Human Services and is administered by individual states. Information about coverage is available from a hospital social worker or a local public health or social services office.

- The Federal Government also administers the Hill-Burton Program, through which many medical facilities and hospitals provide free or low cost care. Hill-Burton hospitals receive government construction and modernization funds and are required by law to provide some services to people who cannot afford to pay. For eligibility information call 1–800–638–0742.

- If a cancer patient or his or her spouse is, or has been a member of the Armed Forces, the U.S. Department of Veterans Affairs (VA) may be able to help with health care costs. The VA provides hospital care covering the full range of medical services. Treatment is available for all service-related conditions and some nonservice-related ones.

- The Civilian Health and Medical Program of the Department of Veterans Affairs is a medical benefits program for dependents of veterans through which the VA provides payment for medical services and supplies obtained from civilian sources. Any VA health care facility can provide information about these programs.

- The Federal Government's Civilian Health and Medical Programs of the Uniformed Services (CHAMPUS) helps pay for civilian medical care for spouses and children of active-duty Uniformed Services personnel, retired Uniformed Services personnel and their spouses and children, and spouses and children of active-duty or retired active-duty personnel who have died. Information about CHAMPUS is available from the CHAMPUS Advisor/Health Benefits Advisor at your nearest Uniformed Services medical facility, or write to: Information Office of CHAMPUS, Aurora, CO 80045.

- The American Cancer Society (ACS) offers counseling, transportation and rehabilitation programs.

- The Leukemia and Lymphoma Society offers service programs, and provides some financial aid, to eligible patients who have leukemia, lymphoma or multiple myeloma. The local office is listed in your telephone directory.

- Groups such as the Salvation Army, United Way, Lutheran Social Services,

Jewish Social Services, the Lions Club, Associated Catholic Charities, as well as churches and synagogues sometimes provide financial help.

- If you are having problems with your insurance company or if you need insurance, see state insurance commissions, below.

- There is more information on finances and cancer in Chapter 27, Living With Cancer.

American Association of Retired Persons (AARP)
601 E Street, NW
Washington, DC 20049
202–443–2277
Provides legislative advocacy, programs such as Medicare/Medicaid assistance and the Breast Cancer and Mammography Awareness information campaign for people 50 or older. Wide range of membership benefits including *Modern Maturity* magazine and Medicare supplementary insurance.

Blue Cross and Blue Shield Association
676 North St. Clair Street
Chicago, IL 60601
312–440–6000
Provides information on Blue Cross/Blue Shield coverage offered in every state, including the availability of annual open enrollment periods.

Communicating For Agriculture Inc.
2626 East 82nd Street, Suite 325
Bloomington, MN 55425
612–854–9005
A national rural organization, open to all, offering up-to-date information on high-risk insurance pools. Since 1975 has served as a strong advocate

for the establishment of these state-run high risk pools.

Disabled American Veterans
807 Main Avenue, SW
Washington, DC 20024
202–554–3501
A national organization, serving veterans and their dependents. Approximately 3,000 chapters offer counseling, educational materials, support groups, transportation, conferences and a newsletter. Aids veterans exposed to nuclear weapons testing who have since developed a cancer caused by radiation.

Health Insurance Association Of America (HIAA)
1201 F Street, Suite 500
Washington, DC 20004
202–824–1600
www.hiaa.org
A trade association representing major health insurance companies. Offers consumer publications about health insurance, long-term care insurance and Medicare supplement insurance.

Medicare Hotline
800–MEDICAR (800–633–4227)
www.medicare.gov
The toll-free number offers information about local services. Web site gives information on health plans, nursing homes, Medigap policies,

participating doctors and prescription drug assistance.

Medical Information Bureau Incorporated (MIB)
PO Box 105
Essex Station
Boston, MA 02112
617–426–3660
www.mib.com
Association of US and Canadian life insurance companies aims to prevent insurance fraud. Can supply copy of your medical records so that you can verify the information in them and correct any inaccuracies. Call MIB first to find out the type of information it requires to process your request.

National Association of Insurance Commissioners (NAIC)
2301 McGee, Suite 800
Kansas City, MO 64108–2604
816–842–3600
www.naic.org/consumer.htm
This phone number or Web site will direct you to your state's insurance commission. Contact your state insurance commission if you feel you are being treated unfairly by your insurance company.

The National Insurance Consumer Helpline
800–942–4242
Provides information on all types of insurance. A joint project of the American Council on Life Insurance, the Health Insurance Association of America, and the Insurance Information Institute.

National Underwriter Company
505 Gest Street
Cincinnati, OH 45203
513–721–2140
Publishes annual guide "Who Writes What in Life and Health Insurance."

National Viatical Association
1030 Fifteenth Street, Suite 870
Washington, DC 20005
800–741–9465
www.nationalviatical.org
This group provides information on predeath purchases of life insurance policies.

Pension and Welfare Benefits Administration (PWBA)
U.S. Department of Labor, Room N–5619
200 Constitution Avenue, NW
Washington, DC 20210
202–219–8141
www.dol.gov/do/pwba
PWBA deals with integrity of pensions, health plans and other employee benefits; enforces your rights under COBRA to continued health insurance coverage and provides information about how to enforce your rights to equal job benefits under ERISA.

State Insurance Commissions and Health Insurance for the Difficult to Insure

The state insurance commission can help you if you are having insurance problems or feel you are being treated unfairly by your insurance company. In addition, a number of states currently sell comprehensive health insurance to state residents with serious medical conditions who are unable to find a company to insure them. Contact your state Department of Insurance to find out whether or not your state is selling such insurance or what assistance they can offer.

ALABAMA
Insurance Department
201 Monroe Street, Suite 1700
Montgomery, AL 36104
334–269–3550

ALASKA
Division of Insurance
550 West 7th Avenue
Suite 1560
Anchorage, AK 99501–3567
907–269–7900

ARIZONA
Department of Insurance
2910 North 44th Street, Suite 210
Phoenix, AZ 85018–7256
602–912–8400

ARKANSAS
Department of Insurance
1200 West 3rd Street
Little Rock, AK 72201–1904
501–371–2600

CALIFORNIA
Department of Insurance
300 Capital Mall, Suite 17
Sacramento, CA 95814
916–492–3500

COLORADO
Division of Insurance
1560 Broadway, Suite 850
Denver, CO 80202
303–894–7455

CONNECTICUT
Department of Insurance
PO Box 816
Hartford, CT 06142–0816
860–566–7410

DELAWARE
Department of Insurance
Rodney Building
841 Siler Lake Boulevard
Dover, DE 19904
302–739–4251

DISTRICT OF COLUMBIA
Department of Insurance & Securities
  Reg.
Government of the District of
  Columbia
810 First Street NE, Suite 701
Washington, DC 20002
202–727–8000

FLORIDA
Department of Insurance
State Capitol, PL11
Tallahassee, FL 32399–0300
850–413–2804

GEORGIA
Department of Insurance
Two Martin Luther King, Jr. Drive
704 West Tower
Atlanta, GA 30334
404–656–2056

HAWAII
Division of Insurance
Department of Commerce and
  Consumer Affairs
250 S. King Street, 5th Floor
Honolulu, HI 96813
808–586–2790

IDAHO
Department of Insurance
700 West State Street, 3rd Floor
Boise, ID 83720–0043
208–334–4250

ILLINOIS
Department of Insurance
320 North Washington, 4th Floor
Springfield, IL 62767–0001
217–782–4515

INDIANA
Department of Insurance
311 West Washington Street,
  Suite 300
Indianapolis, IN 46204–2787
317–232–2385

IOWA
Insurance Division
330 E. Maple Street
Des Moines, IA 50319
515–281–5705

KANSAS
Insurance Department
420 Southwest Ninth Street
Topeka, KS 66612–1698
785–296–7801

KENTUCKY
Department of Insurance
PO Box 517
Frankfort, KY 40602–0517
502–564–6027

LOUISIANA
Department of Insurance
1702 N. 3rd Street

Baton Rouge, LA 70802
255–342–5423

MAINE
Bureau of Insurance
Department of Professional and
  Financial Regulations
State House Station #34
Augusta, ME 04333–0034
207–624–8475

MARYLAND
Insurance Administration
525 St. Paul Place
Baltimore, MD 21202–2272
410–468–2000

MASSACHUSETTS
Division of Insurance
One South Station, 4th Floor
Boston, MA 02110
617–521–7301

MICHIGAN
Office of Financial and Insurance
  Services
611 West Ottawa, 2nd Floor North
Lansing, MI 48933–1020
517–335–3167

MINNESOTA
Department of Commerce
85 7th Place East, Suite 500
St. Paul, MN 55101–2198
612–296–6025

MISSISSIPPI
Insurance Department
501 Northwest Street
Woolfolk State Office Bldg., 10th Floor
Jackson, MS 39201
601–359–3569

MISSOURI
Division of Insurance
301 West High Street, Suite 530
Jefferson City, MO 65102
573–751–4126

MONTANA
Department of Insurance
840 Helena Avenue
Helena, MT 59601
406–444–2040

NEBRASKA
Department of Insurance
The Terminal Building, Suite 400
941 O Street
Lincoln, NE 68508
402–471–2201

NEVADA
Division of Insurance
788 Fairview Drive, Suite 300
Carson City, NV 89710–2319
775–687–4270

NEW HAMPSHIRE
Insurance Department
56 Old Suncook Road
Concord, NH 03301
603–271–2261

NEW JERSEY
Department of Insurance
20 West State Street, CN 325
Trenton, NJ 08625
609–633–7667

NEW MEXICO
Insurance Division
1120 Paseo de Peralta
Santa Fe, NM 87504–1269
505–827–4601

NEW YORK
Department of Insurance
Agency Building #1
One Commerce Plaza
Albany, NY 12257
518–474–4567

NORTH CAROLINA
Department of Insurance
PO Box 26387
Raleigh, NC 27611
919–733–3058

NORTH DAKOTA
Department of Insurance
600 East Boulevard
Bismarck, ND 58505–0320
701–328–2440

OHIO
Department of Insurance
2100 Stella Court
Columbus, OH 43215–1067
614–644–2856

OKLAHOMA
Department of Insurance
2401 NE 23rd St., Suite 28
Oklahoma City, OK 73107
405–521–2828

OREGON
Department of Insurance
350 Winter Street, NE, Room 440
Salem, OR 97310–3883
503–947–7980

PENNSYLVANIA
Insurance Department
1326 Strawberry Square,
  13th floor
Harrisburg, PA 17120
717–783–0422

RHODE ISLAND
Department of Business
  Regulation
233 Richmond Street, Suite 233
Providence, RI 02903–4233
401–222–2223

SOUTH CAROLINA
Department of Insurance
303 Arbor Lake Drive, Suite 1200
Columbia, SC 29223
803–737–6212

SOUTH DAKOTA
Division of Insurance
Department of Commerce and
  Regulations

118 West Capitol Avenue
Pierre, SD 57501–2000
605–773–4104

TENNESSEE
Department of Commerce and
  Insurance
Davy Crockett Tower, 5th Floor
500 James Robertson Parkway
Nashville, TN 37243–0565
615–741–2241

TEXAS
Department of Insurance
333 Guadalupe Street
Austin, TX 78701
512–463–6464

UTAH
Department of Insurance
3110 State Office Building
Salt Lake City, UT 84114–1201
801–538–3800

VERMONT
Department of Banking and
  Insurance
89 Main Street, Drawer 20
Montpelier, VT 05620–3101
802–828–3301

VIRGINIA
State Corporation Commissioner
PO Box 1157
Richmond, VA 23218
804–371–9694

WASHINGTON
Office of Insurance Commissioner
PO Box 40255
Olympia, WA 98504–0255
360–725–7100

WEST VIRGINIA
Division of Insurance
PO Box 50540
Charleston, WV 25305–0540
304-558-3354

WISCONSIN
Office of Commissioner of Insurance
PO Box 7873
Madison, WI 53707–7873
608–267–1233

WYOMING
Insurance Department
Herschler Building
122 West 25th Street
Cheyenne, WY 82002–0440
307–777–7401

Index